ORAL PHARMACOLOGY FOR THE DENTAL HYGIENIST

Mea A. Weinberg, D.M.D., M.S.D., R.Ph.
Cheryl Westphal, R.D.H., M.S.
New York University College of Dentistry

James Burke Fine, D.D.S.
Columbia University College of Dental Medicine

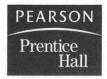
PEARSON

Prentice
Hall

Upper Saddle River, New Jersey 07458

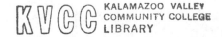

Library of Congress Cataloging-in-Publication Data

Weinberg, Mea A.
  Oral pharmacology for the dental hygienist / Mea A. Weinberg,
James Burke Fine, Cheryl Westphal.
    p. ; cm.
  Includes bibliographical references and index.
  ISBN-13: 978-0-13-049286-9
  ISBN-10: 0-13-049286-8
  1. Dental pharmacology.   2. Clinical pharmacology.
3. Dental hygienists. I. Fine, James Burke. II. Westphal, Cheryl.
III. Title.
  [DNLM: 1. Dentistry.   2. Pharmaceutical Preparations.
3. Dental Hygienists.   4. Drug Therapy—adverse effects.
5. Pharmacology. QV 50 W423o 2008]
  RK701.W45 2008
  615'.10246176--dc22

                           2007028398

Notice:
The author[s] and the publisher of this volume have taken care that the information and technical recommendations contained herein are based on research and expert consultation, and are accurate and compatible with the standards generally accepted at the time of publication. Nevertheless, as new information becomes available, changes in clinical and technical practices become necessary. The reader is advised to carefully consult manufacturers' instructions and information material for all supplies and equipment before use, and to consult with a healthcare professional as necessary. This advice is especially important when using new supplies or equipment for clinical purposes. The author[s] and publisher disclaim all responsibility for any liability, loss, injury, or damage incurred as a consequence, directly or indirectly, of the use and application of any of the contents of this volume.

Publisher: Julie Levin Alexander
Assistant to Publisher: Regina Bruno
Executive Editor: Mark Cohen
Associate Editor: Melissa Kerian
Editorial Assistant: Nicole Ragonese
Media Editor: John J. Jordan
Managing Production Editor: Patrick Walsh
Production Liaison: Cathy O'Connell
Production Editor: Bruce Hobart, Pine Tree Composition
Manufacturing Manager: Ilene Sanford
Manufacturing Buyer: Pat Brown

Design Coordinator: Maria Guglielmo-Walsh
Cover Designer: Wanda España
Director of Marketing: Karen Allman
Marketing Manager: Harper Coles
Marketing Assistant: Wayne Celia
Marketing Specialist: Michael Sirinides
Media Production: Stephen Hartner
Composition: Pine Tree Composition, Inc.
Printer/Binder: Courier Westford
Cover Printer: Phoenix Color Corporation

Pearson Prentice Hall™ is a trademark of Pearson Education, Inc.
Pearson® is a registered trademark of Pearson plc.
Prentice Hall® is a registered trademark of Pearson Education, Inc.

Pearson Education Ltd., *London*
Pearson Education Australia Pty. Limited, *Sydney*
Pearson Education Singapore, Pte. Ltd.
Pearson Education North Asia Ltd., *Hong Kong*
Pearson Education Canada, Ltd., *Toronto*

Pearson Educación de Mexico, S.A. de C.V.
Pearson Education—Japan, *Tokyo*
Pearson Education Malaysia, Pte. Ltd.
Pearson Education, Upper Saddle River, New Jersey

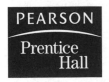

10 9 8 7 6 5 4 3 2
ISBN 0-13-049286-8
ISBN-13 978-0-13-049286-9

Contents

Preface

There is a significant amount of information about pharmacology in the medical/dental field about which it is important for the student and dental clinician to be cognizant. Pharmacology stands alone as a basic science but application of this information to dentistry must be applied to clinical settings to allow for the management of certain medical/dental conditions. This textbook studies the principles of pharmacology and their application to dental hygiene practice.

This textbook was written to (1) help students understand the fundamentals of pharmacology, (2) understand about the different medications their dental patient is taking, (3) show that many medications have adverse oral side effects, and (4) show there is a connection among medicine, pharmacology, and dentistry.

Oral Pharmacology for the Dental Hygienist is divided into sections. Section I reviews the basic concepts of pharmacology. Section II reviews the classifications of medications related directly to dentistry. Section III reviews categories of drugs that the dental patient may be taking. Section IV reviews Special Topics that are of interest to the dental clinician and Section V contains the appendices.

Within most chapters are boxed in "Patient Guidelines" sections that pertain to a specific drug that has oral side effects and explains how the patient can be instructed in how to maintain optimum oral health while taking that drug. "Rapid Dental Hints" remind students about key information or a task that should be performed related to the topic discussed. Additionally, there are Fun Facts found within many chapters that provide whimsical information about the disease or medications. "Quick Drug Guides" at the end of each chapter provide an easy reference to the drugs discussed within the chapter. Special sections on dental drug–drug interactions and prescriptions for common dental conditions are included. Trade names of drugs are in parentheses following the generic name. An extensive glossary should be used while reading the chapters.

The lastest information on treatment of patients on bisphosphonates is discussed in the Special Topic Section. In April 2007, the American Heart Association revised the guidelines for antibiotic prophylaxis in the prevention of infective endocarditis (IE). These current guidelines are presented.

We hope this book will serve as a helpful text for all dental practitioners.

Mea A. Weinberg, DMD, MSD, RPh
Cheryl Westphal, RDH, MS
James Burke Fine, DDS

Contributors

Elvir Dincer, D.D.S.
Assistant Professor
Department of Dental Hygiene
Eugenio Maria de Hostos Community College of The
City of University of New York
Bronx, New York
(Chapter 10: Flourides in Dental Practice)

Adrienne Lynn Ligouri, B.S.B.E., M.D., M.P.H.

Mt. Sinai School of Medicine
New York, New York
(Chapter 10: Fluorides in Dental Practice)

Robert S. Schoor, D.D.S.
Associate Professor
Director of Postgraduate Periodontics
Department of Periodontology and Implant Dentistry
New York University College of Dentistry
New York, New York
(Chapter 9: Sedation and General Anesthetics)

Cheryl Westphal, R.D.H., M.S.
Clinical Associate Professor
Assistant Dean for Allied Health Programs
Director, Dental Hygiene Program
New York University College of Dentistry
New York, New York
(Chapter 10: Fluorides in Dental Practice)

Reviewers

Jonathan R. Abraham, DDS
Adjunct Professor, Dental Hygiene
Community and Technical College at West Virginia
University
Montgomery, West Virginia

Michael R. Bye, M.D.
Acting Director, Pediatric Pulmonary Medicine
Morgan Stanley Children's Hospital of New York
Presbyterian
Professor of Clinical Pediatrics, Columbia University
New York, New York

Kathy Conlin, RDH, CCRN, MS
Assistant Professor, Dental Hygiene
Eastern Washington University
Spokane, Washington

Dennis Connaughton, DMD
Instructor, Dental Programs
Brevard Community College
Cocoa, Florida

Elvir Dincer, DDS
Assistant Professor, Dental Hygiene
Hostos Community College
Bronx, New York

Diane Ellis, RDH, MS
Professor, Dental Hygiene
Tunxis Community College
Farmington, Connecticut

Tami Grzesikowski, RDH
Dean, Dental Hygiene
St. Petersburg College
St. Petersburg, Florida

Carol Haggerty, MD, DDS
Assistant Professor, Dental Programs
Santa Fe Community College
Gainesville, Florida

Steven R. Jacobsen, DDS
Associate Clinical Specialist, Dental Hygiene
University of Minnesota
Minneapolis, Minnesota

Joleen Lee, AS, BS, MEd
Associate Professor, Dental Health
University of Bangor
Bangor, Maine

Angela Monson, RDH, MS
Assistant Professor, Dental Hygiene
Minnesota State University—Mankato
Mankato, Minnisota

Diane R. Samsel, RDH, BS, MS
Assistant Professor, Dental Hygiene
Rock Valley College
Rockford, Illinois

Donal Scheidal, DDS
Associate Professor, Dental Hygiene
University of South Dakota
Vermillion, South Dakota

Rebecca J. Sullivan, EdM, RDH
Professor, Allied Health
Tunxis Community College
Farmington, Connecticut

Lourdes Vazquez, RDH, MS
Assistant Professor, Dental Hygiene
Wichita State University
Wichita, Kansas

Ken Whitley, MS, RN
Instructor, Allied Health
Western Kentucky University
Bowling Green, Kentucky

Chapter **1**

Introduction to Clinical Pharmacology

GOAL: To introduce the basic concepts of pharmacology upon which the practice of dental pharmacotherapeutics is based and to familiarize the student with various pharmacology terminologies.

EDUCATIONAL OBJECTIVES

After reading this chapter, the reader should be able to:

1. Describe the role of pharmacology in the dental hygiene process of care.
2. List and utilize the various online and computer drug references.
3. Discuss various federal drug laws and their impact on drug regulation.
4. List and discuss different types of undesirable drug effects.
5. Identify the various types of pharmaceutical preparations.
6. Describe common routes of drug administration.

KEY TERMS

Food and Drug Administration (FDA)
Pharmacology
Pharmacology references
Drug laws
Drug effects
Drug administration

INTRODUCTION

Although the history of *pharmacology* goes back only a few hundred years, medicines derived from plants, animals, and minerals have been used to treat diseases for thousands of years. Until the end of the nineteenth century, most medicines came from naturally occurring fresh plants including herbs and flowers. For example, morphine is derived from the poppy flower, and marijuana from the cannabis plant. Although these medicaments may have a therapeutic or healing effect, many substances exert a toxic effect.

Drug development has grown substantially since ancient times. Today, most drugs are no longer naturally derived but are made synthetically in laboratories; however, substances with complex structures may still be obtained from various sources. For example, cardiac glycosides used in the treatment of heart failure are derived from the *digitalis purpurea* (foxglove) plant, heparin (inhibits blood clotting; an anticoagulant) is derived from animal tissues, and insulin from gene technology. Herbal medicines such as kava, garlic, and dong quai, although not regulated by the government, are derived from plants.

History of Pharmacology

The history of pharmacology is summarized in the following table:

Table 1-1 Pharmacology History Timeline

- 1825: The first journal of pharmacology published was the Journal of Philadelphia College of Pharmacy, which changed its name to American Journal of Pharmacy in 1835 and was published well into the twentieth century.
- 1828: Friedrich Wohler introduced organic chemistry to the world.
- 1847: Rudolf Buchheim established the first department of pharmacology at the University of Dorpat in Estonia, which was part of Russia during this time.
- Oswald Schmiedeberg (1838–1921) is recognized as the founder of modern pharmacology.
- 1890: John Jacob Abel became the first chair in pharmacology in the United States at the University of Michigan.
- 1926: John Jacob Abel isolated epinephrine from the adrenal gland and made the first preparation of pure crystalline insulin.

Did You Know?

Raw opium is taken from the poppy flower and processed into codeine and morphine.

TERMINOLOGY

Pharmacology is defined as the biomedical study of the interaction of chemical substances with living systems, including cells, tissues, and organisms. The term pharmacology is derived from the Greek words *pharmakos,* which means "drug," "medicine," or "poison"; and *logos,* which means "study." The subject of pharmacology is an expansive topic that ranges from how drugs enter and travel throughout the body to the responses they produce. *Drugs* are substances or chemical agents that affect biologic or living systems that *do not create new physiological responses;* rather, they alter normal processes either by stimulating (increasing) or by depressing (decreasing) the function of the cell. While most drugs today are synthetic, *biologics* are agents that are naturally produced in an animal or human body. Examples of biologics are vaccines, blood and blood components, antibodies, and interferon. *Alternative drug therapy* includes herbs, vitamins, minerals, dietary supplements, and natural extracts.

There are five major subgroups of pharmacology: pharmacokinetics, pharmacodynamics, pharmacotherapeutics, pharmacogenetics, and toxicology.

Pharmacokinetics describes the way the body affects the drug including absorption, distribution, metabolism, and excretion. *Pharmacodynamics* is the action a drug has on a specific target of action in the body, including the drug's mechanism of action, receptor interactions, dose–response relationship, and therapeutic and toxic reactions. *Posology* is the study of the dosages of medicines and drugs. *Therapeutics* is the branch of medicine that deals with the treatment of disease. Drugs are used to prevent, diagnose, and treat diseases. *Pharmacotherapeutics* describes the part of science that deals with the use of drugs in the prevention, diagnosis, and treatment of diseases. For dental professionals, the fields of pharmacology and therapeutics are connected. *Pharmacogenetics* is the convergence of pharmacology and genetics that deals with genetic factors that influence an organism's response to a drug. For example, some individuals are termed "slow acetylators" and "fast acetylators," relating to the breakdown of an antituberculosis drug called isoniazid (INH). This is a form of genetic variation where some people cannot break down this drug as fast as others. The terms pharmacogenomics and pharmacogenetics are used interchangeably. *Toxicology* is the scientific study of poisons, chemical pollutants, and the undesirable effects of drugs on living cells, tissues, and organisms. A poison is any substance detrimental to health that may result in incapacitation, illness (e.g., cancer), or death.

PHARMACOLOGY: THE DENTAL HYGIENE PROCESS OF CARE

Many new classifications of drugs have been introduced in the last decade. Over 1.5 billion prescriptions are filled annually in the United States. The majority of the elderly take multiple medications, which is referred to as polypharmacy. The dental hygienist in the dental hygiene process of care begins with assessment of all medications the patient is currently taking and considers drugs that might be prescribed in the course of treatment. The names, dosages, mechanisms of action, and interactions with other drugs and herbal supplements are all critical in planning the treatment phase of dental hygiene care. The medical history must be reviewed at each visit to confirm the proper drug dosage regimen or indicate any changes in medications or drug interactions. In planned care, the prognosis and diagnosis given the drug history is taken into consideration. Certain medications' effects on oral tissue may affect the planned outcome of dental hygiene care. Risk assessment will include side effects of the medications or possible emergency situations. Implementation of educational and therapeutic services requires knowledge of the prescription and over-the-counter therapies available to the dental hygienist. Use of fluorides, analgesics, chemotherapeutics, local anesthetics, and nitrous oxide require full understanding of the pharmacological effects of these products/drugs.

RDH Rapid Dental Hint

If a medical consultation is required from your patient's physician, be sure that the patient is getting it from the physician who is taking care of that condition.

SOURCES OF DRUG INFORMATION
Printed Resources

Many books and journals are available for **pharmacology references.** Table 1–2 lists selected sources. It should be noted that all information available online should be viewed with caution; only reputable sites should be used.

Many publications are updated monthly or yearly; however, many are not and may not contain the latest medications. Some popular printed text information are the *USP DI* (Thomson Publishing Corporation), *Drugs Facts and Comparison* (Wolters Kluwer Health Company), and *AHFS Drug Information* (American Hospital Formulary Service). The *PDR*® (*Physician's Desk Reference;* Thomson PDR, Montvale, NJ; www.pdr.net) is written in cooperation with participating drug manufacturers and the U.S. Food and Drug Administration (FDA), and is published annually. Other clinical information products from *PDR*® include the *PDR*® *Monthly Prescribing Guide*™, the mobile *PDR*®, the *PDR*® *Pharmacopoeia Pocket Dosing Guide,* the *PDR*® *for Nutritional Supplements, PDR*® *for Herbal Medicines,* and the *PDR*® *Guide to Drug Interactions, Side Effects, and Indications.*

Dental drug resources, including the *ADA Guide to Dental Therapeutics,* the *Drug Information Handbook* (Lexi-Comp), and *Mosby's Dental Drug Reference, are* listed in Table 1–2.

RDH Rapid Dental Hint

Remember to have some type of drug reference book or PDA with you in the clinic or office for quick reference.

Computer Resources

Personal digital assistants (PDAs), which are handheld computer devices, are rapidly becoming popular for recording and storing patient information, calculating appropriate drug doses, and providing databases of medication information.

There are many software resources that are available, including MedTeach (American Society of Health System Pharmacists), Epocrates (http://www.epocrates

Table 1-2   Selective Resources for Pharmacology

Dental Drug References	Medical/Pharmacy Drug References	Journals (not all are listed):
ADA Guide to Dental Therapeutics (American Dental Association) *Dental Drug Reference with Clinical Implications* (Lippincott Williams & Wilkins) *Drug Information Handbook* (LEXI-COMP) *Mosby's Dental Drug Reference*	*American Hospital Formulary Service (AHFS) Drug Information* *Remington's Pharmaceutical Sciences* *Physicians' Drug Reference (PDR)*® (hardcopy, palm pilot, electronic, CD ROM) *PDR*® *Pharmacopoeia Pocket Dosing Guide* *United States Pharmacopeia Drug Information* (USP DI) *Handbook of Nonprescription Drugs* (American Pharmaceutical Association) *Tarascon Pocket Pharmacopoeia* *Drug Facts and Comparison* *Merck Manual*	*U.S. Pharmacist* *Drug Topics* *Pharmacy Times* *Hospital Pharmacy* *Journal of the American Pharmacists Association* *Journal of Clinical Pharmacology* *Journal of Clinical Pharmacy and Therapeutics* *Journal of Clinical Psychopharmacology* *Journal of Pharmacokinetics and Pharmacodynamics* *Journal of Pharmacy and Pharmacology* *Journal of Pharmacy Practice and Research* *Pharmacogenetics and Genomics* *Pharmacological Reviews* *Pharmacoepidemiology and Drug Safety* *Therapeutic Drug Monitoring* *World of Drug Information*

Web Sites	Newsletters
www.ada.org www.medscape.com www.refdesk.com www.pdr.net www.pol.net www.cp.gsm.com www.medecinteractive.com www.nursepdr.com www.rxlist.com www.uspharmacist.com www.fda.gov/medwatch www.micromedex.com www.nhlbi.nih.gov/guidelines/index.htm www.ashp.org www.nlm.nih.gov/medlineplus/druginteraction.html www.nclnet.org (drug-food interactions) www.drugdigest.com www.drugs.com www.mosbydrugconsult.com	***The Medical Letter*** www.medletter.com *Journal Watch* www.jwatch.com

.com), and MedFacts (http://medfacts.info.com) that can be uploaded on the computer or PDAs such as the Palm Pilot.

Additionally, over the past years many textbooks and reference books have included CD-ROMs, which can store a lot of information that complements the written material.

Online Resources

Journals provide the most recent information on medications and therapies. Over 3,000 domestic and international journals and scientific literature are available online at http://www.medline.com and http://www.pubmed.com. Medscape (http://www.medscape.com) is a medically and pharmaceutically based website that offers up to date information on medicine and pharmacology. Other websites are listed in Table 1–1.

REGULATION AND CLASSIFICATION OF DRUGS

Development of New Drugs and Drug Safety

Until the nineteenth century, there were few standards or guidelines to protect the public from drug misuse. In those days there were many medicinal concoctions that, although nontoxic, were not effective. Early drug remedies included heroin for asthma and coughs, and rattlesnake oil for rheumatism. Codeine use started in the late nineteenth century and with that started the problem of addiction to these home remedies.

In 1820, The *U.S. Pharmacopoeia* (*USP*) was the first publication of drug standards in the United States. The USP listed the standards of drug purity and strength and directions for synthesis of all drugs. In 1975, the USP and the *National Formulary (NF),* published by the American Pharmaceutical Association (APhA), became one publication called the *U.S. Pharmacopoeia-National Formulary* (*USP-NF*), which is still published with regular updates. The USP label is found on many medication containers verifying the exact ingredients found within the container.

In the early 1900s, the United States started to develop and enforce tougher **drug laws** to protect the public from deceitful and unsafe methods practiced by medicine manufacturers. From this developed the first federal Food and Drug Act, signed into law by President Theodore Roosevelt in 1906. The act was amended in 1912, and an even stronger Food, Drug, and Cosmetic Act passed in 1938.

Did You Know?

In 1202, King John of England proclaimed the first English food law, the Assize of Bread, which prohibited adulteration of bread with such ingredients as ground peas or beans.

The United States Federal Food, Drug, and Cosmetic Act (FD&C) was a set of laws passed by Congress in 1938 that gave authority to the **Food and Drug Administration (FDA)** to regulate the safety of food, drugs, and cosmetics. These laws required drug labeling to include a list of ingredients and prohibited manufacturers from making false and misleading claims. For example, Dr. Flint's Quaker Bitters was a vegetable remedy for dyspepsia, constipation, sick headache, dizziness, and "low spirit." It was claimed that Bromoseltzer would cure all headaches (Figure 1–1). Refer to http://americanhistory.si.edu/

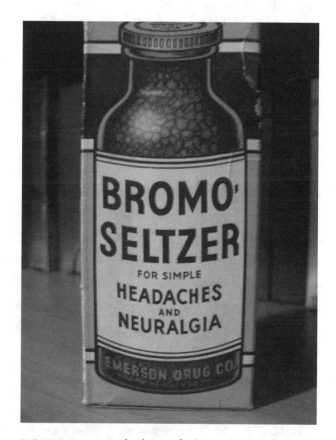

FIGURE 1–1   Early claims of relieving headaches with Bromoseltzer.

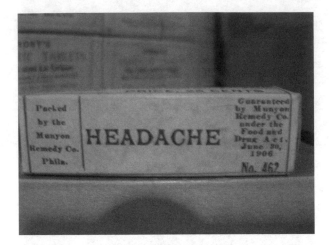

FIGURE 1–2 This headache remedy was "guaranteed" by the drug company; 1906.

collections/group_detail.cfm (National Museum of American History, Washington, DC).

From 1906 to 1918 manufacturers could label their products with the "guarantee" that their medicine complied with the new food and drug law (Figure 1–2). The 1906 law required manufacturers to label their products if any contained alcohol, cocaine, heroin, morphine, opium, cannabis, chloroform, or chloral hydrate (Figure 1–3). A complete listing of all ingredients was not required until 1938.

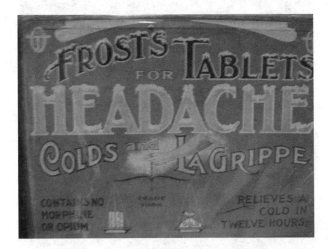

FIGURE 1–3 Tablets for headaches; on label it says it does not contain morphine or opium.

In 1968, the Electronic Product Radiation Control provisions were added to the FD&C. There are nine FD&C certified color additives used in foods in the United States and many D&C color additives used only in drugs or cosmetics. The FD&C made the certification of food color additives mandatory (e.g., FD&C Yellow No. 5). Since 1938, there have been many amendments to the Federal Food, Drug, and Cosmetic Act. Some amendments include:

Infant Formula Act, 1980

Orphan Drug Act, 1983

Drug Price Competition and Patent Term Restoration Act, 1984

Prescription Drug Marketing Act, 1987

Prescription Drug User Fee Act, 1992

Dietary Supplement Health and Education Act, 1994

Food and Drug Administration Modernization Act (FDAMA), 1997

Food Allergen Labeling and Consumer Protection Act, 2004

Rapid Dental Hint

FD&C Red No. 3 is erythrosine (tetraiodofluorescein), which is a cherry-red synthetic coal-based fluorine dye added to plaque-disclosing solutions/tablets. Question your patients regarding allergy to erythrosine.

Table 1–3 Important Drug Acts and Regulations in the United States

- 1902: Congress passed the Biologics Control Act to control the quality of serums and other blood-related products.
- 1906: The Pure Food and Drug Act of 1906 gave the government control over the labeling of medicines.
- 1912: The Sherley Amendment prohibited the sale of drugs labeled with false therapeutic claims that were intended to cheat the consumer.
- 1930: The Food, Drug, and Insecticide Administration was shortened to *Food and Drug Administration (FDA)* under an agricultural appropriations act. Today, before a new drug is introduced into the general population it must be approved by

the Food and Drug Administration, which is a federal regulatory body. The drug must meet specific criteria of efficacy and safety.

- 1938: The Food, Drug, and Cosmetic Act (FDCA) was the first law that required evidence of safety of a drug and truthfulness in labeling before it is marketed to the general public.

- 1952: The Food, Drug, and Cosmetic Act has had many amendments. One of them is the Durham-Humphrey amendment. This amendment clarified prescription and nonprescription drugs. Prescription drugs must say "Caution: Federal law prohibits dispensing without a prescription."

- 1962: The Kefauver-Harris amendment required drug manufacturers to provide proof of the effectiveness of their drugs, as well as their safety, before approval. The law was signed by President John F. Kennedy. Before this law, drug manufacturers only had to prove their products were safe. With this law, they had to prove the new drug was both safe and effective. Informed consent was obtained by patients in the studies and adverse drug reactions were reported to the FDA.

- 1983: The Orphan Drug Act, an amendment to the FDCA, allows drug manufacturers to make drugs for the treatment of rare disease. These drugs are made in small quantities and hold no monetary gains for the manufacturer. Thus, the federal government would allow these drug manufacturers to have tax benefits and other incentives.

- 1986: Congress passed the Childhood Vaccine Act, which authorized the FDA to acquire information about patients taking vaccines, to recall biologics, and to recommend civil penalties if guidelines were not followed.

- 1992: Regulations were published by the FDA to accelerate drug approval for new drugs used to treat life-threatening conditions, including acquired immunodeficiency syndrome (AIDS).

- 1992: Congress passed the Prescription Drug User Fee Act, which required that manufacturers of nongeneric drugs pay fees to help improve the drug review process.

- 1994: Congress passed the Dietary Supplement Health and Education Act, which requires clear labeling of dietary supplements. This act gives the FDA the power to remove supplements that pose a significant risk to the public.

- 1997: The Food and Drug Administration Modernization Act reauthorized the Prescription Drug User Fee Act and gave the FDA authority to accelerate the approval process for critically needed drugs. Instead of waiting approximately 15 months for approval, the drug would be approved in as little as 6 months. This act represents the largest reform effort of the drug review process since 1938.

- 2005: The Omnibus Reconciliation Act was passed, which protects direct-to-consumer drug advertising.

Did You Know?

Federal controls over the drug supply began with inspection of imported drugs in 1848.

Labeling Requirements for Over-the-Counter Drugs

Over-the-counter (OTC) drug package label is required (Code of Federal Regulations) to have "drug facts" labeling appear on the outside container or wrapper of the retail package, or if there is no outside container, on all surfaces of the immediate container or wrapper. This labeling is intended to help the consumer understand how to use the product. The "drug fact" labeling (Figure 1–4) contains the following: active ingredient(s), purpose, use(s), warning(s), allergy alert, do not use, directions, other information, inactive ingredients and questions or comments (with phone numbers).

STAGES OF APPROVAL FOR THERAPEUTIC AND BIOLOGIC DRUGS

All new drugs and biologics must first undergo rigid studies in animals and humans before gaining approval for use by the public. The Prescription Drug User Fee Act (PDUFA), first enacted in 1992, was designed to make the drug approval process faster and more efficient by providing the FDA with more funding through user fees from drug sponsors; however, income from the PDUFA is restricted to use for preapproval activities and not for postmarket monitoring.

Therapeutic drugs and biologics are reviewed in four different steps: preclinical investigations, clinical investigations, review of new drug applications (NDA), and postmarketing surveillance.

Did You Know?

The Federal Trade Commission regulates the label on the juice you drink for breakfast, the cosmetics you apply, and the contact lenses you place in your eyes.

Drug Facts
Active ingredient (in each caplet) **Purpose**
Acetaminophen 500 mg... Pain reliever/fever reducer

Uses temporarily relieves minor aches and pains due to:
- headache
- muscular aches
- backache
- arthritis
- the common cold
- toothache
- menstrual cramps
- temporarily reduces fever

Warnings
Alcohol warning: If you consume 3 or more alcoholic drinks every day, ask your doctor whether you should take acetaminophen or other pain relievers/fever reducers. Acetaminophen may cause liver damage.

Do not use
- with any other product containing acetaminophen

Stop use and ask a doctor if
- new symptoms occur
- redness or swelling is present
- pain gets worse or lasts for more than 10 days
- fever gets worse or lasts for more than 3 days

If pregnant or breast-feeding, ask a health professional before use.
Keep out of reach of children.
Overdose warning: Taking more than the recommended dose (overdose) may cause liver damage. In case of overdose, get medical help or contact a Poison Control Center right away. Quick medical attention is critical for adults as well as for children even if you do not notice any signs or symptoms. ➡

Drug Facts (continued)

Directions
■ **do not take more than directed (see overdose warning)**

adults and children 12 years and over	■ take 2 caplets every 4 to 6 hours as needed ■ do not take more than 8 caplets in 24 hours
children under 12 years	do not use this adult Extra Strength product in children under 12 years of age; this will provide more than the recommended dose (overdose) of TYLENOL® and may cause liver damage

Other information
■ **do not use if carton is opened or neck wrap or foil inner seal imprinted with "Safety Seal®" is broken or missing**
■ store between 20–25°C (68–77°F)
■ see end panel for lot number and expiration date

Inactive ingredients
cellulose, corn starch, FD&C red #40, hypromellose, magnesium stearate, polyethylene glycol, sodium starch glycolate, titanium dioxide

Questions or comments?

FIGURE 1–4 Example of "drug facts" labeling on the box of an OTC drug.

Preclinical investigations must be performed before clinical studies are done on humans. Extensive laboratory research is performed on animals and human and microbial cells cultured in the laboratory. Generally, two or more species (one rodent, one nonrodent) are tested because a drug may affect one species differently from another. Results must be submitted to the FDA before phase 1 clinical trials begin.

Phases of Clinical Human Studies

Clinical human studies occur in three phases (Figure 1–5):

Phase 1 Trials
This is the first time that a drug is administered in a human being. Healthy subjects receive a single dose of a specific drug and are monitored. The primary purpose of Phase 1 trial is to determine a proper and safe dose of the drug; however, any toxicity should be reported.

Did You Know?

Dental manufacturers must get FDA approval for the safety and efficacy of a therapeutic agent, such as fluoride, in their products before they can be released to the market.

New Drug Development Timeline

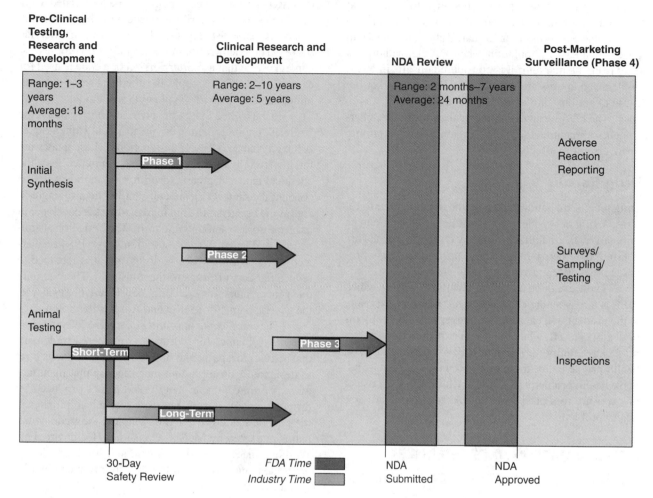

FIGURE 1–5   A new drug development timeline with the four phases of drug approval.

Phase 2 Trials

After safety of the drug has been documented, another group of human subjects with the specific disease for which the drug is intended are given the drug and monitored. These clinical trials are often longterm. This phase of studies also determines the common short-term side effects and risks associated with the drug. Clinical testing is an important part of drug evaluations because of the variability of response among people.

Approval for marketing may be accelerated if a drug is proven to be effective and without serious side effects. The approval process is delayed when a drug has concerns and precautions.

Before drug testing can proceed an NDA must be submitted.

Phase 3 Trials

Review of the New Drug Application (NDA) This phase begins only if the other phases have proven reasonably that the drug is safe and effective. The FDA is allowed 6 months to initially review an NDA. If it is approved, the testing goes to the final phase. If the NDA is rejected, the approval process stops until further notice. It takes about 17–24 months for an NDA to be reviewed. The FDA will not approve an NDA until the new drug is proven "safe and effective."

Postmarketing Surveillance   This is the fourth and final stage of drug approval that monitors the actual use of the drug in dental/medical practice. The purpose of this phase is to monitor for harmful or adverse **drug effects** in a larger population. The FDA can withdraw a drug from the market if it is considered unsafe. In 1997, Seldane, an antihistamine, was taken off the market because of serious cardiac events and death.

The FDA receives comments from the public, pharmaceutical manufacturers, and organizations pertaining to adverse drug effects.

Drug Recalls

Drug recalls are actions taken by the manufacturer to remove a drug or products from the market. Recalls can be initiated by the manufacturer or by the FDA. Recalls are continuously being reported; an up-to-date list is provided at www.fda.gov/opacom/7alters.html.

There are three classes of recalls: Class I, in which there is a reasonable chance that the use of or exposure to the product will cause serious adverse health problems or death; Class II, when the use or exposure to a product may cause temporary or medically reversible adverse health problems, or there is little chance of serious adverse health problems; and Class III, in which the use of or exposure to a product is not likely to cause adverse health problems.

DRUG NAMES AND PROPERTIES
Chemical/Generic/Trade Drug Names

Drugs often have several names. Every drug is given three names: a chemical name, a generic (nonproprietary) name, and a trade or brand name (proprietary name). There are more than 10,000 brand and generic varieties of drugs.

The *chemical name,* which is usually long and complicated, refers to the chemical makeup of the drug and defines the unique molecular structure. When a drug is first discovered it is given a chemical name, which is assigned using the nomenclature conventions of the International Union of Pure and Applied Chemistry (IUPAC). Several correct names may be formulated using these rules, but ordinarily the accepted chemical name will be the name listed by the Chemical Abstracts Service (CAS). The chemical name is usually too complex for general use so that a shorter version or a code is used for easy reference. For example, the chemical name of acetaminophen is N-(4-hydroxyphenyl) acetamide.

In the United States, the *generic name,* which is the "official" preferred name, comes from the United States Adopted Names (USAN) designations. These names are far less complicated and easier to pronounce than the chemical name. A generic drug formulation is one that contains the same therapeutically active chemical ingredients as the brand name drug marketed by the developer in the same dosage amounts and form. The Drug Price Competition and Patent Term Restoration Act of 1984 accelerated the approval of generic drugs, and was intended to reduce the cost of drugs to the consumer. There is only one generic name for each drug developed. For example, the generic name for Motrin and Advil is ibuprofen.

The *trade name* or *brand name* (also referred to as proprietary name) for a drug is a registered trademark that belongs to a particular drug manufacturer and is used to designate a drug product marketed by that manufacturer. A drug can have many brand names produced by different manufacturers. For example, acetaminophen is the generic name for Tylenol, which is the trade name, and is marketed by McNeil Consumer Healthcare, Fort Washington, PA. Nuprin, Motrin, and Advil are different trade names for ibuprofen that are produced by different manufacturers.

Generic drugs are generally less expensive than the brand name drugs. In the United States, a drug developer is given a patent on a drug, which includes exclusive rights to name and market that drug for 17 years after an NDA is submitted to the FDA. Unfortunately, this keeps the drug cost high, because there is no competition. After 17 years, the patent expires and competing manufacturers may sell a generic version of the drug, which is a chemical equivalent, but is usually less expensive.

Did You Know?

About 1,000 drugs have been designated as orphan drugs, and 200 orphan drugs have been approved by the FDA.

Did You Know?

The word *official* as used in the United States Pharmacopeia is synonymous with *pharmacopeial, USP,* and *compendial.*

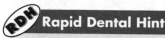

Rapid Dental Hint

Patients may not understand the differences in trade and generic names of many drugs such as analgesics. You may need to educate your patients about these products.

Look Alike–Sound Alike Drugs

Many drugs have similar-looking but quite different generic names, which can cause errors in reading them on a prescription or on a patient's medical history. Most medication errors can be avoided by reviewing carefully the patient's medication history and referring to sources for drug information. (Table 1–4)

Table 1–4 Examples of Look Alike–Sound Alike Drugs

	Look Alike–Sound Alike Drugs 1		*Look Alike–Sound Alike Drugs 2*	
Brand Name	Ativan	Atarax	Celebrex	Celexa
Generic Name	Lorazepam	Hydroxyzine	Celecoxib	Citalopram
Indication	Anti-anxiety	Anti-anxiety	Analgesic	Antidepressant

DRUG EFFECTS

Drug effects are classified as summarized in Table 1–5.

Drugs can be extremely beneficial, lengthening life and improving its quality by reducing symptoms and improving health. Unfortunately, all drugs have adverse effects and can potentially cause injury and even death.

Responsible drug therapy requires knowing not only the efficacy of a particular drug but what combinations and conditions might aggravate a situation. In addition, the dental hygienist should be aware of unexpected reactions, such as allergies, that may occur.

Therapeutic effect is the desired and beneficial pharmaceutical effect that a drug exerts at the target site of action. For example, the primary therapeutic effect of diphenhydramine (Benadryl; an antihistamine) is to reverse allergic reactions.

Table 1–5 Drug Effects

Therapeutic effects
 • Intended pharmacologic effect at target organ
Adverse drug events (ADEs)
 • Type A
 • Type B
Adverse drug reactions (ADRs)
 • Side effects
  ▪ Side effects are dose-related and predictable and affect nontarget organ sites
   • Beneficial effects
   • Adverse effects
 • Toxic reactions
  ▪ Dose-dependent and predictable
  ▪ Affects non-target organs
 • Allergic reactions
  ▪ Not dose-dependent and are unpredictable
 • Idiosyncratic reactions
  ▪ Genetically related abnormal drug response

An *adverse drug event (ADE)* is defined as an injury that results from the use of a drug or dietary supplement. Adverse drug events are classified as predictable (expected) and unpredictable reactions. The FDA categorizes a serious adverse event, related to drugs or devices, as one in which the patient outcome is death, life-threatening, hospitalization, disability, congenital anomaly, or required intervention to prevent permanent impairment or damage. Type A adverse drug events that may lead to death are usually the result of toxicity, including prescribing too much of a correct drug (overdose) for the patient's age or weight, prescribing a drug contraindicated for the patient's condition, providing the correct drug by the wrong route or too quickly, and drug interactions. These reactions are usually predictable and preventable. Type B adverse drug events are rare and generally dose independent and are related more to the individual's response and genetic differences (e.g., some individuals are slow metabolizers of drugs degraded by certain enzymes and may be at risk for serious drug toxicity). Type B reactions are unpredictable and unpreventable.

Determining the actual frequency of fatal ADEs is difficult because they are based on self-reporting; therefore, problems occur in deciding the accuracy of the number of fatal cases and the number of patients receiving the drug.

On the other hand, an *adverse drug reaction (ADR)* has been defined by the World Health Organization (WHO) as "an effect which is noxious and unintended, and which occurs at doses used in man for prophylaxis, diagnosis, or therapy." *This term is restrictive because it only considers incidents where use of the drug is appropriate,* and excludes many situations caused by medication errors. Adverse drug reactions are not predictable and are unintentional because it is not known that a reaction will occur. Harm is directly caused by the drug at normal doses, during normal use. Examples of ADRs are the development of a rash after taking penicillin, and bleeding from the stomach after taking corticosteroids or nonsteroidal anti-inflammatory drugs (Table 1–6).

The FDA has an Adverse Event Reporting System (AERS), which is a computerized information database designed to support the marketing safety surveillance program for all approved drug and therapeutic biologic products. The FDA receives adverse drug reactions reports from manufacturers as required by regulation. Healthcare professionals and consumers send reports voluntarily through the MedWatch program (www.fda.gov/medwatch). These reports become part of the database. In 2007, the FDA's Center for Drug Evaluation and Research (CDER) introduced a Web-based self-learning tutorial called FDA MedWatch and Patient Safety, which is obtained at www.connectlive.com/events/fdamedwatch. This tutorial reviews the FDA's MedWatch program.

A recent analysis of almost 500 case reports concerning fatal ADEs reported that 34 percent were type A and 66 percent were type B. The causes were: 58 percent adverse drug reactions, 17 percent drug errors, and 6 percent drug interactions.

In 1998, a reported adverse drug reaction in a 39-year-old woman ultimately contributed to the FDA withdrawal of terfenadine (Seldane), an anti-allergy drug. When Seldane was taken in excess or with the antifungal drug ketoconazole (Nizoral) or erythromycin, heart problems (ventricular arrhythmias) and even death resulted in some patients.

Adverse drug reactions are classified as adverse effects, toxic reactions, allergic reactions, and idiosyncratic reactions. Side effects of a drug are additional drug actions at therapeutic levels that can be beneficial or adverse. *Side effects are dose related and predictable and*

Table 1–6 Common Serious Adverse Drug Reactions.

Adverse Drug Reaction	*Drug Classification*	*Drug(s)*
Bleeding from the stomach	Nonsteroidal anti-inflammatory drugs	Aspirin, ibuprofen, naproxen
	Corticosteroids (anti-inflammatory)	Prednisone
Sleepiness, drowsiness, sedation	Antidepressants	Amitriptyline, fluoxetine
	Anti-anxiety drugs	Diazepam
	Antihistamines (allergies)	Diphenhydramine
Liver damage	Analgesics	Acetaminophen
	Antituberculosis drugs	Isoniazid (INH)

(Adapted from *Merck Manual,* 18th ed.)

are clinically evident at nontarget organ sites. For example, minoxidil (Loniten, Rogaine) was originally indicated as an antihypertensive drug, with a side effect of growing hair. Rogaine is a product for alopecia (hair loss) that is applied topically to the scalp; this is a beneficial side effect.

Rapid Dental Hint

Always be aware of side effects of a drug. Listen to what your patients say about what happens when he or she takes the prescribed medicine. Quite often a patient may complain of stomach problems (e.g., diarrhea) while taking an antibiotic. This is a side effect of the antibiotic that needs to be addressed.

Adverse effects (also referred to as side effects) are undesirable side effects that develop because drugs are not *totally* selective in their actions. Every medication has potential adverse effects. Generally, adverse effects are dose related: the higher the dose, the greater adverse effects. For example, adverse effects of diphenhydramine are xerostomia, urinary retention, nausea, diarrhea, and drowsiness, which require little to no change in patient management. Categories of adverse effects are usually listed by body systems, including gastrointestinal, endocrine, sense, nervous system, and hematologic.

Toxicity or toxic reaction is defined as permanent damage to cell or tissue on a microscopic or macroscopic level. Acute toxicity results in an overdose when an individual dose is too large and is taken at one time. One example is the development of seizures from excessive lidocaine. Chronic toxicity occurs when the dose effects accumulate and are sometimes difficult to detect, since they may take years to develop. Toxic reactions are predictable, dose dependent, and may be clinically evident at nontarget organ sites. An example of drug toxicity is acetaminophen (Tylenol) overuse, which can lead to liver damage.

A drug *idiosyncrasy* is an unexplained, uncharacteristic response to a drug caused by hereditary factors or genetic differences. These reactions are beginning to be understood through pharmacogenetics. One example of this type of pharmacogenetic condition is seen in the X-linked genetic trait of a deficiency in the red blood cell enzyme glucose-6-phosphate dehydrogenase (G6PD). These patients can develop drug-induced hemolytic anemia after primaquine (for malaria) therapy.

The development of an *allergic response* requires a foreign substance called an antigen to enter the body that causes the body to produce antibodies in response to the antigen. Unlike other adverse reactions, *allergies are not dose related and are unpredictable.* The allergic response occurs when a complex is formed between the antigen and antibody which produces an allergic reaction. Generally, the foreign substance that acts as an antigen is a macromolecule (e.g., protein). Since drugs are not proteins, in order to cause an allergic response, the drug will have to bind irreversibly with some body protein. Once the antibody forms in the body to this drug-protein complex the antibody will subsequently react with the drug alone. An allergic response can range from a mild rash to an anaphylaxis, which is life threatening. Identifying a true drug allergy can be challenging. A true allergy versus a side effect of a drug must be differentiated. For example, a patient reported an upset stomach when ibuprofen was taken. This is an adverse effect, not an allergic reaction. A common drug allergy is to penicillin: 10 percent of the population is allergic to penicillin, including amoxicillin. Other drug allergies include pyrophosphate (anticalculus ingredient in toothpastes), cephalosporins, and sulfa drugs (sulfonamides such as Septra and Bactrim).

Drug reactions commonly manifest with dermatologic symptoms. The most common skin manifestation is an erythematous, maculopapular rash that appears within one to three weeks after drug exposure, originates on the trunk, and eventually spreads to the limbs. Oral manifestations of allergy may be evident as erythematous, vesicular, or ulcerative mucosa.

Mutagenic effects are caused by drug induced damage to DNA (deoxyribonucleic acid). The display of damage is evident in the children from these parents. Essentially, it is an heritable genetic defect. This is distinguished from a *teratogenic defect,* which refers to the drug-induced damage that develops in the fetus. Mutagenic effects depend on when the drug exposure occurred during the DNA replication cycle. It can be a minor error where the damage occurred in only one base pair, or a major error where there is an abnormal protein or no protein produced.

An example of a teratogenic drug is thalidomide, which was originally marketed as a nonaddictive sedative, but its use was discontinued due to severe teratogenic properties. Today it is being used in the treatment of oral mucosal diseases such as severe major aphthous stomatitis in HIV-infected patients and erythema nodosum.

DRUG INTERACTIONS

Certain drugs given concurrently with another drug, herbal supplements, or food can cause a drug interaction that can be clinically significant and cause adverse/toxic side effects. There are many different mechanisms of drug interactions, which are further discussed in Chapter 4. For example, when tetracycline is taken with milk, it forms a complex that prevents absorption of the drug, and thus makes it ineffective as an antibiotic. Food can inhibit or delay absorption of certain antibiotics (e.g., azithromycin, metronidazole). Often a specified time interval must exist between taking certain drugs with foods or with one another.

DRUG ADMINISTRATION

Pharmaceutical Preparations

A chemical substance becomes a medication only after it is put into a *dosage form*. The dosage form is specific for the intended drug use and ease of handling. There are liquid and solid dosage formulations.

Liquid Dosage Formulations

Solutions are a homogenous mixture of two or more substances. They are generally liquid, but it is possible to have a mixture that is a solid. An example is chlorhexidine gluconate mouthrinse.

A suspension is a two-phase system that consists of solid particles dispersed in a liquid, solid, or gas. An example is amoxicillin suspension. An emulsion is a mixture of two liquids that do not usually mix, such as oil and water. One liquid is held in suspension in the other with the aid of an emulsifier. A syrup is an aqueous (water) solution of sugar, which may contain medicinal or flavoring agents. An example is cough syrup. Elixirs are clear, sweetened liquids that contain alcohol. An example is dexamethasone elixir.

Solid Drug Formulations

Solid formulations are easier to manufacture and are easy to store in a pharmacy. At least 70 percent of all prescriptions are solid dosage forms, known as tablets and capsules. These formulations are cheaper, and easier to store and dispense. Once ingested, tablets must disintegrate or break apart and capsules must open before absorption occurs from the gut or gastrointestinal (GI) tract (e.g., duodenum or small intestine). *Enteric-coated* tablets (e.g., aspirin, erythromycin) have a layer, such as wax or a cellulose acetate polymer, on the outside of the tablet that protects the stomach lining from exposure to these acidic drugs.

Sustained- or *extended-release* formulations release the active drug over an extended period of time so that dosing exposure to the drug is continuous over a defined period of time. Abbreviations for extended-release drugs include CR (controlled-release), LA (long-acting), XL, XR (extended release), SR (slow-release), or CRT (controlled-release tablets).

The newest formulation of medications is *orally disintegrating tablets,* which are designed to dissolve rapidly when placed on the tongue and leave an easy-to-swallow residue that is dispersed into the saliva and is then swallowed. The disintegration times are generally less than one minute but they do not have a faster onset of action. This is ideal for patients who have trouble swallowing pills.

Ointments are solid or semisolid fatty preparations intended for external use and which soften or melt at body temperature. Pastes are ointment-like mixtures of medicinal substances made into a smooth paste. An example is Orabase dental paste.

Suppositories are solid forms of drugs in various shapes created for insertion into the orifices of the body (except the mouth) and which melt or soften at body temperature.

Routes of Drug Administration

A drug enters the bloodstream by absorption from its site of administration. The route of administration influences the degree and rate of drug absorption. Routes of **drug administration** are broadly divided into *enteral, parenteral,* and *topical* (Table 1–7).

Enteral Administration

The enteral route of administration involves the drug being absorbed from the GI tract and includes oral, sublingual, buccal, and rectal.

The oral route (PO) is the most common, acceptable, and convenient route for the patient. When prescribed, it is often written as PO, which refers to taking the medication by mouth.

Drugs taken by the sublingual (under the tongue) or buccal (between the cheek and tongue) routes are absorbed directly through the oral mucosa.

Rectal administration (PR) of drugs in a suppository form are necessary when a drug is too irritating to the stomach; if the patient is vomiting or nauseated, or cannot swallow well; or for a local effect (e.g., lesions of the

Table 1–7   Routes of Drug Administration: Advantages and Disadvantages

Route	Advantages	Disadvantages	Examples
Enteral			
Oral (PO)	Most common route of administration; convenient, easy to administer	Unpredictable absorption from the gastrointestinal tract; poor adherence to schedule dosing; patient must be conscious	Capsules, liquids, tablets; antibiotics for dental indications, Periostat (doxycycline 20 mg) for chronic periodontitis
Sublingual (SL)	Provides a rapid drug response	Low doses must be given	Nitroglycerin tablets for angina (heart condition)
Buccal	Provides a rapid drug response	Low doses must be given	Testosterone buccal system
Parenteral			
Intravenous (IV)	Drug injected directly into blood stream; 100 percent of drug administered is absorbed; rapid onset	Once injected, drug cannot be retrieved	Medical emergency drugs, such as antibiotics
Intramuscular (IM)	Good absorption	Must select an appropriate injection site away from bone, large blood vessels, and nerves; soreness at site of injection. Massage injection site.	Drugs given IM include meperidine (Demerol) for severe pain, hepatitis B vaccine
Subcutaneous (SC, SQ)	Good absorption, but slower than intramuscular; avoids enzymes in the liver that would break the drug down.	Doses must be small in volume	Dental anesthetic solution, insulin
Intradermal	Easy to give to patients who cannot take the drug orally; avoids enzymes in the liver that would break the drug down	Only small volumes can be injected	Tuberculin (tuberculosis) test
Topical			
Transdermal	Dosing over extended period of time; low dosage of drugs	Cannot give large volume of drug and not a rapid response	DentiPatch, nitroglycerin patch and ointment, oral contraceptive patch, nicotine patches (for smoking cessation)
Subgingival	Localized effect to oral mucous membrane, gingival crevice, skin	Only treats localized areas	Controlled-release antimicrobials (Atridox, Arestin, PerioChip)
Epicutaneous	Localized effect on the skin	Only treats localized areas	Topical anesthetics, ointments, creams
Inhalation	Rapid drug response; local effect to the lungs or general effect as with general anesthetics	Cannot give large volumes of drug	General anesthetics, moderate sedation drugs, oxygen, asthma drugs

rectum or colitis). This is a very common route for infants and children.

Parenteral Administration

There are five parenteral routes of drug administration: (1) intravenous; (2) intramuscular; (3) subcutaneous; (4) intradermal; and (5) intrathecal. The first four are shown in Figure 1–6.

The parenteral route delivers drugs via a needle into the skin layers, subcutaneous tissue, muscle, CSF (cerebral spinal fluid), or veins, with the needle angled at different degrees, depending on the type of injection. This route is more invasive than enteral or topical administration and requires good aseptic technique.

Intravenous (IV) injection of a drug is administered directly into the circulation via a vein, so it is used for

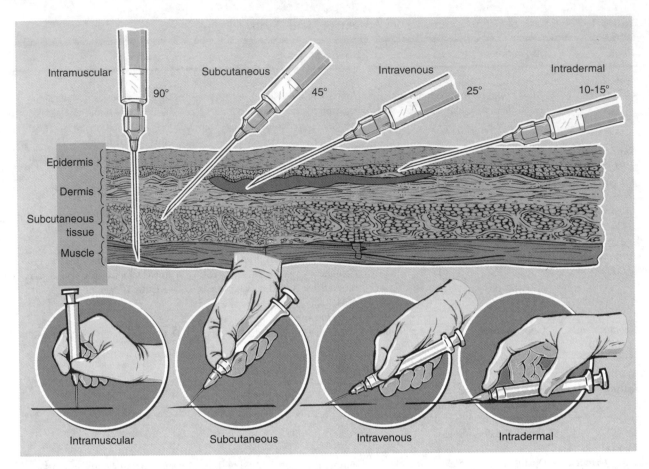

FIGURE 1–6   Different routes of parenteral drug administration.

emergency situations when it is critical to get the drug into the blood as quickly as possible. Since the drug is injected directly into the blood, this route offers the fastest onset of drug action. It is easy to control the rate of drug administered, which results in predictable blood levels. This is the most common route to administer antibiotics and fluid replacement solutions to critically ill patients.

Intramuscular (IM) injections are administered into the layers of skeletal muscle beneath the skin, including the deltoid muscle of the arm or gluteus muscle of the buttocks. Absorption is rapid and uniform since there are many blood vessels in muscles and the drug passes through capillary walls to enter the bloodstream. Irritating drugs can be administered by this route. One example of IM drug administration is the hepatitis B vaccination.

Subcutaneous (SC) administration of a drug involves the injection of liquid into the connective tissue under the skin. This route cannot be used for irritating drugs or if a large volume of the drug solution must be

administered. Examples of drugs given SC include dental anesthetics and insulin.

An intradermal injection is made directly into the dermis layer of the skin, which is below the epidermis. Intradermal injections are given to test for allergic reactions and when performing the tuberculin skin test with purified protein derivative (PPD).

An intrathecal injection, which is a less common parenteral route of administration, is delivered into the CSF, which bathes the spinal cord and is used primarily for spinal anesthesia. An epidural given for childbirth is an example of intrathecal drug injection.

Topical Administration

Topical administration refers to the application of drugs to the surface of the body directly where action is desired. Examples include the skin, mucous membranes of the gingiva (local anesthetics), eyes, ears, and the gingival crevice of teeth, mouth, and throat. When dental drugs are applied topically into the gingival crevice, it is referred to as *subgingival application.* This route is used in dentistry to administer topical anesthetics such as Oraqix and antimicrobials such as Arestin, Atridox, and PerioChip. The intention of topically applied drugs is to produce a local effect at the site of administration; however, they may be absorbed and produce systemic effects.

Inhalation administration is used for drugs that are inhaled through the mouth or nose and are used to treat asthma or rhinitis, diabetes, and for general anesthesia and moderate sedation; nitrous oxide and oxygen is most commonly delivered by this route.

Ophthalmic administration of drugs is used to treat local conditions of the eye and surrounding area including infections, dryness, glaucoma, and dilation of the pupil during an eye exam. Ophthalmic drugs are available in the form of drops, irrigations, ointments, and medicated disks.

Otic administration of drugs is used to treat local conditions of the ear. Otic drugs include drops and irrigations.

Intranasal administration of drugs is used for both local and systemic effects. Nasal spray formulations of corticosteroids are used to treat allergic rhinitis. Nasal drops are also available.

Transdermal administration is the application of a medicated adhesive patch to the skin that delivers a time-released dose of medication through the skin into the bloodstream. Examples include the nicotine patch for smoking cessation, scopolamine for motion sickness, contraceptive patches, nitroglycerin for angina, antidepressant patches (Emsam), and DentiPatch, which is a topical pre-anesthetic (lidocaine) that is applied to dry gingival tissues.

DENTAL HYGIENE NOTES

Since dental hygienists play a pivotal role in clinical pharmacology in the dental practice, they should have an understanding of the fundamentals of drug therapy. Establishing a good reference library is important to allow the hygienist to look up and verify the medications that their patients are taking. Hygienists should be able to converse with patients about medications prescribed for them, including reviewing potential adverse effects, drug interactions, and how to take the medication. A thorough medical history should be reviewed with the patient, including any prescription, over-the-counter products, and herbal supplements. The hygienist should reference any prescribed medications given to the patient to determine if there are any drug interactions with the current medications/herbal products that they are taking.

KEY POINTS

- Medication use impacts the dental hygiene process of care.
- Pharmacology is an integral part of dental care.
- It is important to know the medications that the dental patient is taking and how they impact the dental hygiene process of care.
- Have a few good, up-to-date resources (e.g., reference books or computerized references) for use at chairside during patient assessment.
- Every drug has three names: chemical, generic, brand.

BOARD REVIEW QUESTIONS

1. Which of the following routes of drug administration are dental anesthetics given? (p. 15)
   a. Subcutaneous
   b. Oral
   c. Buccal
   d. Sublingual

2. Which of the following routes of administration applies to Atridox? (p. 15)
   a. Oral
   b. Transdermal
   c. Subcutaneous
   d. Topical

3. Which of the following governmental agencies is responsible for approval of drugs? (pp. 5, 6)
   a. FDA
   b. EPA
   c. CIA
   d. SIA

4. Which of the following drug names refers to the structural makeup of a drug? (p. 10)
   a. Trade
   b. Proprietary
   c. Nonproprietary
   d. Chemical

5. Which of the following terms describes the development of constipation after a patient started taking acetaminophen with codeine after a tooth extraction? (p. 13)
   a. Toxicity
   b. Allergy
   c. Idiosyncrasy
   d. Side effect

SELECTED REFERENCES

Avorn, J. 1997. Putting adverse drug events into perspective. *Journal of the American Medical Association* 277:341–342.

Bates, D. W., and L. Leape. 2000. "Adverse drug reactions." In *Melmon and Morrelli's Clinical Pharmacology,* 4th ed. edited by S. F. Carruthers, B. B. Hoffman, K. L. Melmon, and D. W. Nierenberg, New York: McGraw-Hill. 1223–1256.

Belgado, B. S. 2000. Drug information centers on the Internet. *Journal of the American Pharmaceutical Association* 41:631–632.

Cohen, J. S. 1999. Ways to minimize adverse drug reactions. Individualized doses and common sense are key. *Postgraduate Medicine* 106:163–168;171–172.

deShazo, R. D., and S. F. Kemp. 1997. Allergic reactions to drugs and biologic agents. *Journal of the American Medical Association* 278:1895–1906.

Gossel, T. A. 1998. Pharmacology back to basics. *U.S. Pharmacist* 23:70–78.

Gossel, T. S. 1998. Exploring pharmacology. *U.S. Pharmacist* 23:96–104.

Hansten, P. D., and J. R. Horn. 1996. Drug interactions. *Drug Interactions Newsletter* 16:893–904.

Kelly, W. N. 2001. Can the frequency and risks of fatal adverse drug events be determined? *Pharmacotherapy* 21(5):521–527.

Kramer, J. M, and A. Cath. 1996. Medical resources and the Internet: Making the connection. *Archives of Internal Medicine* 156:833–842.

Kuehn, B. M. IOM: overhaul drug safety monitoring. *Journal of the American Medical Association* 296(17):2075–2076.

Levine, R. R. 1996. *Pharmacology: Drug Actions and Reactions,* 5th ed. New York: Parthenon.

McCaffery, K. 2003. Fluoride and dermatitis. *Journal of the American Dental Association* 134:1165.

Pratt, W. B, and P. Taylor. 1990. *Principles of Drug Action: The Basis of Pharmacology,* 3rd ed. New York: Churchill Livingstone.

Riedl, M. A, and A. M. Casillas. 2003. Adverse drug reactions: Types and treatment options. *American Family Physician.* 68:1781–1790.

WEB SITES

www.pdr.net
www.fda.gov
www.drugs.com
www.rxlist.com
www.fda.gov/cder
www.medscape.com

Chapter **2**

Prescription Writing

GOAL: To provide an understanding of prescription writing in the dental practice.

EDUCATIONAL OBJECTIVES

After reading this chapter, the reader should be able to:

1. Identify the various parts of a written prescription.
2. Develop clinical skills for prescription writing.
3. Discuss how to avoid errors in prescription writing.
4. Discuss issues related to writing prescriptions for controlled substances.
5. Identify common Latin abbreviations used in prescription writing.
6. Discuss the concept of generic substitution.

KEY TERMS

Prescription
Metric system
Prescription drugs
Over-the-counter (OTC) drugs
Controlled dangerous substances (CDS)
Bioequivalence
Medication errors

INTRODUCTION

Once a patient has been evaluated and diagnosed, the dental clinician may have the patient take certain medication(s) as part of therapy. A **prescription** is the prescriber's order to dispense a specific drug for the patient. Selection of a drug of choice depends on the characteristics of the patient and the clinical condition. The patient should be instructed on how to take the medication they are prescribed. Once a patient takes the prescribed medication, the dental clinician must monitor drug effects. For example, an antibiotic is prescribed for an endodontic infection. The patient reports the development of diarrhea. This situation must be assessed and appropriate treatment rendered. For instance, the antibiotic may need to be taken with food to prevent gastrointestinal discomfort. This information should be conveyed to the patient and the situation should still be monitored.

Goals of Prescription Writing

The goals of effective prescription writing are to:

1. Give an order for prescription medications to be dispensed to the patient.
2. Communicate with the pharmacist to minimize errors in dispensing.
3. Comply with any rules that govern prescribing and that could affect the patient's ability to obtain the drug.

PARTS OF THE PRESCRIPTION

Before the pharmacist fills a prescription, all parts of the prescription must be correctly written. The pharmacist must also determine if there is a contact number for the prescriber.

The different parts of the prescription are as follows (Figure 2–1):

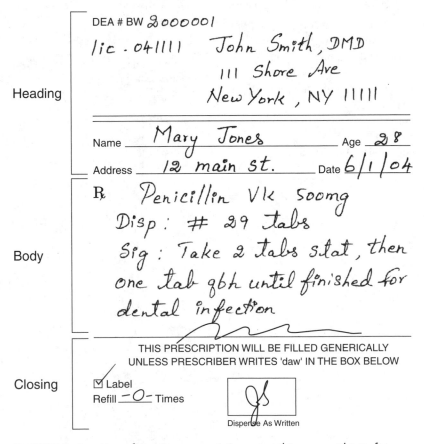

Heading

DEA # BW 2000001
lic. 041111 John Smith, DMD
111 Shore Ave
New York, NY 11111

Name _Mary Jones_ Age _28_
Address _12 main st._ Date _6/1/04_

Body

℞ Penicillin VK 500mg
Disp: # 29 tabs
Sig: Take 2 tabs s.tat, then one tab q6h until finished for dental infection

Closing

THIS PRESCRIPTION WILL BE FILLED GENERICALLY
UNLESS PRESCRIBER WRITES 'daw' IN THE BOX BELOW

☑ Label
Refill _–0–_ Times

Dispense As Written

FIGURE 2–1 Part of a written prescription prescribing an antibiotic for a dental infection.

Rapid Dental Hint

Dental hygienists should review prescriptions for accuracy and review instructions with their patients on proper taking of the medication.

1. Heading: Prescriber and patient information, including the prescriber's name, address, and telephone number; and the patient's name, address, and age. The patient's age is very important and unfortunately is frequently omitted. Knowing the patient's age will ensure the proper dose. The date the prescription was written is important for record-keeping and because some drugs are not valid beyond a specific period or before a certain monthly date.
2. Body: Contains the symbol *Rx*, drug name (generic or brand name; see the following discussion), strength (should be written in metric units; some clinicians use apothecary—see the following discussion), and quantity to be dispensed (written as Disp: #; reflects the anticipated duration of therapy), the dosage, and complete directions for use (written as Sig: Take 2 tabs PO).
3. Closing: Contains the prescriber's signature, Drug Enforcement Administration (DEA) number (the DEA number may also be in the heading), refill information, and the check-off box to label with drug name. The expiration date for the drug must be printed on the label. Additionally, any other labeling instructions should be on the container, including warnings such as "may cause drowsiness" or "take with food." A pharmacist cannot refill a prescription medication without authorization from the prescriber.

The prescriber is required by law only to write for drugs that pertain to his/her profession. All parts of a prescription must be written properly in order for a pharmacist to fill it. This includes the number of refills allowed, label, and the age of the patient. The name of the drug, indication for use, and duration of therapy should be written on the prescription, which will be transcribed by the pharmacist onto the label on the medication container. For example, if penicillin VK were prescribed for a dental infection, it should be written on the prescription that the antibiotic should be taken for 7 days, or take until finished, and that it is for a dental infection (see Figure 2–1).

Units of Measurement

There are different units of measurement that are used in the pharmacy to measure, weigh, and mix drugs: the metric system, avoirdupois system, and apothecary system.

The **metric system** of measures was formulated in France and first used in the United States in 1866. The metric system is the official system of weights and measures used by Navy Pharmacy Department for weighing and calculating pharmaceutical preparations. Each table of the metric system contains a definitive unit. For instance, the *meter* is the unit of length, the *liter* is the unit of volume, and the *gram* is the unit of weight. Table 2-1 lists some units of measure in the metric system. Today, most prescribers and pharmacies use the metric system.

The *apothecary system* (Table 2–2), which is becoming obsolete, uses old measures of weights and volumes such as grains (gr). It is important not to abbreviate when using the apothecary system to prevent confusion between "grains" and "grams." Most clinicians use the metric system when writing prescriptions; however, some still use the apothecary system (Figure 2–2). Since 1980, the USP (United States Pharmacopoeia) and NF (National Formulary) allow the simultaneous use of both the metric and apothecary systems to report the quantity of active ingredients present in a drug product labeling. An example is quinidine sulfate 200 mg (3.086 grains).

Did You Know?

The word prescription stems from the Latin term which means "to write before."

Table 2–1 Metric System: Measure of Weight and Volume

Weight (the basic unit of weight is the gram)
1 kilogram (kg) = 1000 gram (g)
1 gram   = 1000 milligrams (mg)
             = 100 centigrams (cg)
             = 10 decigrams (dg)

Volume (the basic unit of volume is the liter)
1 liter (L) = 1000 milliliters (mL)
            = 100 centiliters (cl)
            = 10 deciliters (dl)

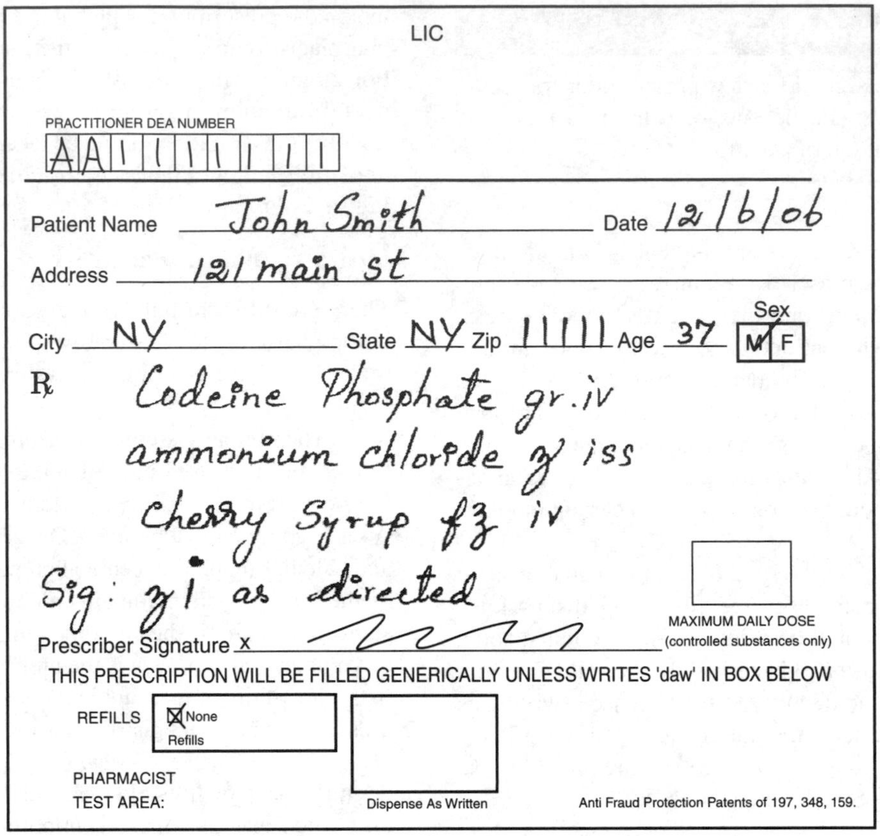

LIC

PRACTITIONER DEA NUMBER

A A | | | | | | |

Patient Name _John Smith_ Date _12/6/06_

Address _121 main st_

City _NY_ State _NY_ Zip _| | | | |_ Age _37_ Sex M F

R

Codeine Phosphate gr.iv

ammonium chloride ʒ iss

Cherry Syrup fʒ iv

Sig: ʒ i as directed

Prescriber Signature X _____

MAXIMUM DAILY DOSE
(controlled substances only)

THIS PRESCRIPTION WILL BE FILLED GENERICALLY UNLESS WRITES 'daw' IN BOX BELOW

REFILLS ☒ None
Refills

PHARMACIST
TEST AREA: Dispense As Written Anti Fraud Protection Patents of 197, 348, 159.

FIGURE 2–2 Apothecary measure of weights were often used for prescription writing, especially for compounding. This is an example of a prescription using the apothecary system for a cough syrup that the pharmacist must mix (compound).

Table 2–2 Apothecary System

Weight (the basic unit of weight is the grain.)
One grain (gr) = 0.065 grams
       (g) = rounded to 60 milligrams (mg)
    20 grains = 1 scruple (Ɔ)
    3 scruples = 1 dram (ʒ)
    8 drams = 1 ounce (ʒ)
    12 ounces = 1 pound (lb)
Volume (the basic unit of volume is the minim)
    60 minims = 1 fluidram
    8 fluidrams = 1 fluidounce
  16 fluidounces = 1 pint (pt)
    2 pints = 1 quart (qt)
    4 quarts = 1 gallon (gal)

The *avoidupois* or household *system* of weights is used in the United States for ordinary commodities. This system defines terms such as ounce, teaspoonful, and tablespoonful.

Latin Abbreviations

Common abbreviations used in prescription writing are listed in Table 2–3.

Did You Know?

In ancient times, the symbol Rx was a symbol for the Roman god Jupiter, who blessed each prescription to ensure its purity.

Table 2–3 Common Latin Abbreviations

ac	before meals
AM	morning
bid	twice a day
cap	capsule
dis	dispense
prn	as needed
q	every
qd	every day
h	hour
hs	at bedtime
qh	every hour
q8h	every 8 hours
qid	4 times a day
pc	after meals
PM	afternoon
stat	at once
sig	write on label
tid	3 times a day
po	orally (by mouth)
Rx (recipe)	take thou a recipe; prescription
qs	a sufficient quantity
tab	tablet
gtts	drops
od	right eye
os	left eye
NR	no refills
mL	milliliter

 Rapid Dental Hint

Since some over-the-counter herbs or vitamins can affect blood clotting levels, the dental hygienist should ask their patients about these.

PRESCRIPTION AND NONPRESCRIPTION DRUGS

In the United States there are two classes of drugs: **prescription** and **over-the-counter (OTC).** Prescription drugs require a written prescription or a telephone order to the pharmacy and can only be prescribed by a dentist, physician, podiatrist, or veterinarian. In some states dental hygienists, specialized pharmacists, nurses, physician assistants, and optometrists can prescribe drugs. Prescription drugs have the federal legend statement, Rx Only. Nonprescription drugs are medications that can be obtained OTC or without a prescription. Dental hygienists should record a patient's prescription and OTC drug use.

The Food and Drug Administration regulates both prescription and OTC drugs. In 1992, the OTC Drugs Advisory Committee was created to assist the FDA in reviewing OTC drugs. An OTC drug review, which started in 1972, is a three-phase process that involves an advisory panel review, tentative final monograph publication, and a final monograph publication. A drug with OTC approval must be able to be safely self-administered.

Although nonprescription drug use has many positive aspects including cost, ease of access, and availability to the patient, there are many drawbacks such as improper use of drugs or improper indications that are potentially harmful to the individual. A consumer must be able to determine whether a drug is appropriate for his or her given condition.

In 1983, the topical prescription drug hydrocortisone was the first drug approved for OTC sales, after which many other drugs followed. Other examples include cimetadine (Tagamet) and famotidine (Pepcid) for ulcers; naproxen sodium (Aleve) and ketoprofen (Actron); which are analgesics; and clotrimazole (Gyne-Lotrimin), which is an antifungal.

CONTROLLED DANGEROUS SUBSTANCES

The Harrison Narcotics Act of 1914 established the first drug abuse legislation in the United States due to the high incidence of abuse of heroin, which was available over-the-counter. This act regulated the distribution and use of all narcotics.

Habit-forming drugs are classified according to their abuse potential for addiction and dependency and are placed in *schedules* by the Federal Drug Enforcement Administration (DEA). Controlled substances have the potential to cause dependency, which is defined as the psychological or physiological need for a drug or substance. These drugs have restrictions and are called **controlled dangerous substances (CDS).**

In the United States, controlled substances are drugs whose use is restricted and accounted for by the Controlled Substances Act of 1970 and later revisions. The Controlled Substances Act is also called the Comprehensive Drug Abuse Prevention and Control Act. Thus, the use of dangerous substances is controlled under federal law but differs from state to state.

Hospitals and pharmacies must register with the DEA to purchase controlled drugs. Prescribers are assigned a number by the DEA in order to write prescriptions for controlled substances. This number is written on all prescriptions for controlled substances.

There are five categories of controlled substances:

- Schedule I (C-I)
- Schedule II (C-II)
- Schedule III (C-III)
- Schedule IV (C-IV)
- Schedule V (C-V)

Schedule C-I drugs have the most abuse potential and are not used clinically. Schedule C-II drugs are highly abused. Schedule C-III drugs are less abused, and Schedule C-IV are even less abused. Schedule C-V drugs (e.g., cough syrups that contain codeine) have a very low abuse level.

Prescriptions for Schedule II drugs cannot be refilled. In some states there are special requirements that the pharmacist must fulfill with regard to dispensing Schedule II drugs, whereas prescriptions for schedule III, IV, and V drugs can only be refilled five times within 6 months (Table 2–4).

In dentistry, controlled drugs are primarily used for dental and orofacial pain control and for sedation. For example, acetaminophen with codeine (Tylenol with codeine No. 1, 2, 3, 4) and acetaminophen with hydrocodone (Vicodin) are both C-III narcotics indicated for pain. Diazepam (Valium) and other drugs in this class that are used to calm the anxious dental patient are listed as C-IV drugs, but in many states these drugs are regulated as C-II medications. Although nitrous oxide, which is referred to as laughing gas, has a high potential for abuse, it is not scheduled.

Triplicate Prescription

Triplicate prescription programs were developed in an effort to decrease the diversion of prescription medications to illicit markets. States with such laws (e.g., Texas) require prescribers to write prescriptions on special triplicate forms for all Schedule II drugs, including narcotic analgesics, barbiturates, and stimulants. If a prescription for a Schedule II drug is phoned or faxed to the phar-

Did You Know?

Until 1937, marijuana was legal in the United States for all purposes. In 1970, marijuana was placed in Schedule I. In the late 1990s attention was focused on making marijuana legal for medical purposes only. In some states (e.g., Oregon), marijuana can be prescribed for reducing nausea and vomiting in cancer patients receiving chemotherapy.

macy, it must be followed up within 72 hours with a written copy of the prescription. The prescriber keeps one copy of the prescription for 5 years and sends two copies with the patient to the pharmacist. The pharmacist keeps one copy and forwards the third to a specified state agency where the prescription is used to track the prescriber's prescribing practices and the patient's use of controlled substances.

DRUG CONTAINER AND PACKAGE INSERT

Prescription drugs are controlled by the U.S. Food and Drug Administration. The FDA Modernization Act of 1997 (FDAMA) required that before dispensing, the labels of prescription drug products (drug container) contain the symbol statement "Rx only" instead of the "Caution: Law prohibits dispensing without prescription." The Rx only statement and the package insert (PI) are part of the packaging requirements for all prescription drugs. The package insert is literature written about the drug that accompanies all prescription drugs and is negotiated between the drug manufacturer and the FDA. The PI describes the chemical nature, indications for which the drug has been officially approved by the FDA, contraindications, warnings, adverse reactions, drug interactions, dosage and administration, and how it is supplied. All PIs are published in the *PDR*® (Thomson, Montvale, NJ).

Beginning June 2006, the FDA required a major revision to the format of information in the PIs. Any new drug or new indication for a drug already on the market must include the newly reformatted labeling. The changes in the labeling include the addition of a section titled Highlights, which is a half-page summary at the start of the labeling that summarizes key information. In

Table 2–4 Drug Schedules (Controlled Drugs)

Drug Schedule	Abuse Potential	Drug Examples	Pharmacist Filling*
C-I	Highest	No safe medical use; medical research, hashish, PCP, LSD, heroin	These drugs are not filled in a pharmacy.
C-II	High	Safe medical use; some narcotics, stimulants, and depressants. Cocaine, morphine, methadone, methamphetamine, oxycodone (Percodan/Percocet), methylphenidate (Ritalin), meperidine (Demerol).	Must have a prescription. Some states (e.g., Texas) require triplicate prescription blanks. Telephone prescription for limited amounts may be filled in an emergency, but written in ink or typed; signed prescription must be sent (postmarked) to the pharmacist within 72 hours. A fax is accepted but the prescription cannot be dispensed until the written prescription is received. Federal law states that if the prescription is written, there are no quantity limitations. No refills allowed.
C-III	Moderate	Acetaminophen with codeine (Tylenol with codeine), acetaminophen with hydrocodone (Vicodin), anabolic steroids	Written or oral prescription allowed. May not refill more than five times within 6 months after the date on the prescription. Must be filled within 6 months of the date the prescription was written. An allowable excess of a 30-day supply may only be refilled once.
C-IV	Low	Triazolam (Halcion; sedative), chloral hydrate, propoxyphene (Darvon), phenobarbital, benzodiazepine (Valium, Xanax); in some states (e.g., New York, Texas) these drugs are classified as C-II.	Written or oral prescription allowed. May not refill more than five times within 6 months. Must be filled within 6 months of the date the prescription was written. An allowable excess of a 30-day supply may only be refilled once.
C-V	Lowest	Cough medicines that contain codeine	May be prescription or OTC. If OTC, no more than 8 oz of codeine can be dispensed in a 48-hour period to any one person. The pharmacist is required to keep a bound book that shows the name of the preparation, date of the purchase, quantity sold, and the name and address of the purchaser.

*Dispensing and prescription writing of controlled substances is federally regulated, but differs from state to state. Since the law is different in various states, only the federal law rules are listed in this textbook. The student is encouraged to review the laws in their state.

addition, the new labeling will include a table of contents following the Highlights section that will have hyperlinks to the pertinent text referenced in the table. This is an accommodation to the movement toward e-prescribing (electronic prescription writing). Information about the labeling change is posted at www.fda.gov/cder/regulatory/physLabel/default.htm. The labeling change was needed because the FDA decided that the existing labeling is too complicated, too long, and makes it too difficult to find important information.

BLACK BOX WARNING

In the United States, the FDA can require a pharmaceutical company to place a black box warning on the label of a prescription drug or in the package insert, at the start of the labeling. A black box warning means that medical studies have shown that the drug causes a significant risk of serious or even life-threatening adverse effects. A black border is placed around the text of the warning. Refer to www.fada.gov/Medwatch/safety/2006/safety06.htm.

Some examples of black box warnings include:

- March 2, 2006: Asthma long-acting beta$_2$-agonist including salmeterol xinafoate (Serevent Diskus) and fluticasone propionate/salmeterol xinafoate (Advair Diskus). These drugs may increase the risk of asthma-related death.
- October 15, 2004: Antidepressants (selective serotonin reuptake inhibitors and some atypical antidepressants) may result in increased suicidal thoughts and behavior ("suicidality") in children and adolescents.
- April 11, 2005: Elderly patients with dementia-related psychosis treated with atypical antipsychotic drugs such as aripiprazole (Abilify), risperidone (Risperdal), olanzapine (Zyrexa), and quetiapine (Seroquel) are at an increased risk of death compared to a placebo.
- November 17, 2004: Depo-Provera, a contraceptive injection, carries a high risk of significant loss of bone density with long-term use.
- September 28, 2006: Lamotrigine (Lamictal), a drug for seizure disorders and bipolar disorder, is not indicated for use in patients below the age of 16 years because of development of a potentially life-threatening rash.
- July 26, 2001: OxyContin is an opioid agonist and a Schedule II controlled substance with an abuse liability similar to morphine. OxyContin tablets are *not* intended for use as a prn (as needed) analgesic. OxyContin tablets are a controlled-release oral formulation of oxycodone hydrochloride indicated for the management of moderate to severe pain when a continuous, around-the-clock analgesic is needed for an extended period of time.
- June 17, 2002: Valproic acid (Depakene) has many black box warnings: (1) can cause hepatic failure resulting in fatalities, especially children under two years of age; (2) can produce teratogenic effects such as neural tube defects; and (3) cases of life-threatening pancreatitis have been reported in both children and adults.

LABELED AND OFF-LABEL USES OF DRUGS

The FDA approves a drug to be used for specific purposes. These approved indications or *labeled uses* are listed on the package insert in the drug box. Drugs may also be prescribed for a different purpose from which it is originally intended, also known as *off-label use*. Diphenhydramine (Benadryl) is indicated for reduction of symptoms of allergy, but may be used off label as a sleeping pill or for the relief of motion sickness.

BIOEQUIVALENCE AND BIOAVAILABILITY: GENERIC DRUG SUBSTITUTION

Once the patent protection for an FDA-approved brand name drug expires, generic products often become available. Bioavailability and bioequivalence of drug products and drug product selection have emerged as critical issues in pharmacy and dentistry over the last few decades when prescribing by generic drug name. Prescribing generic drugs offers the pharmacist flexibility in selecting the drug to be dispensed and the patient possible savings.

Concern about lowering medication costs has resulted in an increase in the use of generic drug products versus brand name drugs. The extraordinary growth of the generic pharmaceutical industry and the large quantity of multisource products has provoked some questions among healthcare professionals and consumers regarding the therapeutic equivalency of these products.

The availability of different formulations of the same drug substance given at the same strength and in the same dosage form creates a challenge to healthcare professionals. Are generic drug products as good as brand name drugs? Are the generic drugs bioequivalent? The answer to both of these questions, according to the FDA, is yes. Thus, a dentist may write a prescription for tetracycline by its generic name, or may prescribe it under

---

Did You Know?

About half of all prescriptions written in the United States are for drugs that can be substituted for a generic product.

the brand names Sumycin, Doryx, or Vibramycin. No matter what name is used, each drug must meet the same FDA standards for tetracycline.

Bioequivalence of a drug is a pharmaceutical equivalent or alternative that contains an identical amount of the active drug as the brand name drug and does not show differences in the rate and extent of absorption. According to FDA regulations, a generic copy of a brand name drug must contain identical amounts of the same active drug ingredient in the same dosage form and route of administration and meet standards for strength, purity, quality, and identity. *However, the inactive ingredients such as bindings, fillers, and flavorings may be different even within the same manufacturer but different batches.* These ingredients and the manufacturing process can cause clinical variability in the rate and extent of liberation of a drug from the dosing unit (e.g., tablet, capsule) and its subsequent absorption. Bioequivalence must be proved for any new form of a drug, including new dosage forms or strengths of an existing trade name drug.

The key factor when comparing brand name drugs with their generic equivalents is the bioavailability of the two drugs. Essentially, it should be determined if the two drugs get to the target tissue and act equally. Legally (FDA requirements), bioequivalence of different batches of a drug can vary by up to 20 percent, but such a difference does not alter the efficacy or safety of the drug. *Sometimes generic substitution is not appropriate either because standards for comparison have not been established or the actions of generic drugs may not be the same (efficacy) in everyone.*

The FDA annually publishes a book called *Approved Drug Products with Therapeutic Equivalence Evaluations* (known as the Orange Book) which lists the trade name drugs that are generically interchangeable.

 Rapid Dental Hint

Patients may ask about the differences between generic and brand name drugs. For example, is there is a difference between ibuprofen and Advil or Motrin? Be able to explain.

A basic issue the prescriber should consider in deciding how to prescribe a drug available generically is whether there is a loss of drug efficacy or increase in toxicity when a patient is changed from one generic formulation to another.

In most states, pharmacists are allowed to or must substitute the cheaper generic drug for a prescribed trade name drug; however, the prescriber can specify on the prescription to dispense the brand name only. The purpose for generic drug substitution is that it is cheaper for the patient. Some states (including Florida, Kentucky, and Missouri) have a list of trade name drugs that pharmacists are not allowed to substitute generically and must be dispensed as the prescriber wrote on the prescription.

 Rapid Dental Hint

The dental hygienist who is reviewing a prescription for fluoride tablets should be sure it is age-, dose-, and quantity-appropriate for the child.

Rapid Dental Hint

When reviewing premedication, the dental hygienist should ensure that patients take the correct dosage and at the right time before dental services are provided.

OTHER FACTORS ASSOCIATED WITH PRESCRIPTION WRITING
Safety of Prescription Pads

Sometimes prescriptions are stolen and forged, especially for illegal prescribing of narcotics because they are cheaper and safer than street drugs. Many states require the prescriber to obtain preprinted prescription pads directly from the state that the prescriber is licensed or from approved printing manufacturers. Prescription pads should not be left unattended.

Patient Adherence

Patient adherence to the prescribed drug regimen is an important part of treatment success. Adherence implies taking a drug in the way it was prescribed or, in the case of OTC drugs, following the instructions on the label. Patient noncompliance can include not taking the medication at all, taking it at the wrong time, taking it the wrong way, or not taking it for the recommended period.

> **Rapid Dental Hint**
>
> Patient education is important for patient adherence to the drug regimen. Review with patients how and when to take drugs prescribed to them.

How to Reduce Medication Errors

The best way to avoid prescribing or **medication errors** is to write in ink and clearly (print, not script) or electronic transmission. Bad penmanship does not make for a better doctor. It is best to avoid abbreviations to avoid misinterpretations. Open-ended statements such as Take as directed or As needed should not be written. Prescriptions written for patients should be copied into the patient's chart. The number of refills should be entered on the prescription and well as the dose and dose frequency.

The FDA has started a national education campaign that focuses on eliminating the use of potentially harmful abbreviations by prescribers. The campaign addresses the use of error-prone abbreviations in all forms of communication, including written prescriptions, computer-generated labels, medication administration records, pharmacy or prescriber computer order entry screens, and commercial medication labeling, packaging, and advertising (go to: www.fda.gov/cder/drug/MedErrors).

As the number of generic products continues to increase, patients, clinicians and pharmacists must be aware of medication appearance. Patients may not question a change in the color of a generic pill that they have been taking for years only to find out that that was not the intended medication. Thus, to avoid errors patients should know what their medication looks like and be educated to always question any change in its appearance. Pharmacies should consider software that allows a description

of the medication's appearance to be printed on the label (New Jersey Board of Pharmacy, April 2007).

> **Rapid Dental Hint**
>
> Review prescriptions for accuracy. Make sure the writing is legible and there are no abbreviations.

Electronic Prescribing

Many states presently allow some form of electronic transmission of prescriptions, which reduces errors in reading handwritten prescriptions. In this process, the prescription is electronically transmitted via a database exchange, which is usually a computer or PDA, or email converted to fax to the patient's pharmacy. The prescription is then filled from the electronically transmitted order. The dentist is usually required to keep a written record of what is prescribed.

GUIDANCE IN PRESCRIBING
Prescribing for Children

Many drug dosage formulas have been suggested (e.g., Clark's and Yong's rules) that assume incorrectly that the adult dose is correct and that the child is a small version of the adult. It is recommended that instead of using of the "rules," pediatric doses should be calculated from age, body-weight, or body-surface area (BSA), which is the preferred method. If using body-weight, the following formula is used:

$$\frac{\text{Child's weight in Kg (kilograms)}}{70} \times \text{adult dose}$$

or

$$\frac{\text{Child's weight in lbs}}{150} \times \text{adult dose}$$

Safety in Pregnancy

The FDA developed a system assigning all drugs a letter designation that indicates safety for use during pregnancy and lactatation. The primary concern with giving certain drugs to pregnant women is that drugs are potential *tera-*

Table 2–5 Food and Drug Administration (FDA) Pregnancy Categories

Safety Category	Definition	Drugs
A	Studies on humans fail to show a risk to the fetus or pregnant woman. Lowest risk.	Levothyroxine (thyroid), potassium, ferrous (iron) sulfate, folic acid
B	Animal studies have not shown a risk to the fetus but there are no human studies in pregnant women.	Acetaminophen, lidocaine ibuprofen, erythromycin, chlorhexidine gluconate, azithromycin (Zithromax), penicillin, amoxicillin, metronidazole, clindamycin, insulin
C	Animal studies have shown a risk to the fetus but no human studies on pregnant women have been done.	Isoniazid (for tuberculosis), carbamazepine (Tegretol), fluoride, antidepressants (Zoloft, Prozac), clarithromycin (Biaxin), antihistamines (Allegra), acetaminophen with hydrocodone (Vicodin), acetaminophen with codeine, propranolol, aspirin (D if full dose; give in third trimester)
D	There is evidence that the drug may cause fetal damage, but in life-threatening situations, benefits for use in pregnant women may be acceptable despite the risk to the fetus. A "warning" will be printed on the label.	Phenytoin (Dilantin; for seizures), tetracyclines antibiotic, anti-anxiety drugs (Valium, Xanax), warfarin (anticoagulant)
X	Studies in animals or humans have shown risk to the fetus and woman. The drug is contraindicated in women who are, or may become, pregnant.	Estrogens

*Note: Many references do not have a classification for nitrous oxide.

togens that may cause harm to the embryo or fetus by causing alterations in the formation of cells, tissues, and organs. Drug-induced teratogenic changes only occur during organ formation. During dental therapy, it is safest to prescribe to pregnant patients drugs that do not affect the embryo or fetus.

The categories are listed as A, B, C, D, and X. Category A is at lowest risk for harming the fetus because medical studies have not demonstrated that the drug is a risk to the fetus or pregnant women. Category D drugs (e.g., tetracycline) have been shown through medical studies to cause harm to the fetus and/or pregnant woman and should not be given. Category X drugs (e.g., estrogens) are contraindicated in women who are, or may become, pregnant. Some drugs, such as cimetidine (Tagamet; for ulcers), alcohol, and tetracycline are contraindicated in nursing women since they pass through breast milk and can cause harm to the nursing baby. Many dental drugs with A, B, and some C designations

can be used safely in pregnant and lactating women. Table 2–5 lists safety categories with drug examples.

DENTAL HYGIENE NOTES

As of 2005, Oregon was the first and only state to allow dental hygienists limited prescription writing for fluoride and antimicrobial agents (e.g., gels, rinses). This change in the practice of a dental hygienist may become more prevalent and full knowledge of prescription writing may fall within the scope of practice. It is also important for the dental hygienist to be able to understand how a prescription is written because patients may ask questions about drugs that the dentist prescribed or drugs they are taking. Before a prescription is given to the patient, the dental hygienist should reference the drug and review the mechanism of action, adverse side effects, how to take the medication, and if there are any drug–drug, drug–herb, or drug–food interactions.

KEY POINTS

- The prescription should be written clearly.
- Prescriptions should state the dose, frequency of administration, and the age of the patient.
- Do not abbreviate words.
- Communicate with the patient on how to take the medication.
- Document in the chart that the medication was reviewed with the patient and that they understood how to take the medication.
- Successful pharmacotherapy depends on patient adherence.
- Different systems of measurement have been used in pharmacy: metric, apothecary, and household.

SELECTED REFERENCES

Hisle, J.M. 2001. Throw away the prescription pad? Debate over electronic prescription and fulfillment. *Medical Crossfire* 3:47–56.

Katzung, B.G. 2004. *Basic and Clinical Pharmacology* 9th ed. New York: Lange Medical Books/McGraw-Hill.

Marek, C.L. 1996. Avoiding prescribing errors: A systematic approach. *Journal of the American Dental Association* 127:617–623.

New Jersey Board of Pharmacy. October 2006. Newsletter.

WEB SITES

www.pdr.net
www.aphanet.org
www.rxlist.com
www.gsm.com
www.FDA-News.com
www.fda.gov/cder/drug/MedErrors

BOARD REVIEW QUESTIONS

1. Which of the following dental drugs cannot be refilled at the pharmacy? (pp. 23–24)
   a. Tetracycline
   b. Percocet
   c. Tylenol with codeine No. 3
   d. Vicodin

2. Compared to the brand name drug, a generic name drug is usually: (pp. 26–27)
   a. Cheaper.
   b. Longer acting.
   c. More expensive.
   d. More effective.

3. Which of the following abbreviations stands for "twice a day"? (p. 23)
   a. bid
   b. tid
   c. qid
   d. qh

4. Which of the following is important when writing a prescription? (p. 20)
   a. Avoid abbreviations when possible.
   b. Use as many abbreviations as possible.
   c. Do not write the dosage on the prescription.
   d. Always write Take as directed.

5. The Latin abbreviation hs means: (p. 23)
   a. At bedtime.
   b. After meals.
   c. In the right eye.
   d. As needed.

Chapter 3

Fundamentals of Drug Action

GOAL: To provide an understanding of the basic principles of what the body does to drugs and the action of drugs on the body.

EDUCATIONAL OBJECTIVES

After reading this chapter, the reader should be able to:

1. Compare the differences between pharmacodynamics and pharmacokinetics.
2. Describe the characteristics of drug molecules.
3. Describe the mechanisms of drug absorption through the various membranes in the body.
4. Describe absorption through the different routes of drug administration.
5. Describe the drug–receptor interaction.
6. Distinguish between a loading dose and a maintenance dose.
7. Describe the various factors involved in the biological variations of drug dosing.

KEY TERMS
Pharmacokinetics
Bioavailability
Drug dose
Pharmacodynamics
Drug receptor
Enterohepatic recirculation

PHARMACOKINETICS

Pharmacokinetics describes how a drug gets to the site of action. The amount of drug in the body at any given time is determined by for processes, abbreviated ADME:

1. Absorption
2. Distribution
3. Metabolism (biotransformation)
4. Elimination or excretion

Figure 3–1a shows factors affecting the onset, duration, and intensity of a drug effect. The ultimate goal of pharmacokinetics is to have the drug reach the site of action in adequate concentrations to produce a pharmacological effect prior to elimination from the body. A *two-compartment model* describes a representation of the pharmacokinetic behavior of many drugs after oral administration. It shows the absorption of drugs into the central compartment (e.g., blood), distribution into the peripheral component (e.g., tissues), and elimination from the central component (Figure 3–1b).

Characteristics of Drug Molecules

In order for drugs to cause a pharmacologic action, they need to achieve an adequate concentration in their target tissues. Drug molecules move around the body in two ways: in the bloodstream (over long distance) and molecule by molecule (over short distance). The rate of diffusion of a substance depends mainly on its molecular size: Large molecules diffuse more slowly than small ones. Many drugs fall within the molecular weight range of 200–1,000. Drugs in this range are large enough to allow selectivity of action and small enough to allow adequate movement between compartments. Drugs are mainly small, simple molecules (e.g., amino acids, alcohols, acids), carbohydrates, lipids, or proteins.

Usually drugs enter the body far from the intended site of action. In order to get to the organ/tissue where it will have a pharmacologic effect, the drug must be absorbed and transported through the bloodstream (systemic circulation).

Absorption

So how does the drug get into the blood? A drug must be in solution to be absorbed and distributed in the body. Liquid dosage forms, such as injectables and cough syrups, are already in solution and are immediately available for absorption and transport. The drug passes through the GI tract (usually the upper part of the duodenum or small intestine), where most absorption occurs into the blood.

The Movement of Drugs Across Cell Membranes

Cell Membranes/barriers   Before a drug is absorbed into the blood it must pass through many *cell membranes* or tissue barriers to get to the organ/tissue where the drug will exert its pharmacological effect. Generally, a drug will be better absorbed in the small intestine than the stomach because the small intestine has a larger surface area. The final destination of a drug is referred to as the *site of drug action*.

Cell membranes form the barriers between different compartments in the body; the structure of cell membranes of the tissues in the body is illustrated in Figure 3–2. Cell membranes are composed of two layers of lipids referred to as the biphospholipid layer with highly polar (water-soluble) heads of the molecules oriented outward and the nonpolar (fat-soluble) chains of fatty acids inside the membrane. Embedded in the membrane are proteins with small aqueous (water) holes, channels, or pores throughout. Thus, the cell membrane acts as a lipid barrier and allows lipid-soluble (*lipophilic*) drugs to penetrate cell membranes more easily by diffusion. Drugs that are water soluble (*hydrophilic*) do not diffuse easily in the lipid layer and either pass through the aqueous pores or are prevented from entering the cell and thus are contained outside.

Optimally, a drug should have some degree of both lipid and water solubility: water solubility to go through fluids to get to the cell, and lipid solubility to get through the cell membrane. Lipid solubility is one of the most important determinants of the pharmacokinetic characteristics of a drug.

An orally administered drug passes down the esophagus into the gastrointestinal tract (small intestine), where it must cross the gastrointestinal mucosa (single-cell layered epithelium) into the blood before being distributed to the target tissue/organ (site of action). This is referred to as the *intestinal mucosa/blood barrier.* Intravenous drugs avoid absorption barriers by entering the bloodstream immediately upon administration.

The *placenta barrier* filters out some substances that can harm the fetus, but allows other substances, including alcohol, to cross.

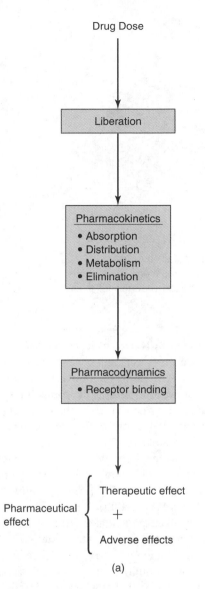

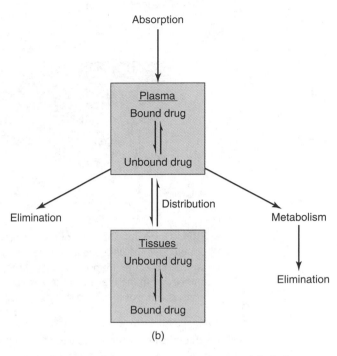

FIGURE 3-1b A two-compartment model of pharmacokinetics.

FIGURE 3-1a Generalized scheme showing the contribution of absorption, distribution, metabolism, elimination, and drug–receptor binding of drugs.

Sublingually or buccally administered drugs must go through the epithelium of the oral mucosa (tongue or buccal mucosa) before entering the blood and being distributed to the site of action (Figure 3–3). This barrier is referred to as the *oral mucosa/blood barrier.*

Once the drug enters the blood, it is transported to the various tissues in the body where it will exert its pharmacological effect(s). The drug must then go through another barrier, the membrane between the blood and the tissue, called the *blood/tissue barrier.* The structure of

capillary cell membranes is different in different areas in the body. The permeability or passage of drugs through the capillary wall is dependent upon the features of the endothelial cells lining the capillaries; for instance, the capillary endothelial cells of the pancreas have pores or openings allowing easy passage of the drug. If the drug is intended to go to the brain, the drug must pass through the capillaries of the brain (*blood/brain barrier*). The cell membrane of the brain is very lipid, so that water soluble substances/drugs cannot enter the brain. Only small molecular size, lipid-soluble drugs such as general anesthetics (e.g., thiopental), and anti-anxiety drugs get through the brain cell membrane very easily.

Absorption How do drugs penetrate cell/tissue membranes? Substances move through cell membranes by passive diffusion, facilitated diffusion, or active transport:

1. Most drugs are absorbed by *passive diffusion* across a cell barrier and into the circulation. The rate of diffusion is proportional to the concentration gradient (Figure 3–3); the rate of absorption increases as long as the concentration outside (blood)

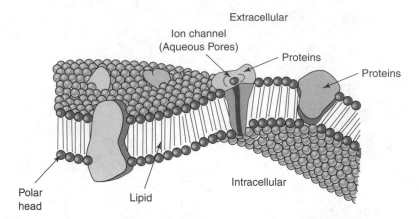

FIGURE 3–2   Diagram of a cell membrane. The cell membrane is a double layer of phospholipid molecules with highly polar heads oriented outward and the nonpolar chains of fatty acids inside the membrane. Embedded in the membrane are proteins that include ion channels for the transport of water-soluble drugs.

the cell is greater than the concentration inside the cell (GI fluids). If the concentration outside equals the concentration inside, an equilibrium exists in which net movement of the substance stops. As described earlier, lipid-soluble drugs dissolve through the cell membrane while smaller, water-soluble drugs pass through the cell membrane via water channels or pores. No energy is used by the cell during passive diffusion.

2. *Facilitated diffusion* occurs when a carrier such as a protein is necessary to get a drug that is too large and/or too polar to diffuse across a lipid membrane. By definition, diffusion is a passive process that does not require energy in moving the drug across the cell membrane. Sugars, penicillin, and aspirin are transported in this way.

3. *Active transport* involves the use of carrier proteins to move drugs against the concentration gradient with expenditure of energy. This is not a common process of absorption and is limited to drugs structurally similar to endogenous substances such as vitamins (e.g., vitamin B_{12}), sugars, and amino acids.

4. *Pinocytosis* involves the engulfment of fluids or particles by a cell. The cell membrane traps the substance, forming a vesicle that will detach and move to the interior of the cell. This process involves energy expenditure and plays a minor role in drug movement.

Effect of pH on Absorption of Weak Acids and Bases   Most drugs are either weak acids or bases (Table 3–1) and are present in solution as both ionized & nonionized forms. Ionization is the formation of ions from neural molecules and involves the removal or addition of one or more electrons (a function of the electrostatic charge of the molecule).

The ionized form, which has low lipid solubility and has an electric charge, cannot easily cross a lipid membrane. The nonionized form is usually lipid soluble and readily crosses cell membranes. Thus how much of the drug changes to the ionized form will depend on the pK_a of the drug and the pH of the solution. The pH refers to the concentration of the H^+ ions. The pK_a of a drug is related to the equilibrium that the drug has with its ionized form and is the pH at which the drug is 50 percent ionized and is a constant value. Generally, the pK_a of weak acids is 3–5 and weak bases is 8–10.

The Henderson-Hasselbalch equation is used to calculate the pH of the environment or surrounding fluid which determines the ratio of nonionized drug to ionized drug if the drug is a weak acid or base. This equation is used primarily by drug manufacturers for determining the solublities of drugs. The Henderson-Hasselbalch equation for a weak acid is:

$$pH = pK_a + \log \frac{\text{concentration of nonionized drug}}{\text{concentration of ionized drug}}$$

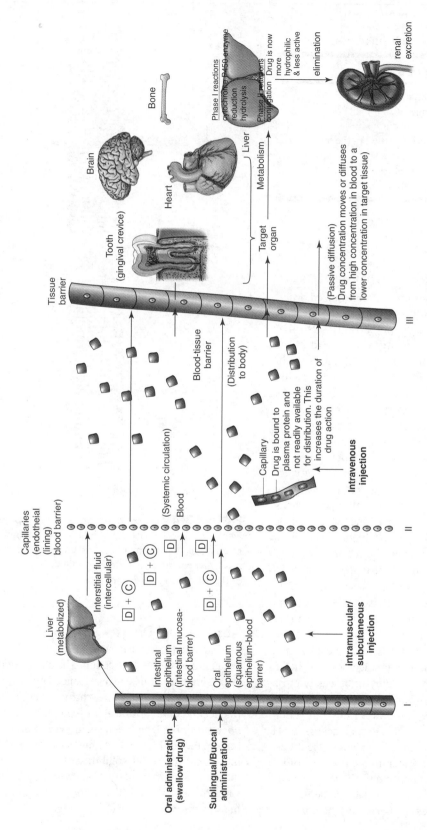

FIGURE 3–3 Absorption of a drug through cell membranes into the blood stream (systemic circulation). The drug has to go through many tissue–blood barriers to get to the final site of action. The tissue–blood and blood–tissue barriers are: After swallowing a drug it goes from the GI tract (gut or small intestine) into the blood (I), then from the blood through the blood–tissue barrier (II) to the site of action (organ or tissue). This is another blood–tissue barrier (III). D = drug; C = carrier.

35

Table 3–1 Weak Acids and Weak Bases

Weak Acids	Weak Bases
Aspirin	Caffeine
Penicillin V	Codeine
Phenytoin	Erythromycin
Tetracycline	Pilocarpine (used in the treatment of dry mouth)
	Local anesthetics
	Diazepam (Valium)

and for a weak base is:

$$pH = pK_a + \log \frac{\text{concentration of ionized drug}}{\text{concentration of nonionized drug}}$$

Drugs that are weak acids (e.g., aspirin- pK_a 4.4, penicillin- pK_a 2.5) will be mostly nonionized at the acidic pH of the stomach (pH 1.4), allowing it to be absorbed readily. In theory, weak acids are more readily absorbed from the stomach than weak bases (Figure 3–4). On the other hand, drugs that are weak bases (e.g., erythromycin, codeine, and morphine) will be more nonionized at the pH of the basic small intestine (pH 6–7) and ionized in the stomach. The nonionized portion of the drug shows great lipid solubility and therefore greater absorption in the small intestine. However, regardless of the pH and ionization, most drug absorption, even weak acids, usually occurs in the small intestine, which has the greatest surface area. Enteric-coated tablets (e.g., aspirin, erythromycin) have a layer, such as wax or a cellulose acetate polymer, on the outside of the tablet that protects the stomach lining from exposure to these acidic drugs.

Local anesthetics are weak bases. The closer the pK_a of local anesthetics are to the local tissue pH (pH 7.4), the more nonionized the drug is and the faster it will be absorbed with a quicker onset of action. The lower pK_a means that a greater fraction of the molecules exist in the nonionized form in the body, so they more easily cross nerve membranes, leading to faster onset. For example lidocaine, with a pK_a of 7.9, has a faster onset of action than bupivicaine, with a pK_a of 8.1. If the local tissue pH is more alkaline and closer to the pK_a values of the drugs, the onset of action would be faster. In the presence of inflammation, the local tissue environment becomes acidic. Thus there is less local anesthetic (basic) in the ionized form that is required to cross the nerve cell membrane.

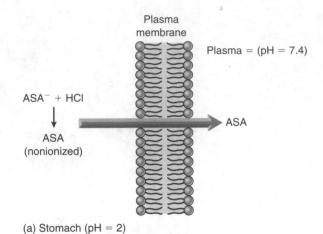

(a) Stomach (pH = 2)

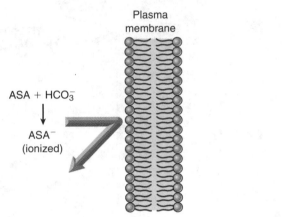

(b) Small intestine (pH = 8)

FIGURE 3–4 Effect of pH on drug absorption. (a) A weak acid such as aspirin (ASA) is in a noninonized form in an acidic environment and absorption occurs; (b) in a basic environment, aspirin is mostly in an ionized form and absorption is prevented.

Absorption of Drugs

It is important to know the way in which drugs are absorbed because this affects drug action. The choice of the route of drug administration is also influenced by drug absorption.

Factors altering absorption Factors that can influence the **bioavailability** or the *rate and extent of drug absorption into the blood* include the route of administration, blood flow to the organ, surface area of the small intestine, lipid/water solubility of the drug, salt form of the drug, and drug interactions with other drugs, herbal supplements, or food. The following factors are involved in absorption:

1. The more vascular (increased blood flow) an organ (e.g., brain and kidney), the greater the rate of absorption. There is a high rate of absorption from the small intestine due to an increased blood flow to the area. Nitroglycerin is administered under the tongue because it is more rapidly absorbed. Fat tissue receives less blood flow, allowing the accumulation of the drug to occur more slowly.

2. The small intestine has a large surface area due to microvilli present on its surface. This feature increases the rate and efficacy for absorption. Drugs administered in aqueous solution are more rapidly absorbed than those given in solid form or suspension.

3. The salt form of the drug [e.g., hydrochloride (HCl) is the salt form of tetracycline] affects absorption and stability of the drug. Salts differ in their solubility profiles. Generation of a salt form of a drug is done to enhance its solubility. For example, when manufactured, local anesthetics are poorly soluble in water; however, when combined with an acid to form a salt, they can be combined with sterile water or saline.

4. Drug absorption is affected by gastric emptying (a drug being absorbed from the small intestine into the blood), which may be delayed by certain foods, and concurrent drug–food administration. For example, if a drug is a weak base it is best absorbed in the more alkaline pH of the small intestine. If it is delayed from leaving the stomach, the drug cannot reach its site of action of absorption. Fatty foods tend to delay gastric emptying.

Rapid Dental Hint

Remind patients not to eat large amounts of fatty foods at meals if taking erythromycin or codeine.

Absorption via different routes of drug administration ORAL: Most orally administered drugs are in the form of tablets or capsules. Once a tablet is swallowed (Figure 3–5), it travels down the esophagus into the stomach, where the active ingredient in the drug is *liberated* from its dosage form by *disintegration* into smaller particles and then dissolved so these will be in solution with the gastric fluid. This is similar to a sugar cube placed in coffee; it must disintegrate into small par-

ticles, which will then dissolve. A capsule must open before it undergoes dissolution.

Absorption usually occurs in the small intestine, which is ideal for absorption because of its large surface area. A drug given orally has low bioavailability; little absorption occurs until the drug enters the small intestine. Oral drugs must be absorbed through two barriers—epithelial cells and blood vessel walls—in order to enter the blood.

Rapid Dental Hint

Absorption of antibiotics used in dentistry may be affected by food; discuss with patients how foods affect the antibiotic being taken.

Once absorbed into the blood, the drug is carried to the liver through the hepatic portal vein (Figure 3–1; Table 3–2); however, absorption may be slow and how much will be absorbed cannot be predicted. Generally, when mixed with certain drugs food may decrease the availability of the drug to bind to the absorbing surface of the GI tract, decreasing the amount absorbed. The temperature of food also influences drug absorption; hot food slows the emptying of the stomach, while cold food enhances gastric emptying.

Particle size and formulation have major effects on absorption. Drugs from different manufacturers have different plasma concentrations because of difference in particle size. Capsules may remain intact for many hours after ingestion in order to delay absorption. Tablets with a enteric coating are designed to delay absorption.

Gut pH plays an important role, as it affects how much of the drug is in the unionized form and thus how much of the drug is fat soluble and will be absorbed. Theoretically, weakly acidic drugs, such as aspirin, are more nonionized in the stomach and should be more readily absorbed there; the intestines favor absorption of weak bases. However, *regardless of pH, most drug absorption occurs in the small intestine because of its greater surface area.*

Other factors affecting absorption of orally administered drugs, such as tetracycline and ciprofloxacin, include minerals (e.g., iron, calcium, magnesium) that form insoluble complexes in the intestinal tract, which slows down absorption. This limitation can be avoided by taking the drug one hour before or two hours after having dairy or minerals.

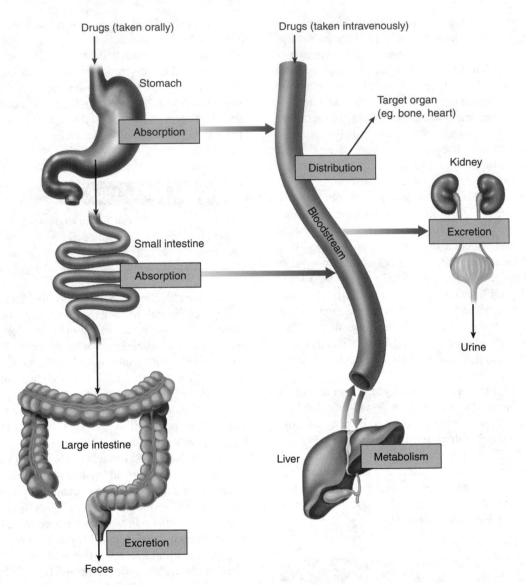

FIGURE 3–5 Movement of a drug through the body (pharmacokinetics): absorption, distribution, metabolism and excretion.

Rapid Dental Hint

Recognize that the elderly and children require dose adjustments.

Another disadvantage of the oral route is that all drugs that are taken orally must pass through the liver via the hepatic portal vein prior to reaching general circulation (Figure 3–6). This is called *hepatic first-pass metabolism* or *first-pass effect*. If liver enzymes rapidly inactivate the drug, only small amounts of active drug will enter the blood and eventually the site of action. To avoid first-pass effect, drugs are IV, IM, or sublingual so the blood supply from these areas does not pass through the liver. When the oral dose of a drug is much larger than the intravenous dose it might have poor absorption and indicate that the drug has a high first-pass effect. Some drugs with a high first-pass metabolism include morphine—a narcotic analgesic—norepinephrine, and nortriptyline—an antidepressant.

Sublingual: The major advantage to administering a drug through the oral mucosa (versus swallowing) is that a higher initial concentration of the drug is reached in the bloodstream and at the site of action because these drugs do not pass through the hepatic circulation (portal vein). Nitroglycerin for acute angina attacks is an example of a drug administered sublingually.

Rectal: Absorption is often unreliable and erratic, but rapid, and these drugs undergo relatively little first-pass metabolism in the liver.

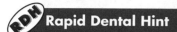

Rapid Dental Hint

Placing nitroglycerin under the tongue is effective due to the vascular nature of the floor of the mouth.

Parenteral: Unlike enterally administered drugs, parenteral administration of drugs bypasses the gastrointestinal tract.

IV: Intravenous administration of a drug is made directly into the circulation through a vein, bypassing absorption barriers. Most drug used in anesthesia are given by this route, which provides a reliable and rapid onset of action. An intravenously administered drug has 100 percent bioavailability because the entire drug enters the bloodstream (refer to Table 3–3).

SC: In subcutaneous administration, because the drug is injected into the connective tissue under the skin absorption is slow but uniform, because circulation is slow. The rate of absorption depends greatly on the site of injection and on local blood flow.

Table 3–2 Summary of Drug Action: Common Routes of Administration

Oral

1. Tablet/capsule (e.g., tetracycline) is taken by mouth with a glass of water.
2. Tablet goes through the esophagus.
3. Into the stomach where a tablet is disintegrated (broken up) and a capsule opens up and the active ingredients in the drug are dissolved. An enteric-coated tablet is disintegrated in the duodenum (small intestine), not the stomach, because the drug is acid liable and will irritate the stomach.
4. Drug goes into the small intestine, where most drugs are absorbed.
5. The drug must cross the intestinal mucosa–blood barrier. Lipid-soluble drugs are absorbed more easily because the intestinal barrier is a lipid membrane.
6. After absorption from the small intestine, the drug goes through the portal vein into the liver.
7. As drugs go through the liver on its way to the blood, some will extensively be metabolized and inactivated before becoming available to the body (first-pass metabolism) in the liver.
8. From the liver, the transformed drug goes through capillary (blood vessel) barriers via the superior vena cava into the bloodstream for distribution in the body.
9. Drugs that are highly protein bound in the plasma will be found primarily in the plasma and cannot exert pharmacological actions. For example, 98 percent of warfarin, a anticlotting agent, is 98 percent bound to plasma proteins. Thus, only 2 percent of the drug is free and will interact with receptors.
10. After the drug exerts its pharmacologic action, it will either be eliminated unchanged if it is a hydrophilic drug or metabolized in the liver (by liver enzymes) to a water-soluble form that will be readily eliminated from the body (e.g., excreted via the kidneys in the urine).
11. Some drugs (large, polar drugs; estrogens, rifampicin, digitoxin, phenytoin) undergo enterohepatic recirculation, where they are excreted from the liver into the bile, then reabsorbed from the intestine, returned to the liver and eliminated in the bile.
12. Drugs that are sufficiently lipid soluble are more readily absorbed and distributed orally. However, lipid-soluble drugs must first be converted in the liver into water-soluble metabolites that can be excreted by the kidneys.

Intravenous

1. A drug is injected directly into the blood and is rapidly distributed to the tissues.
2. In the blood, some drugs are extensively protein bound.
3. First-pass metabolism is eliminated.
4. There are no barriers to absorption; 100 percent bioavailablity.
5. After distrubution, the drug is excreted in the urine by glomerular filtration.
6. Enterohepatic circulation: metabolism by the liver and elimination in the bile.

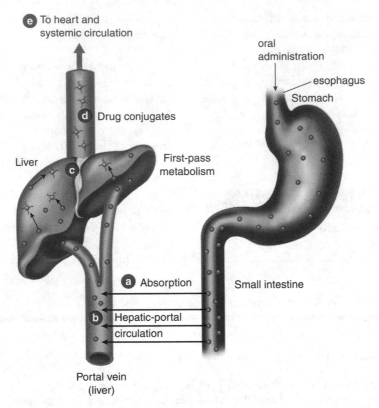

FIGURE 3–6   First-pass metabolism (biotransformation). Absorption of an orally administered drug.

IM: With an intramuscular injection, the drug is delivered into muscle. Absorption is rapid and uniform because there are many blood vessels in muscles. Thus only the capillary (blood barrier) separates the drug from the blood. The drug goes deep into muscles and close to blood vessels, where it will be rapidly absorbed. Massaging or heating the area of injection increases the blood flow. The rate of absorption depends greatly on the site of injection and on local blood flow.

Intrathecal: When a rapid effect is required, as in spinal anesthesia, drugs are injected directly into the subarachnoid space of the spinal cord.

Topical: The major barrier to absorption from topical administration is the top layer of skin, called the *stratum corneum,* which blocks both lipid and water-soluble substances. The exception to this is cortisone, which can be absorbed through the skin, stored in lower layers, and eliminated through the kidney. If the skin is damaged or

Table 3–3   Metabolism of Drugs: Features of Phase I and II

Phase I Modification of drug involving P450 enyzmes	*Phase II Involves synthetic conjugation reactions*
Carried out in the liver	Conjugated (linked) with highly water-soluble compounds
If still fat soluble after going through Phase I, the drug will continue and may be subject to Phase II metabolism.	

abraded, absorption of topical substances increases. If a substance is massaged into the affected area, absorption rate increases due to increased circulation. An occlusive (pressure) dressing placed over the topical substance or pressure applied over the affected area increases absorption.

Antimicrobial agents (e.g. Atridox, Arestin) when administered subgingival into the gingival crevice are absorbed through the sulcular epithelium.

Rapid Dental Hint

Delivery of the topical anesthetic reaches the nonkeratinized sulcular epithelium, which increases its absorption.

Inhalation: Substances can be absorbed through nasal passages or directly through the trachea. There is rapid absorption due to the presence of many capillaries in the respiratory tract. Thus, a systemic effect is achieved. It is difficult to monitor doses, and certain drugs may be irritating to the respiratory tract.

Intradermal: Intradermal administration is not intended for systemic effect, although it is a parenteral delivery. It is used for tests such as the tuberculin Mantoux skin test. To restrict the amount of absorption the needle is held almost parallel to the skin, so it penetrates only the top layers of the skin in the forearm. Absorption is very slow. Emla, which is a eutectic mixture of local anesthesia that is given prior to venipuncture, is also delivered transdermally.

Transdermal: Drugs delivered by patch therapy must be lipid soluble to pass through the layers of the skin for absorption, and are typically more concentrated than in other dosage forms. Some drugs that are administered transdermally such as nitroglycerin are intended to have systemic effects.

Distribution

Once a drug is present in the bloodstream, it is distributed throughout the body fluids to tissues and organs that it is physically able to penetrate (Figures 3–1, 3–6). After the drug leaves the blood it is distributed to the extracellular fluid [all body fluids outside of the cells; includes plasma, interstitial fluid (between cells) and lymph] or enters the cells (intracellular space)]. The time it takes for this to occur is called the *distribution phase*. The volume of fluid in which a drug is able to distribute is referred to as *volume of distribution,* or V_d. This is a useful term for understanding where the drug goes and for drug calcula-

tions. Drug absorption and distribution are important because it is through these two processes that the effective concentration of the drug is reached at the site of action. A low V_d indicates that the drug's distribution is restricted to a particular compartment, either plasma or other extracellular fluids. A large V_d indicates that the drug is concentrated intracellularly (within the cells), resulting in low plasma levels.

Many weak bases have an extremely large V_d because of *ion trapping*. Weak bases are less ionized within plasma than they are within cells because of the difference in pH. When a weak base diffuses into a cell, a larger part is ionized in the more acidic fluid inside the cell. This prevents its passage across the cell membrane into the surrounding fluid and results in a large V_d.

Factors Affecting Drug Distribution   To produce the required effect on the tissue or organ there must be an adequate dosage of the drug. A loss of drug concentration may occur during this distribution phase due to many factors:

1. Absorption across various lipid membranes and into body fat: Membrane affinity refers to the drug's attraction to cell membranes in the body. Hydrophilic drugs such as insulin do not have the capacity to penetrate lipid cell membranes; they are entirely distributed in the extracellular fluid. On the other hand, lipophilic drugs (e.g., general anesthetics, alcohol) have the capacity to cross lipid cell membranes and are more evenly distributed in all fluids.

   To be distributed to the site of action drugs must pass between cells via capillary beds. The capillary system surrounding the blood–brain barrier permits only very lipid-soluble drugs and drugs with small molecular weight to enter the brain. In addition to being a lipid barrier, the placental barrier allows only such drugs (most drugs are smaller than 1,000 molecular weight) to pass.

2. Many drugs are bound to plasma proteins (proteins, commonly albumin, found in the plasma): While in the bloodstream, drugs may either exist in the *free form* or be bound to the many proteins, primarily albumin (Figure 3–7), which is referred to as *plasma protein binding*. The degree of protein binding depends upon the concentration of the drug present in the blood and the affinity of a drug to that protein. Plasma protein binding decreases the distribution of the drug from the plasma to the intended site of action. Protein binding does not play

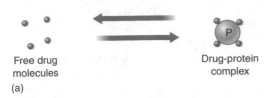

Free drug molecules

Drug-protein complex

(a)

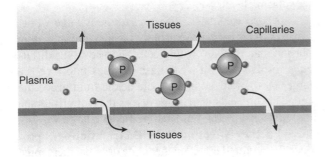

(b)

FIGURE 3-7 Plasma protein binding and drug availability. (a) Drug exists in a free state or bound to plasma protein; (b) drug–protein complexes are too large to cross membrane.

a significant role in pharmacokinetics until it reaches or exceeds 80 percent. The elderly have less protein available for drug binding so that drug administration is unpredictable.

Binding is generally reversible and the number of binding sites on the protein is limited, so two drugs with similar chemical structures may bind to the same site on the protein and compete. Administration of a second drug having a higher affinity for the same binding sites will displace the other drug from the site, elevating the free concentration of the displaced drug which can result in toxic levels of the drug. Warfarin (an anticoagulant drug that prevents blood clotting) is an example of a highly plasma protein bound drug. After being administered, 99 percent of the drug is bound to plasma proteins and only 2 percent of free warfarin molecules interact with receptors. Drugs such as nonsteroidal anti-inflammatory drugs (e.g., ibuprofen), fluoxetine (Prozac), and gemfibrozil (a lipid-lowering drug) displace warfarin from the drug-protein complex, thus raising blood levels of warfarin and increasing the risk of bleeding. These highly protein bound drugs have a low V_d. This effect is short lived because the increased free drug will accelerate drug biotransformation and elimination.

Rapid Dental Hint

Patients on warfarin require a medical consultation from their physician.

To summarize, *drugs that are plasma protein bound are in an inactive state; only the free drug is active.*

3. Blood flow: The greater the blood flow to an organ, the greater the rate of distribution of the drug to that organ Thus, drugs will be distributed faster to the heart, kidneys, and brain than to the skeletal muscle, adipose tissue, and skin, which have a much lower blood flow.

Drug Elimination

Immediately after a drug is administered, the body begins to eliminate it. There are two major processes of drug elimination: *biotransformation* and *excretion* (both usually occur in combination). Renal excretion is elimination through the kidneys in the urine. Other routes of excretion include bile, feces, skin sweat, saliva, or lungs.

Biotransformation (Metabolism) To be eliminated readily from the body, a drug must be in a water-soluble form. Drugs are eliminated either as the original parent compound, referred to as *unchanged,* or as a drug *metabolite,* where the drug molecule must be chemically altered or biotransformed. Although some drugs are biotransformed by enzymes in the plasma, kidney, lungs, intestinal mucosa, and other tissues, the liver is the primary site of drug biotransformation (Figure 3–1). Generally, polar drugs that are not biotransformed are excreted unchanged in the urine. Lipophylic drugs must be biotransformed before elimination so as not to be reabsorbed from the kidneys back into the blood, prolonging the duration of drug action. Thus, a lipid-soluble drug must become less lipophilic and more water soluble to be easily eliminated by the kidneys.

Some drugs are *prodrugs* because when orally administered they are inactive, but become active after biotransformation in the liver. Prodrugs are usually better absorbed than an active metabolite. Examples of orally administered prodrugs include codeine, which is biotransformed to the active morphine, levodopa (for Parkinson's disease) that needs to be metabolized in the liver to dopamine in order for it to be active, benazepril (Lotensin, an antihypertensive drug) and losartan (Cozaar, another antihypertensive drug). Lithium (a bipolar–manic depressive drug) is not metabolized and continues to be active until eliminated unchanged in the urine.

Phases of drug biotransformation There are two phases of biotransformation: Phase I and Phase II (Table 3–3). The purpose of *Phase I biotransformation* is to change a lipid-soluble drug to a more polar metabolite, which involves metabolic reactions including oxidation, hydrolysis, and reduction pathways. The type of biotransformation a drug undergoes depends upon the chemical groups attached to the parent drug molecule.

Oxidative reactions are the most common type of Phase I metabolism. In these reactions, the liver uses enzymes to make lipid-soluble drugs more water soluble or hydrophilic. These hydrophilic *metabolites* are filtered more easily into the kidney tubules than lipophilic drugs. These microsomal enzymes or *cytochrome P450 enzymes* are located primarily in the endoplasmic reticulum of the liver. When a drug is introduced into this system, it combines with oxidized P450, forming a drug–P450 complex. Since these enzymes have a low substrate (the drug that is being metabolized) specificity, only a small number of different enzymes are required to metabolize lipid-soluble substances. There are many different P450, enzymes including:

CYP3A4: This is the most common enzyme that metabolizes many drugs used in dentistry. Some drugs that are metabolized by CYP34 include lidocaine (a local anesthetic), erythromycin and clarithromycin (Biaxin).

CYP2D6: This enzyme metabolizes codeine (a narcotic), fluoxetine (Prozac), and propranolol (heart medication).

CYP2C9: This enzyme metabolizes ibuprofen (Advil).

There are certain drugs that will either inhibit (decrease action) or induce (increase action) of these CYP enzymes. For example, grapefruit juice inhibits the CYP3A4 metabolism of alprazolam (Xanax, an anti-anxiety drug), resulting in elevated serum levels of alprazolam.

Other less common forms of Phase I biotransformation include hydrolysis and reduction. Hydrolysis involves other liver enzymes that break down bonds or linkages in certain drugs containing esters and amides to increase its water solubility for increased elimination.

If a metabolic product of Phase I biotransformation is sufficiently water soluble, the kidneys may excrete it. If it is still fat soluble, enough to be reabsorbed from the kidneys back into the blood, it may be subject to *Phase II biotransformation*. In this process molecules on the drug or metabolite from Phase I are conjugated or linked with highly water-soluble compounds such as glucuronic acid (through glucouronide formation), sul-

fate, acetyl coenzyme A or acetate (through acetylation), or glycine in the liver to make a more water-soluble product. A drug must possess a suitable linking group for conjugation to occur. Often conjugation occurs as a second metabolic step following hydroxylation.

Factors that may influence an individual's ability to metabolize drugs include:

1. Genetics: Enzymes present in the liver are genetically determined and may either have lesser or greater amount of enzymes which breakdown the drugs.
2. Age: In the older individual, first-pass metabolism may be reduced, resulting in increased absorption of drugs. Also, in the older individual there may be a reduced capacity to eliminate drugs.
3. Disease: Liver or kidney disease may reduce metabolism and elimination of drugs, resulting in increased drug levels in the body.

Excretion   The most common route for drug excretion is through the kidney in the urine. Hydrophilic drugs are easily excreted by the kidney; patients with impaired kidney function have a reduced ability to eliminate hydrophilic drugs.

Drug clearance is the volume of plasma from which the drug is completely removed from the body per unit of time. The amount eliminated is proportional to the concentration of the drug in the blood.

To understand the process of renal excretion it is necessary to understand the anatomy of the kidneys (Figure 3–8). The kidneys consist of an outer zone (cortex) and an inner zone (medulla). The kidney is composed of a million or so nephrons, which are the functional units of the kidney. A nephron consists of a tubule, about 3 centimeters (cm) long, closed at one end and communicating with a collecting duct at the other. The closed end is enlarged to form a thin-walled bag called a glomerular capsule surrounding the glomerulus, which consists of loops of fine capillary blood vessels connected to an arteriole of the renal artery. Blood is filtered through the kidneys to remove unwanted waste substances. The capsule is the collecting unit for the fluid filtered from the blood circulated through the kidney.

Renal excretion Plasma containing the drug and other substances is forced through the capillary blood vessels and into the glomerular capsule. Large molecules in the plasma such as proteins and cells are filtered out and remain in the blood. The resultant fluid that enters the capsule is called *glomerular filtrate*. About 25 percent of

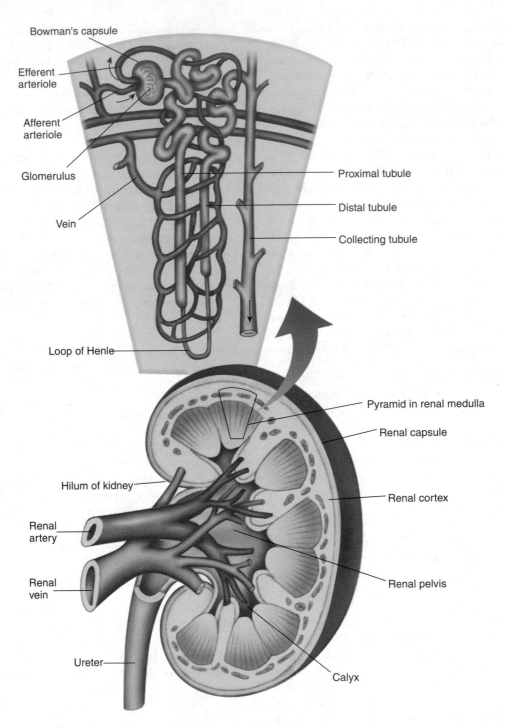

FIGURE 3–8   Anatomy of the kidney.

plasma that enters the kidney is filtered, and 75 percent is unfiltered. Drugs that are not highly plasma protein bound, the free drug, will have a high rate of *glomerular filtration.*

Some substances not removed by filtration because they are too large are eliminated by *active tubular secretion,* which requires energy, into the urine. Besides active secretion, selective *passive reabsorption* of some drugs useful to the body such as water, glucose, and salts back into the blood takes place in the tubule. Additionally, a hydrophilic drug is excreted in the urine readily and will not be reabsorbed, while a lipophilic drug will be reabsorbed from the tubule back into the blood (passive diffusion) because it needs to be converted into metabolites before it is excreted.

The excretion rate is also dependent upon whether the drug is a weak acid or weak base. Weak acids are less ionized in an acidic environment. Thus, to increase the rate of excretion and reduce the chances of reabsorption of weak acids, the acid has to be ionized by increasing the pH of the urine; this can be done by administration of sodium bicarbonate. On the other hand, weak bases are less ionized as the pH of the urine increases.

Biliary excretion In addition to renal excretion, some drugs are excreted in the bile by a process called biliary excretion. Bile, a fluid secreted by the liver, concentrates in the gallbladder and helps to breakdown fats and eliminates wastes and drugs in the body. Liver cells have active transport mechanisms for excreting high molecular weight acids and bases and others. Bile is then transported to the small intestine via the bile duct, then reabsorbed into the bloodstream, then back into the liver by enterohepatic recirculation to be available for elimination (Figure 3–9). These recirculating drugs are

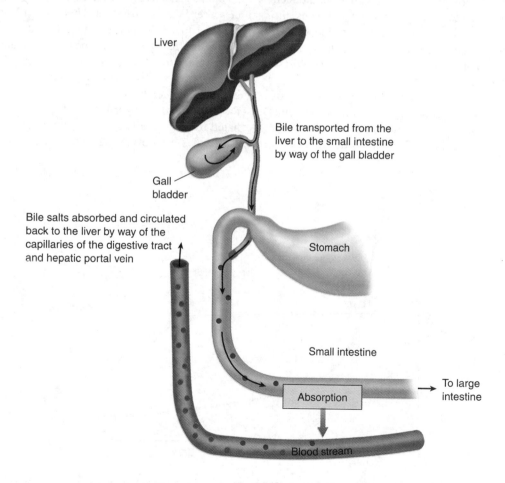

FIGURE 3–9 Illustration of enterohepatic recirculation. Certain drugs are secreted into bile and eventually are eliminated in the feces (versus the urine).

eventually metabolized by the liver and excreted into the kidneys; however, the part of the drug that is not recirculated continues in the bile and eventually is eliminated in the feces. Drugs subjected to enterohepatic circulation are excreted more slowly and have a prolonged duration of action. Examples of drugs that undergo enterohepatic circulation are cardiac glycosides (digoxin; treatment of heart conditions such as congestive heart failure) and tetracyclines.

Table 3–2 reviews the pharmacokinetics of some common routes of drug administration.

Clinical Pharmacokinetics   *Elimination Rate constant and half-life*   Most drug elimination follows *first-order* kinetics: A constant percent of drug is eliminated from the body per each unit of time (Figure 3–10). That is to say, after a drug is given orally it will be absorbed by passive diffusion and the blood levels attained will be proportional to the dose administered. Thus, the greater the dose administered, the larger the blood level concentration. As the drug is eliminated from the body, the concentration of the drug in the plasma will decrease equally over time.

There are exceptions to this rule. At high doses of some drugs (such as alcohol and aspirin), the enzyme system for biotransformation and elimination becomes saturated or overloaded and clearance is determined by how fast these pathways can work. The metabolic pathways work to their limit and cannot increase this rate even if the amount of drug delivered to them is increased. This means that the drug will be metabolized at a constant rate in spite of the amount of drug present. This is referred to as *zero-order kinetics,* in which drug elimination is at a constant rate in spite of the amount of drug present (Figure 3–11).

Half-life (t½) of elimination is the time it takes for the concentration of the drug in the blood to fall to half (50 percent) of its original value. It is an indicator of how long a drug will produce its effect in the body and defines the time interval between doses. It takes about 4–5 half-lives for a drug to be considered eliminated from the body.

For example, if the elimination t½ of a drug is 20 minutes, 50 percent of it remains in the blood 20 minutes after IV administration. This is a mathematical calculation that is important for adequate drug dosing. Penicillin VK is given four times a day but amoxicillin is given three times a day, because amoxicillin has a longer t½ in the body (1.3 hours) so it does not have to be administered as frequently as penicillin (30 minutes). The larger the t½ value, the longer it takes for a drug to be eliminated from the body. Doxycycline, a tetracycline antibiotic, has a t½ of 18–22 hours so it only has to be

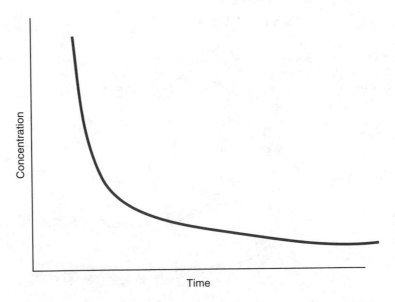

FIGURE 3–10   Most drugs exhibit first-order elimination, in which the rate of drug elimination is equivalent to the drug concentration in the blood.

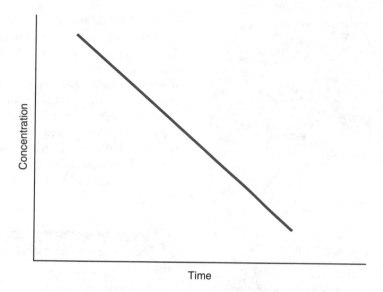

FIGURE 3–11 If drug elimination mechanisms become saturated, a drug may exhibit zero-order elimination.

taken once a day after a twice-a-day loading dose on the first day. Drugs with very short half-lives, such as aspirin (t½ = 15 to 20 minutes) must be given every 3 to 4 hours. If a patient has renal or hepatic disease, the plasma half-life of a drug will increase, and the drug concentration may reach toxic levels. In these patients, drugs must be given less frequently, or the dosages must be reduced.

Drug Administration

Single Dose Kinetics

Plasma Drug Concentration Curve   After a single dose of drug is administered, the plasma concentration increases as the drug is absorbed. It reaches a peak or maximum concentration as absorption is completed and then decreases as the drug is eliminated (Figure 3–12). In most cases, except for rapid IV administration, drug distribution and absorption occur simultaneously.

Bioavailability   Bioavailability is the rate and the extent to which a drug is absorbed into the systemic circulation. The bioavailability of orally administered drugs is of special concern because it can be reduced by many factors, including the rate and extent of disintegration and dissolution, food, pH, and the effect of intestinal and liver enzymes. It is expressed as a percentage, so a drug delivered intravenously has 100 percent bioavailability because the entire amount of drug enters the bloodstream.

Multiple Dosing Kinetics

Drug Accumulation and the Steady State Principle   If a drug that is eliminated by first-order kinetics is administered repeatedly or intermittently (e.g., amoxicillin—1 cap every 8 hours for a dental infection), the average plasma concentration of the drug will increase or accumulate until it reaches a plateau or a steady-state plasma drug concentration (Figure 3–13). *Steady-state plasma concentration* refers to the point at which the rate of drug administration is equal to the rate of drug elimination. The steady-state drug concentration depends on the drug dose administered and on the t½ of the drug. If the dose is doubled, the steady-state concentration is also doubled. When given at regular intervals, a drug reaches the steady-state level after approximately four to five half-lives.

Pharmacotherapeutics

Drug Dosing

Drug dose is defined as the quantity of drug administered. Dose size and dose regimen that is determined for an individual should compensate for any unusual properties of disposition that a drug may have. For example, if a drug exhibits a high rate of absorption, small doses of the drug are necessary to prevent high peak blood levels. If a drug exhibits a high rate of elimination, then more frequent doses are needed to maintain effective blood levels. Few drugs are administered as a single dose. The purpose

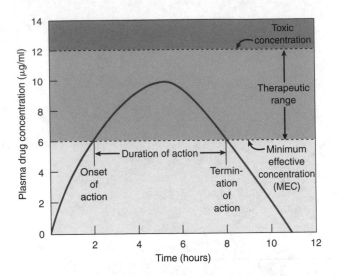

FIGURE 3-12   Graph showing oral administration of a single-dose drug. The time of onset is 2 hours and the end of drug action is 8 hours. This means that the drug has a duration of action of 6 hours. The plasma t½ is about 4 hours (time it takes to decrease its concentration by one-half, or 50 percent).

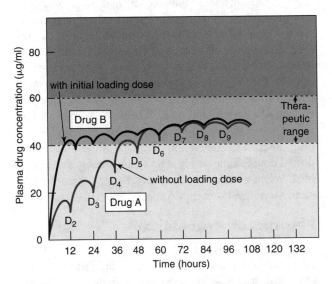

FIGURE 3-13   How repeated doses (D) of a drug causes an accumulation of drug in the blood. Eventually, a plateau is reached where the level of drug in the blood is maintained continuously with the therapeutic range. Drug A and drug B are administered every 12 hours but drug B reaches the therapeutic range faster because a loading dose of drug B was given but not with drug A.

of a *loading dose,* which is a large initial dose, is to rapidly establish a therapeutic plasma drug concentration (Figure 3–13). A large loading dose may be required initially in order to achieve a rapid response in situations that are life threatening. Subsequent doses, referred to as maintenance doses, are reduced. A maintenance dose maintains a desired steady-state plasma drug concentration. For example, for a dental infection penicillin VK is prescribed: 1,000 mg of penicillin VK is given immediately as a loading dose to obtain high initial blood levels, followed by 500 mg four times a day as a maintenance dose.

 Rapid Dental Hint

While reviewing the medical history ask the patients for drug dosage.

Therapeutic Drug Responses

There are two plasma drug levels that are important in pharmacokinetics: the *minimum effective concentration* (MEC), which is the amount of drug required to produce a therapeutic effect, and the *toxic concentration,* which is the level of drug that will result in serious adverse effects (Figure 3–12). If an individual has a toothache and takes half an aspirin tablet, the plasma level will remain below the MEC and there will not be a therapeutic effect of pain relief. By taking 2–3 tablets, the plasma level of aspirin is increased into the therapeutic range with pain relief. If more than 3 tablets are taken, adverse effects will occur, resulting in toxic plasma concentration. This could be at zero-order kinetics at this point.

The *therapeutic range* or the *margin of safety* is the concentration of the drug in the plasma between the MEC and the toxic concentration. The goal to achieve a maximal response is to keep the plasma concentration in the therapeutic range. Some drugs such as warfarin and digoxin have a narrow therapeutic range, so that even a small amount above the therapeutic range can cause toxicity; penicillin has a wide margin of safety and is virtually nontoxic, even in large doses.

Adjustment of Dosage

Certain conditions may reduce the clearance of drugs, which requires an adjustment of dosage.

Children and the Elderly Children and the elderly require lower drug doses than other individuals due to differences in their response to drugs. In neonates, the toxicity of drugs may be increased by delayed excretion or removal of the drug from the body because the organ systems are not yet developed. It is particularly important that the strengths of capsules or tablets be stated. Liquid preparations are especially suitable for young children; however, they may contain sucrose, which is a risk factor for caries. The elderly may have increased sensitivity to many commonly used drugs because the organs metabolize and excrete less efficiently.

Renal and Liver Impairment Liver disease, including hepatitis and cirrhosis, may alter the response to drugs in many different ways. Drug prescribing should be kept to a minimum in all patients with severe liver disease, and sufficient information must be available to provide treatment guidelines. Certain drugs are contraindicated or require a reduced dose in patients with impaired liver function.

The use of drugs in patients with reduced kidney function (e.g., patients on dialysis) may produce toxicity because of impaired elimination from the body. The level of renal function must be determined before adjustment of doses. Either the drug dose remains the same but the dosing interval is increased or the dose is reduced while keeping the same dosing interval. Tetraycycline antibiotics are contraindicated in patients with kidney disease because the half-life is increased from about 10 hours to 57–108 hours.

Renal and liver function should be checked before prescribing any drug. Many problems can be avoided by reducing the dose or by using alternative drugs.

PHARMACODYNAMICS

In the first section of this chapter, we reviewed how a drug gets to the site of action and what the body does to the drug. In this section, we will review **pharmacodynamics,** which describes the actions a drug has on the body and involves drug–receptor interactions, mechanism of drug action, drug response, and the dose–response relationship.

Drug–Receptor Interaction

In order to initiate a physiological response, most drugs must first bind to a receptor. A **receptor,** usually a protein, is any structural component of a cell to which a drug

binds in a dose-related manner and produces a response. The drug attaches to the receptor in a way similar to a lock and key (Figure 3–14). This type of *direct (specific) drug reaction* is the most common reaction involving drug–receptor interactions on the cell. One cell may have hundreds of receptor sites; the action of the drug is due to a change in the conformation of the receptor proteins where the drug attaches. Drugs bind to their receptor by forming Van der Waal's forces or ionic bonds (most common) with the receptor site. These bonds are reversible and weak, allowing the drug to leave the receptor easily as its tissue concentration decreases. A drug must possess an affinity or attachment to the receptor and have efficacy, which is a measure of the ability to the drug to induce a positive change in the function of the receptor. Signal transduction occurs when the drug binding to the receptor causes a chain of biochemical events that leads to a pharmacologic or physiologic effect such as lowering blood pressure or muscle contraction.

There are many different types of receptors (Table 3–4). Receptors will allow binding of either a drug that is administered into the body or an endogenous substance that is synthesized and released within the body, such as

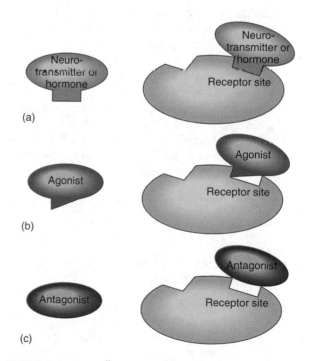

FIGURE 3–14 Illustration of a receptor on the surface of a cell with the drug.

Table 3–4   Types of Drug Receptors

Drugs and endogenous substances bind to these receptors to initiate a drug action and therapeutic response.

Receptor
Receptors for hormones and neurotransmitters
- Adrenergic receptors
- Muscarinic receptors
- Nicotinic receptors
- Insulin receptors
- Histamine receptors

Membrane transport proteins
- Ion channels
- Transporters for neurotransmitters

Enzymes
- Cyclooxygenase
- Carbonic anhydrase
- DNA polymerase
- Human immunodeficiency virus (HIV) protease
- Tyrosine kinsase (for insulin)

Protein synthesis-regulating receptors

(Adapted from: Brenner, G.M., 2000. *Pharmacology*. W.B. Saunders: Philadelphia, p. 27)

a neurotransmitter (e.g., acetylcholine) found in the central nervous system or a hormone such as insulin, thyroid, steroids, or histamine. Receptors are usually macromolecules composed of proteins, carbohydrates, and glycoproteins. A *ligand* is a molecule or drug that binds to a receptor to form a larger complex.

Some drugs (e.g., emollients, alcohol, general anesthetics, and hypnotics) do not act upon receptors, but act in an *indirect* or *nonspecific drug reaction*. Instead of relying on a receptor for drug action, these drugs saturate the water or lipid parts of the cell. The extent of drug action is proportional to the degree of drug saturation at the site of action within the cell. By reaching a certain level of saturation at a specific site on the cell, drug action occurs.

Drug Classifications in the Drug–Receptor Complex

There are three types of drug–receptor complexes: agonist, antagonist and partial agonist. All of these types of drugs have an affinity for the receptor but they differ in what they cause the receptor to do. An *agonist* is a drug that rapidly combines with a receptor to initiate a response and rapidly dissociates or releases from the receptor; it has a high efficacy. An *antagonist* is a drug that

binds to the receptor but does not dissociate and has no positive response or efficacy. It blocks the reaction of an agonist and is referred to as a blocking drug. A *partial agonist* binds to the receptor and produces a mild or submaximal therapeutic response and may inhibit the action of an agonist when given concurrently, acting like an antagonist. A *competitive antagonist* is a drug which occupies a significant proportion of the receptors and thereby prevents them from reacting maximally with an agonist. A noncompetitive antagonist may react with the receptor in such a way as not to prevent agonist–receptor combination but to prevent the combination from initiating a response, or it may act to inhibit some subsequent event that leads to the final overt response.

Dose–Response Relationships

New drugs must be tested in clinical trials. The outcome of treatment can be plotted as response vs. log dose, where the response of the drug is measured in one of two ways: graded dose–response curve or quantal dose–response curve. The relationship between the concentration of a drug at the receptor site and the degree of the response is called the dose–response relationship.

In graded dose–response relationships, the response obtained with each dose is described in terms of a percentage of the *maximal response* and is plotted against the *log dose* of the drug (Figure 3–15). As the dose of the drug is increased, there is a gradual, progressive increase in the response until a maximum effect is seen. The drug causes a response with each dose and the maximal response is produced when all of the functional receptors are occupied and less of a response is seen when 50 percent of the functional receptors are occupied. Most drugs follow this *dose–response curve*. The patient's response obtained at different doses of the drug can be observed and measured. For example, after administration of a sleep-inducing drug such as a barbiturate, ataxia is the first response seen, followed by sleep.

In *quantal dose–response relationships*, the response seen with each dose of a drug exhibits an all-or-none effect. For example, a sedative will cause either sleep or death.

Potency, Efficacy, and the Ceiling Effect

Potency refers to the dose required to produce a therapeutic effect. It is usually expressed in terms of the median *effect dose (ED$_{50}$)*, which is the dose of the drug required to produce the desired clinical effect in 50 percent of test

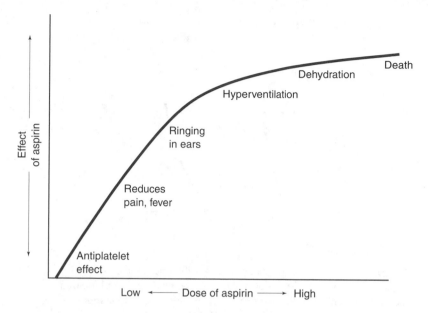

FIGURE 3–15   Dose–response relationship. As the dose of the drug increases a maximal response or plateau is reached. Increasing the drug dose produces no additional therapeutic response.

animals. The potency of a drug varies inversely with a drug's ED_{50}. For example, a drug whose ED_{50} is 5 mg is ten times more potent than a drug whose ED_{50} is 50 mg. Potency is determined by the affinity of a drug for its receptor.

Efficacy is the ability to produce a therapeutic effect regardless of the dose. Potency and efficacy often describe the success of drug therapy. For example, just knowing that 10 mg of morphine administered subcutaneously produces relief from pain tells us little about morphine's potency; it tells us only the dose required to produce a given intensity of response. However, 1.5 mg of hydromorphone or 120 mg of codeine, administered by the same route, is as effective as 10 mg of morphine in relieving the pain induced by the same stimulus, but morphine is less potent than hydromorphone and more potent than codeine. All three drugs have the same efficacy since they all produce a biologic effect (Figure 3–16).

The *ceiling effect* of a drug occurs when the therapeutic response cannot be increased with a higher dose of the drug. For example because of its ceiling effect and poor bioavailability, increased doses of buprenorphine, a drug used in the management of opiate addiction, does not produce increased effects after a certain point, or ceiling. In fact, high doses of the drug can actually precipitate withdrawal symptoms in opiate-addicted individuals. Aspirin and NSAIDs also have a ceiling effect.

Toxicity

The ratio of a drug's toxic dose to its therapeutic dose is termed the *therapeutic index (TI)*. A safe drug will have a high therapeutic index. The *median effective dose (ED$_{50}$)* is the drug dose that produces 50 percent of the maximum possible response in test animals. The dose at which 50 percent of test animals die is called the *lethal dose (LD$_{50}$)*. Since a drug does not have a single toxic effect and has many therapeutic effects, it is not possible to have a list of a drug's TI; it must be calculated. The calculation is done by the following equation: $TI = LD_{50} \div ED_{50}$. A "safe" drug will have a high TI (generally at least 10). For example, the effective dose of drug A is 20 mg, and 50 mg is the average lethal dose. Thus, the TI is $50 \div 10 = 5$. This means that it would take an error in magnitude of approximately five times the average dose to be lethal to the patient.

Pharmacogenetics: Factors That Modify the Effects of Drugs

Biological Variation

Biological variation explains the different responses seen among individuals within the same population, given the same dose of a drug. Certain factors are responsible for individual variation. For instance, body weight will

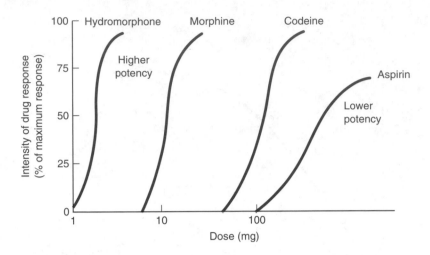

FIGURE 3–16   Effect-log dose curve for the analgesic action of three narcotics and aspirin. Hydromorphone is more potent than morphine and codeine, regardless of the response level at which they are compared.

influence drug dosing. Generally, when dealing with most adults drug adjustment of dose to body weight is not really necessary. However, dose adjustment is necessary if the body weight is outside the normal adult range or if a potent drug with a small margin of safety is given. Smaller females may require a lower dose than males.

It is important to recognize the physiologic responses that change with age. In very young children, liver enzymes are underdeveloped, resulting in a deficiency in enzyme function. The renal tubular system is not completely developed and there is a deficiency in active excretion. Also, the blood flow through the kidneys is slower. Thus, a lower drug dose may be necessary.

In the elderly there is a deterioration of drug removal processes and a decrease in responsiveness of receptor sites. This makes it difficult to adjust the dose. Additionally in the elderly there are decreases in renal function, body cell mass, liver enzyme activity, and metabolic activity.

There are certain enzyme deficiencies that are hereditary and may affect drug dosing. Some individuals may show slow or fast acetylation of certain drugs such as isoniazid (INH; antituberculosis drug) that is metabolized by acetylation.

The presence of disease may alter the drug response. Any disease which affects the liver or kidney will increase or extend the duration of drug action. There may also be changes in receptor site sensitivity. The most obvious example of this is aspirin. Aspirin will reduce fever in an individual with fever, but does not reduce body temperature in an individual without fever.

An *idiosyncratic response* is an unusual effect of a drug that is possible with any drug or individual.

Some individuals are unusually responsive and are called *intolerant* or *hyperresponsive*. One factor involved in this response distribution is adaptation. *Adaptation* is a homeostatic adjustment that may occur during a continued or prolonged presence of a drug. The body adjusts itself and minimizes the effects of the drug.

Tolerance is the need for increasing amounts of drug to obtain the same therapeutic effect. For instance, progressive, small increases in the amount of alcohol are needed to cause the same effect. Tolerance does not occur universally and is a long-term reduction in response (e.g., weeks or months). An individual may develop tolerance to a certain drug and not to others.

There are two types of tolerance. In the first type, drug disposition tolerance occurs when the adaptive response alters the rate of drug disposition. The rate of metabolism is increased, resulting in a decrease in drug concentration at a given time. This is usually seen with short-acting barbiturates. The other type of tolerance is cellular tolerance, commonly seen with narcotics such as codeine. A reduced analgesic response is seen with the same dose but as tolerance develops, the response to the depression effect is not decreased; thus the drug may accumulate until lethal. *Tachyphlaxis,* a very rapid development of tolerance, is a rapid decreasing response (within hours or days) with repeated administration of the same dose of drug at short intervals. In dental practice, tachyphlaxis to local anesthetics may develop. For example, a local anesthetic is administered to a dental patient. Once the nerve function returns to its preinjection state and the patient requires more anesthetic because of pain, the duration and intensity of anesthesia with reinjection is greatly diminished. Thus, successive doses of the anesthetic will be less effective than those given previously.

Placebo Response

A *placebo* is a treatment that is similar to the active medication except that it does not contain the active drug. Placebos are usually required as control in FDA clinical trials. Often, an individual given a placebo will report experiencing effects that would have been expected when receiving the active drug. This is called the placebo effect and is a measurable, observable, or felt improvement in health not attributable to treatment. The placebo effect can also be a psychological or physiological reaction, having confidence in the drug.

DENTAL HYGIENE NOTES

In order to produce their desired pharmacologic and biologic effects, most drugs must interact with a receptor on/in a cell and initiate a series of physiologic events. The receptor site is the site of action of a drug.

Pharmacodynamics deals with the events of drug action; it explains what the drug does to the body. In order for the drug to produce this action, it must be absorbed through various tissue membranes, be distributed to the various tissues and organs, and be metabolized to a water-soluble form so that it can be eliminated from the body. Pharmacokinetics determines the drug concentration at the site of action.

To understand the mechanisms of drug action and the clinical use of therapeutic agents for the prevention, diagnosis, and treatment of disease, it is important to understand the basics of pharmacology that have been presented in this chapter.

Many orally administered drugs (e.g., propranolol, a cardiac drug) lose some activity due to first-pass metabolism through the liver. Only the nonionized form of

Rapid Dental Hint

The dental hygienist plays an integral part of the dental team. Understanding the general principles of pharmacology is important when dealing with dental patients. The medical and drug history of patients must be reviewed. Drug–drug interactions can be recognized if the clinician has an understanding of the various mechanisms of pharmacokinetics and pharmacodynamics.

weak acids and bases is lipid soluble and more easily absorbed from the small intestine. Morphine and lidocaine undergo extensive first-pass metabolism, which prevents them from being administered orally.

A drug will absorb through cell membranes by passive diffusion more easily if it is lipophilic. Many drugs are bound to plasma proteins to a limited extent, but some (e.g., warfarin, an anticoagulant drug) are extensively bound (more than 95 percent), which limits distribution to tissues and organs. Many drugs are biotransformed (metabolized) before elimination from the body. Drugs are eliminated from the body either unchanged or as water-soluble metabolites. Lipid-soluble drugs must be biotransformed to more water-soluble metabolites. A loading dose is given to establish an initial therapeutic plasma drug concentration. A lower, maintenance dose follows to maintain therapeutic plasma drug concentrations.

KEY POINTS

- Pharmacokinetics is the study of how drugs are handled by the body.
- Pharmacodynamics is the study of how the body responds to drugs, the mechanism of action.
- A drug exerts a pharmacologic effect or response.
- Drugs are absorbed into the blood in the nonionized, lipid-soluble form.
- All drugs are eventually eliminated by the body by either hepatic biotransformation or renal excretion, or a combination of both.
- Liver cytochrome P450 enzymes are involved in many drug–drug interactions.
- Lipid solubility is one of the most important determinants of the pharmacokinetic characteristics of a drug; rate of absorption can be predicted from knowledge of a drug's lipid solubility.

- Highly ionized drugs cannot pass lipid membranes.
- Drugs are absorbed in the nonionized, lipid-soluble form. The unionized portion of the drug shows great lipid solubility and therefore greater absorption.
- Nonionized drugs can cross lipid membranes freely.
- Most drugs are either weak acids or weak bases.
- Acids are most highly ionized at a high pH (e.g., an alkaline environment such as the intestines).
- For weak acids, the more acidic the environment, the less ionized the drug and the more easily it crosses lipid membranes.
- Bases are most highly ionized in an acidic environment (e.g., the stomach).
- Water-soluble (hydrophilic) drugs are excreted through the kidney in the urine.

BOARD REVIEW QUESTIONS

1. Nitroglycerin is not given orally because it: (pp. 37–38)
   a. Has a bad taste.
   b. Dissolves slowly in the mouth.
   c. Has a high first-pass metabolism.
   d. Undergoes absorption in the stomach too quickly.

2. Displacement of a drug from plasma albumin binding sites would usually be expected to: (pp. 41–42)
   a. Decrease the amount of distribution.
   b. Increase blood levels of the drug.
   c. Decrease the metabolism of the drug.
   d. Increase the metabolism of the drug.

3. Which of the following routes will a drug follow after intravenous administration? (pp. 41–42)
   a. Vein, general circulation, liver, kidney
   b. Esophagus, stomach, small intestine, liver, kidney
   c. Liver, small intestine, kidney
   d. Vein, liver, general circulation, kidney

4. Which of the following features describes antagonist drugs? (p. 50)
   a. Binds to the same receptor sites as agonist drugs.
   b. Binds to the receptor to reduce the actions of the agonist.
   c. Have a greater affinity to the receptor than agonists.
   d. Have a lesser affinity to the receptor than agonists.

5. Which of the following reasons explains the rationale for giving a loading dose for an antibiotic? (p. 48)
   a. Maintains a desired steady-state plasma level.
   b. Attains the desired blood level immediately.
   c. Decreases premature clearance of the drug.
   d. Increases the rate of drug metabolism.

6. In order for an orally administered drug to be absorbed into the blood, it must pass through: (pp. 32–33)
   a. Three barriers: epithelial cells + blood vessels + brain
   b. Two barriers: epithelial cells + blood vessel
   c. One barrier: blood
   d. No barrier: drug does directly into blood

7. All of the following statements are true about lipid soluble drugs *except* one. Which one is the exception? (pp. 34–37)
   a. Readily absorbed through blood vessel wall
   b. Slowly absorbed through cell membrane
   c. Goes through the blood–brain barrier
   d. Can be given by inhalation

8. Which of the following reasons explains why an intravenously administered drug such as an antibiotic achieves very high initial blood concentration levels? (pp. 37–39)
   a. Drugs made of small molecules
   b. Drugs have a high pH
   c. No barrier to absorption
   d. Expensive to give

9. Which of the following statements is true regarding absorption of local anesthetics? (p. 36)
   a. Lidocaine (pK_a 4) is not absorbed easily through lipid membranes.
   b. Lidocaine (pK_a 7.7) has a fast onset because the tissue pH is close to the pKa.
   c. Bupivicaine (pK_a 8.3) has a faster onset than lidocaine.
   d. Bupivicaine (pK_a 7.7) has a slow onset of action because it is highly unionized.

10. Which of the following terms is related to the amount of drug administered? (p. 47)
    a. Dose
    b. Response
    c. Agonist
    d. Toxicity

SELECTED REFERENCES

Barker, L. and L. Bromley. 2002. Pharmacology 2—Pharmacokinetics. Update in *Anesthesia* 15:25–36.

Brenner, G. M. 2000. *Pharmacology.* Philadelphia: W.B. Saunders, pp. 9–31.

Flexner, C. 1999. Pharmacokinetics for physicians—A primer. www.medscape.com/viewarticle/408238.

Gossel, T. A. 1998. Pharmacology: Back to basics. *U.S. Pharmacist* 23:70–78.

Gossel, T. S. 1998. Exploring pharmacology. *U.S. Pharmacist* 23:96–104.

Lazo, J. and K. Parker. 2005. Pharmaco Kinetics, Pharmacodynamics: The dynamics of drug absorption, distribution, action and elimination. IN: Goodman & Glman's *The Pharmacological Basis of Therapeutics.* Eds. Brunton L, Lazo J, Parker K. 11th Ed. McGraw-Hill Publishing, NY.

Levine, R. R. 1996. Pharmacology: Drug Actions and Reactions, 5th ed. New York: Parthenon.

Pratt, W. B. and P. Taylor. 1990. *Principles of Drug Action: The Basis of Pharmacology,* 3rd ed. New York: Churchill Livingstone.

WEB SITES

www.fda.gov
www.medscape.com

Chapter 4

Drug Interactions in Dentistry

GOAL: To provide knowledge of the current concepts of drug interactions in dentistry.

EDUCATIONAL OBJECTIVES

After reading this chapter, the reader should be able to:

1. Differentiate between pharmacokinetic and pharmacodynamic drug interactions.
2. Explain how drug–drug, drug–disease, drug–food, and drug–herbal interactions affect patients.
3. Identify common drug–drug, drug–disease, and drug–food interactions.

KEY TERMS

Adverse drug reactions (ADRs)
Drug interaction
Risk factors
Cytochrome P450 enzymes

DRUG–DRUG INTERACTIONS

With increasing number of patients taking multiple medications (polypharmacy), the potential for **adverse drug reactions (ADRs)** with other medications and foods is an increasing concern. The estimated incidence of clinical drug–drug interactions ranges from 3 to 5 percent in patients taking a few medications to as much as 30 percent in patients taking at least 10 different drugs.

A drug–drug **interaction** occurs when the pharmacological or clinical response to the administration of a drug combination is different from that anticipated from the known effects of the two drugs when given alone. Although most drug interactions are unwanted, some may be desirable. For example, a drug–drug interaction may occur if a patient is taking an anti-anxiety drug such as alprazolam (Xanax) before a dental procedure and diphenhydramine (Benadryl), an antihistamine for allergies. When taken together, these two drugs cause excessive sedation and fatigue, resulting in an additive interaction. An antagonistic interaction may occur when a patient is taking both penicillin (a bactericidal antibiotic) and azithromycin (a bacterostatic antibiotic). The bacteriostatic antibiotic interferes with the actions of the bactericidal antibiotic.

It is important to note that it is impossible to review or mention all drug interactions that may occur even in medications that are prescribed in your dental office. It is recommended that dental clinicians have a drug interaction handbook, online or computer references, available for review in the clinic or office (Table 4–1).

Rapid Dental Hint

It is wise to have access to a drug reference to look up any drug interactions that could occur with a drug prescribed to your patients. Review with your patients.

Risk Factors

There are certain **risk factors** that increase the incidence of a drug interaction. Risk factors are classified into medication factors and patient factors (Table 4–3). Drug interactions are usually rated according to severity of the interaction. These rating are intended to assist the clinician in deciding if the interaction is potentially life threatening or if it only causes mild effects that will not change the clinical status of the patient (Table 4–4).

Table 4–1   Drug Interaction Resources

Online References
- www.medscape.com/drugchecker
- www.rxlist.com
- www.gsm.com
- www.pdr.net

Software Programs used with PDAs
- iFacts
- Lexi-Interact
- Mosby's Drug Consult
- Mobile Micromedex
- ePocrates Rx v. 6.0

Table 4–2   Types of Drug Interactions

There are five main types of interactions:

Interaction	*Definition*
Pharmacokinetic	A change in the pharmacokinetics of one drug caused by the interacting drug
Pharmacodynamic	A change in the pharmacodynamics of one drug caused by the interacting drug
Addition	The effect of two or more drugs when administered together is the same as if the drugs were given separately.
Synergism	The effect of two or more drugs when administered together is greater than if the drugs were given separately; may produce responses equivalent to overdosage.
Antagonism	The effect of two or more drugs when administered together is less than when the drugs are given separately.

Pharmacokinetic Mechanisms

Pharmacokinetic drug interactions affect the absorption, distribution, metabolism, or elimination of the drugs.

Absorption

Usually when a drug is affected by absorption this involves the presence of a food or supplement that forms drug complexes, resulting in decreased absorption into the blood. Other factors affecting absorption include gastric pH and changes in gastrointestinal motility that alter

Table 4–3 Risk Factors for Drug Interactions

Medication Factors	Patient Factors
Use of drugs that are highly protein bound. When one drug is highly bound to plasma proteins and a second drug is given that is also highly protein bound, the drugs will compete for the same binding site. This may result in the displacement of one of the drugs from the protein, resulting in increased free drug in the blood.	Very young and elderly (metabolism is different)
Use of drugs with a narrow margin of safety (or low therapeutic index) that require frequent blood level testing (e.g., digoxin, warfarin, theophylline)	Male versus female
Chronic drug therapy Drugs that induce or inhibit hepatic microsomal enzymes	Comorbid illnesses (patients with many illnesses) Decreased liver and kidney function

transit time within the intestines, delaying absorption. Food alters the rate of absorption of many antibiotics. Most antibiotics should be given on an empty stomach (1 hour before or 2 hours after meals) except penicillin V, amoxicillin, doxycycline, and minocycline.

Examples of drugs or foods that decrease or delay absorption of another drug given concurrently are:

Tetracycline + antacids

Tetracycline + dairy products

Ciprofloxacin + food

It is recommended that food/antacids be spaced 2 hours apart.

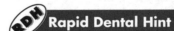

Rapid Dental Hint

Food affects the absorption of many drugs your patients are taking or will be taking. Review any potential drug–food interaction with your patients.

Distribution

Distribution drug interactions deal with two or more drugs that are highly bound to plasma proteins in the blood. Remember that drugs that are bound to plasma proteins are not active; only drugs that are not bound to

Table 4–4 Rating of Drug Interactions

Severity Rating	Documentation Rating
Major: Potentially life threatening or causing permanent body damage	Established: Proven with clinical studies to cause an interaction
Moderate: Could change the patient's clinical status and require hospitalization	Probable: Very likely to cause an interaction
Minor: Only mild effects are evident or no changes seen	Suspected: Supposed to cause an interaction, but more clinical studies are required
	Possible: Limited data proven
	Unlikely: Not certain to cause an interaction

plasma proteins (so-called free drugs) are active. If two drugs have an affinity for the same binding site on the protein molecule in the blood, they may compete for that binding site and one drug will displace the other drug from the protein molecule. Drugs that are most susceptible to this interaction are warfarin (Coumadin), phenytoin (Dilantin), nonsteroidal anti-inflammatory drugs (e.g., ibuprofen) and sulfa (sulfonamide) drugs.

Metabolism

Metabolism-type drug interactions occur primarily due to metabolism of drugs. Few drugs are eliminated from the body unchanged in the urine. Most drugs are metabolized or chemically altered to a less lipid-soluble compound which is more easily eliminated from the body. One way of metabolizing drugs involves alteration of groups on the drug molecule via the **cytochrome P450 enzymes** (Table 4–5). These enzymes are found mostly in the liver, but can also be found in the intestines, lungs, and other organs. Each enzyme is termed an isoenzyme, because each de-

rives from a different gene. There are more than 30 cytochrome P450 enzymes present in human tissue.

A *substrate* is a drug that is metabolized by a specific CYP450 isoenzyme. An *inhibitor* is a drug that inhibits or reduces the activity of a specific CYP450 isoenzyme. An *inducer* is a drug that increases the amount and activity of that specific CYP450 isoenzyme.

Drug interactions can occur when a drug that is metabolized and/or inhibited by these cytochrome enzymes is taken concurrently with a drug that decreases the activity of the same enzyme system (e.g., an inhibitor). The result is often increased concentrations of the substrate. Another scenario is when a substrate that is metabolized by a specific cytochrome enzyme is taken with a drug that increases the activity of that enzyme (e.g., an inducer). The result is often decreased concentrations of the substrate.

Some substrates are also inhibitors for the same enzyme, probably due to competitive inhibition of enzyme activity. Some inhibitors affect more than one isoenzyme and some substrates are metabolized by more than one isoenzyme.

Table 4–5   *Common Cytochrome P450 Drug Interactions in Dentistry*

Enzyme	*Substrate Drug**	*Inhibitor Drug*§	*Inducer Drug*¶	*Notes*
CYP1A2	Caffeine **Antiasthmatic:** Theophylline **Alzhemier's disease:** Tacrine (Cognex) **Tricyclic antidepressants:** Amitriptyline (Elavil) Imipramine (Tofranil) **Antidepressants: SSRIs** [e.g., fluvoxamine (Luvox)] **Antipsychotics:** Clozapine (Clozaril) Haloperidol (Haldol)	**SSRIs:** Fluvoxamine (Luvox) **Fluroquinolones:** Ciprofloxacin (Cipro)	Tobacco (smoking) **Antiulcer:** Omeprazole (Prilosec) **Antiseizure:** Phenytoin (Dilantin)	If possible, do not give a substrate with an inducer or inhibitor if they will interact; if necessary to give, then observe the therapeutic and adverse effects.
CYP3A4	**Local anesthetic:** Lidocaine **Antibiotics:** Erythromycin Clarithromycin (Biaxin) **Calcium channel blockers:** Amlodipine (Norvasc) Diltiazem (Cardizem) Felodipine (Plendil)	**Grapefruit juice** (lasts about 24 hours) **Antibiotics:** Erythromycin Clarithromycin **Antifunguals:** Ketoconazole (Nizoral) fluconazole (Diflucan) itraconazole (Sporanox) **Antidepressants:** Fluvoxamine (Luvox)	**Trigeminal neuralgia:** Carbamazepine (Tegretol) **Antiseizure:** Phenytoin (Dilantin) **Barbiturates:** Phenobarbital **Antituberculosis:** Rifampin (Rifadin, Rimactane)	If possible, do not give a substrate with an inducer or inhibitor if they will interact; if necessary to give, then observe the therapeutic and adverse effects.

(continued)

Enzyme	Substrate Drug*	Inhibitor Drug§	Inducer Drug¶	Notes
	Nifedipine (Adalat, Procardia) Verapamil (Calan, Isoptin) **Antidepressants:** Sertraline (Zoloft), trazodone (Desyrel), nefazodone (Serone) **Benzodiazepines:** Diazepam (Valium) Midazolam (Versed) Triazolam (Halcion) **Cholesterol-lowering drugs (statins):** Atorvastatin (Lipitor) Lovastatin (Mevacor) Simvastatin (Zocor) **Anticoagulant:** Warfarin (Coumadin) **Antihistamine:** Fexofenadine (Allegra) **Corticosteroid:** Hydrocortisone **Antidiabetics:** Glyburide (Glynase, Micronase) **Antirejection drugs:** Cyclosporine **Hormones:** Estradiol Progesterone **HIV protease Inhibitors:** Ritonavir (Norvir) Saquinavir (Invirase) Indinavir (Crixivan) Nelfinavir (Viracept) **Antigout** Colchicine	Nefazodone (Serzone) **H₂ receptor blocker:** imetadine (Tagamet)		
CYP2C9	**Nonsteroidal anti-inflammatory drugs:** Ibuprofen (Motrin, Advil) Naproxen sodium (Aleve) Celecoxib (Celebrex) **Antiseizure:** Phenytoin (Dilantin) **Anticoagulant:** Warfarin (Coumadin)	**Antibiotics:** Metronidazole (Flagyl) **Antifungals:** Fluconazole (Diflucan) Ketoconazole (Nizoril)	**Antituberculosis:** Rifampin	If possible, do not give a substrate with an inducer or inhibitor if they will interact; if necessary to give, then observe the therapeutic and adverse effects.

Substrate: A drug that is metabolized by an enzyme system.

§*Inhibitor:* A drug that decreases the activity of the enzyme which may decrease the metabolism of the substrate and generally lead to increased drug effect.

¶*Inducer:* A drug that will stimulate the synthesis of more enzymes enhancing the enzyme's metabolizing actions. Inducers increase metabolism of substrates, generally leading to decreased drug effect.

Rapid Dental Hint

Drug interactions via cytochrome P450 enzymes are very common. Review Table 4–5 and Hersh, E.V. 2004. Drug interactions in dentistry. *JADA* 135:298–309.

Table 4–5 reviews common dental drug–drug interactions occurring with different cytochrome P450 isoenzymes. Cytochrome is abbreviated as CYP followed by an Arabic numeral, a letter, and another Arabic numeral. The major isoenzymes responsible for most drug metabolism are: CYP1A2, CYP2C9, CYP2C19, CYP2D6, CYP2E1, and CYP3A4.

Many cytochrome P450 enzyme drug interactions involve erythromycin. Clarithromycin (Biaxin) is a potent inhibitor of CYP3A, increasing the serum levels of calcium channels blockers such as nifedipine (Procardia). These drugs should not be given together. Selection of another antibiotic such as azithromycin (Zithromax) is recommended. Lovastatin (Mevacor) and simvastatin (Zocor), cholesterol-lowering drugs, undergo extensive first-pass metabolism by CYP3A4; clarithromycin and erythromycin inhibit CYP3A4, resulting in increased serum levels of the anticholesterol drugs, which may lead to acute renal failure. It should be noted that there are fewer interactions with azithromycin because it is not metabolized by the cytochrome P450 enzymes.

Another type of drug–drug interaction involves metronidazole inhibiting the activity of enzymes, other than liver cytochrome enzymes, responsible for the metabolism of warfarin, resulting in increased warfarin plasma levels.

Elimination/Excretion

Interactions can occur when drugs compete for the same transport system in the renal tubules. This mechanism can be used to enhance therapy, or it can result in drug toxicity.

Another type of elimination interaction occurs between oral contraceptives and antibiotics. Oral contraceptives need to be activated in the intestines by the gastrointestinal flora. Some antibiotics such as tetracyclines and amoxicillin disrupt this intestinal flora, decreasing the enterohepatic circulation and effects of the contraceptive. Rifampin, an antituberculosis drug, stimulates estrogen metabolism, resulting in decreased effectiveness of oral contraceptives.

Pharmacodynamic Mechanisms

Pharmacodynamic interactions result from an antagonistic or additive drug effect. An example of an antagonistic effect is when a nonsteroidal anti-inflammatory drug (NSAID) such as ibuprofen (Motrin, Advil) is given to a patient after a dental procedure who is already taking a diuretic such as furosemide (Lasix) for congestive heart failure. Ibuprofen may inhibit the actions of the diuretic in excreting sodium, which causes fluid to be retained; the congestion may worsen. An example of an additive or synergistic effect is when an NSAID is given to a patient already taking aspirin or warfarin: There is an increased risk of bleeding.

DRUG-FOOD INTERACTIONS

Grapefruit Juice

Grapefruit juice in large quantities (32 oz. or more a day) can inhibit CYP3A4 enzyme in the small intestine and increase blood levels of drugs metabolized by this pathway. This interaction only occurs with the juice and not the fruit itself. This effect has been shown to be due to flavonoids in the grapefruit juice.

Caffeine

Caffeine is present in coffee, tea, cola sodas, and medications. Ciprofloxacin (Cipro), an antibiotic, inhibits the metabolism of caffeine thus increasing blood levels.

Dairy Products/Calcium Foods

Dairy products and foods (e.g., orange juice, some breads) containing calcium chelate (binds to) tetracycline and fluroquinolone (e.g., ciprofloxacin, levofloxacin) preventing the absorption of these drugs and thus making them ineffective. To minimize this interaction the drug should be taken at least 2 hours before or 6 hours after the calcium.

Alcohol

There are many drug interactions with alcohol. Any drugs that affect the central nervous system (e.g., antidepressants, antianxiety drugs, antihistamines) when taken with alcohol with increase the central nervous system effects (e.g., sedation, respiratory depression, drowsiness). Use

Table 4–6 Clinically Significant Drug–Drug Interactions in Dentistry

Note: Most drug–drug or drug–food interactions occur when two or more drugs are taken at the same time. To avoid these interactions most drug dosing is spaced so as not to administer them concurrently. If in doubt, the patient's physician should be contacted.)

Antibiotics

Drug	Interacting Drug	Effect	What To Do?
Doxycycline (including 20 mg doxycycline, Atridox)	Antacids (magnesium hydroxide/aluminum hydroxide), iron (ferrous sulfate) penicillins	Decreased doxycycline absorption into the blood Interferes with bactericidal effect of penicillins	Space 1 hour before or 2 hours after meals. Do not take at same time; take penicillin a few hours before doxycycline.
Minocycline (including Arestin)	Warfarin	Increased anticoagulant effect	Monitor patients for enhanced anticoagulant effects; warfarin dosage may need adjustments.
	Oral contraceptives	May interfere with contraceptive effect	May not be clinically significant; some sources say to use alternative methods of birth control.
	Phenytoin (Dilantin)	Decreased serum doxycycline levels	Either switch to another antibiotic or monitor.
Tetracycline	Antacids (magnesium hydroxide/aluminum hydroxide), calcium-containing products, iron (ferrous sulfate)	Decreased doxycycline absorption into the blood	Do not take concurrently.
	Warfarin	Increased anticoagulant effect	Minimal risk; monitor patients for enhanced anticoagulant effects.
	Penicillins	Interferes with bactericidal effect of penicillins	Do not take at same time; take penicillin a few hours before the doxycycline.
	Digoxin	Digoxin is partially metabolized by bacteria in intestine; increased digoxin blood levels	Either switch antibiotic or monitor for increased serum digoxin levels.
	Oral contraceptives	May interfere with contraceptive effects	May not be of clinical significance; some sources recommend to use alternative birth control
Penicillins	Erythromycin, tetracyclines	Decreased effectiveness of penicillin	Do not take at same time; give the penicillin a few hours before the tetracycline.
	Probenicid (Benemid): drug for gout	Inhibits penicillin excretion	Can take together; make sure penicillin levels are not excessive.
	Oral contraceptives (including ampicillin)	May interfere with contraceptive effects	May not be clinically significant; some say to use alternative birth control methods.
Erythromycin Clarithromycin	Theophylline	Increased theophylline levels	Avoid together; contact physician; reduce theophylline dosage to avoid toxicity.
	Carbamazepine (Tegretol)	Increased carbamazepine levels	Avoid concurrent use.

Drug	Interacting Drug	Effect	What To Do?
	Statins: atorvastatin (Lipitor); simvastatin (Zocor)	Increases statin levels (increased myopathy, including muscle pain)	Either switch to azithromycin or to another statin drug like lovastatin (Mevacor) or pravastatin (Pravachol).
	Oral contraceptives	Interfere with contraceptive effects	Some sources recommend alternative birth control.
	Digoxin (Lanoxin)	Increased digoxin levels (see increased salivation and visual disturbances) Increased	Switch antibiotic to penicillin. Monitor for signs of digoxin toxicity or switch antibiotic.
	Cyclosporine	Cyclosporine toxicity	Cyclosporine doses may need reduction.
	Ergot alkaloids [e.g., ergotamine (Bellergal-S, Cafergot)] (for migraine headache)	Toxic ergot levels (ergotism; pain, tenderness, and low skin temperature of extremities)	Use azithromycin or another antibiotic.
	Midazolam (Versed)	Increased sedation	Avoid combination; use alternative drugs.
	Disopyramide (Norpace)	Prolongation of QTc interval	Switch to another antibiotic or monitor for development of arrhythmias.
	Warfarin	Increases anticoagulant effect	Switch to azithromycin (Zithromax) or monitor for anticoagulant effects; contact physician. Switch to azithromycin (Zithromax).
Fluroquinolones (Cipro)	Oral hypoglycemics	Increases hypoglycemic effects	Space apart the antacid and antibiotic.
	Antacids, iron (decrease absorption of the drug) Caffeine	Decreases fluroquinolone effect Increase caffeine effects	Do not take together
Clindamycin (Cleocin)	Neuromuscular blockers (succinylcholine)	Increased neuromuscular blocking effect	Since most dental patients are not taking these drugs, there is no special precautions.
Metronidazole (Flagyl)	Alcohol	Severe disulfiram-like reaction with headache, flushing and nausea	Avoid alcohol.
	Warfarin	Inhibits warfarin metabolism; increased anticoagulant effect	Contact physician; adjustment of warfarin dosage.
	Lithium	Lithium excretion, inhibited resulting in toxic levels	No need to avoid concurrent use.

Analgesics

Drug	Interacting Drug	Effect	What To Do?
Aspirin and nonsteroidal anti-inflammatory drugs (NSAIDs) (ibuprofen, naproxen)	Anticoagulant (e.g., warfarin)	Additive anticoagulant effects (increased bleeding)	Avoid concurrent use/contact patient's physician.
	Angiotensin-converting enzyme (ACE) inhibitors (e.g., enalapril, captopril); beta-blockers, angiotensin II receptor blockers (ARBs)	Decrease antihypertensive response (lowers blood pressure). Short-term course (5 days) may not significantly increase blood pressure	Interaction causes lowering of blood pressure. Monitor blood pressure. Use alternative analgesic such as acetaminophen or narcotic after 5 days or more of use of NSAIDs.

(continued)

Drug	Interacting Drug	Effect	What To Do?
	Lithium	Inhibits renal clearance of lithium	Monitor or avoid.
	Oral antidiabetic drugs (occurs with aspirin)	Increases hypoglycemic effects	Limited importance.
	Furosemide (Lasix)	Decreased diuretic effect	Monitor patient.
	Venlafaxine (Effexor)	Possible serotonin syndrome	Avoid concurrent use.
	Phenytoin (Dilantin)	Decreased hepatic phenytoin metabolism (increased serum levels)	No special precautions.
Acetaminophen	Alcohol	Increase incidence of hepatotoxicity (liver disease)	Contraindicated in alcoholics; avoid taking together.
	Warfarin	Increased anticoagulant effect	Avoid concurrent use of adjustment of warfarin dosage.

Sympathomimetics

Drug	Interacting Drug	Effect	What To Do?
Epinephrine (contained in local anesthetics)	Beta-blockers Nonselective ($\beta_1\beta_2$) such as propranolol (Inderal), nadolol (Corgard), timolol (Blocadren) and sotalol (Betapace)	Elevated blood pressure	Epinephrine should be used cautiously. Limit the amount used to 0.04 mg (two cartridges of 1:100,000).
	Selective beta-blockers (β_1) such as atenolol (Tenormin), metoprolol (Lopressor), acebutolol (Sectral) and betaxolol (Kerlone)	No elevation in blood pressure	No concerns.
	Tricyclic antidepressants	Hypertension (enhances sympathomimetic effects)	Treat similar to the cardiac patient; maximum amount is two cartridges of EPI 1:100,000.
	Cocaine	Increased heart contraction leading to death	Do not use cocaine if the patient used cocaine within 24 hours.
Levonordefrin (contained in mepivicaine)	Nonselective beta-blockers (e.g., propranolol, nadolol)	Stimulates alpha-receptors on heart tissue, causing an increase in blood pressure; limit use of vasoconstrictor	Minimize the amount of levonordefrin.
	Tricyclic antidepressants (e.g., imipramine, amitriptyline)	Enhanced sympathomimetic effects	Avoid use of levonordefrin.

Anti-anxiety drugs (benzodiazepines)

Drug	Interacting Drug	Effect	What To Do?
Diazepam (Valium), alprazolam (Xanax)	Grapefruit juice + midazolam (Versed) or triazolam (Halcion)	Inhibits CYP3A4 enzyme, decreasing metabolism of these drugs thus increasing blood levels	The duration of effect of grapefruit juice—do not take juice while on these drugs.
	Cimetidine (Tagamet)	Inhibits diazepam elimination Increases CNS depression	Little clinical importance.
	Opioids (narcotics; codeine, hydrocodone)	Increases CNS depression	Avoid taking together.
	Clarithromycin with midazolam (Versed)	Increased sedation	Avoid combination; use alternative drugs.

Table 4–7 Clinically Significant Drug–Food Interactions in Dentistry

Dental Drug	Food	What To Do?
Tetracycline	Dairy products, (e.g. milk, yogurt) (Forms a calcium/tetracycline complex which inhibits tetracycline absorption)	Space 1 hour before or 2 hours after meal.
Doxycycline (Vibramycin), minocycline (Minocin) Ciprofloxacin (Cipro)	Dairy products (only 30% decrease in bioavailability) Caffeine (decreases absorption of the drug) Food (e.g. orange juice fortified with calcium) and dairy (increases absorption of the drug)	No special management, can take with dairy. Space 1 hour before or 2 hours after the calcium containing supplement or food
Erythromycins	Food (decreases absorption of the drug)	Take drug 1 hour before or 2 hours after.
Azithromycin (Zithromax)	Food (decreases absorption of the drug)	Take 1 hour before or 2 hours after meals.
Amoxicillin	Food decreases absorption	Take 1 hour before or 2 hours after meals.

Table 4–8 Clinically Significant Drug–Disease Interactions in Dentistry

Dental Drug	Condition	What To Do?
Clindaymicn (Cleocin)	Ulcerative colitis, Crohn's disease, pseudomembranous enterocolitis	Do not give clindaymcin; remember, this antibiotic is given for infective endocarditis prophylaxis if patient is allergic to penicillins.
Tetracyclines (doxycycline, minocycline)	Pregnant and lactating women Children under 8 years	Do not give to these patients.
Clarithromycin	Prolonged QT interval Ventricular arrhythmias	Do not give to these patients.
Erythromycin	Cardiac arrhythmias Liver disease Prolonged QT interval	Do not give to patients with these conditions.
Penicillins	Infectious mononucleosis Pseudomembranous enterocolitis Renal disease	Do not give to these patients. Do not give to these patients. Reduce dosage or don't give depending on severity.
Metronidazole (Flagyl)	Central nervous system disorder, epilepsy, lactating mother	Do not give; substitute another antibiotic.
Ciprofloxacin (Cipro)	Achilles tendonitis, pseudomembranous enterocolitis	Do not give; substitute another antibiotic.
NSAIDs (e.g., Aleve, Motrin) Aspirin	Gastrointestinal bleeding (ulcers), nasal polyps with asthma, blood coagulation disorder, pregnancy	Do not give; give acetaminophen.
Epinephrine	Narrow angle glaucoma, dilated cardiomyopathy Hypertension, diabetes, hyperthyroidism	Do not give to these patients. Use with caution; limited quantities.

of acetaminophen with alcohol increases the incidence of heptotoxicity.

Drug–Disease Interactions

A drug–disease interaction refers to a patient that has an allergy to a certain drug or a systemic disease that would contraindicate the use of a drug. For example, a patient with ulcerative colitis should not be prescribed clindamycin (Table 4–5).

DENTAL HYGIENE NOTES

Simply knowing that a patient is taking interacting drugs is not sufficient to prevent serious adverse outcomes. If the interacting drug combination is necessary, the prescriber must be prepared to manage the interaction to minimize the risk of an adverse event. Effective management usually includes assessment of the likely time course of the drugs' interaction. Drug–drug and drug–food interactions are common causes of treatment failure, adverse events, and possible death. Although dental hygienists do not prescribe drugs, they are an integral part of clinical pharmacy. Dental patients who are taking medications should be monitored for drug interactions. Many drugs that dentists prescribe—including antibiotics, antifungals, antivirals, and analgesics—may be involved in many interactions. Before a prescription is given to the patient, a thorough review of the medications the patient is taking and a review of the medication the patient will be taking is necessary. After writing down all of the medications the patient is taking, go to the computer and research to see if there are any drug–drug or drug–food interactions. Additionally, tell the patient how to take the medication that the dentist prescribed (e.g., with or without food, take with yogurt etc.). Tables 4–6 through 4–8 review some commonly encountered drug interactions. Not all interactions can be listed, and it behooves the dental clinician to review all medications the patient is currently taking and any medications newly prescribed by the dentist to identify any interactions among these drugs.

KEY POINTS

- Be aware that there are many drug–drug, drug–food, drug–herbal supplement and drug–disease interactions.

- Take a complete drug (prescription, OTC and herbal supplement) and medical history on every patient.
- Look up any interactions that may occur with the medications or disease condition.
- Before any dental medication (e.g., analgesics, antibiotics, NSAIDs) are prescribed to the patient look up to see that there are not any significant interactions with that drug.

BOARD REVIEW QUESTIONS

1. Which of the following types of drug interactions occurs when an antacid is taken with doxycycline? (pp. 57–58)
   a. Absorption
   b. Distribution
   c. Metabolism
   d. Excretion

2. If a patient has nasal polyps and is sensitive to aspirin, which of the following drugs should not be administered? (p. 65)
   a. Erythromycin
   b. Acetaminophen
   c. Ibuprofen
   d. Doxycycline

3. Which of the following drugs is contraindicated in a patient with Achilles tendonitis? (p. 65)
   a. Ciprofloxacin
   b. Penicillin
   c. Azithromycin
   d. Clarithromycin

4. Which of the following drugs should not be taken with alcohol? (p. 63)
   a. Ciprofloxacin
   b. Metronidazole
   c. Epinephrine
   d. Digoxin

5. Which of the following types of drug interactions occurs when aspirin and warfarin are taken concurrently? (p. 57)
   a. Addition
   b. Synergism
   c. Antagonism
   d. Pharmacodynamics

SELECTED REFERENCES

Anastasio, G. D., K. O. Cornell, and D. Menscer. 1997. Drug Interactions: Keeping it straight. *Am Fam Physician* 56:883–894.

Brown, C. H. 2000. Overview of drug interactions. *U.S. Pharmacist* 25(5):HS-3–HS-30.

Cupp, M. J. and T. S. Tracy. 1998. Cytochrome P450: New nomenclature and clinical implications. *Am Fam Physician* 57:107–114.

Hansten, P. D. and J. R. Horn. 2005. *The Top 100 Drug Interactions: A Guide to Patient Management.* Edmonds, WA: H& H Publications.

Haas, D. A. 1999. Adverse drug interactions in dental practice: Interactions associated with analgesics—Part III in a series. *JADA* 130:397–406.

Hersh, E. V. 1999. Adverse drug interactions in dental practice: Interactions involving antibiotics—Part II of a series. *JADA* 130:236–251.

Hersh, E.V., and P. A. Moore. 2004. Drug interactions in dentistry: The importance of knowing your CYPs. *JADA* 135:298–311.

Hulisz, D. 2007. Food-Drug interactions. Which ones really matter? *US Pharmacist* 32(3):93–98.

Marek, C. 1966. Avoiding prescribing errors: A systematic approach. *JADA* 127:617–623.

Moore, P. A. 1999. Adverse drug interactions in dental practice: Interactions. *JADA* 130:541–554.

WEB SITES

www.PDR.net
www.gsm.com
www.medwatch.com
www.rxlist.com

Chapter **5**

Drugs for Pain Control

GOALS:

- To educate dental hygienists on the pathophysiology, treatment, and patient management for oral pain.
- To gain an understanding of the basic principles of drug abuse.

EDUCATIONAL OBJECTIVES

After reading this chapter, the reader should be able to:

1. Discuss the concepts of dental pain.
2. Discuss the commonly used pharmacologic agents used for the treatment of orofacial pain.
3. Identify drug–drug interactions that pertain to dental treatment.
4. Describe the classification of narcotic analgesics.
5. Discuss when a narcotic versus a nonnarcotic analgesic is indicated for dental patients.
6. Discuss screening methods to detect potential patients with a chemical dependency.

KEY TERMS

Orofacial pain
Nociceptive pain
Neuropathic pain
Substance P
Cyclooxygenase
Prostaglandins
Opioid
Narcotics
Dependency

INTRODUCTION

Medications to selectively decrease pain perception are used extensively in dentistry. These medications are termed analgesics. Analgesics are indicated for the relief of acute and chronic dental/orofacial pain, postoperative pain, and preoperative pain to reduce expected pain after the dental procedure (e.g., periodontal surgery).

NEUROPHYSIOLOGY OF PAIN

Pain Components

There are two parts to pain: sensory which is the actual painful stimulus, and the reaction to pain, which is the emotional response to pain. The reaction to pain is more important than the actual pain stimulus in controlling pain. *The emotional response to pain originates from the central nervous system, while the stimulus comes from the peripheral nervous system.* This distinction is important because analgesics used to treat pain will target the peripheral pain, central pain, or both.

Pain can be acute or chronic, depending upon when it started. Acute pain has a short time course and is usually simple to evaluate and treat. Chronic pain has an undetermined time course with a more complex evaluation. Treatment is not as successful as with acute pain.

Types of Pain

Classification: Orofacial Pain

Orofacial pain is classified into **nociceptive** and **neuropathic pain;** acute and chronic (Table 5–1).

Nociceptive acute orofacial pain Pain that arises from a stimulus (e.g., injury to tissues), bone, joint, muscle, or connective tissue, that is outside of the central nervous system produces nociceptor pain. Examples of nociceptive orofacial pain include pulpitis (inflammation of the pulp), pericoronitis, exposed dentin, post-periodontal surgery, post-oral surgery, and maxillary sinusitis. Nociceptor pain is classified into somatic pain, which produces sharp, localized sensations, or visceral pain, which is a generalized dull, poorly localized, throbbing or aching pain. Visceral pain is associated with a phenomenon called referred pain, which detects the painful stimulus in areas removed from the site where the pain originated. For example, an individual having a heart attack has pain referred to the jaw and arm. A dental patient has pain in the maxillary sinuses which was pain referred from the maxillary molar area.

The process of pain transmission begins when *nociceptors* (located at the end of nerves within peripheral body tissue) are stimulated by noxious stimuli such as tissue damage (e.g., gingiva, bone, pulp). This is normal pain in response to injury to the body. The nerve impulse signaling the pain is sent to the spinal cord along two types of sensory neurons, called Aσ and C fibers. The Aσ fibers signal sharp, well localized pain and the C fibers conduct dull, poorly localized pain.

Once pain impulses reach the spinal cord, neurotransmitters such as acetylcholine send the message along to the next neuron. At this neuron a protein called **substance P** is responsible for continuing the pain message and signals the brain to feel pain. Substance P may be affected by other chemical called endogenous opioids, which include endorphins, enkephalins, and dynorphins. These substances may alter or change sensory information at the spinal cord (Figure 5–1).

Nociceptive pain prevents an individual from using injured parts of the body because further damage can occur. The concept of blocking nociceptors with local anesthetics allows for dental procedures to be performed

Table 5–1   Nociceptive and Neuropathic Pain

Nociceptive Acute Pain	Neuropathic Chronic Pain
Toothache (pulpitis)	Trigeminal neuralgia
Dental surgery (extractions, periodontal surgery, orthodontic surgery)	Post-herpetic neuralgia
	Oral dysesthesia (burning mouth)
Mucosal lesions (aphthous ulcers, herpetic lesions)	Migraine headache
	Atypical facial pain
	Drug-induced nerve damage
Maxillary sinusitis	Fibromyalgia
Other: arthritis (joint), cancer	Peripheral neuropathy

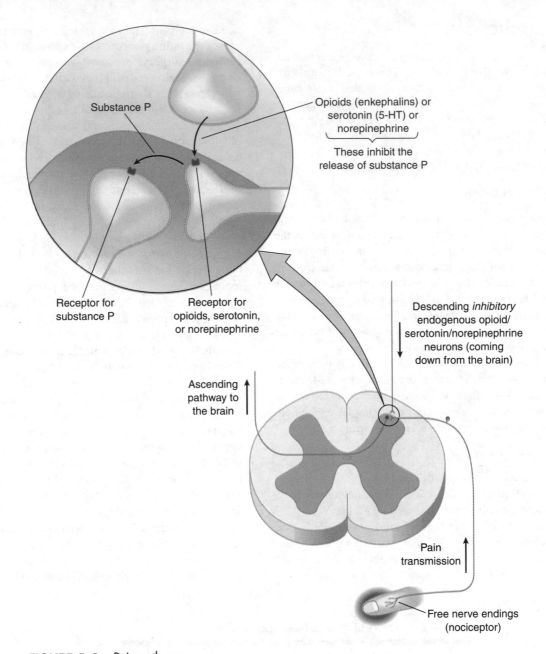

Substance P

Opioids (enkephalins) or
serotonin (5-HT) or
norepinephrine

These inhibit the
release of substance P

Receptor for
substance P

Receptor for
opioids, serotonin,
or norepinephrine

Descending *inhibitory*
endogenous opioid/
serotonin/norepinephrine
neurons (coming
down from the brain)

Ascending
pathway to
the brain

Pain
transmission

Free nerve endings
(nociceptor)

FIGURE 5–1 Pain pathway.

without causing pain. Nondental-related examples of no-ciceptive pain include backaches, sprains, sports/exer-cise injuries, broken bones, and arthritis (joint pain).

Because pain signals begin at nociceptors located within peripheral body tissues and continue through the CNS, there are several targets where medications can work to stop pain transmission. Control of nociceptive

pain is usually accomplished with nonnarcotics (e.g., as-pirin, acetaminophen), nonsteroidal anti-inflammatory drugs (NSAIDs) at the peripheral level, and opioids (nar-cotics) at the central level within the CNS.

Neuropathic Orofacial pain Neuropathic oro-facial pain does not serve any biologic function. It is so-cially and psychologically destructive, and often leads to depression. Neuropathic pain differs from nociceptive pain in that neuropathic pain is caused by damage to nerve tissue. Neuropathic pain is not associated with specific pain receptors as is nociceptive pain, but originates anywhere in the nervous system (peripheral or central). Factors that cause neuropathic pain include injury, infection, and surgery. This is a persistent and severe pain that may be burning, sharp, or stabbing, similar to "pins and needles." There is often a delay in the onset of pain (days to months) after the initial injury. The prevalence of neuropathic pain is high after general surgery and maxillofacial trauma and surgery. Examples of neuropathic pain include orofacial neuralgias such as trigeminal neuralgia or tic doloureux, diabetic peripheral neuropathy (nerve damage secondary to diabetes mellitus), postherpetic neuralgia, carpal tunnel syndrome, and oral dysesthesia (burning mouth). Trigeminal neuralgia is a disorder of the fifth cranial (trigeminal) nerve that causes episodes of intense stabbing, shock-like pain in the areas of the face where the branches of the nerve are distributed—lips, eyes, nose, scalp, forehead, upper and lower jaw. Postherpetic neuralgia is pain that sometimes follows resolution of acute herpes zoster and healing of the zoster rash. Phantom tooth pain is experienced in the area of a missing tooth after extraction. Tooth allodynia is a condition in which an ordinarily nonpainful (nonnoxious) stimulus such as a light touch induces pain. Tooth hyperalgesia is increased response to a noxious stimulus. Treatment includes tricyclic antidepressants, analgesics, and anticonvulsants.

DRUG THERAPY FOR DENTAL PAIN

Treatment for *nociceptive dental pain* is not as complicated as it is for neuropathic pain. Nonsteroidal anti-inflammatory drugs (NSAIDs) or acetaminophen (Tylenol) is adequate for mild to moderate acute pain control. More intense nociceptive chronic pain may also respond well to narcotic analgesics.

Medications for *chronic neuropathic orofacial pain* include gabapentin (Neurontin) and pregablin (Lyrica), which are antilepileptic drugs that enhance neuronal stability which results in pain relief, the 5% lidocaine patch, calcium channel blockers, and tricyclic antidepressants. The problems that cause neuropathic pain are not reversible, but some improvement may be possible with proper treatment.

The following sections review the fundamentals of nonnarcotic analgesics, nonsteroidal anti-inflammatory drugs (NSAIDs), opioid analgesics, antiepileptics, and tricyclic antidepressants. Dosage adjustments may be necessary in renal and hepatic impairment and in the elderly.

Nonnarcotic Analgesics

Drugs used for the treatment of mild to moderate nociceptive acute dental pain include nonnarcotic analgesics (aspirin, acetaminophen) and nonsteroidal anti-inflammatory drugs (NSAIDs). Aspirin and NSAIDs are anti-inflammatory (reduce inflammation associated with pain) with analgesic (pain relief) and antipyretic (reduce fever) properties. Acetaminophen has no peripheral anti-inflammatory activity.

Prostaglandin Synthesis Pathway: Peripheral Inflammation

Pain is provoked when a variety of substances (e.g., histamine, prostaglandins, leukotrienes, and bradykinin) are released or injected into the tissues after trauma (surgery, cut, or infection). The prostaglandin synthesis pathway explains the inflammatory events that occur locally after tissue trauma/damage (Figures 5–2 and 5–3). These events occur in all tissue cells found in the body.

Any slight trauma to a nerve fiber stimulates an enzyme called phospholipase A_2, which breaks off arachidonic acid from the phospholipids bound in the cell membrane. Arachidonic acid enters two metabolic pathways: In the first pathway, an enzyme called **cyclooxygenase** breaks down arachidonic acid into **prostaglandins** (PGE_2) *prostacyclin* (PGI_2) and *thromboxane* A_2. The second metabolic pathway involves arachidonic acid being metabolized by the lipoxygenase pathway into leukotrienes. Leukotrienes produce bronchoconstriction in allergic reactions. The following topics will all pertain to the arachidonic–cyclo-oxygenase pathway.

The following substances are metabolites of arachidonic acid via the **cylcooxygenase pathway:**

- **Prostaglandins (PGs):** Prostaglandins are fatty acids found in all tissues. Prostaglandins are not stored in the cells, but are synthesized during inflammation. Once released, prostaglandins are metabolized rapidly. The biologic effects of prostaglandins include:
  - PGE_2, which has potent inflammatory properties and is relevated in inflammatory periodontitis

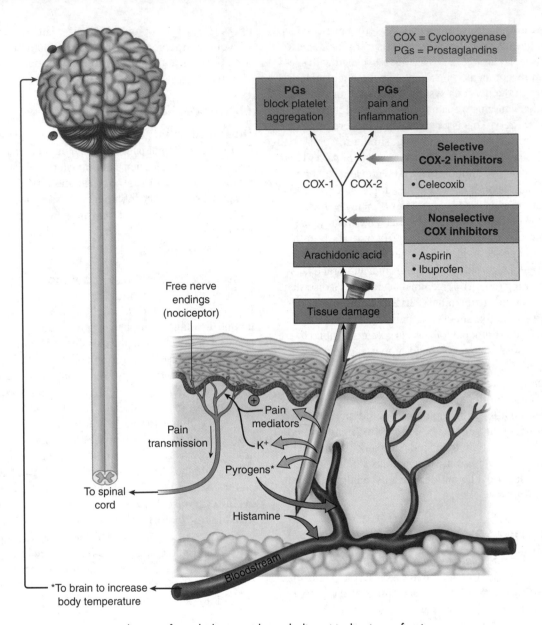

FIGURE 5–2   Pathways of arachidonic acid metabolism: Mechanisms of pain.

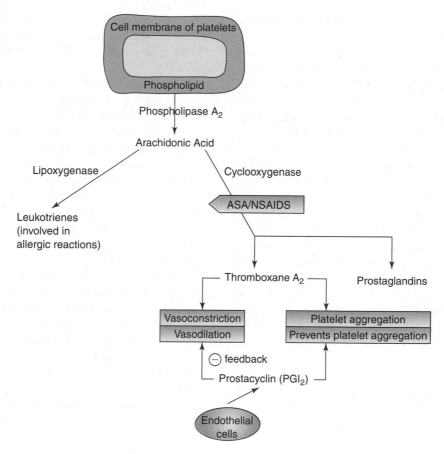

FIGURE 5–3   Aspirin and most other NSAIDs block prostaglandins.

- Production of gastric mucus and reduced production of gastric acid (protective effects)
- Uterine contractions during labor
- PGI_2 (prostacyclin) released from blood vessels and inhibiting platelet (clot) formation,
- Bronchodilation (PGE_2 and PGI_2) and bronchoconstriction ($PGF_2\alpha$)
- Increased renal blood flow
- Reduction in blood pressure
- **Prostacyclin and thromboxane A_2** play a role in regulating the aggregation of platelets. Small breaks in capillaries cause platelets to aggregate (come together), which forms clots.
  - Thromboxane A_2 (TXA_2) is synthesized and found in platelets. When released from platelets, it is a potent vasoconstrictor of blood vessels and *induces* platelet aggregation or clumping and prevents bleeding.

- Prostacyclin (PGI_2), which is synthesized and present in endothelial cells in blood vessel walls, has the opposite function of thromboxane A_2. It prevents platelet aggregation (clumping) and prolongs bleeding time. It is through the generation of prostacyclin that the healthy vessel wall is able to resist the life-threatening deposition of platelets. This is a homeostatic process whereby both thromboxane A_2 and prostacyclin balance each other without one substance being produced excessively and not the other.

Cyclooxygenase   Currently, three cyclooxygenase isoenzymes are known: COX-1, COX-2, and COX-3. COX-1, an endogenous enzyme normally found in most body cells, is responsible for tissue homeostasis and is considered a "housekeeping" enzyme. COX-1 is normally found in the gastrointestinal tract, kidneys, and platelets. Under the influence of *COX-1,* prostaglandins maintain and protect the gastric mucosa (lining of the stomach), maintain normal platelet function (aggregation and homeostasis) through the formation of thromboxane A_2 and prostacyclin (PGI_2), and regulate renal blood flow.

On the other hand, *COX-2* is produced only during inflammation and is found only in low amounts in the tissues. Thus, the objective of using anti-inflammatory drugs is to reduce the inflammation which is caused by COX-2, but ideally the drug should not affect COX-1, which is a protective substance. The analgesic properties of aspirin and other nonsteroidal anti-inflammatory drugs (NSAIDs) such as ibuprofen (Advil, Motrin, Nuprin) are due to inhibition of cyclooxygenase but these drugs are not selective for COX-2; thus there are many adverse side effects due to the inhibition of COX-1, which serves a protective role. Celebrex, an NSAID that selectively inhibits COX-2, minimizes the adverse effects seen with inhibition of the protective COX-1; there is less gastrointestinal upset because the gastric mucosa is kept intact.

NONNARCOTIC ANALGESICS

Salicylates

Salicylic Acid Derivatives (aspirin)

Aspirin (acetylsalicylic acid; abbreviated as ASA) is a component of the bark of the willow tree. In the fifth century B.C., the Greek physician Hippocrates used this substance. In 1899, Bayer marketed this substance with the trade name "Aspirin." Aspirin was introduced in the United States in 1925, and Bayer lost a law suit to keep Aspirin as a trade name.

Aspirin is a nonnarcotic analgesic drug with anti-inflammatory and antipyretic (reduces fever) actions. According to the National Drug Code, which is part of the Center for Disease Control (www.cdc.gov/nchs/datawh/nchsdefs/ndc_dtc.htm, Table XI), aspirin is considered to be a nonnarcotic analgesic and not a nonsteroidal anti-inflammatory drug (NSAID) because of its common use for cardiac therapy; however, many references may include aspirin as being an NSAID because of its anti-inflammatory properties. Most of aspirin's effects are due to its interruption of prostaglandin synthesis via blockade primarily of COX-1 rather than COX-2 enzymes.

Therapeutic Indications for Aspirin

Analgesia: Aspirin acts primarily peripherally at the site where the pain originates (e.g., pain produced at a tooth). For example, when someone has a toothache, bradykinin (a vasodilator that stimulates nerve endings of pain fibers) is released from the injured tissue. This stimulates pain receptors in the area. Prostaglandins, which are also released from the inflamed tissue, *increase the sensation of this pain* but do not cause the pain itself. Aspirin will not eliminate the pain; it only decreases the sensitivity to pain. Aspirin is indicated for mild to moderate pain, with an onset of action of about 30 minutes.

Aspirin has a *ceiling effect* whereby increasing the dose does not produce increased effects after a certain point (Figure 5–4). For example, an average weight individual will take 650 mg (two 325 mg tablets) of aspirin for mild to moderate pain following periodontal debridement. Let's say that this amount of aspirin does not take the individual out of pain; however, increasing the dosage to three or four tablets will not be effective in increasing the analgesic effect and may even cause more adverse effects. Thus, if two tablets of aspirin are ineffective in the relief of pain, a more potent alternative drug should be used.

Anti-inflammation: Aspirin has anti-inflammatory proprieties because it blocks the formation of PGE_2, which has a potent inflammatory effect. This attribute allows for treatment of arthritic conditions. The optimal anti-inflammatory dose of aspirin is 3.6–5.4g/day, which is higher than the analgesic dose, which is a maximum of 4g/day. Inflammation causes pain, which is relieved by the analgesic action of aspirin quickly, but the other features of inflammation such as swelling and difficulty in moving joints, may take about a week to be relieved.

Antipyretic: Aspirin's antipyretic actions reduce abnormal high body temperature (fever) but do not alter normal body temperature. Aspirin affects body temperature through the action on the hypothalamus in the brain. A decrease in temperature occurs by causing vasodilation (increased blood flow to surface by dilating blood vessels), which causes an increase in respiration. This results in an increase in the evaporation of water and increased sweating. Thus aspirin does not reduce heat production, but increases heat loss through sweating.

┌─ **Did You Know?** ─────────────────────

Bayer Aspirin was the first drug to be marketed in tablet form.

└──

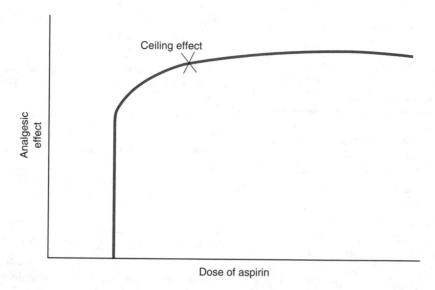

FIGURE 5–4   Ceiling effect of aspirin. A plateau is reached where increasing the dose of aspirin will not create more analgesic/anti-inflammatory effects.

Uricosuric effects: Aspirin increases the excretion of uric acid, which is used in the treatment of gout, an arthritic condition of an imbalance in uric acid metabolism. In gout, too much uric acid is produced, which is deposited in joints. Aspirin is usually not used for this condition because very high doses are required.

Antiplatelet effects: Until the early 1980s, aspirin was used exclusively as an anti-inflammatory, analgesic, and antipyretic drug for short periods of time. Clinical studies in the 1980s documented that aspirin in low doses also was a platelet aggregation inhibitor. Because of its role in prevention of clots, aspirin in low doses is used as antiplatelet therapy in the prevention of heart attack and stroke in individuals who previously have had a heart attack or stroke (secondary prevention), but whose cardiovascular disease is stabilized. Clinicians have been reluctant to recommend low-dose aspirin in patients who are relatively healthy, without any cardiovascular conditions.

In the gastrointestinal tract and blood, aspirin breaks down into salicylate (salicylic acid) and acetic acid. It is the acetic acid that *irreversibly* covalently binds to COX-1 in platelets, while salicylate has analgesic and anti-inflammatory actions. This binding prevents the formation of thromboxane A_2, resulting in a decrease in the ability to form clots and increase bleeding time, which lasts for the life of the platelet because the platelet is incapable of resynthesizing new cyclo-oxygenase enzyme.

In order to make more enzymes, new platelets must be formed, which takes about 7 days. It is controversial whether to stop taking aspirin 7–10 days before dental surgery that will cause bleeding (e.g., extractions, periodontal/implant surgery).

The antiplatelet effect of aspirin lasts for the lifetime of a platelet, about 7–10 days. This occurs because the effect of aspirin on cyclooxygenase enzymes in platelets is irreversible, so bleeding will occur until new platelets are formed. It may not be necessary to discontinue aspirin; however, if the patient is taking aspirin prophylactically and has no previous heart conditions, discontinuing aspirin is acceptable. Consult with the patient's physician before any action is taken. Effective local hemostatic measures should be taken.

Recent research advocates continuing use of aspirin to prevent emboli (see Jeske, A.H. and G.D. Suchko. 2003. Lack of scientific basis for routine discontinuation or oral anticoagulation therapy before dental treatment. *JADA* 134:1492–1497); and Ardekian, G. et al. 2000. *JADA* 131(3):331–335.).

 Rapid Dental Hint

Many dental patients take aspirin daily without the supervision of a physician.

Did You Know?

Early 20th Century advertisements for Bayer aspirin noted, "does not affect the heart." Today, aspirin is well known for its cardiovascular benefits for recurrent heart attack and stroke prevention.

At the same time aspirin inhibits the formation of thromboxane A_2 in the platelets via inhibiting COX-1, the synthesis of PGI_2 in the blood vessels walls is inhibited by COX-2. Do these seem like opposite actions? Yes, but aspirin causes inhibition of thromboxane A_2, resulting in inhibition of platelet aggregation resulting in bleeding because it is a more potent inhibitor of COX-1 than COX-2. So, low doses (as low as 40 mg but up to 81— "baby aspirin"— to 100 mg/day or 325 mg every other day) of aspirin inhibits platelet aggregation and prolongs bleeding time, while high doses (arthritis doses 3 to 6 g per day) may have no effect or shorten bleeding time because high doses prevent the formation of prosta-cyclin.

Rapid Dental Hint

One baby aspirin contains 81 mg of aspirin.

Pharmacokinetics Orally administered aspirin is absorbed rapidly, mostly from the upper small intestine, but also (a small part) from the stomach. Concentrations are found in the blood within 30 minutes, with peak concentration by 2 hours. It is metabolized in the liver to salicylic acid. Salicylates are excreted in the urine.

Rapid Dental Hint

Tell patients not to suck on aspirin tablets; this causes white lesions on the buccal mucosa.

Adverse Effects Therapeutic doses of aspirin can cause gastric irritation and contribute to gastrointestinal bleeding and peptic ulcers. These gastrointestinal side effects are due to COX-1 inhibition, which decreases GI mucosal defense mechanisms and increases gastric acid secretion. This leads to ulceration. Inhibition of prostaglandins decreases gastric mucous production and increases gastric (hydrochloric) acid pro-

duction. Aspirin is formulated as enteric coated tablets to avoid these problems.

Nausea and vomiting is due to a central action that stimulates the chemoreceptor trigger zone (CTZ) in the CNS and a peripheral action by direct irritation of the GI tract.

Salicylates can alter carbohydrate metabolism resulting in hypoglycemia (low blood sugar), which in some diabetics taking medications (e.g., insulin) can cause a loss of control of blood sugar.

Aspirin may cause renal dysfunction (decrease renal elimination), especially in patients with pre-existing renal disease or congestive heart failure. Aspirin inhibits renal prostaglandin production, which causes water retention and decreased renal blood flow.

Aspirin may produce hemolytic anemia in certain racial groups (e.g., Egyptians), who do not have the enzyme glucose-6-phosphate dehydrogenase, responsible for inactivating certain metabolites of aspirin inside red blood cells.

Patient Instructions Enteric coated tablets and extended-release preparations will reduce absorption in the stomach, which can prevent stomach irritation and ulcers and allow the tablet to break up and dissolve in the small intestine. Buffered aspirin is another type of formulation to avoid irritating effects on the stomach. Buffered aspirin may make the immediate area more basic, which will speed dissolution of the aspirin and may reduced GI irritation. Additionally, instruct patients to swallow aspirin in an upright position with a full glass of water to minimize stomach upset and to allow for more absorption in the small intestine and to ingest it in an upright position, which will allow it to pass more easily down the esophagus, preventing esophageal irritation.

Absorption into the blood from the small intestine is delayed if aspirin is taken with food, which will also help to minimize irritation.

Rapid Dental Hint

Aspirin comes in many different strengths and formulations:
Chewable tabs: 81 mg
Enteric coated tabs: 81, 165, 325, 500, 650, 975 mg
Sustained release (SR) tabs: 650, 800 mg
Tabs: 81, 325, 500 mg
Suppositories:120, 200, 300, 600 mg

Aspirin Toxicity and Treatment of Overdose

Excessive doses of aspirin produce many toxic effects. Aspirin in high doses (600–900 mg) stimulates the depth and rate of respiration (hyperventilation).

Salicylism, which is manifested as ringing in the ears or tinnitus and vertigo (loss of equilibrium/severe dizziness) occur in doses of only 300–600 mg and can lead to deafness. Onset of chronic salicylism may be insidious especially in the elderly, who may consume an increasing amount over several days to alleviate the pain of arthritis.

Shock, coma, and respiratory and renal failure and ultimately death occur after ingesting 2000–3000 mg.

Aspirin is more toxic to children than adults. In a child, toxicity is seen with 1 g (1,000 mg) and a lethal dose is 10 g. Treatment of an overdose is initiated by stopping absorption by gastric lavage and activated charcoal. Intravenous administration of sodium bicarbonate counteracts the metabolic acidosis. Finally, vitamin K is administered to compensate for prothrombin anemia, seen following toxicity.

Precautions/Contraindications

Aspirin should be used with caution and is contraindicated in patients with renal disease, gastric ulcer, and bleeding tendencies. The minimal effective dose should be used in the elderly because they are more susceptible to GI bleeding and acute renal insufficiency.

Certain individuals with a history of nasal polyps and asthma are at risk of developing bronchoconstriction if aspirin is taken. The association between asthma, nasal polyps, and aspirin intolerance is know as Samter's triad. Almost one out of four people with nasal polyps has an intolerance to aspirin. Aspirin and NSAIDs should be used with caution in asthmatics and avoided in asthmatics with nasal polyps. About 10 percent of patients with asthma are intolerant to aspirin and NSAIDs. Asthmatic patients who take aspirin are at risk of developing severe, even fatal, exacerbations of asthma. Aspirin should be avoided in asthmatics with a history of aspirin-induced bronchospasm.

Reye's syndrome is primarily a children's disease, although it can occur at any age. Using aspirin to treat viral illnesses, including chicken pox or flu, increases the risk of developing Reye's syndrome. Symptoms of Reye's syndrome include repetitive vomiting, lethargy, headache, fever, convulsions, even death. The cause of Reye's syndrome is unknown; a preceding viral illness is seen in most cases.

Drug–Drug Interactions

There are many drug–drug interactions with aspirin. A careful patient interview and medical history review can prevent unexpected interactions.

- Aspirin inhibits PGE_2, which increases insulin secretion. In diabetics, aspirin increases the hypoglycemic response of oral antidiabetic drugs (e.g., sulfonylureas). Consult with the patient's physician.
- Alkalinizing agents such as antacids can reduce salicylate levels.
- Aspirin interferes with the diuretic effect of thiazide or loop diuretics (flurosemide) because it inhibits renal prostaglandin production, which causes water retention. This will decrease the actions and effectiveness of the diuretic.
- By inhibiting cyclo-oxygenase, aspirin prevents the formation of prostaglandins, which have vasodilation effects. This *may* decrease the hypotensive ef-

Guidelines for Patients Taking Aspirin

- Ask patients why they are taking aspirin (e.g., for pain, or as a blood thinner to prevent heart problems).
- Ask patients if their physician knows they are taking aspirin
- Ask patients if they are taking "baby" aspirin (81 mg) or regular strength aspirin (325 mg).
- Determine if aspirin will cause increased bleeding during the dental procedure.
- You may need to consult with the patients' physician.
- Remind patients not to put aspirin directly on the tooth or gums because it may cause an "aspirin burn" on the tissue which clinically looks white.

fects of antihypertensive medications, including angiotension converting enzyme inhibitors: ACE inhibitors (e.g., Vasotec), diuretics (e.g., hydrochlorothiazide), and beta-blockers (e.g., Tenormin, Inderal). However, low-dose aspirin may not interfere with these antihypertensives (refer to Zanchetti A., L. Hansson, G. Leonetti, KH. Rahn et al. 2002. Low-dose aspirin does not interfere with the blood pressure–lowering effects of antihypertensive therapy: *J Hypertension* 1015–1022.)

RDH Rapid Dental Hint

Patients may be taking vitamin E and aspirin, both blood thinners. Ask patients about all medications taken.

- There is an increased risk of bleeding when aspirin is taken with anticoagulants, due to its effect on platelet aggregation. Aspirin and warfarin bind to the same plasma proteins and can displace warfarin from these plasma protein–binding sites, causing bleeding (remember that drugs that are plasma protein bound are inactive and those drugs that are displaced from these sites are highly active).
- Alcohol should not be taken with aspirin because both act as gastric irritants.
- The use of aspirin with other NSAIDs should be avoided because of increased risk for GI bleeding or decreased kidney function.
- Drug–herbal interactions include: white willow, dong quai, chamomile, ginseng, ginger, and red clover. Taking these herbal supplements with aspirin may cause increased bleeding.

Did You Know?

Caffeine, a stimulant included in many OTC analgesics for "headaches," helps the analgesic (aspirin, acetaminophen) work better. This is a contradiction; caffeine is a common cause of headaches because caffeine is a vasodilator.

Drug Profile Aspirin

Aspirin (acetylsalicylic acid, ASA) inhibits prostaglandin synthesis via inhibiting cyclo-oxygenase-1 and cyclo-oxygenase-2 enzymes, involved in the production of pain, fever, and inflammation. It inhibits thromboxane A_2, involved in anticoagulation (antiplatelet effect; inhibits blood clots). For this reason, aspirin is given in low doses (81 mg) to reduce the risk of mortality following heart attacks and to reduce the incidence of strokes.

Aspirin may cause gastrointestinal bleeding because of its antiplatelet effects. Aspirin should not be given to children with fever, chicken pox, or flu-like symptoms because of its association with Reye's syndrome.

Other Salicylate-Like Drugs

Diflunisal (Dolobid) is a derivative of salicylic acid but is not converted to salicylic acid. It is a more potent anti-inflammatory than aspirin, and it is an inhibitor of cyclo-oxygenase. It does not have antipyretic activity because it penetrates the CNS poorly. It is used primarily as an anti-inflammatory in arthritis. It has been used for dental pain. Diflunisal is absorbed almost completely after oral administration, with significant analgesia occurring within 1 hour and peak blood levels by 2 to 3 hours. Profound analgesia last from 8 to 12 hours. It is extensively bound to plasma proteins. Side effects are few, and it causes fewer and less intense gastrointestinal and antiplatelet effects than does aspirin. Diflunisal is useful for dental pain starting with a loading dose of 1 g followed by 500 mg twice a day. It is indicated for mild to moderate pain.

RDH Rapid Dental Hint

Low-dose aspirin is taken by many patients with or without it being prescribed by a physician for prevention of cardiovascular disease and stroke. Older patients should be questioned about aspirin use, including the amount taken.

Acetaminophen

Acetaminophen (Tylenol), a nonnarcotic analgesic, is a derivative of para-amino phenol. Acetaminophen is a poor inhibitor of cyclooxygenase in the tissues, so its anti-inflammatory effects are less potent than aspirin and NSAIDs. A major difference between aspirin and acetaminophen is its lack of effect on platelet function and less (or no) gastric irritation. Acetaminophen is primarily used as an analgesic and antipyretic. Studies have shown that NSAIDs are more effective than acetaminophen alone for the relief of acute dental pain. It has a pregnancy category B and is safe to use during pregnancy.

Pharmacokinetics

Acetaminophen is rapidly and almost completely absorbed from the GI tract into the blood stream. After ingestion, it reaches peak blood levels in about 30 to 60 minutes. It is not highly bound to plasma proteins, so that there is no interaction with drugs that are highly plasma protein bound such as warfarin. It is extensively metabolized in the liver and distributed to most tissues. Little is excreted unchanged in the urine, which means that it undergoes conjugation to glucuronic acid followed by kidney excretion.

Adverse Effects

Acetaminophen overdose is the leading cause of acute liver failure, even if alcohol is not taken concurrently. The maximum safe dose for adults of acetaminophen should not exceed 4 grams or 4,000 mg (e.g. eight 500 mg tablets) over a 24-hour period, with higher doses increasing the risk of liver damage. Acetaminophen has a narrow margin of safety so that the difference between a therapeutic dose and a toxic one is very small. The toxic dose is only 7 grams taken all at once.

Acetaminophen is supplied as 500 mg caps; 160, 325, 500 and 650 mg tabs. Long-term use (more than 10 days) is not recommended. Acetaminophen overdose is treated with acetylcysteine (Mucomyst), which can prevent or reduce hepatotoxicity.

Effects on the GI tract are few to none. Common side effects include skin rash and allergic reactions, which can develop into a drug-induced fever. Acetaminophen is metabolized into methemoglobin, which can result in methemoglobinemia (decreased capacity of red blood cells to carry oxygen).

Drug Profile Acetaminophen

The exact mechanism of acetaminophen's ability to reduce pain is not clear. It reduces fever by direct action in the central nervous system. Acetaminophen and aspirin are equally effective in relieving pain and reducing fever. It is good for the treatment of fever in children and for the relief of mild to moderate pain when aspirin is contraindicated.

When taken in toxic doses, acetaminophen may cause liver damage. The maximum dose per day is 4,000 mg (4 grams). Alcohol should not be taken with acetaminophen. It is safe to give during pregnancy.

There is some evidence that long-term use of acetaminophen is associated with an increased risk of renal dysfunction.

Drug Interactions

A significant interaction occurs between alcohol and acetaminophen. Both ethanol and acetaminophen are metabolized by CYP2E1. If there is enough ethanol to occupy the CYP2E1 enzyme, then it is not available to metabolize acetaminophen into n-acetyl-p-benzoquinone imine or NAPQ1, which are responsible for its toxic effects. Thus it may be worse for someone to discontinue drinking alcohol while taking acetaminophen; however, it has also been reported that there is an increased risk of hepatotoxicity with excessive alcohol use (more than three drinks per day).

Carbamazepine (Tegretol), phenytoin (Dilantin), and rifampin may increase the risk of chronic hepatotoxicity.

NONSTEROIDAL ANTI-INFLAMMATORY DRUGS

Although aspirin is separately classified as a non-narcotic analgesic there are many similarities with nonsteroidal anti-inflammatory drugs (NSAIDs). The difference between the two types of drugs is that NSAIDs do not have the same antiplatelet effect.

Ibuprofen and Ibuprofen-Like Drugs

Mechanism of Action Ibuprofen, the prototype NSAID, and other NSAIDs function to inhibit prostaglandin synthesis (primarily PGE_2) by inhibiting the cyclo-oxygenase enzymes resulting in a reduction of inflammation. However, similar to aspirin, they inhibit both COX-1 and COX-2, resulting in many adverse effects because COX-1 has a protective role on the GI mucosa and kidneys. Inhibition of COX-2 in tissues is responsible for the anti-inflammatory effects of NSAIDs.

Analgesic: Has an indirect analgesic effect by inhibiting the production of prostaglandins and does not directly affect hyperalgesia or the pain threshold.

Anti-inflammatory: Most of the anti-inflammatory effects of NSAIDs are due to inhibition of COX-2 rather than COX-1.

Fever: NSIADs are antipyretic by suppressing the synthesis of prostaglandins, specifically PGE_2 near the hypothalamus.

Antiplatelet effects: Inhibition of COX-1 also inhibits the production of thromboxane A_2, which prevents platelet aggregation. NSAIDS *do not covalently* bind to the cyclo-oxygenase enzymes and *do not irreversibly* inhibit platelet function as aspirin. *Thus, unlike aspirin, ibuprofen and the other NSAIDS are not used to prevent heart attacks and strokes;* however they still cause increased bleeding and for this reason aspirin and NSAIDs should not be taken together.

Indications All NSAIDs are antipyretic, analgesic (mild to moderate acute pain) and anti-inflammatory. NSAIDs are primarily used as anti-inflammatory drugs in the treatment of various forms of arthritis (Table 5–2). NSAIDs are not indicated for prophylaxis against heart attacks and strokes.

Adverse Effects Adverse gastrointestinal effects are similar to aspirin: increased stomach irritation, bleeding, and ulcer formation (Table 5–3). As with aspirin, there is a high risk for ulcer development in patients taking a corticosteroid (e.g., prednisone), and previous GI problems. In these high-risk patients, concurrent administration of an antiulcer drug such as a proton pump inhibitor [e.g., esomeprazole (Nexium) or omeprazole (Prilosec)] may help prevent the development of gastric ulcers from NSAIDs use. Misoprostol (Cytotec) is a prostaglandin E_2 analog and is approved for prophylaxis against NSAID-induced ulcers.

Patients should be warned about the potential side effects of aspirin and NSAIDs, and should be asked if they are using any of these products. Since many of these preparations are over the counter and available without a prescription, initially patients may not inform the dental clinician about usage.

Kidney function may be depressed due to inhibition of prostaglandin synthesis, which plays a protective role in kidney function. This problem is reversible within 1–3 days after stopping the NSAID.

It should be noted that there are different preparations of naproxen: naproxen (Naprosyn) and naproxen sodium (Aleve, Anaprox, Anaprox DS). The preparations containing sodium are not recommended for use in patients with hypertension.

Precautions/Contraindications The precautions that were taken for aspirin in patients with asthma and nasal polyps are taken with the other NSAIDs. This reaction rarely occurs in children. Within 20 minutes to 3 hours of taking an NSAID, aspirin-sensitive asthmatics can develop respiratory symptoms such as bronchospasm and respiratory arrest.

Unlike with aspirin, there is no contraindication for giving an NSAID such as children's Motrin to a child with the flu or chicken pox.

Drug Interactions

- NSAIDs may counteract the antihypertensive effects of angiotension converting enzyme inhibitors [ACE inhibitors (e.g., Vasotec), diuretics (e.g., hydrochlorothiazide) and beta-blockers (e.g., Tenormin, Inderal)] by inhibiting formation of prostaglandins. It is important to monitor blood pressure and dosage adjustment may be necessary. This may also cause an increased risk of recurrence of heart failure. NSAIDs should not be used for more than 5 days (refer to: *European Society of Hypertension Scientific Newsletter: Update on hypertension management.* 2003. 4(*17*). Interactions

---

RDH Rapid Dental Hint

Interview your patients concerning the use of aspirin for the prevention of heart attack and stroke and the use of NSAIDs (e.g., ibuprofen) for pain relief. Many patients may not think to tell you that they are taking one or both of these drugs because of increased bleeding tendencies. It is important to fully interview patients about all OTC drugs!

Table 5–2   Analgesics: Nonsteroidal Anti-Inflammatory Drugs—Salicylates and Other Analgesics

Drugs	*Notes*
Nonselective NSAIDs and Salicylates	Most NSAIDs are used in the treatment of mild to moderate pain, arthritis, and dysmenorrhea. Listed below are the NSAIDs used in the treatment of mild to moderate dental pain. Use caution in the concurrent use of an NSAID and ACE inhibitor or beta-blocker in control of hypertension.
Salicylates Aspirin (Ecotrin, Bayer, Halfprin and many more) Diflunisal (Dolobid)	OTC: acute mild to moderate pain, fever, osteoarthritis and rheumatoid arthritis, dysmenorrhea, prophylaxis of stroke and heart attacks, thromboembolic disorders Prescription: acute and long-term relief of mild to moderate pain; dental pain
Choline magnesium trisalicylate (Trilisate)	Not used in dentistry (potential of abnormal coagulation)
Indoles Indomethacin (Indocin) Sulindac (Clinoril)	Primarily for arthritis Not for dental pain
Indole Acetic Acids Tolmetin (Tolectin) Ketorolac (Toradol)	Not for dental pain Prescription: can be used for short-term moderate dental pain
Phenylalkoanoic Acid Derivative Ibuprofen (Advil, Motrin, Nuprin) Ketoprofen (Orudis, Actron) Flurbiprofen (Ansaid) Naproxen (Naprosyn) Naproxen sodium (Anaprox, Anaprox DS, Aleve) Oxaprozin (Daypro) Etodolac (generic)	OTC: prescription; mild to moderate dental pain OTC (Actron): prescription (Orudis); mild to moderate dental pain Prescription: mild to moderate dental pain OTC (Aleve): mild to moderate dental pain Not for dental pain; arthritis Acute dental pain
Napthylalkanone Nabumetone (Relafen)	Not for dental pain; arthritis
Fenamates Meclofenamate (Ponstel) Diclofenac (Voltaren)	Not for dental pain; arthritis Not for dental pain; arthritis
Oxicam Prioxicam (Feldene)	Not for dental pain; arthritis
Highly COX-2 selective NSAIDs Celecoxib (Celebrex)	Unlabeled use for dental pain
Other Analgesics Acetaminophen	OTC: hepatotoxicity with chronic use, especially in alcoholics

between antihypertensive agents and other drugs). Aspirin does not interfere with the actions of antihypertensive medications.

 Rapid Dental Hint

Before recommending an OTC NSAID such as ibuprofen or Aleve to your patients, make sure they are not taking antihypertensive medications.

Table 5–3   Risk Factors for NSAID-Induced Gastrointestinal Ulcers

- Elderly
- Past history of ulcers
- Higher doses of NSAID
- Concurrent use of corticosteroids

Guidelines for Patients Taking NSAIDs (E.G., Ibuprofen)

- Patients should take pill with a full glass of water and with food.
- Patients should not take with aspirin; can take with acetaminophen.

- Aspirin taken with NSAIDs increases the incidence of GI problems and bleeding; these drugs should not be taken together.
- Antacids may decrease the absorption of NSAIDs.
- Patients taking a corticosteroid such as prednisone may be at higher risk for GI ulcers if they also take aspirin or an NSAID.
- NSAIDs decrease renal excretion of lithium, which increases lithium plasma levels.
- All NSAIDs are highly plasma protein bound and have the potential to displace other highly protein bound drugs such as warfarin. (NSAIDs potentiate the anticoagulant effect) and antidiabetic drugs (sulfonylureas) (NSAIDs potentiate the hypoglycemic effects).

Selective COX-2 Inhibitors

While COX-1 is found in most body tissues, COX-2 is primarily found in the brain, kidney, bones, and reproductive organs. Selective cyclo-oxygenase-2 (COX-2) inhibitors were introduced in 1998. Three medications—celecoxib (Celebrex), rofecoxib (Vioxx), and valdecoxib (Bextra)— were marketed originally. These COX-2 inhibitors were intended to provide pain relief comparable to that of traditional NSAIDs but with a decrease risk for adverse gastrointestinal effects of bleeding and ulcerations. However, severe GI adverse events have occurred.

Safety and Adverse Effects   In 2004, the FDA issued a public health advisory in response to clinical studies that found that the COX-2 inhibitors were associated with a significantly greater incidence of thrombotic cardiovascular events (heart attack and stroke), leading to death in some cases. Data collected from clinical studies suggested that high doses and long-term use of these drugs may contribute to these risks. This prompted the FDA to remove rofecoxib (Vioxx) and

valdecoxib (Bextra). Presently, the only selective COX-2 inhibitor on the U.S. market is Celebrex. A box warning highlights the potential for increased risk of cardiovascular events, as well as serious and potentially life-threatening gastrointestinal bleeding. The government has also requested that manufacturers of over-the-counter NSAIDs such as ibuprofen (Advil, Motrin), ketoprofen (Orudis, Actron), and naproxen (Aleve) also revise their labeling to include these risks. It is advised to use the lowest effective dose for the shortest duration to avoid these potentially fatal adverse events.

Since celecoxib is the only selective COX-2 inhibitor on the market, all information in this section will be directed toward this drug.

Mechanism of Action   Celecoxib exerts anti-inflammatory and analgesic effects through the inhibition of prostaglandin synthesis, by binding of the sulfonamide side chain on celecoxib to a site on COX-2 that is not present on COX-1, thus *reversibly* blocking COX-2 activity and preventing the formation of prostacyln (PGI2), which will induce platelet clumping and cause vasoconstriction. Celecoxib and the traditional NSAIDs are equally effective in treating pain and inflammation.

Celecoxib does not inhibit platelet aggregation because platelets contain the COX-1 enzyme and not COX-2. Therefore, celecoxib selectively inhibits the formation of prostacyclin (PGI_2) rather than thromboxane A2.

Contraindications and Drug Interactions   Celecoxib is contraindicated in patients with sulfonamide (sulfa) allergy because of a sulfonamide chain on the drug molecule.

Celecoxib is metabolized by the liver CYP450 cytochromes, specifically CYP2C9, so drugs that inhibit CYP2C9 (fluconazole, fluvastatin—antifungal drugs) may increase celecoxib blood levels. Celecoxib also is an inhibitor of CYP2D6 and thus should not be taken with tricyclic antidepressants or beta-blockers, which are substrates for CYP2D6.

OPIOID ANALGESICS

Introduction

An **opioid** analgesic is a natural or synthetic morphine-like substance used for reducing moderate to severe pain that cannot be controlled with other types of analgesics. Opioids are **narcotics** that act exclusively on the central components of pain and produce analgesia and CNS depression. Several opioids are derived from opium, which was originally isolated from the dried juice of seeds of the Oriental poppy flower in the nineteenth century. Opium contains primarily morphine, codeine, and other substances. These natural substances are called opiates. Narcotic is a general term used to describe morphine-like drugs and can be natural (morphine) or synthetic (meperidine).

Morphine, the prototype narcotic, produces analgesia, drowsiness, and a change in mood and mental clouding, without a loss of consciousness. Other sensory modalities such as touch, vision, and hearing are not impaired at doses that reduce pain. Opiates are water soluble, allowing them to be abused by the parenteral route.

Mechanism of Action

Opioid Receptors

Opioids interact with binding sites in the CNS called opiate receptors, which are diffusely distributed throughout the central nervous system with highest concentrations in the limbic system (Table 5–4). The endogenous peptides, enkephalins, endorphins, and dynorphins are released from neurons in the brain and activate opioid receptors, thereby blocking the transmission of pain impulses. These substances are the body's natural opiates that inhibit painful stimuli.

Did You Know?

If you eat poppy seeds from a bagel, you could have a positive urine test for narcotics!

Table 5–4 Opioid Drugs

Short-Acting Opioid Agonists
- Morphine
- Hydromorphone (Dilaudid)
- Oxycodone (controlled-release OxyContin)
- Hydrocodone (Vicodin, Lorcet, Vicoprofen in combination with a nonnarcotic)
- Codeine
- Meperidine (Demerol)
- Fentanyl (Duragesic patch)

Long-Acting Opioid Agonists
- Methadone
- Levorphanol (Levo-Dromoran)
- Propoxyphene (Darvon)
- Oxymorphone (Numorphan)

Other Opioid Agonists
- Dextromethorphan (used in cough syrups; Robitussin, Sucrets, Vicks, Delsym, Benylin)
- Diphenoxylate (with atropine; Lomotil)
- Loperamide (Imodium; antidiarrheall)
- Tramadol (central analgesic; Ultram)

Mixed Agonist/antagonists
- Buprenophine (Buprenex)
- Butorphanol (Stadol)
- Nalbuphine (Nubain)
- Pentazocine (Talwin)

Antagonists
- Naloxone (Narcan)

Classification of Opioid Receptors

The main opioid receptors are classified as mu (μ), delta (δ) and kappa (κ), depending upon their affinity for the different opioids (Figure 5–5). For example, morphine stimulates both mu receptors and kappa receptors. Other opioids such as pentazocine (Talwin) stimulate the kappa receptors and block the mu receptors. Naloxone (Narcan) is an opioid blocker and inhibits both the mu and kappa receptors. Table 5–5 shows responses produced by activation of specific receptors.

Pharmacokinetics

Opioids are readily absorbed from the GI tract, nasal mucosa, and lungs. They are also absorbed after parenteral

Table 5–5 The Opioid Responses

Response	Mu Receptor	Kappa Receptor
Analgesia	+	+
Decreased GI mobility (Constipation)	+	+
Euphoria	+	−
Miosis (pupil contraction)	−	+
Physical dependence	+	−
Respiratory depression	+	−
Sedation	+	+

injection (e.g., subcutaneous, intramuscular, and intravenous), producing the greatest effect.

Classification

Based on their clinical effectiveness or strength (potency), opioids are classified as:

- Full agonists: strong or moderate in producing an analgesic effect
- Mixed opioid agonist/antagonists: analgesic (relief of pain) effect with some antagonist activity
- Pure antagonists: no analgesic effects; used in opioid overdose

Opioid Agonists: Strong Potency

Morphine

Morphine is the prototype narcotic analgesic that is the standard against which other narcotic analgesics are compared. The main actions of opium are due to its morphine content (9–17%). Morphine binds to the μ and κ receptors to produce strong analgesic effects. In doses of 5 to 10 mg severe pain will be reduced (make it less intense) or eliminated. Morphine increases the pain threshold and increases the capacity to tolerate pain by reducing the emotional component of pain. Essentially, the painful stimulus itself is recognized, but it may not be perceived as painful. The patient may say the pain is still present,

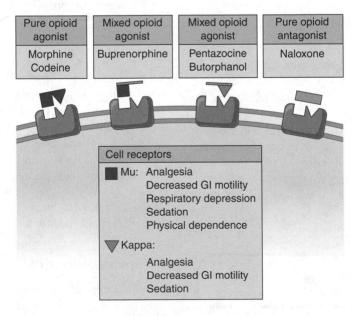

Pure opioid agonist	Mixed opioid agonist	Mixed opioid agonist	Pure opioid antagonist
Morphine Codeine	Buprenorphine	Pentazocine Butorphanol	Naloxone

Cell receptors

■ Mu: Analgesia
Decreased GI motility
Respiratory depression
Sedation
Physical dependence

▼ Kappa:

Analgesia
Decreased GI motility
Sedation

FIGURE 5–5 Opioid receptors.

CHAPTER 5 DRUGS FOR PAIN CONTROL **85**

but they feel more comfortable. Morphine acts not only in the brain, but also in the spinal cord where it is injected directly into the cerebral spinal fluid.

Morphine does not accumulate in tissues because it is not lipid-soluble. It is cleared from the body within 24 hours of the last dose. Excretion is 90% in the urine and 10% in the feces followed by biliary excretion.

Actions and Adverse Effects

Central actions of morphine

- Analgesia
- Drowsiness/sleep
- Cough suppression
- Vomiting (due to stimulation of chemoreceptor trigger zone in the brain)
- Hypotension
- Miosis (papillary constriction due to stimulation of parasympathetic nerves)
- Respiratory depression (in high doses, respiratory depression becomes the major toxic effect and cause of death because no tolerance is developed to respiratory depression)
- Euphoria (ecstasy; develop tolerance rapidly to euphoric actions)
- Increased release of ADH (antidiuretic hormone), which causes urinary retention (an effect on the sphincter)

Peripheral actions

- Constipation (due to stimulation of cholinergic activity in the GI tract); and
- Body warmth/flushing/itchy (due to histamine release)

Indications Morphine sulfate is used for relief of moderate to serious pain due to trauma, postsurgery, cancer, or myocardial infarction. It is usually given intramuscularly or subcutaneously. It is also used as preanesthetic medication before surgery. Morphine is not administered orally because it undergoes extensive first pass inactivation in the liver.

Characteristics Morphine exhibits dependence and drug-seeking behavior which is dose related. The higher the dose and the longer the individual is taking the drug and then stops the drug, the more severe the withdrawal symptoms. Cross-dependence develops between morphine and other opioids such as heroin, methadone, and meperidine. Withdrawal can be suppressed by substituting another one of these drugs for morphine. Tolerance develops to the analgesic, sedative,

and euphoric effects of the drug but not miosis and constipation; as you use the drug, it becomes less effective. Normally a dose of 10 mg will produce strong analgesic effects, but addicts often require up to 250 mg to achieve the same effect. There is a cross-tolerance where an individual will also become tolerant to other narcotics; if morphine does not work, then other narcotics like morphine will not work either. Since there is no tolerance to miosis, a characteristic sign of narcotic use is pinpoint pupils. Because of its high abuse potential, it is not used as an antitussive.

Drug Interactions Any drug that causes CNS depression will potentiate the effects of opioid drugs because they also are CNS depressants. Examples include antihistamines, sedative/hypnotics, alcohol, and psychiatric drugs. Herbals such as kava-kava, valerian, and St. John's wort may increase sedation.

Methadone

Methadone is a long-acting synthetic morphine derivative used orally in the treatment of opioid (usually heroin) addiction or pain. Since it is a narcotic, it can be abused; however, it is used to "wean" patients off narcotics because it does not produce euphoria. A daily dose of 30 to 40 mg of methadone prevents withdrawal symptoms for 24 to 36 hours. Daily doses of at least 65 mg achieve greater tolerance and lower the effects of street heroin doses. Rifampin (for tuberculosis), phenytoin (Dilantin), barbiturates, carbamazepine (Tegretol), and ethyl alcohol accelerate methadone metabolism. Cimetidine (Tagamet), erythromycin, and ketoconazole (Nizoral; antifungal) inhibit methadone metabolism, resulting in elevated serum levels. This type of treatment is done in a methadone maintenance program which is currently restricted to highly regulated, federally licensed programs.

Methadone is also indicated in patients with chronic pain. In 2007, the US Food and Drug Administration (FDA) Issued an adverse event alert concerning reports of death and respiratory depression, and cardiac arrhythmias in patients receiving methadone for chronic pain. These adverse events were probably due to unintentional methadone overdoses, drug interactions, and methadone's cardiac toxic effects. Methadone doses for pain relief is not the same as for opioid withdrawal. Methadone doses should be slowly titrated to an analgesic effect (Health Agencies Update. JAMA 2007;297(4):354). Refer to www.pbm.va.gov/archive/methadonedosing.pdf.

Meperidine

Meperidine (Demerol) is a less effective analgesic than morphine, with half the duration of action [75 mg meperidine IM (intramuscular injection) = 10 mg morphine IM]. It is sometimes used in dentistry. It is metabolized to normeperidine, which can cause convulsions. It does not have antitussive properties. Tolerance, cross-tolerance, dependence and cross-dependence develop with meperidine. No tolerance develops to CNS stimulation. Meperidine should not be used in patients also taking antidepressant monoamine oxidase inhibitors such as selegiline (Eldepryl). There are increased CNS depressant effects when taken with alcohol, and increased sedation when taken with St. John's wort.

Oxycodone and Hydrocodone

Oxycodone (OxyContin) and hydrocodone are semisynthetic morphine derivatives used in the treatment of moderate to severe pain. Vicodin is a combination of hydrocodone and acetaminophen. These have all of the adverse effects of morphine: respiratory depression, antitussive, constipation, and dependence. They are most effective when combined with NSAIDS, aspirin, or acetaminophen. OxyContin has received much media attention because of its high abuse potential. Other opioids are listed in Table 5–4.

Often opioids are combined with nonnarcotic analgesics or NSAIDs into a single tablet to act synergistically to relieve pain, and the dose of narcotic can be kept small to avoid dependence and opioid-related side effects. Examples include hydrocodone/acetaminophen (Vicodin) and hydrocodone/ibuprofen (Vicoprofen).

Fentanyl

Fentanyl (Duragesic) is a semisynthetic opiate that is very potent and lipid soluble and crosses the blood–brain barrier very quickly; thus it is used primarily in anesthesiology. It is also available as a patch (absorbed easily through the skin because it is lipid soluble) or injectable, and is indicated for severe chronic pain when continuous analgesia is required.

Opioid Agonists: Moderate Potency

Codeine

Codeine is a naturally occurring narcotic agonist obtained from the opium poppy but in lesser amounts than morphine. It is much more active orally than other opioid compounds, but is a less potent analgesic than morphine

(120 mg of codeine phosphate IM = 10 mg morphine IM; 200 mg codeine oral = 30–60 mg morphine orally). It causes less respiratory depressant action and constipation, and has less dependence potential. It is a prodrug because its analgesic activity is the result of a conversion to morphine by cytochrome P450 liver enzymes (CYP2D6). Some people respond well to codeine, but some do not because of a deficiency of CYP2D6.

Adverse Effects   Codeine causes less respiratory depression than morphine, but if given in high doses the same degrees of respiratory depression will occur. Additional adverse effects include (as with all narcotics) dizziness, nausea, vomiting, constipation, sedation, and itching.

Indications   Codeine is usually combined with other nonnarcotic drugs such as acetaminophen for the relief of acute nociceptive mild to moderate dental pain, and is not used for treating serve pain. It is also added to many cough syrups as an antitussive. Codeine has the same abuse potential as morphine, but is less potent. The phosphate and sulfate salt forms are available, but the phosphate form is more water soluble and thus is more commonly used. The oral dose of codeine is 60, 30, or 15 mg.

Drug–drug Interactions   There may be an increase in CNS depressant effects if taken with alcohol or other CNS. There may be increased sedation if taken with St. John's wort. Since codeine is metabolized by CYP2D6, any drugs that inhibit this enzyme will increase plasma levels of codeine. Some drugs include selective serotonin reuptake inhibitors (antidepressants) such as Paxil and Prozac, Celebrex, and cimetidine (Tagamet). Because of differences in responseiveness among individuals in the activity of codeine, some clinicians prefer to use hydrocodone.

Propoxyphene   Propoxyphene (Darvon) is a chemical related to methadone and with less analgesic activity than codeine. Usually it is used in combination with acetaminophen to increase its effectiveness in the treatment of moderate pain, but in clinical studies it was found that the combination drug was just as effective as acetaminophen alone. It is not easily abused and lowers the seizure threshold in patients with such disorders.

Other Agonists

Dextromethorphan is an opioid without any analgesic activity but high antitussive effects. It is a component of cough medicines. Some trade names are Benylin, Delsym Vick's, and Robitussin.

Guidelines for Patients Taking Codeine

- Monitor patients for dry mouth; fluoride rinses if indicated.
- Monitor vital signs due to effects of the heart and the respiratory system.
- Causes drowsiness/sedation.

Loperamide (Imodium) is an opioid without analgesic effects but increased smooth muscle tone in the gastrointestinal tract, and is used as an antidiarrheal. It is available over the counter.

Diphenoxylate is an opioid/anticholinergic Schedule V controlled drug that is also used as an antidiarrheal. It is combined with atropine in a product called Lomotil. It can cause severe respiratory depression, coma, and death after overdose in children. It is a Schedule V drug.

Tramadol (Ultram) is a unique analgesic having both opiate and central acting adrenergic qualities. It is an opioid-like drug that is not a controlled substance. It is FDA approved for moderate to moderately severe pain. Tramadol can cause serious neurotoxicity, and is not the first-line drug of choice.

Mixed Agonist/Antagonists

Mixed agonist/antagonists are analgesic drugs that have combinations of full agonist, partial agonist, and antagonists. These parenterally administered drugs are used for preoperative and postoperative analgesia and for analgesia during labor and delivery. Examples include buprenorphine, butorphanol, nalbuphine, and pentazocine. Pentazocine (Talwin) is a kappa receptor agonist with partial agonist activity at mu receptors. It is available in an oral and parenteral form and is used for moderate to severe pain. Butorphanol (Stadol) is available as a nasal spray for migraine headaches (Table 5–4).

Antagonists

Opioid antagonists inhibit the effects of morphine and are used in situations of narcotic overdose, reversing all opioid effects including analgesia. Naloxone (Narcan) and naltrexone (Depade) are not used to reverse non–life threatening effects.

The antagonist drug binds the opioid receptors but exerts no activity (there is no analgesic or antitussive activity, nor is there respiratory depression). For exam-

ple, naloxone (Narcan) binds to all three receptors and blocks the action of the opioid.

Combination Narcotic Analgesic and Nonnarcotic Analgesic

Many opioids are used in combination with a nonnarcotic analgesic such as aspirin, acetaminophen, or ibuprofen to obtain a greater analgesic effect than any of the agents alone and to use less dose of the narcotic. Table 5–6 lists the various narcotic/nonnarcotic analgesic combinations that are used for moderate to severe pain. The disadvantage of using combination therapy is that it increases the risk of adverse effects and drug interactions.

Selection of Agent and Dosage

There are two criteria for the selection of a narcotic drug:

1. Potency and maximal effect: The most potent in maximal effect is morphine; meperidine (Demerol) is intermediate in activity; and codeine and propoxyphene (Darvon) are the least active
2. Duration of action: Morphine has a quick onset and short duration but it is not used orally and thus not used in dentistry; meperidine (Demerol) has a short onset and very short duration; and methadone has a long onset and long duration.

OTHER DRUGS USED FOR OROFACIAL PAIN MANAGEMENT

Besides treating orofacial pain with narcotics, there are other drugs that can be used with fewer adverse effects that patients can taken for longer periods of time. Treatment is usually initiated with one drug, and the dose is increased as needed and tolerated. Medications may be decreased gradually during periods of remission (Table 5–7).

Antiepileptic Drugs

Antiepileptic drugs such as gabapentin (Neurontin) and pregablin (Lycria) are generally well tolerated and effective in chronic orofacial pain management, including postherpetic neuralgia and migraine headaches. Pregabalin (Lycria) has a better pharmacokinetic profile than gabapentin, achieving efficacy at lower doses. The most common adverse effects are peripheral edema, xerostomia, dizziness, and sleepiness. A proposed mechanism of reducing pain is blocking sodium and calcium chan-

Table 5–6   Narcotic/Nonnarcotic Combinations

Formulation	Trade Name	Schedule
Hydrocodone/acetaminophen	Lorcet 10/650 mg	C-III
	Lorcet HD 5/500	
	Lorcet Plus 7.5/650	
	Lortab 2.5/500; 5/500; 7.5/500; 10/500	C-III
	Vicodin 5/500	C-III
	Vicodin ES 7.5/750	
	Vicodin HP 10/660	
Hydrocodone/ibuprofen	Vicoprofen 7.5/200	
Oxycodone/acetaminophen	Percocet 2.5/325; 5/325; 7.5/500; 10/650	C-II
	Roxicet 5/325; 5/500	C-II
	Tylox 5/500	C-II
Oxycodone/ibuprofen (5mg/400mg)	Combunox 5/400	C-II
Oxycodone HCl/aspirin	Percodan 5/325	C-II
	Percodan-Demi 2.5/325	C-II
Acetaminophen/codeine	Tylenol w/ codeine (No. 2, No. 3, No. 4) 300/15; 300/30; 300/60	C-III
Aspirin/codeine/carisoprodol	Soma compound w/codeine 325/16/200	C-III
Dihydrocodeine/aspirin	Synalgos-DC 16/356 (contains 30 mg caffeine)	C-III
Propoxyphene/acetaminophen	Darvocet 50/325	
Propoxyphene/aspirin/caffeine	Darvon compound 65/389/32.4	C-IV
Acetaminophen/butalbital/caffeine/codeine	Fioricet w/ codeine	C-III
Aspirin/butalbital/caffeine/codeine	Fiorinal w/codeine	C-III

Table 5–7   Pharmacologic Treatment Options for Orofacial Chronic Pain

Drug	Dose	Notes
Tricyclic antidepressants: Amitriptyline (Elavil) Desipramine (Norpramine) Nortriptyline (Pamelor)	25 mg at bedtime and tritrate (adjusting the dose until the desired effect is achieved) every 3 days up to 20–100 mg/day. Therapeutic effects seen in about 1–2 weeks.	Vasoconstrictor interactions: use EPI cautiously—no more than two cartridges of 1:100,000. Avoid levonordefrin (in mepivicaine)
Gabapentin (Neurontin)	300 mg at bedtime and tritrate by 300 mg every 3–7 days to a maximum of 1,900–3,600mg/day. Wait about 2 weeks for therapeutic effect	Adverse effects include xerostomia
Pregablin (Lyrica)	Doses start at 50 mg tid	Adverse effects include xerostomia, peripheral edema
Lidocaine patch (Lidoderm 5%)	One patch daily on for 12 hours; off for 12 hours. Up to four patches	Lidocaine HCl is being delivered; no special precautions
Carbamazepine (Tegretol) Oxycarbazepine (Trileptal)	Carbamazepine: 100mg bid on day 1, increase by not more than 200 mg/day Oxycarbazepine: 300 bid	Xerostomia, blood disorders (carbamazepine)

nels and enhancing the inhibitor effects of gamma-aminobutyric acid (GABA).

Carbamazepine (Tegretol) was the first antiepileptic drug approved for neuropathic pain associated with trigeminal neuralgia. The starting daily dose is low, ranging from 100 to 400 mg/day. Some adverse effects include blood disorders such as lekcopenia or agranulocytosis (decrease in the number of white blood cells) or aplastic anemia (bone marrow stops producing blood cells). Oxycarbazepine (Trileptal), a form of carbamazepine, has fewer adverse effects and risks of toxicity, but must be taken in higher doses to provide adequate pain control. Doses begin at 300 mg bid and is gradually increased to achieve pain control.

Lamotrigine (Lamictal) for trigeminal neuralgia acts by blocking sodium channels. A serious life-threatening rash has been reported as well as cleft lip/palate in newborns.

Tricyclic Antidepressants

Tricyclic antidepressants (TCAs), including amitriptyline (Elavil), clomipraime (Anafranil), desipramine (Norpramin), and nortriptyline (Pamelor) have been used to treat neuropathic pain. Many mechanisms of reducing pain include blocking the reuptake of norepinephrine and serotonin back into the nerve endings and blockade of sodium channels. Anticholinergic side effects are common, including xerostomia, blurred vision, and urinary retention. Doses used are less than when used for depression.

The SSRIs (selective serotonin reuptake inhibitors) are not as effective as the TCAs in treating neuropathic pain.

Lidocaine Patch

Lidocaine, an amide local anesthetic, is available in a patch (Lidoderm 5% patch) and is indicated for relief of pain associated with postherpetic neuralgia. It is absorbed into the superficial layers of intact skin so there is systemic absorption, but this most likely will not be an additive affect in the dental patient receiving lidocaine local anesthetic. The patch can be used for a maximum of 4 days; one patch is applied daily for 12 hours, then off for 12 hours.

Lidoderm is contraindicated in patients with a history of sensitivity to local anesthetics (amide type). Excessive dosing (e.g., applying Lidoderm to larger areas or for longer than the recommended wearing time) could result in increased absorption of lidocaine and high blood concentrations leading to serious adverse effects.

Calcium Channel Blockers

Calcium channel blockers are heart medications such as nifedipine (Procardia). These drugs reduce the activity of the nociceptive pathways and block calcium from going into the nerve so that substance P is not released.

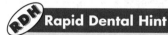

Rapid Dental Hint

Remember: Before any drugs are prescribed to your patients, reference the drug.

SUBSTANCE ABUSE AND DEPENDENCY

Drug (substance or chemical) dependency and abuse are major public health problems; many patients seen in the dental office or clinic are dependent on or abuse drugs or alcohol. Drug **dependency** (formerly called drug addiction) is when a patient feels the absolute need for a drug or will experience withdrawal symptoms if the drug is taken away. Tolerance may develop whereby more and more of the drug must be taken to achieve the desired effect. The individual finds it is difficult to discontinue and cannot quit. If the person does stop taking the drug, they will undergo withdrawal symptoms characterized by painful physical and/or mental suffering. Drug abuse refers to the recurrent and frequent use of a drug or substance that causes physical or mental harm or impairs social behavior (for example, a substance abuser cannot function at work, school, or home, or drugs will be used in situations that are physically hazardous, e.g., driving a car under the influence).

Recognizing Drug Abuse Patients

The dental hygienist should recognize and screen those patients who are currently abusing drugs and alcohol as well as those who are recovering from substance abuse and dependency. Some patients may not reveal that they currently have or have had a history of drug abuse. Thus, dental hygienist should be aware of signs and symptoms of drug abuse (Table 5–8).

Patients may request a second prescription for a narcotic for many reasons, including "The pills fell into the sink" or "My dog ate them."

Table 5–8   Signs and Symptoms of Drug Abusers

Symptoms of drug abuse depend on the drug being abused:
- Alcoholics may have facial (especially nose) "spider veins," odor of alcohol on their breath, liver disease, weight changes, abusive behavior, and difficulty concentrating.
- Cocaine users may have chronic sniffles due to vasconstrictive properties, increased alertness, euphoria, excitation, increased blood pressure, and pulse rate.
- Marijuana users have an increased appetite and may be disoriented.
- Depressant drugs users (barbiturates, benzodiazepines) may show slurred speech, disorientation or behavior similar to an alcoholic but without the alcohol breath, shallow respiration, clammy/sweating skin, and dilated pupils.
- Amphetamine and LSD users have illusions and hallucinations, and an altered perception of time.
- Narcotics abusers (e.g., heroin, hydrocodone, oxycodone, morphine) appear as euphoric with dilated pupils. They are usually show drowsiness, respiratory depression and nausea, clammy/sweaty skin.

Central nervous system stimulants produce excitatory effects in the central nervous system, characterized by increased wakefulness and alertness and feelings of increased initiative and ability and depression of appetite. Excessive dosage, particularly when administered intravenously, produces a delirious or psychotic state. Examples of central nervous system stimulants include amphetamines and cocaine.

Narcotic analgesics relieve pain, induce sedation or sleep, and elevate mood—particularly when it is depressed—and act as cough suppressants. A high degree of tolerance and severe physical and psychological dependence usually develops with prolonged or repeated use. There are reportedly between 1 and 2 million Americans abusing opioids, including heroin. The dental hygienist must be wary of patients requesting these types of drugs.

These drugs are taken orally, sniffed, injected subcutaneously or intravenously, and smoked (opium). Examples of more commonly abused narcotic analgesics include: opium, morphine, heroin, codeine, meperidine, and methadone.

Cannabis is a drug derived from the hemp plant *cannabis sativa.* Cannabis is smoked (marijuana), occasionally ingested (hashish), or sniffed. In high doses it produces clearly hallucinogenic effects.

Common long-term adverse effects of opioids include xerostomia, constipation, and papillary constriction. Sniffing cocaine causes irritation and drying of the nasal mucosa. Those who take intravenous opioids will have puncture marks on their arms.

Only about 20 percent of heroin addicts are receiving treatment with methadaone, naltrexone, clonidine, or levo-alpha-acetyl-methadol (LAAM). Withdrawal syndrome is severe and uncomfortable for the individual.

Methadone is a long-acting oral opioid that does not produce euphoria (ecstasy) like the other opioids. LAAM is similar to methadone, but it has a longer duration of action, which allows patients to visit treatment programs less frequently. Clonidine is a α_2-adrenergic agonist that decreases withdrawal symptoms by decreasing the sympathetic output responsible for many withdrawal symptoms such as sweating, diarrhea, intestinal cramping, and nausea. Overdose can cause death by respiratory depression.

Buprenorphine (http://www.usdoj.gov/ndic/pubs10/10123/index.htm) is the latest drug approved for the management of opiate addiction. There are two formulations: buprenorphine (Subutex), used in the initial stages of therapy, and buprenorphine and nalxone (Suboxone), used in the maintenance stage. While most commonly used to treat heroin addiction, it is also used to treat addiction to OxyContin and Percoet. Physicians must become certified by attending a special training course and submitting their qualifications to the Substance Abuse and Mental Health Services Administration (SAMHSA).

Buprenorphine is a derivative of thebane, an extract of opium. It is a partial agonist and thus can produce the euphoria, analgesia, and sedation associated with opiates, but to a lesser degree than full opiate agonists such as morphine and heroin. Buprenorphine has a ceiling effect. High doses can actually precipitate withdrawal symptoms in opiate addicted patients.

Buprenorphine is administered under the tongue via a small syringe and is absorbed through the sublingual mucous membranes. A flexible dosing schedule allows for better compliance. The nalxone contained in Suboxone prevents it from being abused because naloxone will precipitate withdrawal symptoms.

There are several advantages of using buprenorphine versus methadone. Buprenorphine is prescribed in a physician's office rather being dispensed in a clinic, as needed with methadone. It is also obtained from a local pharmacy. Methadone abuse is increasing throughout the Northeast region and contributes to many overdose deaths.

Patients asking for medications that are addicting, including opiates and anti-anxiety drugs, should be evaluated for a dependency problem. Some patients may request a certain pain medication after periodontal surgery or extractions that they say works best for them. The dental hygienist should be aware that if the dental procedure is not too traumatic or painful and the patient requests a narcotic such as Percodan or Vicodin, this patient may have a drug problem. Patients who are recovering from substance abuse should not be prescribed drugs that will have the potential for abuse or addiction. This includes alcohol containing mouthrinses such as Listerine or chlorhexidine gluconate (Peridex, PerioGard). Nonalcoholic rinses (e.g., Rembrandt, Oral-B) are recommended.

Alternative drugs to prescribe to patients either currently experiencing or recovering from chemical dependency for certain conditions related to dentistry include for pain control, instead of giving a narcotic, recommend acetaminophen and/or a NSAID such as ibuprofen or naproxen.

DENTAL HYGIENE NOTES

The World Health Organization (WHO) provides a stepladder for the treatment of pain.

Mild Pain	Moderate Pain	Severe Pain
Aspirin	APAP/codeine	Morphine
Acetaminophen	APAP/hydrocodone	Methadone
NSAIDs	APAP/oxycodone	Levophanol
+/- adjuncts	APAP/dihydrocodeine	Fentanyl
	Tramadol	Oxycodone
	+/- adjuncts	+/- adjuncts

APAP = acetaminophen.
(Adapted from World Health Organization. 1996): Cancer Pain Relief, with a Guide to Opioid Availability.

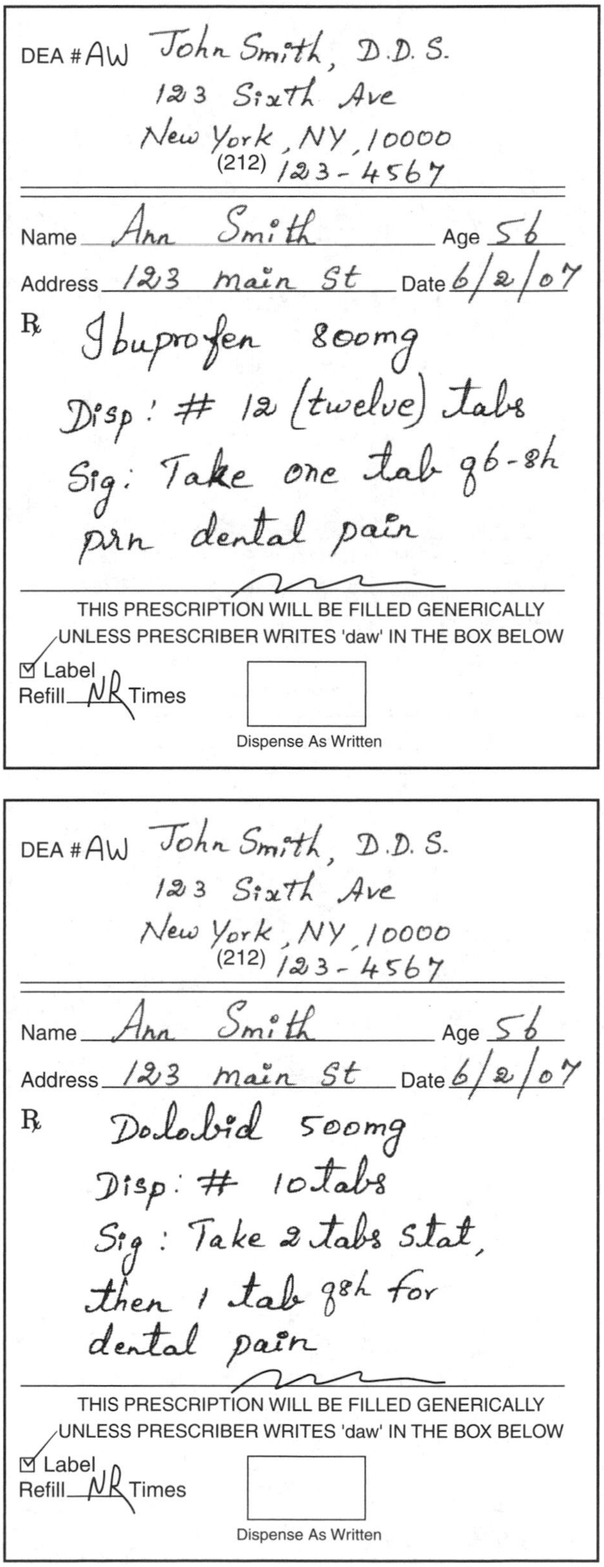

Dental pain is an acute nociceptive pain that in most cases can be managed as mild to moderate pain

FIGURE 5-6 Prescriptions for common analgesics used in dentistry.

DEA #AW   John Smith, D.D.S.
123 Sixth Ave
New York, NY, 10000
(212) 123-4567

Name   Ann Smith   Age 56
Address 123 main St   Date 6/2/07
℞
      Celebrex   100mg
      Disp : 12 Capsules
      Sig : Take one Cap
            bid

THIS PRESCRIPTION WILL BE FILLED GENERICALLY
UNLESS PRESCRIBER WRITES 'daw' IN THE BOX BELOW
☑ Label
Refill NR Times   [ ]
                    Dispense As Written

DEA #AW   John Smith, D.D.S.
123 Sixth Ave
New York, NY, 10000
(212) 123-4567

Name   Ann Smith   Age 56
Address 123 main St   Date 6/2/07
℞ Combunox
      Disp : # 21 (twenty-one) tabs
      Sig : Take one tab q6-8h
      for not more than 7 days
      prn dental pain

THIS PRESCRIPTION WILL BE FILLED GENERICALLY
UNLESS PRESCRIBER WRITES 'daw' IN THE BOX BELOW
☑ Label
Refill NR Times   [ ]
                    Dispense As Written

DEA #AW   John Smith, D.D.S.
123 Sixth Ave
New York, NY, 10000
(212) 123-4567

Name   Ann Smith   Age 56
Address 123 main St   Date 6/2/07
℞ (OTC)
      Aleve 220mg
      Take one Caplet
      q8-12 hrs

THIS PRESCRIPTION WILL BE FILLED GENERICALLY
UNLESS PRESCRIBER WRITES 'daw' IN THE BOX BELOW
☑ Label
Refill NR Times   [ ]
                    Dispense As Written

DEA #AW   John Smith, D.D.S.
123 Sixth Ave
New York, NY, 10000
(212) 123-4567

Name   Ann Smith   Age 56
Address 123 main St   Date 6/2/07
℞
      Tylenol No. 3
      Disp : # 16 (sixteen) tabs
      Sig : Take one tab q4-6h
      prn dental pain

THIS PRESCRIPTION WILL BE FILLED GENERICALLY
UNLESS PRESCRIBER WRITES 'daw' IN THE BOX BELOW
☑ Label
Refill NR Times   [ ]
                    Dispense As Written

FIGURE 5-6   (continued)

DEA # AW

John Smith, D.D.S.
123 Sixth Ave
New York, NY, 10000
(212) 123-4567

Name Ann Smith Age 56
Address 123 main St Date 6/2/07

R℞ Naproxen 250mg
Disp : # 12 tabs
Sig: Take 2 tablets
initially, then one tab
q6-8h for dental pain

THIS PRESCRIPTION WILL BE FILLED GENERICALLY
UNLESS PRESCRIBER WRITES 'daw' IN THE BOX BELOW

☑ Label
Refill NR Times

Dispense As Written

DEA # AW

John Smith, D.D.S.
123 Sixth Ave
New York, NY, 10000
(212) 123-4567

Name Ann Smith Age 56
Address 123 main St Date 6/2/07

R℞ Vicoprofen
Disp: # 12 tabs
Sig : Take one tab q4-6h
prn dental pain

THIS PRESCRIPTION WILL BE FILLED GENERICALLY
UNLESS PRESCRIBER WRITES 'daw' IN THE BOX BELOW

☑ Label
Refill NR Times

Dispense As Written

DEA # AW

John Smith, D.D.S.
123 Sixth Ave
New York, NY, 10000
(212) 123-4567

Name Ann Smith Age 56
Address 123 main St Date 6/2/07

R℞ Etodolac 400mg
Disp: # 12 tabs
Sig : Take one tab q6-8h
prn for dental pain

THIS PRESCRIPTION WILL BE FILLED GENERICALLY
UNLESS PRESCRIBER WRITES 'daw' IN THE BOX BELOW

☑ Label
Refill NR Times

Dispense As Written

DEA # AW

John Smith, D.D.S.
123 Sixth Ave
New York, NY, 10000
(212) 123-4567

Name Ann Smith Age 56
Address 123 main St Date 6/2/07

R℞ Anaprox 275 mg
Disp : # 12 tabs
Sig : Take two tabs Stat,
then one tab q6-8h prn
dental pain

THIS PRESCRIPTION WILL BE FILLED GENERICALLY
UNLESS PRESCRIBER WRITES 'daw' IN THE BOX BELOW

☑ Label
Refill NR Times

Dispense As Written

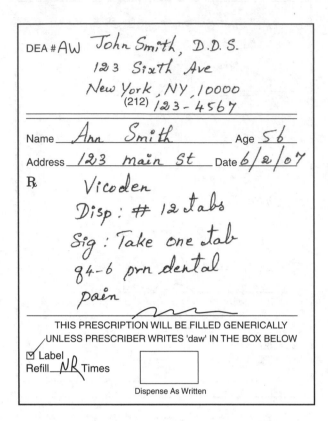

DEA # AW   John Smith, D.D.S.
            123 Sixth Ave
            New York, NY, 10000
              (212) 123-4567

Name Ann Smith   Age 56
Address 123 main St   Date 6/2/07
℞
        Vicoden
        Disp: # 12 tabs
        Sig: Take one tab
        q4-6 prn dental
        pain

THIS PRESCRIPTION WILL BE FILLED GENERICALLY
UNLESS PRESCRIBER WRITES 'daw' IN THE BOX BELOW
☑ Label
Refill NR Times
                    Dispense As Written

FIGURE 5–6 (continued)

using either a NSAID or, for more moderate pain, a short-acting narcotic/nonnarcotic combination containing oxycodone or codeine.

Aspirin and the NSAIDs have a ceiling effect whereby increased doses do not produce increased effects after a certain point. Opioids do not have a ceiling effect; thus all opioids, regardless of their potency, actually provide the same amount of analgesia. The dose can be titrated (administration of small incremental doses) to achieve maximum pain relief.

Neuropathic pain—such as trigeminal neuralgia, postherpetic neuralgia, entrapment neuropathy (e.g., carpal tunnel syndrome), and phantom limb pain—is chronic, difficult to treat, and is often resistant to therapy but may respond to anticonvulsants (e.g., gabapentin), tricyclic antidepressants, or lidocaine patch. Studies are ongoing testing the efficacy and safety of opioid agonists in the treatment of neuropathic pain of nonmalignant origin.

Samples of common prescriptions of NSAIDs and narcotics are given in Figure 5–6.

KEY POINTS

- Prostaglandins are created by cells and act only in the surrounding area before they are broken down.
- Prostaglandins control many body functions (protective).
- COX-1 serves a protective function in the body: Inhibition of COX-1 is associated with adverse GI effects and inhibition of platelet aggregation.
- COX-2 is only associated with inflammation.
- Aspirin for prevention of heart attack and stroke used in low doses (81 to 100 mg/day or 325 mg every other day) causes inhibition of thromboxane A_2, which results in prevention of platelet aggregation and increases bleeding.
- Aspirin in high arthritic doses (more than 6g/day) causes inhibition of prostacyclin, which has the opposite effect of thromboxane A_2 and causes platelet aggregation.
- NSAIDs and aspirin have a ceiling effect; there are no additional benefits in taking more than a certain dose.
- Some caution is necessary in administering NSAIDs to patients who are being treated for hypertension and asthma.
- Selective COX-2 inhibitors have a cardiovascular warning effect.
- Opioids are the drugs of choice for severe pain.
- Opioid narcotic analgesics have an abuse potential and all are controlled substances except for tramadol.
- For orofacial pain, long-term use of narcotics is not recommended because of abuse potential and many adverse effects.
- Cocaine users, or patients who you suspect to be abusers, are at increased risk of developing myocardial infarction and cardiac arrhythmias. Avoid the use of epinephrine.
- Patients with a history of drug addiction most likely require more analgesia.
- If possible, nonnarcotic analgesics should be prescribed/recommended to patients with addictions.
- There may be abnormal liver function in alcoholics, decreased metabolism of local anesthetics, and increased bleeding time. Avoid acetaminophen.

BOARD REVIEW QUESTIONS

1. Which of the following substances are prostaglandins formed from (pp. 71–72)?
   a. Arachidonic acid
   b. Endorphins
   c. Enkephalins
   d. Norepinephrine

2. Which of the following dosages of aspirin is recommended for men to prevent stroke and heart attack (pp. 75, 76)?
   a. 81 mg/day or twice a week
   b. 325 mg every 3 months
   c. 650 mg/day
   d. 3g/day

3. Opioids are recommended for patients whose nociceptive pain is considered to be (p. 82):
   a. Mild to moderate
   b. Moderate
   c. Moderate to severe
   d. Intermittent

4. Which of the following drugs is indicated for the treatment of trigeminal neuralgia (p. 89)?
   a. Phenytoin
   b. Acetaminophen
   c. Carbamazepine
   d. Lidocaine

5. Which of the following toxic effects occur with high doses of morphine (pp. 84, 85)?
   a. Cardiac failure
   b. Respiratory depression
   c. Muscle paralysis
   d. Allergic reaction

6. Which of the following opioids is considered to be a moderate agonist (p. 86)?
   a. Methadone
   b. Morphine
   c. Oxycodone
   d. Codeine

7. Which of the following opioids is used for heroin addiction (p. 90)?
   a. Fentanyl
   b. Hydrocodone
   c. Naloxone
   d. Buprenorphine

8. All of the following are adverse effects of codeine except one. Which one is the exception (p. 86)?
   a. Itching
   b. Respiratory depression
   c. Antitussive
   d. Diarrhea

9. Which of the following drugs has a ceiling effect (p. 74–75)?
   a. Codeine
   b. Morphine
   c. Aspirin
   d. Methadone

10. Neuropathic pain usually responds well to all of the following drugs except one. Which is the exception (pp. 87–89)?
    a. Anticonvulsants
    b. Tricyclic antidepressants
    c. Topical analgesics
    d. Aspirin
    e. Opioids

11. Celecoxib is contraindicated in patients allergic to (p. 82):
    a. Sulfa
    b. Aspirin
    c. Penicillin
    d. Erythromycin

12. Which of the following drugs should be used with some caution in a patient that is taking enalapril (Vasotec) (pp. 80, 81)?
    a. Lithium
    b. Penicillin
    c. Ibuprofen
    d. Codeine

13. Most of the selective COX-2 inhibitors drugs have been taken off the market because of increased risk of (p. 82):
    a. Thrombotic cardiovascular events
    b. Duodenal and gastric ulcer formation
    c. Anaphylactic reactions
    d. Asthmatic attacks

14. Which of the following adverse effects is commonly seen in patients taking ibuprofen? (p. 80)
    a. Gastrointestinal bleeding
    b. Hair loss
    c. Sedation
    d. Xerostomia

15. Which of the following substance is responsible for platelet aggregation? (p. 72)
    a. PGE$_2$
    b. PGI$_2$
    c. Thromboxane A$_2$
    d. COX-2

SELECTED REFERENCES

Aghabeigi, B. 1992. The pathophysiology of pain. *Br Dnet J* 173:91–97.

Ardekian, L., R. Gaspar, M. Peled, B. Brener, D. Laufer. 2000. Does low-dose aspirin therapy complicate oral surgical procedures? *JADA* 131(*3*):331–335.

Benoliel, F., Y. Sharav, M. Tal, E. Eliav, Management of chronic orofacial pain: Today and tomorrow. *Compendium* 2003;24:909–927.

Berdine H. J., C. K. O'Neil. Neuropathic pain pathophysiology, treatment and patient management. *US Pharmacist,* Supplement to December 2003.

Campbell, C. L., S. Smyth, G. Montalescot, et al. 2007. Aspirin dose for the prevention of cardiovascular disease. A systematic review. *JAMA,* 297: 2018–2024.

Eisenberg, E., E. D. McNicol D. B. Carr. Efficacy and safety of opioid agonists in the treatment of neuropathic pain of nonmalignant origin. *JAMA* 2005:293;3043–3052.

European Society of Hypertension Scientific Newsletter: Update on hypertension management. 2003; 4(17).

Haas, D. A. Adverse drug interactions in dental practice: Interactions associated with analgesics. Part III in a series. *JADA* 1999:130:397–407.

Jones, E. M., D. Knutson, D. Haines. Common problems in patients recovering from chemical dependency. *Am Fam Physician* 2003;68:1971–1978.

Kittelson, L. Substance abuse. Chicago, 2006. In *ADA Guide to Dental Therapeutics,* 3rd ed.: ADA Publishing. pp. 569–578.

Lancaster, T., D. W. Wareham, J. Yaphe. 2003. Postherpetic neuralgia. *Am Fam Physician* 67:1557–1558.

Noble, S. L., B. S. King, J. Olutade. 2000. Cyclo-oxygenase-2 enzyme inhibitors: Place in therapy. *Am Fam Physician* 61:3669–3676.

Page, R. L. II. Weighing the cardiovascular benefits of low-dose aspirin. *Pharmacy Times.* ACPE Program ID Number 290-000-05-017-H01.

Ridker P. M., Cook N. R., Lee I. M., Gordon D., Gaziano M., et al. A randomized trial of low-dose aspirin in the primary prevention of cardiovascular disease in women. *New Engl J Med* 2005;352:1293–1304.

Rosenberg, R. N. *Pain Arch Neurol* 2003;60:1520.

Sachs, C. J. Oral analgesics for acute nonspecific pain. *Am Fam Physician* 2005;71:913–918.

Schwartzman R. J., Crothusen J., Kiefer T. R., Rohr P. Neuropathic central pain. *Arch Neurol* 2001;58:1547–1551.

Zagaria M. A. E. Pain assessment in older adults. *US Pharmacist* 2006; 31(5):30–36.

Zanchetti A., Hansson L., Leonetti G., Rahn K. H. et al. Low-dose aspirin does not interfere with the blood pressure lowering effects of antihypertensive therapy. hypertens 2002: 1015–1027

Zuniga J. R. The use of nonopioid drugs in management of chronic orofacialpain. *J Oral Maxillofac Surg* 1998; 56:1075–1080.

WEB SITES

www.ncbi.nlm.nih.gov
www.pharmacytimes.com
www.uspharmacist.com
www.usdoj.gov/ndic/pubs10/10123/index.htm

QUICK DRUG GUIDE

Nonnarcotic Analgesics

Salicylates and Salicylate Derivatives

- Aspirin (Ecotrin, Bayer, Halfprin and many more)
- Diflunisal (Dolobid)
- Choline salicylate; magnesium salicylate (Trilisate)

Nonsteroidal Anti-Inflammatory Drugs (NSAIDs)

Indoles

- Indomethacin (Indocin)
- Sulindac (Clinoril)

Indole Acetic Acids

- Tolmetin (Tolectin)
- Ketorolac (Toradol)

Phenylalkoanoic Acid Derivative

Ibuprofen (Advil, Motrin)
- Ketoprofen (Orudis)
- Flurbiprofen (Ansaid)
- Naproxen (Naprosyn) Naproxen sodium (Anaprox, Aleve)
- Oxaprozin (Daypro)

Napthylalkanone

- Nabumetone (Relafen)

Fenamates

- Meclofenamate (Ponstel)
- Diclofenac (Voltaren)

Oxicam

- Prioxicam (Feldene)

COX-2 selective NSAID

- Celecoxib (Celebrex)

Other Nonnarcotic Analgesics

- Acetaminophen

Opioid (Narcotic) Analgesics

Short-Acting

- Morphine
- Hydromorphone (Dilaudid)
- Oxycodone (controlled-release OxyContin)
- Hydrocodone (only in combination with a nonnarcotic)
- Codeine
- Meperidine (Demerol)
- Fentanyl (Duragesic patch)

Long-Acting

- Methadone
- Levorphanol (Levo-Dromoran)
- Propoxyphene (Darvon)
- Oxymorphone (Numorphan)

Other Opioid Agonists

- Dextromethorphan (used in cough syrups; Robitussin, Sucrets, Vicks, Delsym, Benylin)
- Diphenoxylate (with atropine; Lomotil)
- Loperamide (Imodium; antidiarrheall)
- Tramadol (central analgesic) (Ultram)

Mixed Agonist/antagonists

- Buprenophine (Buprenex)
- Butorphanol (Stadol)
- Nalbuphine (Nubain)
- Pentazocine (Talwin)

Antagonists

- Naloxone (Narcan)

Drugs for Orofacial Pain

Tricyclic antidepressants

- Amitriptyline (Elavil)
- Desipramine (Norpramine)

Anesthetic

- Lidocaine patch (Lidoderm 5% patch)

Antiepileptics

- Gabapentin (Neurontin)
- Pregablin (Lyrica)
- Carbamazepine (Tegretol)
- Oxycarbazepine (Trileptal)
- Lamotrigine (Lamictal)

Narcotic/Nonnarcotic Combinations

Formulation	Trade Name	Schedule
Hydrocodone/acetaminophen	Lorcet 10/650 mg Lorcet HD 5/500 Lorcet Plus 7.5/650	C-III
	Lortab 2.5/500; 5/500; 7.5/500; 10/500	C-III
	Vicodin 5/500 Vicodin ES 7.5/750 Vicodin HP 10/660	C-III
Hydrocodone/ibuprofen	Vicoprofen 7.5/200	
Oxycodone/acetaminophen	Percocet 2.5/325; 5/325; 7.5/500; 10/650	C-II
	Roxicet 5/325; 5/500	C-II
	Tylox 5/500	C-II
Oxycodone/ibuprofen (5mg/400mg)	Combunox 5/400	C-II
Oxycodone HCl/aspirin	Percodan 5/325	C-II
	Percodan-Demi 2.5/325	C-II
Acetaminophen/codeine	Tylenol w/ codeine (No. 2, No. 3, No. 4) (300/15; 300/30; 300/60)	C-III
Aspirin/codeine/carisoprodol	Soma compound w/codeine 325/16/200	C-III
Dihydrocodeine/aspirin	Synalgos-DC 16/356 (Contains 30mg caffeine)	C-III
Propoxyphene/acetaminophen	Darvocet 50/325	
Propoxyphene/aspirin/caffeine	Darvon compound 65/389/32.4	C-IV

Acetaminophen/butalbital/caffeine/codeine Fioricet w/ codeine C-III	*Aspirin/butalbital/caffeine/codeine* Fiorinal w/codeine C-III

Chapter **6**

Antimicrobial Drugs

GOAL: To introduce the concepts of systemic and locally applied antibiotics and antimicrobials in the treatment of bacterial infections, including dental infections.

EDUCATIONAL OBJECTIVES

After reading this chapter, the reader should be able to:

1. List the classifications of the different antibiotics including penicillins, cephalosporins, tetracyclines, macrolides, fluroquinolones, and nitroimidazoles.
2. Understand the concept of bactericidal versus bacteriostatic antibiotics.
3. Describe adverse effects of the various antibiotics.
4. Explain the use of antibiotics in periodontics, implants, oral surgery and endodontics.
5. Discuss the rationale for use of topical agents used in dentistry.

KEY TERMS
Antibiotic
Bactericidal
Bacteriostatic
Dental infection

ANTIMICROBIAL AGENTS
Antimicrobial Activity

Louis Pasteur's concept of symbiosis incorporates the cooperative efforts of two organisms of any kind. For example, we live in a symbiotic relationship with microorganisms in the gut (gastrointestinal tract). The opposite of symbiosis is asymbiosis, in which two organisms create substances harmful to each other.

Antibiotics are substances produced by living organisms (e.g., microorganisms) which are harmful to other organisms. Essentially, antibiotics are asymbiotic. Antibiotics are either natural or semisynthetic. There are two broad classifications of antibiotics based on whether they kill bacteria (**bactericidal**) or inhibit bacterial multiplication (**bacteriostatic**).

The *spectrum of activity* of an antibiotic indicates the range of bacteria the antibiotic affects. Narrow-spectrum antibiotics are active against some gram-positive pathogens, whereas broad-spectrum antibiotics are effective against a wider range of bacterial pathogens, including many gram negatives. Extended-spectrum antibiotics act in between a narrow and broad spectrum. Ideally, antibiotics should be concentrated at the site of infection.

Adverse Effects

Ideally an antibiotic should be selective. Unfortunately, this is rarely the case. Antibiotics often have significant side effects (Table 6–1). These may include:

1. Bacterial resistance to the antibiotic
2. Superinfections
3. Gastrointestinal effects (nausea, vomiting, diarrhea)
4. Allergic reactions
5. Photosensitivity
6. Drug interactions

Did You Know?

In ancient times, honey from a bee was thought to have antibiotic properties and was used to heal ulcers and burns, and later to treat gunshot wounds.

Antimicrobial Resistance

Antibiotic use promotes development of antibiotic-resistant bacteria, rendering the antibiotic ineffective against the bacterium, and allowing progression of the infection. The bacteria continue to multiply and survive despite concentrations of an antibiotic that should be lethal to them.

Normally, four situations can occur when bacteria are exposed to an antibiotic:

1. The antibiotic kills the bacteria (bactericidal).
2. The antibiotic weakens, disables, and decreases its growth (bacteriostatic), thus making it easier for the host's own natural defenses to kill the bacteria.
3. The bacteria will not be affected by the antibiotic (e.g., bacteria are not sensitive to the antibiotic: wrong antibiotic for the bacteria).
4. Resistance has developed.

Antimicrobial resistance is an increasing problem worldwide. The danger is that when antibiotics are used unnecessarily, they will not be effective if administered later on for a serious bacterial infection. The resultant, untreated infection may result in significant morbidity and/or mortality.

The development of antibiotic resistance is both natural (inherent) and acquired. Bacteria have a certain *inherent resistance* to certain antibiotics. For example, a gram-negative bacterium may have an outer cell membrane that is impermeable to the antibiotic and the organism may lack a transport system that brings the antibiotic into the cell. This is why whenever possible a culture and sensitivity test is performed on bacterial samples from tissue specimens or spaces (e.g., periodontal pocket). When such specimens are available, it is important to use the antibiotic to which the organism is sensitive. Resistance in the micro-organisms (not the host) occurs most commonly due to either inadequate amount of antibiotic, or inadequate duration of therapy. Resistance among the normal inherent organisms may also occur when antibiotics are given in the absence of bacterial infection. When these organisms subsequently cause a clinical infection, the usual antibiotics will not be effective. Bacteria require high concentrations of an antibiotic to kill them if they are less sensitive to that antibiotic. Additionally, in some cases the antibiotic may kill some bacteria but some may survive; the survivors have usually developed resistance to that antibiotic.

Table 6-1 Penicillins

Drug	Mechanism of Action	Adverse Effects	Drug Interactions	Patient Instructions
Natural penicillins; Narrow spectrum *Penicillin V (Pen-vee K, V-cillin K, Veetids)* *Penicillin G injectable*	Bactericidal— inhibiting bacterial cell wall synthesis, thus killing the bacterium Pencillin V: 500 mg qid	Allergic skin reactions (anaphylaxis), nausea, vomiting, diarrhea (could be pseudo-membranous colitis). Superinfection by multiresistant bacteria or yeasts (e.g, vaginal candidiasis or vaginitis, stoma-titis, glossitis)	Probenicid (antigout) inhibits excretion of penicillin, thus increasing blood levels. Food increases breakdown in stomach. Bacteriostatic drugs (e.g., erythromycin, tetracyclines) may interfere with the bactericidal effects of penicillin. Avoid concurrent use (space the doses apart).	To reduce incidence of superinfection take penicillin with yogurt or acidophilus gel-caps. The patient may experience stomatitis (sore mouth) or glossi-tis (sore tongue) due to fungal overgrowth. If this occurs, they should call the office immediately. Best taken on empty stomach (empty stomach is defined as 1 hour before or 2 hours after meals) because absorption of the drug is decreased with food, but if GI upset take with food and a full glass of water to prevent esophagitis (inflammation of the esophagus).
Aminopenicillins: Broad spectrum *Amoxicillin (Amoxil, Trimox)* *Ampicillin (Omnipen)*	Amoxicillin: 500 mg tid	Less diarrhea with amoxicillin than ampicillin. Ampicillin is not usually prescribed in dentistry.	Possible interaction with oral contracep-tive. Avoid concurrent use with bacterio-static drugs.	Can be taken with food. See above
Beta-lactamase inhibitors *Amoxicillin + calvulante (Augmentin)* *Ampicillin + sulbactam (Unasyn)* *Piperacillin + tazobactam injectable*		More severe gastroin-testinal upset because of clavulanic acid.	See above	Must be taken with food because of the clavulanic acid.
Penicillinase resistant *Dicloxacillin (Dycill)* *Nafcillin (injectable)* *Oxacillin (Bactocill)* *Cloxacillin (cloxacillin)*	Not used in dentistry	See above	See above	Take on an empty stomach.
antipseudomonal penicillins: Extended spectrum (all injectables) *Carbenicillin (Geocillin)* *Ticarcillin (Ticar)* *Mezlocillin (Mezlin)* *Piperacillin (Pipracil)*	Not used in dentistry	See above	See above	Take on empty stomach.

Acquired antibiotic resistance can be produced either through a mutation or conjugation. A *mutation* is a genetic transformation that takes place under the influence of an antibiotic. A spontaneous mutation or change in the bacterial chromosome imparts resistance to a particular drug. The antibiotic kills the nonmutants, but those mutants which are resistant to the antibiotic survive and replicate.

Another form of antibiotic resistance is the transfer or exchange of resistance genes (DNA) from one bacterium to another, known as *genetic exchange.*

An *active efflux system* in some types of bacteria "pushes" the antibiotic out of the cell, allowing the bacterium to resist that antibiotic.

Adaptation is a *nongenetic transformation,* but there is genetic capability. For example, *penicillinase* is an enzyme that breaks down the antibiotic penicillin and is secreted only in the presence of penicillin. Penicillinase is produced by certain bacterial strains such as *Staphylococcus aureus.* Penicillinase breaks up the β-lactam ring on the penicillin molecule, rendering the penicillin inactive.

Treatment resistance may develop if:

1. The diagnosis was not made promptly.
2. Inadequate doses were prescribed.
3. The patient did not take the prescribed antibiotic at the prescribed dose for the prescribed amount of time.

Misuse resistance occurs when antibiotics are taken indiscriminately. Antibiotics target only bacteria, not viruses. Thus, antibiotics should not be used against the flu; the common cold; most sore throats; most episodes of "bronchitis" in children; and most cases of fever without a definite source. To help prevent antibiotic-resistant infections, patients should be encouraged to throw away any unused antibiotics, not to take an antibiotic that is prescribed for someone else, and take the antibiotic the way it was prescribed. Many cases of resistance are found in hospital settings where the patient is either immunocompromised or elderly.

Superinfections

Superinfections occur when a broad-spectrum antibiotic causes eradication of micro-organisms that are part of the normal flora (bacteria that normally live in these areas) of the gastrointestinal (GI) tract, oral cavity, respiratory tract, or vaginal area. This reduction/elimination of normal bacterial flora allows for the growth of other organisms such as fungi. If this occurs, treatment with antifungal medication is necessary. Oral superinfections include sore mouth (stomatitis) or tongue (glossitis). To help prevent superinfections some suggest acidophilus in the form of yogurt or gelcaps to replace the normal flora.

Gastrointestinal Problems

Antibiotics commonly affect the GI tract either by direct irritation or indirectly by changing the normal GI flora, resulting in nausea, vomiting and/or diarrhea. Antibiotic-associated *pseudomembranous colitis* occurs when there is an overgrowth of the bacteria *Clostridium difficile,* which secretes a toxin that causes severe inflammation of the bowel wall. It is characterized by watery diarrhea and abdominal cramping.

If the antibiotic can be taken with food, then symptoms may be less likely to occur. Some find benefit if the antibiotic is taken with *Lactobacillus acidophilus,* a beneficial bacteria found normally in the intestines. Antibiotic use may reduce these "good," bacteria causing GI distress.

Allergic Reactions

Some antibiotics may cause an allergic reaction manifested by hives, wheezing, or systemic anaphylaxis. If an allergic reaction occurs, the drug must be discontinued immediately.

Photosensitivity

When taking some antibiotics, some individuals develop an exaggerated sunburn when exposed to the sun. Ciprofloxacin and doxycycline cause such photosensitivity.

Drug Interactions

Antibiotics may interact with other drugs (drug–drug interactions) or with foods (drug–food interactions). These interactions can either increase or decrease serum levels of the antibiotic.

> **Did You Know?**
>
> Fifty million unnecessary antibiotics are prescribed for viral respiratory infections each year in the United States.

Selection

In dental practice, antibiotics are indicated for three primary purposes:

1. Treatment of acute odontogenic/orofacial infections
2. Prophylaxis against infective endocarditis
3. Prophylaxis for patients at risk for infection because of compromised host defense mechanisms

The choice of antimicrobial therapy is based on the morphology and growth of bacteria. This is true whether a dental or medical infection is being treated. Bacteria are classified according to shape (morphology) (e.g., cocci, bacilli) and growth patterns (e.g., aerobic—oxygen; anaerobic—without oxygen). Also, bacteria are classified according to whether a bacterium does or does not retain a certain stain; gram positive or gram negative).

In the majority of dental cases, empirical therapy is practiced, whereby the antibiotic is chosen based on knowledge of the bacterium expected to be causing the **dental infection.** This is based on previous experience by the clinician or other clinicians, and is evidence based, based on the bacteria normally found in such infections. If an unusual infection is suspected or if the patient has recently been on multiple antibiotics, thereby increasing the risk of antibiotic resistance, then culture and sensitivity tests can be performed. This will enable the clinician to choose the proper antibiotic. Samples of dental subginaval biofilms may be sent for culture and sensitivity.

Many prescriptions for antibiotics are inappropriate because they are used for conditions that most likely do not require them. For instance, a dental patient presents with a gingival abscess located on the free gingival margin. If there are no palpable lymph nodes (lymphadenopathy) and no fever, then antibiotics are not necessary. The best treatment for this case is periodontal debridement.

In the medical community, antibiotics are given inappropriately for conditions caused by viruses, such as colds, sore throats, nonspecific fevers, and "bronchitis" in children. Additionally, many broad-spectrum antibiotics (e.g., amoxicillin) are inappropriately given for dental infections. The majority of bacteria in dental infections (e.g., endodontic, periodontic) do not require these broad-spectrum drugs, and penicillin VK is the drug of choice in most dental infections. The FDA points out that antibiotics should be used only to treat bacterial infections, and recommends counseling patients on proper antibiotic use, including taking the antibiotic for the required time.

In Periodontal Therapy

Systemic antibiotics are usually used in patients with aggressive periodontitis because the bacteria with this periodontal disease invade the soft tissue and elude mechanical debridement. Systemic antibiotics are contraindicated in chronic periodontitis and gingivitis. Topical antimicrobial agents (e.g., Atridox, Arestin) are used in patients with localized chronic periodontitis.

In Endodontic Therapy

Antibiotics are not necessary in an uncomplicated endodontic infection or if there is well localized soft tissue swelling without systemic signs of infection such as fever, lymphadenopathy, or cellulitis. Systemic antibiotics are indicated with an endodontic lesion with soft tissue swelling, systemic involvement, or spread of the infection. The drug of choice is penicillin VK.

In Implant Dentistry

A systemic antibiotic as well as an antimicrobial oral rinse may be indicated for implant surgery. Postoperative infections, which usually occur on the third or fourth day after surgery, are treated with drainage and systemic antibiotics such as penicillin VK. Antibiotics are indicated in the treatment of peri-implant infections which are associated with bone loss, suppuration, and increased pocket depths. Antibiotics are not indicated in peri-implant mucositis which involves soft tissue inflammation around the dental implant. If necessary, an antimicrobial mouthrinse such as chlorhexidine gluconate should be used.

BACTERICIDAL ANTIBIOTICS: INHIBITORS OF BACTERIAL CELL WALL SYNTHESIS

Penicillins

Actions

Penicillin was the first antibiotic discovered by Sir Alexander Fleming in 1929, but it did not have a clinical application until 1939. Today, most penicillins are produced from a strain of *P. chrysogenum,* while some are semisynthetically produced. Penicillin G is the prototype natural penicillin and is the most potent. Penicillins are administered orally or parenterally, but never topically because of severe allergic reactions.

Microbial Activity

The β-lactam ring on the penicillin molecule is responsible for the antibacterial activity (Figure 6–1). Penicillins are bactericidal or bacteriostatic depending on the concentration achieved. Penicillins act by inhibiting one or more of the penicillin-binding proteins (PBPs) located on bacterial cell walls of susceptible organisms, rendering the internal part of the bacteria cell vulnerable to the outside environment. This results in cell rupture and death (Figure 6–2). Penicillins are most effective against rapidly multiplying bacteria. Since human cells do not have a cell wall but rather cell membranes, penicillins do not affect human cells.

Spectrum of Activity

Penicillins are primarily effective against gram-positive bacteria (e.g., *Streptococcus pneumoniae*) but also some gram-negative bacteria. *Narrow-spectrum or natural penicillins* (see Table 6–1) are relatively effective against gram-negative bacteria because those organisms have a thick lipopolysaccharide coat which penicillins cannot penetrate. The *broad-spectrum penicillins* (Table 6–1) include the *aminopenicillins* (amoxicillin and ampicillin) and *antipseudomonal penicillins* (e.g., piperacillin, ticarcillin) and are more active against gram-negative bacteria. The *penicillinase-resistant penicillins* (e.g., oxacillin, cloxacillin, dicloxacillin) treat bacteria such as staphylococci that release penicillinase. Other penicillins include *beta-lactamase inhibitors* (e.g., amoxicillin plus clavulanate), *carbapenems* and *monobactams*.

Penicillins are administered orally (PO), intravenously (IV), or intramuscularly (IM). Review Table 6–1 for individual penicillins.

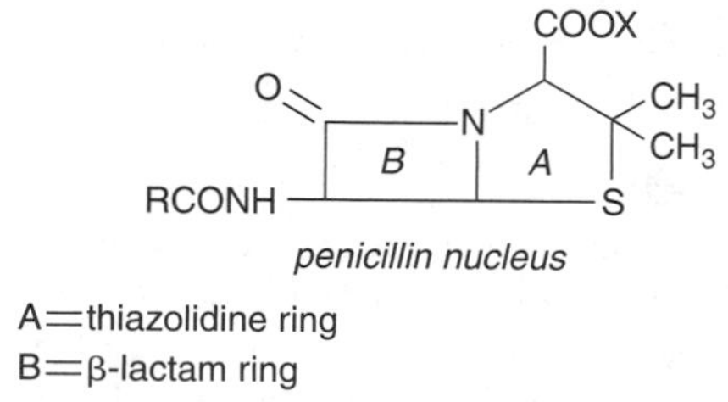

$$O = \quad \quad COOX$$

penicillin nucleus

A = thiazolidine ring
B = β-lactam ring

FIGURE 6–1 Illustration of the penicillin structure. The β-lactam ring gives penicillin its antibacterial activity.

Guidelines for Patients Taking Penicillin V or Amoxicillin

- Instruct patients to take all of the prescribed antibiotic even if they feel better. Take on an empty stomach (1 hour before or 2 hours after meals); amoxicillin can be taken without regard to meals.

- Monitor patients for superinfections.

Penicillin Resistance

Beta-lactamases Natural penicillins (penicillin G and penicillin V) are more potent than semisynthetic penicillins, but natural penicillins are more susceptible to destruction by β-lactamase (penicillinase). This is especially true in a hospital setting, where up to 95 percent of *Staphylococcus aureus* produce penicillinase.

Since amoxicillin (broad-spectrum) is sensitive to breakdown by β-lactamases, clavulanic acid (potassium clavulanate) was combined with amoxicillin to form Augmentin. Clavulanic acid is a weak acid without any antibacterial activity but when added to the amoxicillin molecule the β-lactamase binds to the inactive clavulanic acid molecule and leaves the amoxicillin alone. Since this product contains an acid it should be taken with food, which will lessen the adverse side effects of nausea and diarrhea.

Penicillins may also have a decreased affinity to the penicillin-binding proteins, which are enzymes essential for cell-wall synthesis.

Pharmacokinetics

Absorption of penicillins depends on acid stability in the stomach, but they are primarily absorbed in the duodenum (small intestines). Pipercillin and ticarcillin are not acid stable. Absorption is greatest when penicillins are taken on an empty stomach (i.e., 1 hour before or 2 hours after eating). Amoxicillin is the exception and can be

Did You Know?

Penicillin is a naturally occurring substance and was first grown in bed pans during World War II, when Howard Florey was trying to find enough containers to grow penicillin mold.

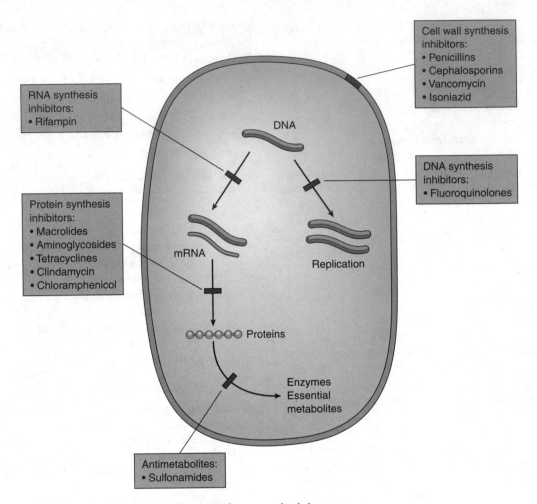

FIGURE 6–2 Mechanism of action of antimicrobial drugs.

taken with food. All penicillins should be taken with a full glass of water to increase absorption from the GI tract.

Amoxicillin is more completely absorbed from the gastrointestinal (GI) tract than ampicillin and thus has fewer GI effects, such as nausea and diarrhea.

Penicillins are eliminated through the kidneys. Thus, in a patient with renal failure, drug dosage must be reduced. The semisynthetic penicillins (oxacillin, dicloxacillin, cloxacillin, and nafcillin) are eliminated through the liver.

Indications

Penicillin VK and amoxicillin are the only two penicillins that are used in dentistry for mild to moderate odontogenic infections (periodontal, endodontic, oral surgery). Bacteria responsible for most odontogenic infections in-

clude *Streptococci,* obligate anaerobes gram-positive cocci (e.g., *Peptostreptococcus*) and obligate anaerobic gram-negative (e.g., *Porphyromonas* or *Prevotella* sp.). Penicillin is effective against strep species and most oral anaerobic bacteria although some *Prevotella* species are resistant. Amoxicillin has limited activity against strep and anaerobes but is effective against *Peptostreptococus,* which is found in periodontitis sites.

Adverse Effects

1. Allergic reaction: Allergic reactions occur in more than 10 percent of the population. Severity of an allergic reaction ranges from a mild rash and fever to severe anaphylaxis, which has a low incidence. Some patients will develop a nonpruritic red rash on the trunk while taking amoxicillin. This is not

a true allergy, and is not a contraindication to further amoxicillin use. This rash is more likely to occur when a patient has infectious mononucleosis.

2. Pseudomembranous colitis: The drug is stopped and metronidazole (PO) is given to the patient. If enteral (PO) administration is not possible, vancomycin (IV) is given.

3. Gastrointestinal upset: Nausea, vomiting, and diarrhea are the most common side effects. These may be due to a direct irritation of penicillin to the GI tract. Most penicillins should be taken on an empty stomach. Amoxicillin can be taken without regard to meals. Augmentin should be taken with food. Oral penicillins may be taken with *Lactobacillus acidophilus* to help replace normal flora and reduce GI distress.

4. Superinfection

5. Seizure activity: Associated with high levels of penicillin

Drug Interactions

There are very few drug–drug interactions of penicillin.

1. Penicillin + a bacteriostatic antibiotic (e.g., tetracyclines, erythromycins): A bactericidal antibiotic requires that the bacteria be multiplying actively to be effective. If a bacteriostatic antibiotic is given concurrently, penicillin will not be as effective.

2. Oral contraceptives: Penicillins may decrease effectiveness of oral contraceptives. One theory is that estrogen (oral contraceptive) undergoes enterohepatic circulation and needs bacteria in the gut to break it down before it reabsorbs. Penicillin prevents this, thus estrogen is poorly reabsorbed and not effective.

3. Colestipol (for hypercholesterolemia): Reduces absorption (into the bloodstream) of penicillins.

4. Food: Increases breakdown of penicillin in the stomach.

5. Probenicid (treatment of gout): Decreases renal (kidney) elimination of penicillins, raising the blood level.

Pregnancy

B, caution during nursing

How Supplied

Penicillin VK (Pen-Vee K, Penicillin VK), tablet; Amoxicillin trihydrate (Polymox, Trimox, Amoxil): capsule, tab; Augmentin: tablet.

Dental Hygiene Notes

Amoxicillin is the standard regimen for antibiotic premedication for infective bacterial endocarditis (IBE). Oral penicillin VK is the drug of choice for mild to moderate endodontic, periodontic and odontogenic infections (e.g., abscess). Amoxicillin is used in skin infections, sinusitis, otitis media, and bite wound infections. For dental infections, amoxicillin should only be used for more serious infections. Penicillin VK is a drug of choice in the treatment of necrotizing ulcerative gingivitis (NUG). Augmentin (amoxicillin + clavulanic acid) is used for resistant strains of bacteria, especially for periodontal patients that are refractory to treatment or have aggressive forms of infection. While amoxicillin has a broader spectrum of activity and penetrates bone well, it is more limited against *Streptococci* and oral anaerobes than penicillin VK. Thus, penicillin VK is a good antibiotic for oral abscesses.

If concurrent use of penicillin plus a bacteriostatic antibiotic is necessary, then the penicillin should be given a few hours before the bacteriostatic antibiotic.

 Rapid Dental Hint

Patients on oral contraceptives should be warned to discuss their options with their obstetrician/gynecologist.

Cephalosporins

Actions

Cephalosporins were isolated at the same time as penicillins were discovered. They have a similar β-lactam ring, which is responsible for its antibacterial activity. Cephalosporins are bactericidal and kill bacteria by inhibiting cell wall synthesis by the same mechanism as penicillins.

There are four generations of semisynthetic cephalosporins; only a few are given orally (Table 6–2). All cephalosporins can be administered without regard to meals but with a full glass of water.

Indications

First-generation oral cephalosporins are ineffective against bacteria that produce beta-lactamase. They are generally used for skin, bone, genitourinary, and respiratory tract infections, otitis media (middle ear infection), and acute prostatitis.

Table 6–2   Cephalosporins

Drug Name	Mechanism of Action	Adverse Affects	Drug Interaction
1st generation Cefadroxil (Duricef) cephalexin (Keflex)	Bactericidal: Inhibits bacterial cell wall synthesis by binding to penicillin-binding proteins (PBPs).	Allergic reaction (hypersensitivity)/ about 10% cross sensitivity with penicillin	Probenicid (antigout) inhibits excretion of penicillin, thus increasing blood levels.
2nd generation Cefaclor (Ceclor) cefprozil (Cefzil) cefuroxime—axetil (Ceftin, Veftin)	Not any more effective than penicillins for dental infections, and more expensive.		Bacteriostatic drugs (e.g., erythromycin, tetracyclines) may interfere with the bactericidal effects of penicillin. Avoid concurrent use (space the doses apart).
3rd generation Omnicef (cefdinir) cefixime (Suprax) cefpodoxime (Vantin) ceftibuten (Cedax)			
4th generation Only injectable			

Second-generation oral cephalosporins are more resistant to beta-lactamase and have a broader spectrum of gram-negative antimicrobial activity than the first-generation cephalosporins. They are used in similar situations as the first generation drugs, and for pelvic inflammatory disease. Cefuroxime, cefproxil, and cefaclor are used for bronchitis, sinusitis, and local soft tissue infections.

Third-generation cephalosporins have even more broad-spectrum antimicrobial activity than the second-generation drugs. They have good antimicrobial activity against *Streptococci*.

The fourth-generation cephalosporin (cefepime; only IV/IM) has broad-spectrum activity against *Escherichia coli* (*E. coli*), *Proteus vulgaris, Salmonella* (food poisoning), *Enterbacter* ssp., *Staphylococci* and *Streptococci*. It is used in neutropenic patients with fever and in severe antibiotic-resistant gram-negative bacterial infections.

Cephalosporins are generally not indicated for endodontic or periodontal infections. The most popular oral cephalosporins used in dentistry are cephalexin and cefadroxil. They have a broad antimicrobial spectrum (aerobes) of activity but they are expensive.

Adverse Effects
Generally, cephalosporins are well tolerated.

1. Allergic reaction: Anaphylaxis occurs within minutes after ingestion of the antibiotic. Clinically there is respiratory distress (e.g., bronchospasm), angioedema (swelling), rash and itching, hypotension. Death is from airway obstruction.
2. There is a 10 percent cross-hypersensitivity reaction with penicillins (10 percent of people allergic to penicillin will be allergic to cephalosporins).
3. Morbilliform (skin) rashes: Clinically these appear as raised, inflamed skin.
4. Superinfection
5. Gastrointestinal: GI distress, including nausea and diarrhea

Drug Interactions
Probenicid: Decreased excretion of cephalosporin

Warfarin: May increase actions of anticoagulants; monitor blood tests (INR/PT)

Pregnancy
B; drug enters breast milk, so caution during lactation

How Supplied
1st generation:

Cefadroxil (Duricef): tab, oral suspension

Cephalexin (Keflex, cap, oral suspension)

2nd generation:

Cefaclor (Ceclor cap, oral suspension)

Efprozil (Cefzil) tab, oral suspension

Cefuroxime—Axetil (Ceftin, Veftin, tab, oral suspension)

3rd generation:

Omnicef (cefdinir cap, oral suspension)

Cefixime (Suprax tab)

Cefpodoxime (Vantin tab, oral suspension)

Ceftibuten (Cedax cap, oral suspension)

4th generation:

Only injectable

Dental Hygiene Notes

Since only a few cephalosporins are administered orally and they are expensive, they are not drugs of choice for dental infections. Additionally, even though they are broader spectrum than penicillins, penicillins are effective against the anaerobic organisms that are usually found in dental infections. Cephalosporins are generally not used for an endodontic or periodontal abscess, but may be used for antibiotic premediation.

Nitroimadazoles

Actions

Metronidazole is specifically effective against obligate or strict anaerobic (live in a pure nonoxygen environment) bacteria. Metronidazole is bactericidal, and its mechanism of action is to bind to and break down bacterial DNA.

Indications

Medical indications include intestinal amoebiasis, trichomoniasis, bacterial anaerobic infections, and giardiasis.

Metronidazole is used in the treatment of necrotizing gingivitis (NUG). Metronidazole in combination with amoxicillin or Augmentin may be effective against refractory and aggressive forms of periodontitis associated with *A. actinomycetemcomitans* and *Porphyromonas gingivalis* infection. Metronidazole is also used for peri-implant infections. Antibiotic resistance to metronidazole is rare, but there are numerous adverse side effects.

Guidelines for Patients Taking Metronidazole

- Inform your patients that this drug is an antibiotic for his/her periodontal condition.
- Avoid alcohol even alcohol-containing mouthrinses.
- A metallic taste may develop.
- Take the medication for the recommended time.

Adverse Effects

Gastrointestinal upset is seen frequently, especially nausea. A metallic taste has been reported, as well as darkened urine.

Drug Interactions

Consumption of alcohol, including use of alcohol-containing mouthrinses, while taking metronidazole results in a reaction which may include headache, flushing, nausea, vomiting, and cramps. The reaction usually lasts for up to 1 hour, though it may continue for a few days after discontinuation of the medication. Alcohol should not be consumed during metronidazole therapy and for at least 3 days after discontinuing the drug. Metronidazole is contraindicated in patients taking lithium (a drug used for manic depression) and cimetidine (an antiulcer drug).

Metronidazole may decrease the metabolism of anticoagulants (e.g., warfarin), which will increase the bleeding effect of the drug.

Pregnancy: B
How Supplied
Metronidazole (Flagyl): cap, tab

Rapid Dental Hint

Patients may be taking metronidazole during periodontal therapy. Remind them not to use any products containing alcohol, even mouthrinses.

Dental Hygiene Notes

Many patients in the dental office may be taking metronidazole for the adjunctive treatment of refractory or chronic periodontitis. It is also used after placement of barrier membranes during periodontal surgery. Thus patients should be counseled on the proper use of metronidazole. Alcoholic beverages are contraindicated, as are mouthrinses containing alcohol. Also, inform the patient that changes in taste perception may occur. Dry mouth and a metallic taste may develop.

Rapid Dental Hint

Review with your patients how to take his or her antibiotic, and possible drug–drug, drug–food interactions, and adverse effects.

Quinolones (Fluoroquinolones)

Actions
Fluoroquinolones are bactericidal because they inhibit bacterial DNA replication. Quinolones are not technically antibiotics because they are totally synthetically produced. Nevertheless, they are frequently referred to as broad-spectrum antimicrobials with good activity against facultative gram-negative anaerobes.

Indications
Acute bacterial sinusitis, acute bacterial chronic bronchitis, pneumonia, skin infections, bacterial conjunctivitis (use eye drops), urinary tract infections, and chronic periodontitis

Adverse Effects
Muscle weakness, muscle pain, phototoxicity, dizziness, convulsions, headache, hallucinations, and possible joint and cartilage damage

Drug Interactions
Ciprofloxacin should be administered with care for patients taking warfarin (anticoagulant), theophylline (antiasthma) or caffeine because it inhibits their metabolism, resulting in increased blood levels. Dairy products (cal-

Did You Know?

In 2001, Cipro and doxycycline were used prophylactically for exposure (inhalation) to the anthrax bacteria. Anthrax is not known to spread from one person to another.

cium), sodium bicarbonate, iron and antacids (magnesium, aluminum) delay absorption so these products should be given 4 hours before or 2 hours after oral administration of a fluoroquinolone. Food does not slow absorption.

Pregnancy: C
How Supplied (Oral Preparations)

Nonfluorinated quinolone—Nalidixic acid (Neggram): tab

Fluorinated quinolones—Ciprofloxacin HCl (Cipro): tab, oral suspension; Norfloxacin (Noroxin): tab; Enoxacin (Pentrex): tab; Lomefloxacin (Maxaquin): tab; Ofloxacin (floxin): tab; levofloxacin (Levaquin): tab; sparfloxacin (Zagam): tab; gatifloxacin (Tequin): tab; moxifloxacin (Avelox): tab; trovafloxacin (Trovan): tab

Rapid Dental Hint

The majority of patients taking a quinolone will most likely be taking it for chronic bronchitis. The air polishing system should not be used, since sodium bicarbonate delays absorption of the drug.

BACTERIOSTATIC ANTIBIOTICS

Macrolides

Actions
Macrolides are usually bacteriostatic, but they may be bactericidal at high doses. Macrolides inhibit the multiplication of bacteria by reversibly binding to the 50S ribosomal subunit of susceptible bacteria and consequently inhibit protein synthesis within the bacterial cell (Figure 6–2). Erythromycin is a type of macrolide. Erythromycins can be used when the patient is allergic to penicillin. Erythromycins are most effective against gram-positive bacteria and some gram-negative strains. Resistance to erythromycin is generally not a problem in short-term therapy. Erythromycin is produced by *Saccharopolyspora erythraea* (Table 6–3).

Azalides are second-generation semisynthetic derivates of erythromycin that have a broader spectrum of action with fewer adverse side effects than the erythromycins. The two drugs in this classification are azithromycin (Zithromax) and clarithromycin (Biaxin). On July 5, 2006, the FDA approved safety labeling revisions to clarithromycin, postmarking reports of colchicine (for gout) toxicity (some fatal) in patients receiving concomitant clarithromycin, especially in the elderly, and some cases in patients with renal insufficiency. Because clarithromycin and other macrolide antibiotics are known to inhibit enzymes for which colchicines are a substrate (e.g., CYP3A), patients receiving both drugs should be monitored for toxicity related to increased colchicines exposure. Dose adjustments should be considered when treating elderly patients with severe renal impairment.

Azithromycin has several unique features which makes it useful in dentistry. It concentrates in phagocytes such as PMNs and macrophages, which contributes to its distribution into inflamed periodontal tissues (gingival connective tissue) in greater amounts than in plasma. In addition, a postantibiotic effect is seen, whereby high antibiotic levels remain after the drug is discontinued. It also has anti-inflammatory effects, and has been used in some lung diseases because of this characteristic.

Telithromycin (Ketek) is the first of a new class of macrolide antibiotics known as ketolides. It has a pregnancy category of C, and has more adverse side effects than erythromycins.

Pharmacokinetics

Erythromycins that are orally administered are absorbed primarily in the duodenum and are widely distributed to most body tissues except the brain. Erythromycin is partly metabolized in the liver and is primarily excreted unchanged via the bile.

Erythromycin base, which is the active form of the drug, is acid-labile and breaks down in stomach acid. To prevent the disintegration or breaking down of the tablet in the stomach, the tablets are coated with a wax or cellulose film (enteric coating). These tablets are referred to as filmtabs. Additionally, the erythromycin base is dispensed as a salt (stearate) or an ester (ethylsuccinate) to decrease irritation caused by acids in the stomach.

Indications

Mild upper and lower respiratory tract infections, pharyngitis, tonsillitis, community-acquired pneumonia, gonorrhea, skin infections, otitis media, acute pelvic inflammatory disease, Legionnaires' disease, Chlamydia infections. Azithromycin is used in the management of aggressive periodontal diseases.

Adverse Effects

Hepatic (liver) dysfunction (mild elevated liver function tests evident as hepatitis, usually with erythromycin es-

tolate), gastrointestinal disturbances (abdominal pain, diarrhea, nausea, vomiting) but the second-generation macrolides have less.

Drug Interactions

Erythromycin and clarithromycin have the potential to inhibit drug metabolism in the liver through inactivation of the cytochrome P450 liver enzymes.

Erythromycin and clarithromycin are inhibitors of CYP3A4 enzymes. Theophylline, carbamazepine (Tegretol), cyclosporine, phenytoin (Dilantin), lovastatin (Mevacor), and simvastatin (Zocor), are metabolized by the CYP3A4 enzymes. Erythromycin or clarithromycin, when taken concurrently with these drugs, significantly decreases their metabolism, resulting in increased blood levels.

Antacids may decrease levels of macrolides. Taking a bactericidal antibiotic such as penicillin with a bacteriostatic antibiotic may interfere with the action of the bacteriostatic antibiotic. Space the dosing of the different antibiotics so that they are a few hours apart.

Capsules of azithromycin should be taken on an empty stomach because food decreases absorption, but tablets can be taken with food.

Pregnancy

Erythromycin, B; clarithromycin, C; azithromycin, B; telithromycin, C

How Supplied

Erythromycin base (E-mycin, tab; ERYC cap; Ery-Tab, tab; Ilotycin tab, PCE tab)

Erythromycin estolate (Ilsosone, tab, cap)

Erythromycin ethylsuccinate (E.E.S. filmtab)

Erythromycin stearate (Erythrocin stearate filmtabs)

Azithromycin (Zithromax tab; cap; oral suspension)

Clarithromycin (Biaxin, tab; tab extended release, oral suspension)

Telithromycin (Ketek, tab)

Dental Hygiene Notes

Many patients seen in the dental office will be taking a form of erythromycin such as azithromycin (Zithromax) or clarithromycin (Biaxin) for many types of infections, including chronic bronchitis. Since these antibiotics are

Table 6-3 Macrolide Antibiotics

Drug	Mechanism of Action	Adverse Effects	Drug Interactions	Patient Instructions
Erythromycin base (E-Mycin, Eryc, PCE, Ery-tab) Erythromycin estolate (Ilosone) Erythromycin ethylsuccinate (E.E.S., Eryped)	Bacteriostatic: Inhibits protein synthesis inside bacterial cells and prevents growth	Erythromycin estolate (hepatitis) Gastrointestinal upset (nausea, vomiting diarrhea—could be pseudomembranous colitis) Rash	Interacts with the P450 liver cytochrome enzymes so there are many drug interactions. Reduces metabolism of resulting in toxic blood levels. Theophylline (for asthma) Carbamazepine (Tegretol—for trigeminal neuralgia) Warfarin (anticoagulant) Triazolam (Halcion; sedative-hypnotic, anti-anxiety) Avoid: Lovastatin (Mevacor) –antihyper-lipidemic drug Simvastatin (Zocor)—antihypertipidemic drug Cyclosporine (Neoral) –antirejection drug for organ transplant	To reduce incidence of super-infection take penicillin with yogurt or acidophilus gelcaps. The patient may experience stomatitis (sore mouth) or glossitis (sore tongue) due to fungal overgrowth. If this occurs they should call the office immediately. Best taken on an empty stomach (empty stomach is defined as 1 hour before or 2 hours after meals) because absorption of the drug is decreased with food. If GI upset, take with food and a full glass of water. Enteric-coated tablets (filmtabs) can be taken with food
2nd generation macrolides (Azalides) Azithromycin (Zithromax-filmcoated) Clarithromycin (Biaxin Filmtabs)		Less gastrointestinal upset	Azithromycin does not interact with the P450 liver cytochrome enzymes, so not associ-ated with the above interactions. Clarithromycin has a lower affinity for P450 hepatic cytochrome enzymes than erythromycin, so it has fewer clinically important drug interactions. Interacts with the P450 liver cytochrome enzymes so there are many drug interactions.	Azithromycin: capsules on an empty stomach (1 hour before or 2 hours after meals) and tablets can be taken without regard to food. Clarithromycin is well absorbed from the GI tract with or without food.

	Reduces metabolism of resulting in toxic blood levels: Theophylline (for asthma) Carbamazepine (Tegretol–for trigeminal neuralgia) Warfarin (anticoagulant) Triazolam (Halcion; sedative-hypnotic, anti-anxiety) Avoid: Lovastatin (Mevacor) – antihyperlipidemic drug Simvastatin (Zocor) – antihypertipidemic drug Cyclosporine (Neoral) – antirejection drug for organ transplant Bactericidal drugs (penicillin, metronida-zole) given concurrently with bacteriostatic may interfere with the actions of the bacteri-cidal drugs.		Can be taken with food.
3rd generation (Ketolides) Telithromycin (Ketek)	Pseudomembranous colitis, liver problems, headache, dizziness	See above	

bacteriostatic at usual doses, care must be taken when deciding on an antibiotic to use for prevention of infective endocarditis. For example, if the patient will be taking amoxicillin, there is a potential drug–drug interaction. In these situations, if concurrent use is appropriate, the bactericidal amoxicillin should be given a few hours before the bacteriostatic drug. Erythromycins may be used for antibiotic premedication in patients allergic to amoxicillin.

Lincomycins

Actions
Clindamycin (Cleocin) is a type of lincomycin that inhibits protein synthesis by binding to the 50S ribosomal subunit on the bacteria. It is effective against most gram-positive organisms and gram-negative bacteria; aerobes (oxygen liking) are resistant to it. Clindamycin is primarily bacteriostatic, but can be bactericidal in high doses. Often dental patients will be taking clindamycin for a dental infection such as periodontal abscess or periodontal disease.

Indications
Acute bacterial exacerbation of chronic bronchitis, acute bacterial sinusitis and community-acquired pneumonia, dental infections, and refractory (resistant to treatment) periodontitis (FDA off-label use)

Adverse Effects
Pseudomembranous colitis (characterized by severe watery diarrhea or blood in the stools), visual disturbances, liver dysfunction

Drug Interactions
No significant drug interactions

Contraindications
Do not give to patients with Crohn's Disease, pseudomembranous enterocolitis or ulcerative colitis.

Pregnancy: B
How Supplied
Clindamycin HCl (Cleocin; cap)

Dental Hygiene Notes
Since the dental patient may be taking clindamycin for an abscess (infection of the tooth or gingival) or for refractory periodontitis, counseling is important. Many references have notoriously linked clindamycin to

pseudomembranous colitis (antibiotic-associated diarrhea). Antibiotic-associated diarrhea can occur with almost any antibiotic, especially if it is broad spectrum. The patient should observe for changes in bowel frequency and discontinue the antibiotic if there is watery diarrhea. The drug may be taken with food to minimize stomach upset, and a full glass of water to prevent esophagitis. Clindamycin may be used in antibiotic premedication.

Tetracyclines

Actions
Tetracyclines as a group are bacteriostatic and broad spectrum, inhibiting bacterial growth and multiplication by inhibiting protein synthesis at the 30S ribosomal subunit (Table 6–4). Two semisynthetic analogues of tetracycline, doxycycline hyclate and minocycline HCl, are broad-spectrum antibiotics, affecting both gram-positive and gram-negative microorganisms. Doxycycline and minocycline, which are slightly more active than tetracycline, have been used in the treatment of *A. actinomycetemcomitans* infections in localized aggressive periodontitis and refractory periodontitis.

Anticollagenase Feature   Tetracyclines have both antibacterial and nonantibacterial properties. Besides affecting bacterial growth, they also affect the host response by inhibiting the production and secretion of collagenase by cells in the body such as polymorphonuclear leukocytes (PMNs). Collagenase is an enzyme responsible for the destruction of collagen, which makes up the connective tissue of the periodontium. This anticollagenase property does not depend on the drug's antibacterial actions. Doxycycline 20 mg tablets (Periostat) is indicated for chronic periodontitis with a mechanism of action to inhibit the production and secretion of collagenase from the white blood cells (PMNs).

Concentration in Gingival Crevicular Fluid Another property of tetracyclines is their ability to concentrate in the gingival crevicular fluid (GCF) at two to four times blood levels following multiple doses. Doxycycline and minocycline also concentrate in higher levels in the GCF than in serum. Tetracyclines exhibit higher substantivity than other antibiotics, which allows binding to root surfaces with a slow release into the GCF. The binding of tetracyclines to calcium ions in the GCF enhances their substantivity. These properties allow the drug to maintain high therapeutic levels in the GCF. It is advantageous for a drug to concentrate in high levels in the

GCF because the GCF bathes the subgingival pocket area where the periodontal pathogens live.

Indications

Chlamydia genital infections, syphilis, travelers' diarrhea, periodontitiis (off-label use)

Adverse Effects

Common adverse side effects of tetracyclines include nausea, vomiting, and diarrhea. Diarrhea results because of changes in bowel flora (bacteria living in GI tract).

Superinfection is common after prolonged use, especially with the broad-spectrum antibiotics. This usually occurs with the broad-spectrum penicillins (e.g., amoxicillin). To help prevent superinfections, acidophilus in the form of yogurt or gelcaps should be taken to replace the acidophilus that was eliminated with the antibiotic. If yogurt is taken with tetracycline HCl, it must be taken 2 hours after the tetracycline dose because the calcium in the yogurt binds to tetracycline and prevents its absorption.

Tetracyclines should be taken with a full glass of water to prevent esophagitis and esophageal ulcers and on an empty stomach (1 hour before or 2 hours after meals). This is due to a direct irritation by tetracycline of the esophagus. It must not be taken with milk.

Gastrointestinal upset is much less severe with the semisynthetic drugs because they are more absorbed from the gastrointestinal tract.

Tetracyclines stain newly formed teeth during enamel deposition and should not be used during the last half of pregnancy or in children up to 8 years of age. A complex is formed with calcium orthophosphate that produces a yellow-gray fluorescent discoloration. Photosensitivity (with doxycycline and tetracycline) results in exaggerated sunburn when patients are exposed to the sun.

Skin hyperpigmentation occurs with ingestion of minocycline but has not been reported for doxycycline.

Drug Interactions

Tetracyclines, except doxycycline and minocycline, should not be taken concomitantly with dairy products because tetracycline binds to calcium, inhibiting its absorption. Tetracycline should be taken on an empty stomach (1 hour before or 2 hours after meals) because food delays its absorption. Doxycycline and minocycline can be taken without regard to meals.

Absorption of all tetracyclines into the bloodstream is delayed with antacids containing aluminum and magnesium, as well as products containing iron.

Tetracyclines, as well as other antibiotics, interfere with the metabolism of oral contraceptives. Estrogens, a component in oral contraceptives, must be metabolized to active form in the stomach by bacteria. Most antibiotics kill or stop the growth of these bacteria, inhibiting estrogen breakdown. Patients must use other forms of birth control while taking tetracyclines.

Tetracyclines, or any other bacteriostatic drug, should not be given together with bactericidal antibiotics such as penicillin, metronidazole, or ciprofloxacin that would interfere with the bactericidal action of that drug.

Isolated cases have been reported of increased warfarin effect (bleeding) with tetracyclines.

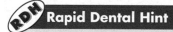

Rapid Dental Hint

Dairy products should not be taken with tetraycycline, but can be taken with doxycycline.

Pregnancy: D

May cause fetal harm with pregnancy and permanent tooth discoloration during tooth development during the last half of pregnancy.

How Supplied

Tetracycline (Sumycin, Achromycin): cap

Doxycycline hyclate (Vibramycin, Vibra-Tabs, Doryx): tab, cap

Periostat (20 mg): tab

Minocycline HCl (Minocin): cap

Dental Hygiene Notes

Some dental patients may be taking a tetracycline for a dental infection, including periodontal disease. The patient should be counseled on how to take the medication and what foods/drugs to avoid while taking it. Tetracyclines should be taken with a full glass of water to prevent esophageal irritation.

Figure 6–3 reviews the prescriptions for common antibiotics used for treating dental infections.

Table 6-4 Tetracyclines

Drug	Mechanism of Action	Adverse Effects	Drug Interactions	Patient Instructions
Tetracyclines	Antimicrobial; inhibits protein synthesis within bacteria anticollagenase. At submicrobial doses (20 mg) tetracyclines inhibit the production and secretion of collagenase (enzyme that breaks down collagen) from the polymorphonuclear leukocytes (PMNs), which prevents bone destruction.	See below	See below	See below
Tetracycline HCl (Sumycin)	Bacteriostatic	Excessive thirst, diarrhea, nausea, vomiting, stomatitis, glossitis, darkened or discolored tongue (fungal overgrowth), hypertrophy of the papillae, photosensitivity	Antacids (magnesium, aluminum) or iron supplements or calcium supplements such as calcium carbonate or dairy products will form a nonabsorbable complex and decrease tetracycline absorption. Bactericidal drugs (penicillin, metronidazole) given concurrently with bacteriostatic may interfere with the actions of the bactericidal drugs. Decreases effectiveness of oral contraceptives; use supplement contraceptive.	Dairy products and antacids should not be taken at the same time
Doxycycline hyclate 20 mg (Periostat) Doxycycline hyclate (Vibramyin, Doryx)	Bacteriostatic	Excessive thirst, diarrhea, vomiting, nausea, stomatitis, glossitis, darkened or discolored tongue (fungal overgrowth), hypertrophy of the papillae, photosensitivity	See above in addition to: Barbiturates, carbamazepine and phenytoin (antiseizure) decreases doxycycline blood levels and effects. Dairy (calcium) causes about a 30% decrease in absorption.	Antacids and iron may markedly impair oral absorption. Milk (dairy products) can be taken concurrently with doxycycline. Food has little effect on absorption.

| Minocycline HCl (Minocin) | Excessive thirst, diarrhea, vomiting, nausea, stomatitis, glossitis, darkened or discolored tongue (fungal overgrowth), hypertrophy of the papillae | Antacids (magnesium, aluminum) or iron supplements or calcium supplements such as calcium carbonate or dairy products will form a nonabsorbable complex and decrease tetracycline absorption. Bactericidal drugs (penicillin, metronidazole) given concurrently with bacteriostatic may interfere with the actions of the bactericidal drugs. Decreases effectiveness of oral contraceptives; use supplement contraceptive. | Antacids and iron may markedly impair oral absorption. Milk (dairy products) can be taken concurrently with doxycycline. Food has little effect on absorption. |

117

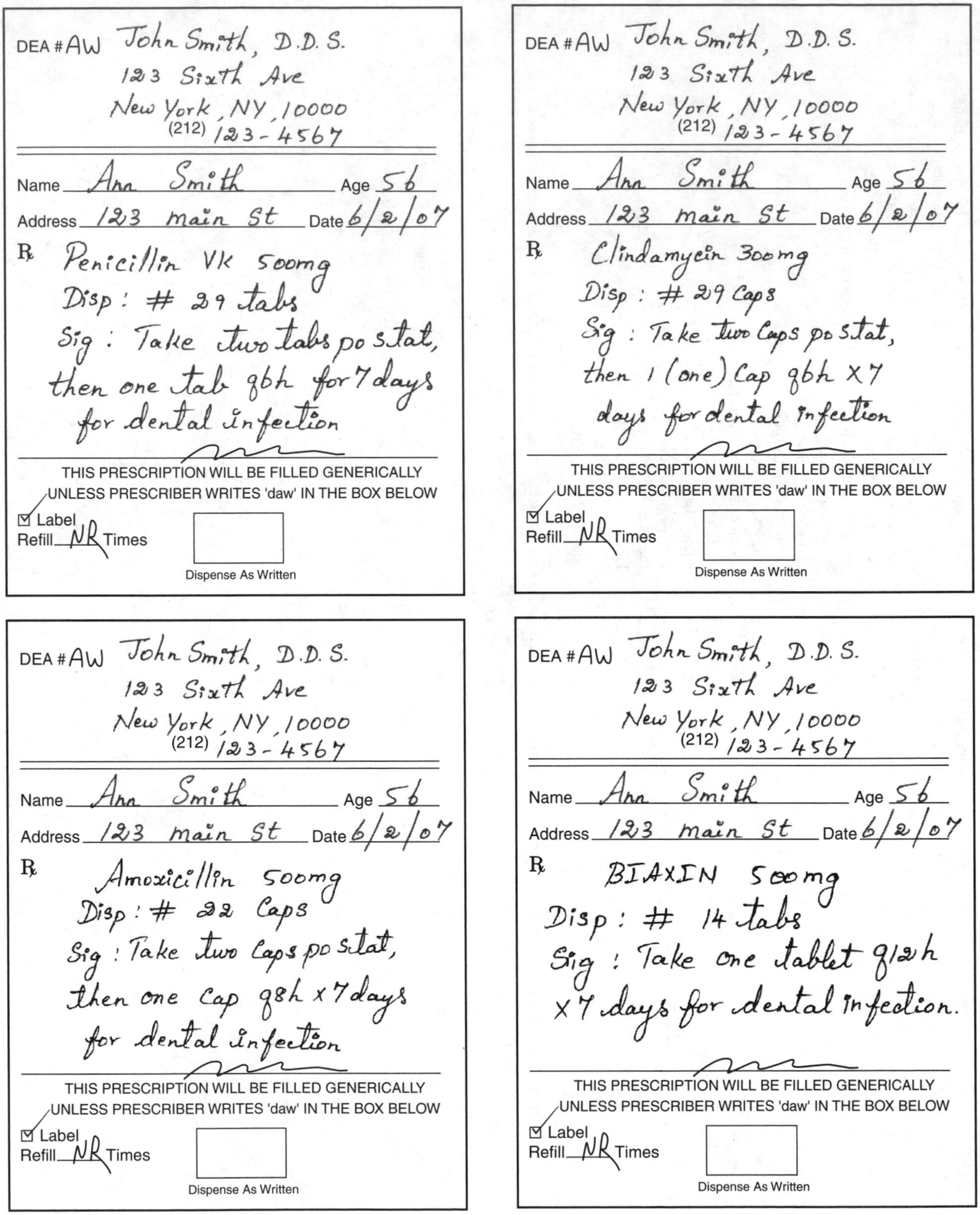

FIGURE 6-3 Sample prescriptions of antibiotics for dental infections.

DEA # AW John Smith, D.D.S.
123 Sixth Ave
New York, NY, 10000
(212) 123-4567

Name Ann Smith Age 56
Address 123 main St Date 6/2/07

R
erythromycin sterate 500 mg
Disp: # 20 tabs
Sig: Take one tab q12h
X 10 days

THIS PRESCRIPTION WILL BE FILLED GENERICALLY
UNLESS PRESCRIBER WRITES 'daw' IN THE BOX BELOW
☑ Label
Refill NR Times

Dispense As Written

DEA # AW John Smith, D.D.S.
123 Sixth Ave
New York, NY, 10000
(212) 123-4567

Name Ann Smith Age 56
Address 123 main St Date 6/2/07

R
PCE 333 mg
Disp: # 30 tabs
Sig: Take 1 tab q8h
X 10 days

THIS PRESCRIPTION WILL BE FILLED GENERICALLY
UNLESS PRESCRIBER WRITES 'daw' IN THE BOX BELOW
☑ Label
Refill NR Times

Dispense As Written

DEA # AW John Smith, D.D.S.
123 Sixth Ave
New York, NY, 10000
(212) 123-4567

Name Ann Smith Age 56
Address 123 main St Date 6/2/07

R
Cipro 500 mg
Disp: # 20 tabs
Sig: Take one tab po
q12h X 10 days

THIS PRESCRIPTION WILL BE FILLED GENERICALLY
UNLESS PRESCRIBER WRITES 'daw' IN THE BOX BELOW
☑ Label
Refill NR Times

Dispense As Written

DEA #AW John Smith, D.D.S.
123 Sixth Ave
New York, NY, 10000
(212) 123-4567

Name Ann Smith   Age 56
Address 123 main St   Date 6/2/07

Rx   Augmentin 500 mg
Disp: # 30 tabs
Sig: Take 1 tab q8h
X 10 days for dental
infection

THIS PRESCRIPTION WILL BE FILLED GENERICALLY
UNLESS PRESCRIBER WRITES 'daw' IN THE BOX BELOW

☑ Label
Refill NR Times

Dispense As Written

DEA #AW John Smith, D.D.S.
123 Sixth Ave
New York, NY, 10000
(212) 123-4567

Name Ann Smith   Age 56
Address 123 main St   Date 6/2/07

Rx   minocycline Hcl 100mg
Disp: # 15 tabs
Sig: Take 2 tabs initially
then 1 tab q12h until
finished

THIS PRESCRIPTION WILL BE FILLED GENERICALLY
UNLESS PRESCRIBER WRITES 'daw' IN THE BOX BELOW

☑ Label
Refill NR Times

Dispense As Written

DEA #AW John Smith, D.D.S.
123 Sixth Ave
New York, NY, 10000
(212) 123-4567

Name Ann Smith   Age 56
Address 123 main St   Date 6/2/07

Rx   doxycycline hyclate 100mg
Disp: # 11 tabs
Sig: Take 1 tab q12h on
first day, then one tab
qd until finished

THIS PRESCRIPTION WILL BE FILLED GENERICALLY
UNLESS PRESCRIBER WRITES 'daw' IN THE BOX BELOW

☑ Label
Refill NR Times

Dispense As Written

DEA #AW John Smith, D.D.S.
123 Sixth Ave
New York, NY, 10000
(212) 123-4567

Name Ann Smith   Age 56
Address 123 main St   Date 6/2/07

Rx   Zithromax 250 mg
Disp: # 7 tabs
Sig: Take 2 tabs qd x 1 day,
then one tab qd x 5 days

THIS PRESCRIPTION WILL BE FILLED GENERICALLY
UNLESS PRESCRIBER WRITES 'daw' IN THE BOX BELOW

☑ Label
Refill NR Times

Dispense As Written

FIGURE 6-3 (continued)

Did You Know?

Tetracycline stain does not respond well to dental bleaching.

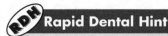 **Rapid Dental Hint**

It is important to remind patients to take all of the antibiotic even if they are feeling better.

MISCELLANEOUS ANTIBIOTICS

Sulfonamides

Actions

Sulfonamides are a synthetic analogue of para-aminobenzoic acid (PABA), which inhibits the synthesis of folic acid from PABA in bacteria. These drugs are also referred to as folate antagonists.

Indications

Prophylaxis of recurrent urinary tract infection (UTI), and *Pneumocystis jiroveci* in AIDS.

Adverse Effects

Gastrointestinal irritation (nausea, vomiting, anorexia), skin rashes, glossitis, stomatitis, photosensitivity, allergic skin rashes in AIDS patients, changes in white blood cells. These drugs are contraindicated if an individual has hypersensitivity to sulfonamides.

Drug Interactions

Increased effects of warfarin

Pregnancy: C
How Supplied

Sulfamethoxazole + trimethoprim (Bactrim): tab

Sulfadiazine (Microsulfon): tab

Sulfamethoxazole (Gantanol): tab

Sulfisoxazole (Gantrisin): suspension, syrup

Trimethoprim (Proloprim): tab

Dental Hygiene Notes

There are no significant dental drug–drug interactions. Patients seen in the dental office taking a sulfonamide are usually taking Bactrim for *P. jiroveci*.

Vancomycin

Actions

Vancomycin HCl binds irreversibly to the bacterial cell wall in a manner slightly different from β-lactams (penicillins). It is primarily active against gram-positive bacteria (e.g., *Clostridium difficile*).

Indications

Antibiotic-associated pseudomembranous colitis.

Adverse Effects

Chills, fever, nausea, "red man syndrome" (hot, red rash)

Drug Interactions

No significant dental drug interactions

Pregnancy: B
How Supplied

Vancomycin (Vancocin): cap 125, 250 mg; oral suspension; IV

Aminoglycosides

Actions

Aminoglycosides have bactericidal activity against gram-negative aerobic bacteria by binding to the interface between the 30S and 50S ribosomal subunits on the bacteria. Anaerobic bacteria are resistant.

Indications

Gram-negative infections: Serious infections of GI, respiratory, and urinary tracts; soft tissue (burns) when other less toxic antimicrobial agents are ineffective; ophthalmic (eye) infections. Streptomycin, a type of aminoglycoside, is a secondary drug used in combination with other drugs in the treatment of tuberculosis when other drugs have failed, or there are drug-resistant organisms.

Adverse Effects

Dizziness, sensation of ringing or fullness in ears, nephrotoxicity (impaired kidney function)

Drug Interactions

Concurrent use with neuromuscular blocking agents may cause respiratory failure.

Pregnancy: C
How Supplied

Neomycin: Topical for minor infections; gentamicin (Garamycin: inj. ophth., topical); tobramycin (Nebcin; inj. ophth.), amikacin (Amikin; inj.)

PREVENTION OF INFECTIVE ENDOCARDITIS

Although its incidence is rare, infective endocarditis (IE) is a critical and potentially lethal condition. The older term, subacute bacterial endocarditis (SBE), is no longer used because IE can be caused by microorganisms other than bacteria. The risk of IE associated with dental procedures makes it an important condition for the dental hygienist to be aware of. Equally important is the need for the hygienist to be thoroughly familiar with its causes and prevention. With proper knowledge of what conditions to recognize, which procedures present a risk, and how to premedicate patients at risk, the chances of a dental procedure resulting in IE may be drastically reduced.

Endocarditis most often is an infection of the valves of the heart. The heart valves are made of avascular tissue. In a healthy heart, the cusps of each valve are washed as blood passes over them with each heartbeat. However, when one of the valves is functioning abnormally, the individual may be susceptible to infection. The avascular nature of the valve tissue enables foreign microorganisms to colonize and literally hide from the immune system. Once bacteria have colonized the valve(s), they proliferate and affect the function of the valve(s). The valve affected most often is the mitral valve or bicuspid valve, on the left side of the heart. Some medical conditions create a higher risk of IE than others. In April 2007, the American Heart Association (AHA) changed the guidelines which were last published in 1997, for patients required to take prophylactic antibiotics. These most recent guidelines are published in *Circulation* April 23, 2007. The new guidelines are aimed at patients who have the greatest risk of a serious infection if they developed a heart infection. For patients requiring antibiotic prophylaxis the same antibiotics and dosing as stated in the previous guidelines are to be followed. Table 6–5 lists the patients that are recommended to have antibiotic prophylaxis. Visit www.ada.org for more information. Patients with congenital heart disease can have complicated circumstance and a consultation with their cardiologist may be needed. The article can be accessed from the Infective Endocarditis link on the American Heart Association website at www.americanheart.org.

According to the new guidelines, patients who have taken prophylactic antibiotics in the past but no longer need them include patients with:

- Mitral valve prolapse
- Rheumatic heart disease
- Bicuspid valve disease
- Calcified aortic stenosis
- Congenital heart conditions such as ventricular septal defect, atrial septal defect and hypertrophic cardiomyopathy.

Bacteremia may be caused by many different dental procedures, but it is important to take into account all conditions that may give rise to bacteria in the bloodstream (bacteremia). Bacteremia has been associated with poor oral hygiene and periodontal or periapical infections. The incidence and magnitude of bacteremia are directly proportional to the degree of oral inflammation and infection. It is therefore essential for patients at risk for endocarditis to establish and maintain the best possible oral health. This is maintained through regular professional care, as well as routine home care. Table 6–6 represents the dental procedures for which prophylaxis is recommended and those for which it is not recommended.

The antibiotic regimen has not changed. Antibiotics for prophylaxis should be administered in a single dose, 30–60 minutes before the procedure. If the dosage of antibiotic is inadvertently not administered before the procedure, the dosage may be administered up to 2 hours after the procedure. The recommendations in Table 6–6 are guidelines, and not a substitute for good clinical judgment. If it is suspected that a patient will bleed during any dental procedure, it is advisable to pretreat. Patients who have not been pretreated and those who are currently

Table 6–5 Conditions Recommended for Prophylaxis Antibiotics

1. Artificial heart valves
2. A history of infective endocarditis
3. Certain specific, serious congenital (present from birth) heart conditions, including
    - Unrepaired or incompletely repaired cyanotic congenital heart disease, including those with palliative shunts and conduits
    - A completely repaired congenital heart defect with prosthetic material or device, whether placed by surgery or by catheter intervention, during the first six months after the procedure.
    - Any repaired congenital heart defect with residual defect at the site or adjacent to the site of a prosthetic patch or a prosthetic device.
4. A cardiac transplant that develops a problem in a heart valve.

Table 6–6   Antibiotic Prophylaxis Recommendations for Dental Procedures

Higher Incidence	*Lower Incidence*
• Dental extractions • Periodontal procedures: surgery, scaling and root planing, probing and recall maintenance • Implant placement and reimplantation of avulsed teeth • Root canal instrumentation when beyond apex (endodontics) • Subgingival placement of antibiotic fibers or strips • Placement of orthodontic bands (not brackets) • Intraligamentary local anesthesia injection • Prophylactic cleaning of teeth and implants	• Restorative dentistry (operative and prosthodontic) • Local anesthetic injections (all except intraligamentary) • Placement of rubber dams • Postoperative suture removal • Placement of removable prosthodontic/orthodontic appliances • Taking oral impressions or radiographs • Fluoride treatment

taking antibiotics for other reasons will be discussed later in more detail. It is important to note that it is not acceptable to pretreat every patient, since prolonged use or misuse of antibiotics may lead to drug resistance. Furthermore, although it can significantly reduce the risk, antibiotic prophylaxis does not eliminate the risk of endocarditis. Clinical judgment is always necessary to evaluate each patient's risk, and close attention should be paid to the patient when risk is suspected. In the future, antibiotic prophylaxis may be eliminated.

Table 6–7 indicates recommended prophylactic antibiotic regimens for oral and dental procedures. The regimens are most effective when given around the time of dental treatment in doses that allow for adequate levels of the drug in the serum before, during, and after the procedure. In order to reduce the development of antibiotic resistance and maintain minimum serum levels for prophylaxis, the regimens are designed to give the patient adequate serum levels of the drug no longer than necessary.

The bacterium most commonly associated with endocarditis following dental and oral procedures is *Streptococcus viridans* (α-hemolytic streptococci). Amoxicillin remains the most recommended antibiotic for endocarditis prophylaxis. Agents such as ampicillin and penicillin V have an equal antimicrobial effect against these α-hemolytic streptococci, but amoxicillin is better absorbed in the gastrointestinal tract and provides higher, more sustained serum levels than the other penicillins.

Table 6–7   Prophylactic Antibiotic Regimens for Oral and Dental Procedures

Situation	*Drug*	*Regimen (to be taken 30 min to 60 min before dental procedure)*
Oral	Amoxicillin	adults: 2.0 g / children: 50 mg/kg
Unable to take oral medications	ampicillin or cefazolin, or ceftriaxone[*]	adults: 2.0 g IM or IV/ children: 50 mg/kg IM or IV adults: 1 g IM or IV/ children: 50 mg/kg
Allergic to penicillins or ampicillan-oral	Cephalexin[*] or clindamycin or azithromycin or clarithromycin	adults: 2 g / children: 50 mg/kg adults: 600 mg / children: 20 mg/kg adults: 500 mg / children: 15 mg/kg
Allergic to pencillins or ampicillan and unable to take oral medications	cefazolin or ceftriaxone[*] or clindamycin	adults: 1 g IM or IV/ children: 50 mg/kg IM or IV. adults: 600 mg IM or IV/ children: 20 mg/kg IM or IV

[*]Cephalosporins should not be given to an individual with a history of anaphylaxis, angioedema, or urticaria with penicillins or ampicillin.

Until 1994, the recommended adult pretreatment dose of amoxicillin for antibiotic prophylaxis was 3.0 g. However, a recent study has indicated that 2.0 g is sufficient to reach adequate serum levels for several hours. Previously, it was recommended that a second dose be given postoperatively. Currently, it has been demonstrated that not only will the initial dose of amoxicillin remain above the minimal serum level for long enough following the procedure, but the inhibitory effect of the drug is sufficient to eliminate the need for a postoperative dose.

Erythromycin, which was originally approved as an effective prophylactic agent for endocarditis in cases of penicillin allergy, is no longer among the recommended agents. Erythromycin can cause severe gastrointestinal upset, and certain formulations (e.g., erythromycin ethylsuccinate) have complicated pharmacokinetics. Instead, second-generation erythromycins, azithromycin, or clarithromycin can be used because they have better absorption and produce much less gastrointestinal upset.

Periodically, patients will present to the dental office for a routine visit during a course of antibiotic therapy with a drug used for endocarditis prophylaxis. Patients receiving antibiotics for other reasons at the time of a routine dental visit who are considered at risk for endocarditis have specific recommendations. Rather than increasing the dose of the drug currently being used, it is advisable to select an agent from a different class of antibiotic. Remember, if you have to choose another antibiotic, it must have the same bactericidal or bacteriostatic activity as the antibiotic taken for prophylaxis. For instance, if the patient is taking tetracycline (a bacteriostatic drug), he or she cannot take amoxicillin (a bactericidal antibiotic), but can take clindamycin, azithromycin, or clarithromycin, all bacteriostatic. If possible, the dental procedure is best postponed until at least 9 to 14 days after completion of the antibiotic. This will allow the normal oral flora to re-establish.

Since repeated use of antibiotics can lead to the emergence of antibiotic-resistant microorganisms in the oral cavity, it is recommended that there be an interval of at least 7 days between dental appointments.

Specific cardiac surgical procedures have varied implications in terms of risk for endocarditis. There is no evidence to suggest that coronary artery bypass surgery introduces risk for endocarditis (see Table 6–5). In the case of prosthetic valve placement, the risk of postoperative endocarditis increases. There is no evidence to suggest that heart transplant patients are at risk for endocarditis, but such patients are subject to an increased likelihood of valve dysfunction and are often treated as moderate-risk patients. Whenever possible, patients who plan to have any cardiac surgery should have a carefully executed dental treatment plan in order to complete any dental work necessary before the cardiac procedure. This may decrease the chance of late postoperative endocarditis.

Patients who have joint replacement surgery are at risk for developing infections of the implanted joints. Bacteria can enter the bloodstream and attach to implanted joints causing an infection at the prosthetic joint. In 2003, the American Academy of Orthopedic Surgeons (AAOS) and the American Dental Association Advisory Statement recommended antibiotic prophylaxis for all patients within the first two years after total joint replacement surgery only. After two years, the recommendation for antibiotic prophylaxis was limited to high-risk or medically compromised/immunosuppressed patients that might place them at increased risk for total joint infection. In 2009, guidelines for patients who have a total joint replacement were updated by the AAOS. The AAOS recommends that clinicians consider antibiotic prophylaxis for all total joint replacement patients prior to any invasive procedure that may cause bacteremia. The guideline is available at http://www.aaos.org/about/papers/advistmt/1033.asp.

Table 6–8 lists recommendations for antibiotic prophylaxis in these patients. Figure 6–4 reviews the prescriptions for each of these antibiotics.

Table 6–8 Suggested Antibiotic Prophylaxis Regimens in Patients at Potential Increased Risk of Hematogenous Total Joint Infection

Situation	Drug	Regimen
Standard general prophylaxis	Cephalexin or amoxicillin	2 g orally 1 h before dental procedure
Patients unable to take oral medications	Cefazolin or Ampicillin	1 g IM or IV 1 h before procedure 2 g IM or IV 1 h before procedure
Allergic to penicillin	Clindamycin	600 mg orally 1 h before procedure
Allergic to penicillin and unable to take oral medications	Clindamycin	600 mg IV 1 h before procedure

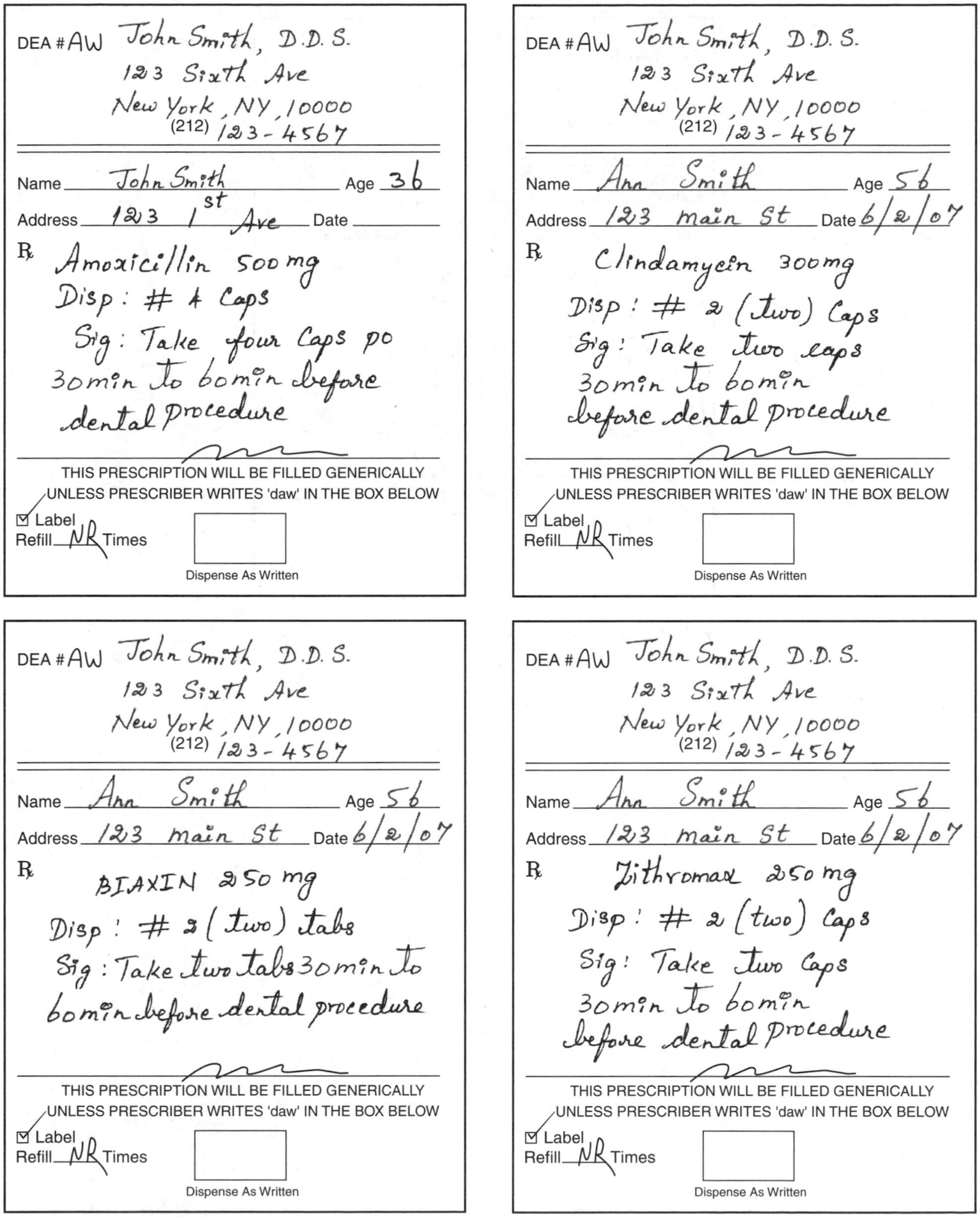

DEA # AW   John Smith, D.D.S.
123 Sixth Ave
New York, NY, 10000
(212) 123-4567

Name _____ John Smith _____ Age 36
Address _____ 123 1st Ave _____ Date _____

℞   Amoxicillin 500 mg
Disp: # 4 Caps
Sig: Take four Caps po
30 min to 60 min before
dental procedure

THIS PRESCRIPTION WILL BE FILLED GENERICALLY
UNLESS PRESCRIBER WRITES 'daw' IN THE BOX BELOW
☑ Label
Refill NR Times

Dispense As Written

DEA # AW   John Smith, D.D.S.
123 Sixth Ave
New York, NY, 10000
(212) 123-4567

Name _____ Ann Smith _____ Age 56
Address _____ 123 main St _____ Date 6/2/07

℞   Clindamycin 300 mg
Disp: # 2 (two) Caps
Sig: Take two caps
30 min to 60 min
before dental procedure

THIS PRESCRIPTION WILL BE FILLED GENERICALLY
UNLESS PRESCRIBER WRITES 'daw' IN THE BOX BELOW
☑ Label
Refill NR Times

Dispense As Written

DEA # AW   John Smith, D.D.S.
123 Sixth Ave
New York, NY, 10000
(212) 123-4567

Name _____ Ann Smith _____ Age 56
Address _____ 123 main St _____ Date 6/2/07

℞   BIAXIN 250 mg
Disp: # 2 (two) tabs
Sig: Take two tabs 30 min to
60 min before dental procedure

THIS PRESCRIPTION WILL BE FILLED GENERICALLY
UNLESS PRESCRIBER WRITES 'daw' IN THE BOX BELOW
☑ Label
Refill NR Times

Dispense As Written

DEA # AW   John Smith, D.D.S.
123 Sixth Ave
New York, NY, 10000
(212) 123-4567

Name _____ Ann Smith _____ Age 56
Address _____ 123 main St _____ Date 6/2/07

℞   Zithromax 250 mg
Disp: # 2 (two) Caps
Sig: Take two Caps
30 min to 60 min
before dental procedure

THIS PRESCRIPTION WILL BE FILLED GENERICALLY
UNLESS PRESCRIBER WRITES 'daw' IN THE BOX BELOW
☑ Label
Refill NR Times

Dispense As Written

FIGURE 6–4   Sample prescriptions of antibiotics for prophylaxis against infective endocarditis.

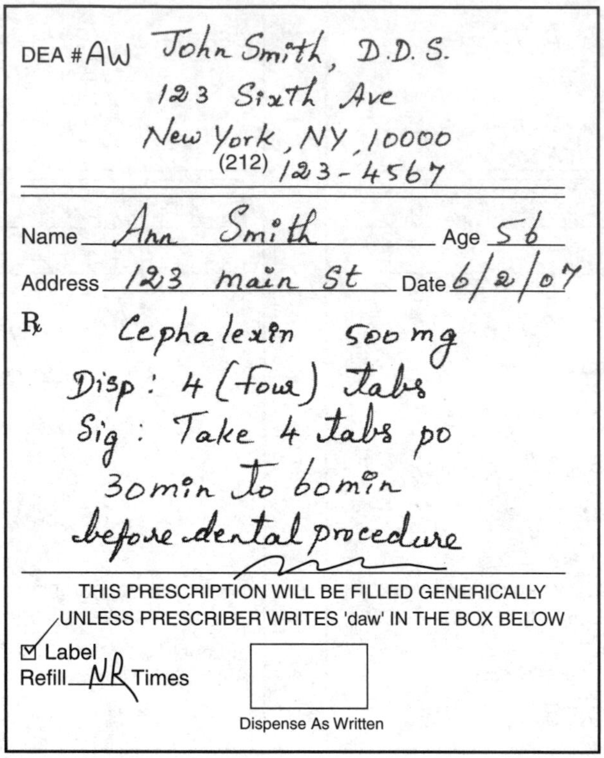

DEA #AW John Smith, D.D.S.
123 Sixth Ave
New York, NY, 10000
(212) 123-4567

Name Ann Smith _____ Age 56

Address 123 main St _____ Date 6/2/07

℞ Cephalexin 500 mg
Disp: 4 (four) tabs
Sig: Take 4 tabs po
30 min to 60 min
before dental procedure

THIS PRESCRIPTION WILL BE FILLED GENERICALLY
UNLESS PRESCRIBER WRITES 'daw' IN THE BOX BELOW

☑ Label
Refill _NR_ Times

Dispense As Written

FIGURE 6–4 (continued)

Dental Hygiene Notes

Although the majority of dental cases are treated empirically with antibiotics that the clinician has used before with good results, the concept of culture and sensitivity should be stressed. Occasionally, a patient with persistent periodontal disease who has been to many dentists and has chronically taken many different antibiotics may come to your office. In these cases, if oral hygiene is adequate, then it is more than likely necessary to culture the patient's subgingival biofilms (plaque) because there may be antibiotic resistance, since the patient is on chronic antibiotics.

ANTIBACTERIAL AGENTS: TOPICAL

Local delivery of antimicrobial agents is either by topical application or by controlled-release devices.

Topical application distributes the agent or drug to an exposed surface such as the teeth and gingiva. The most common route for the supragingival topical delivery of antimicrobial agents is by a mouthrinse, a dentifrice, or an oral irrigator. Subgingival topical delivery of antimicrobial agents is by oral irrigation or the use of controlled-release devices.

Controlled-release delivery devices are placed directly into the periodontal pocket and are designed to release a drug slowly over 24 hours for prolonged drug action. Antimicrobials are delivered into the periodontal pocket by gels, chips, powder, ointments, acrylic strips, or collagen films.

Oral Rinses

Mouthrinses generally are divided into two classifications: therapeutic rinses, used to treat diseases such as gingival diseases, and cosmetic rinses, used to freshen the breath. Indications for using oral rinses are as follows:

1. An addition to home care regimens that have failed to achieve plaque-control goals by other means
2. An addition to periodontal instrumentation
3. When oral hygiene may be inadequate or difficult to accomplish, as in the physically or mentally compromised
4. Following surgical procedures, when brushing and flossing are generally not practical
5. For maintenance of dental implants

Topical antimicrobial agents delivered by a rinse are effective only against supragingival bacteria; no antimicrobial rinse has been shown to be effective against periodontitis because oral rinses do not reach the subgingival area. Mouthrinses may be discontinued if oral health conditions can be maintained without their use.

Antiplaque/Antigingivitis Agents

Antimicrobial agents ideally should inhibit microbial colonization on tooth surfaces and prevent the subsequent formation of plaque. They also should eliminate or suppress the pathogenicity of existing plaque. Antiseptics have a greater potential to prevent the formation of plaque than to resolve established plaque and gingivitis.

An antimicrobial agent relies on two factors for efficacy: the amount of time the agent stays in contact with the target site, and how well the agent gains access to the target site. Substantivity involves the ability of the drug to stay at the target site for longer periods of time, maintaining therapeutic levels. It is ideal to have a drug with high substantivity that will be bound in the oral cavity and released over a period of hours in order to prolong its effects. Lack of substantivity can be overcome by more frequent use of the agent, but this would likely result in noncompliance and undesirable side effects.

Classification of Oral Rinses

Topical antimicrobial oral rinses can be classified as either first- or second-generation agents (Table 6–9). First-generation agents have antibacterial properties with low substantivity and limited therapeutic value in reducing plaque and gingivitis. Examples include phenolic compounds, quaternary ammonium compounds, and peroxide. Second-generation agents have antibacterial properties in addition to substantivity. Chlorhexidine gluconate is an example of a second-generation agent and is currently the only such agent proven to prevent and control gingivitis. It is available in the United States only by

Table 6–9 Antimicrobial Mouthrinses

- Chlorhexidine gluconate 0.12% (Peridex, Periogard)
- Phenolic compounds (Listerine)
- Cetylpyridiunium (Scope, Cepacol)
- Oxygenating agents (Glyoxide)

a prescription. All first-generation mouthrinses are available without a prescription.

In 1986, the American Dental Association (ADA) established guidelines for evaluation of the therapeutic effectiveness of products against gingivitis. For example, studies should be conducted over a minimum of 6 months, two studies with independent investigators should be conducted, and the active product should be used as part of a normal regimen and compared with a placebo or control product.

Most mouthrinses contain alcohol as a flavor enhancer and as a vehicle for the active ingredients. There has been some concern about the association of alcohol in mouthrinses with oral cancer. Studies have yielded inconsistent findings. Some studies document that there is no reason for patients to refrain from use of alcohol-containing mouthrinses, while research from the National Cancer Institute has drawn an association between alcoholic mouthrinse to mouth and throat cancers. In vitro (laboratory) studies of acetaldehyde, a toxic compound produced by alcohol metabolism, showed that acetaldehyde caused changes in gingival fibroblasts (cells involved in oral connective tissue maintenance).

Bisbiguanides

Description and Mechanism of Action Chlorhexidine gluconate (Peridex®, PerioGard®) is a cationic (positively charged) molecule. Originally, chlorhexidine was used in medicine as an antiseptic cream for wounds, as a preoperative skin cleanser, and as a surgical scrub. In 1970, the first study on the ability of chlorhexidine to inhibit the formation of plaque and maintain soft tissue health was released. It was not until 1986 that chlorhexidine became available in the United States by prescription at a 0.12% concentration with an alcohol concentration of 11.6%. It has the ADA seal of acceptance for the treatment of gingivitis.

After rinsing, chlorhexidine (positively charged) is attracted to and attaches to the negatively charged bacterial cell walls, causing lysis or breakage of the cell wall. The contents of the cells leak out. Chlorhexidine enters the cell through the opening, resulting in death of the bacteria. By binding to the pellicle on the tooth surface, chlorhexidine inhibits plaque attachment. Chlorhexidine exhibits substantivity, with approximately 30 percent of the drug binding to oral tissues and the plaque on the teeth, and showing antimicrobial activity for 8 to 12 hours afterward.

Indications Rinsing with chlorhexidine is indicated before, during, and after periodontal debridement to reduce plaque levels and gingival inflammation. Chlorhexidine rinses can improve wound healing and provide better plaque control after periodontal surgery when brushing and flossing is not feasible. Rinsing with chlorhexidine has been shown to decrease the severity of mucositis in patients receiving chemotherapy. Since peri-implantitis is similar to gingivitis, rinsing with chlorhexidine may be effective in implant plaque control.

Usage It is recommended to rinse twice a day for 30 seconds. The positive charge of chlorhexidine causes it to bind to the negatively charged molecules in toothpastes such as fluorides and sodium lauryl sulfate (a detergent), and thus inactivates them. Therefore, it is best to rinse either 30 minutes before or after tooth brushing or rinse very well with water after tooth brushing. Because of this inactivation by anionic compounds, chlorhexidine is not available in toothpaste. Chlorhexidine can be used as an irrigant, but it is usually diluted with water to reduce the incidence of staining. A sample prescription is shown in Figure 6–5.

Adverse Effects Chlorhexidine is relatively safe because it is poorly absorbed from the oral membranes and systemic circulation. The most common adverse side effect is a yellow, brownish extrinsic staining of the teeth, tongue, and restorations within the first few days of use. Staining is more frequent with chlorhexidine than with other agents because of its affinity for oral surfaces. The staining may be associated with food dyes found within certain foods and beverages. This staining is not permanent and can be removed mechanically during professional prophylaxis (stains may not be removed from pits of composite restorations). If the patient is compliant with oral home care, the staining is more likely on proximal tooth surfaces than facial or lingual surfaces. Other adverse side effects include a temporarily impaired taste perception and increased supragingival calculus formation.

Phenolic Compounds

Listerine® is a combination of phenolic compounds or essential oils, including thymol, eucalyptol, menthol, and methyl salicylate, in an alcohol vehicle. The mechanism of action is cell wall disruption, resulting in leakage of intracellular components and lysis of the cell. The original-formula Listerine contains 26.9% alcohol, whereas the Cool Mint, Fresh Burst Listerine and Natural Citrus contain 21.6% alcohol.

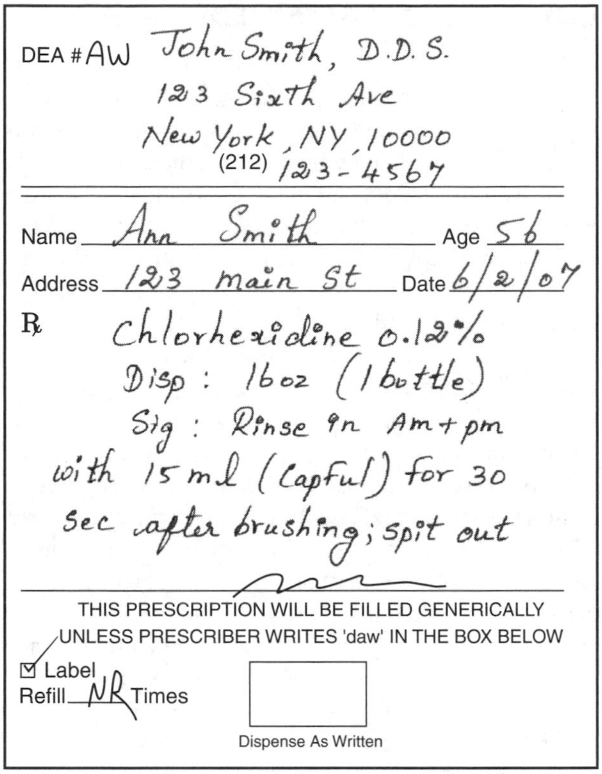

DEA # AW   *John Smith, D.D.S.*
             123 Sixth Ave
             New York, NY, 10000
                  (212) *123-4567*

Name _*Ann Smith*_   Age *56*

Address _*123 main St*_   Date *6/2/07*

℞   *Chlorhexidine 0.12%*
         Disp : 16 oz (1 bottle)
         Sig : Rinse in Am + pm
    with 15 ml (Capful) for 30
    sec after brushing; spit out

THIS PRESCRIPTION WILL BE FILLED GENERICALLY
UNLESS PRESCRIBER WRITES 'daw' IN THE BOX BELOW

☑ Label
Refill _NR_ Times

Dispense As Written

FIGURE 6-5   Sample prescription for Chlorhexidine.

Because of low substantivity, effectiveness is strongly related to the duration of tooth contact. Clinical studies have shown this product significantly to reduce plaque development in patients with minimal plaque levels. Listerine® has been documented to reduce plaque and gingivitis from 20 to 34%; the subjects had pre-existing plaque and gingivitis, and no prophylaxis was performed at the beginning of the study.

Recommendations are to rinse for 30 seconds with 2/3 oz, once in the morning and once at night. Possible adverse side effects include a burning sensation and bitter taste.

Quaternary Ammonium Compounds

Quaternary ammonium compounds are positively charged (cationic) compounds similar to chlorhexidine. They readily bind to oral surfaces and are released more rapidly or lose their activity on binding to the surface. Substantivity is only approximately 3 hours. An increase in bacterial cell wall permeability leads to cell lysis and decreased attachment of bacteria to tooth surfaces. Cetylpyridinium chloride is the active ingredient in Scope® Original and Cepacol. The alcohol concentration is 14% for Cepacol and 18.9% for Scope Original.

Clinical data on plaque reduction and gingivitis control have been relatively inconclusive because of variability in results between studies. Following an initial professional prophylaxis and suspension of all oral hygiene, chlorhexidine was found to be superior to cetylpyridinium in the reduction of plaque. Cetylpyridinium chloride may have some antiplaque action but less effect on gingivitis when used as an adjunct to conventional oral home care. Lack of substantivity limits clinical efficacy. As with chlorhexidine, to obtain the maximum effect, the patient should rinse very well or wait 30 minutes after brushing with a dentifrice before using the rinse. Adverse side effects are similar to those of chlorhexidine, including some staining, calculus formation, and mucosal ulceration.

Oxygenating Agents

Oxygenating agents such as peroxides and perborates have been used in mouthrinse formulations primarily for inflammation of the gingival soft tissues. Since hydrogen peroxide liberates gaseous oxygen, it provides a cleansing action and gentle effervescence for oral wounds. Its antimicrobial effect is directed at anaerobic microorganisms that cannot live in the presence of oxygen, and it has a physical effect on plaque through the bubbling of oxygen as it is released from the peroxide. The Food and Drug Administration has approved its use as a temporary debriding agent in the oral cavity. However, antiplaque/antigingivitis claims are not well supported.

The safety of hydrogen peroxide has been disputed. Long-term use of 3% hydrogen peroxide has resulted in gingival irritation and delayed tissue healing. On the other hand, some studies found that adverse effects from exposure to 3% or less hydrogen peroxide were rare. It was concluded that exposure to less than 3% hydrogen peroxide was safe; however, long-term studies do not demonstrate any additional benefit over regular home career. Because many patients use hydrogen peroxide on a regular basis, the dental hygienist should question patients about their oral home-care practices.

Povidone-Iodine

Povidone-iodine is antibacterial and antiseptic. Its primary use is in the prevention and treatment of surface infections. Often povidone-iodine is combined with hydrogen peroxide as a subgingival irrigant for the reduction of gram-negative microorganisms. Most studies confirm that iodine may be a beneficial adjunctive treatment for the prevention and control of gingivitis when used with optimal oral hygiene self-care procedures; however, iodine can stain teeth, clothing, skin, and restorations.

Fluorides

Fluorides have been used in dentistry primarily for prevention of dental caries by reducing demineralization and enhancing remineralization. Fluoride rinses have not been proven clinically to prevent root caries. Fluoride's role as an antiplaque/antigingivitis agent is less well documented and shows controversial results.

Prebrushing Rinses

Plax®, a prebrushing rinse, contains surfactants such as sodium lauryl sulfate (which functions as a detergent to help loosen and remove plaque), sodium benzoate (a preservative), and tetrasodium pyrophosphate (an anticalculus agent). Studies have shown limited beneficial effects of this agent over rinsing with water alone (Grossman 1988).

Alcohol-Free Mouthrinses

Most mouthrinses contain alcohol as a vehicle to carry other ingredients and as a flavor enhancer. The form of alcohol in the rinse is either ethanol (ethyl alcohol) or a specially denatured (SD) alcohol that is made synthetically. Alcohol can cause drying of the oral mucosal tissues, especially when the agent is used for extended periods of time. Indications for a nonalcoholic mouthrinse include pregnant women, former alcoholics, patients who are taking medications that would additionally dry the mouth, patients taking metronidazole, and patients who prefer to avoid alcohol.

Alcohol-free mouthrinses include:

Chlorhexidine 0.12% alcohol-free rinse (Butler)

Crest Pro-Health Rinse

Rembrandt

Oral B Plaque Rinse

Listermint

BreathRX

CONTROLLED (SUSTAINED)-RELEASE DRUG DELIVERY

The development of site-specific, controlled (sustained)-release delivery systems has provided a further option for antimicrobial therapy by allowing therapeutic levels of a drug to be maintained in the periodontal pocket for prolonged periods of time. If the drug is released from the device past 24 hours, it is called a controlled-release device; if the drug is released within 24 hours, it is called a sustained-release device. Many devices are available in the United States and Europe that incorporate an antimicrobial agent into a specific material (a polymer) that is placed into the periodontal pocket. The active ingredient is then released from the material, which subsequently exerts its antibacterial activity on subgingival bacteria over several days. Then the material is absorbed (dissolves). The concentration of antimicrobials administered in a controlled (sustained)-release device does not enter the bloodstream and thus does not trigger adverse side effects. Types of materials used to incorporate antimicrobial drugs include gels, chips, collagen film, and acrylic strips. Controlled-release drug therapy is used as an adjunct to periodontal debridement and should not replace conventional mechanical therapy. In fact, the American Academy of Periodontology reported that it "would be premature to conclude that insertion of sustained-release antimicrobial systems is as effective as scaling and root planing in all populations of patients." They are indicated for use in recurrent pockets of 5 mm or greater that continue to bleed on probing. The intended results with these devices are gains in clinical attachment levels and reductions in probing depths and bleeding on probing.

Currently in the United States, PerioChip, Atridox, and Arestin are available commercially (Table 6–10). Other controlled-release systems are available in Europe that are not approved for use in the United States.

Resorbable Controlled (Sustained)-Release Devices

Chlorhexidine Gluconate Chip

The PerioChip is a gelatin matrix (bovine origin) containing 2.5 mg of chlorhexidine gluconate. This product received Food and Drug Administration approval in June 1998. PerioChip is indicated for use as an adjunct to instrumentation in maintenance patients with pockets 5 mm or larger that bleed recurrently on probing. A clini-

Table 6-10   Controlled Antimicrobial Drugs Used in Dentistry

- Arestin (microspheres of minocycline HCl)
- Atridox (10% doxycycline hyclate)
- PerioChip (2.5 mg chlorhexidine gluconate)

cal study comparing the efficacy of periodontal debridement alone with that of periodontal debridement plus PerioChip revealed statistically significant reductions in probing depth and gains in clinical attachment in the periodontal debridement plus PerioChip group. However, the magnitude of these changes was small (0.3 mm), so the results are not clinically significant. In this study, mechanical debridement was limited to only 1 hour in patients with moderately advanced periodontitis (5- to 8-mm pockets), which does not seem realistic.

After periodontal debridement, the chip is placed into the periodontal pocket. In contact with subgingival fluids it becomes sticky and binds to the epithelium lining the pocket, so no periodontal dressing is indicated. Its antibacterial action occurs when chlorhexidine is released over 7 to 10 days, after which it resorbs and does not have to be removed. Up to eight chips can be inserted into pockets in one visit. Another round of treatment can be done at 3 months.

Doxycycline Hyclate Gel

Atridox is composed of 10% (42.5 mg) doxycycline hyclate in a gel formulation that is biodegradable and subsequently will reabsorb. The ingredients are available in two syringes (powder and liquid) that are mixed together and injected into the pocket around the entire tooth. The gel form allows for ease of flow, readily adapting to subgingival root morphology. When the gel comes in contact with gingival fluid in the pocket, it solidifies to a wax-like substance.

Atridox is indicated as an adjunct to scaling and root planing procedures in patients with chronic periodontitis. Local anesthesia is not required. Results of therapy are to promote attachment level gain, to reduce pocket depths, and to reduce bleeding on probing. Atridox may also be used in patients who refuse to have periodontal debridement or periodontal surgery, and who are medically, physically, or emotionally compromised.

Levels of doxycycline in the pocket peaked at 2 hours after placement into the pocket, and effective drug levels were maintained at 28 days, although within a few days levels of doxycycline has peaked.

Minocycline Hydrochloride Microspheres

The most recent FDA-approved sustained-release device is Arestin. Arestin is a sustained-release product containing the antibiotic minocycline hydrochloride. Minocycline is a type of tetracycline but it is longer acting over a broader spectrum of antibiotic activity. Each cartridge of Arestin contains 1 mg of minocycline. Arestin is indicated as an adjunct to scaling and root planing procedures for the reduction of pocket depth in patients with chronic localized periodontitis. Studies have shown that scaling and root planing followed by the application of Arestin resulted in a greater percentage reduction in pocket depths (greater than or equal to 2mm) at 9 months compared to scaling and root planing alone.

Dental Hygiene Notes

When using locally applied Arestin or Atridox on certain periodontal patients, the same judgments concerning drug interactions, adverse side effects, and contraindications must be used as if these products were systemically applied. These products are an analogue of tetracycline, and as such, should not be given to pregnant women or children under 8 years of age. Additionally, one must be careful about interactions with oral contraceptives.

Alcohol-containing mouthrinses including Peridex, Periogard, and Listerine should not be used in a patient taking metronidazole (Flagyl). A severe reaction occurs with nausea, vomiting, flushing and faintness.

KEY POINTS

- Indiscriminate use of antibiotics causes bacterial resistance to the antibiotic, whereby the antibiotic becomes ineffective in killing that bacteria.
- Bactericidal antibiotics kill the bacteria.
- Bacteriostatic antibiotics stop the growing and multiplication of the bacteria.
- Stomach problems (e.g., diarrhea) are an adverse effect of most antibiotics; instruct the patient to take acidophilus tablets with the antibiotic.

- Most dental infections do not require broad-spectrum antibiotics.
- Chronic periodontitis does not need antibiotics as part of the treatment.
- Antibiotics primarily used in dentistry are penicillin V, amoxicillin, azithromycin, metronidazole, tetracyclines, and clindamycin.
- Many drug interactions are associated with antibiotics; review the patient's medical history and ask questions.
- Bactericidal and bacteriostatic antibiotics should not be given concurrently.
- Antimicrobial oral rinses include chlorhexidine gluconate, phenolic, and compounds (Listerine).
- Placement of controlled-delivery antimicrobials into the pocket: doxycycline (Atridox) and minocycline (Arestin)
- The same adverse effects, drug interactions, and contraindications that are documented with systemic antibiotics hold for controlled-release antibiotics.

BOARD REVIEW QUESTIONS

1. Which of the following antibiotics can be used for prophylaxis against infective endocarditis if a patient is allergic to penicillin? (p. 123)
   a. Ampicillin
   b. Erythromycin
   c. Azithromycin
   d. Doxycycline

2. Which of the following antibiotics is used to treat Legionnaires' disease? (p. 111)
   a. Penicillin
   b. Amoxicillin
   c. Metronidazole
   d. Azithromycin

3. Which of the following antibiotics is used to treat *Pneumocystis jiroveci* infection in AIDS patients? (p. 121)
   a. Metronidazole
   b. Trimethoprim + sulfamethoxazole
   c. Penicillin
   d. Doxycycline

4. A primary concern for using antibiotics for infections that are not bacterial in nature is that: (p. 101)
   a. Drug-resistant microorganisms could develop.
   b. Drug/drug interactions increase.
   c. Drug dependence will develop.
   d. Significant blood diseases could occur.

5. A patient is taking Biaxin for chronic bronchitis. Which of the following procedures should be followed if the patient has to take amoxicillin for prophylaxis against infective endocarditis? (pp. 121–124)
   a. Discontinue the Biaxin for 4 days before the dental appointment.
   b. Prescribe another drug for chronic bronchitis.
   c. Take the Biaxin a few hours before the amoxicillin.
   d. Don't take the amoxicillin and double the dose of Biaxin.

6. Which of the following drugs is contraindicated while a patient is taking metronidazole for NUG? (p. 109)
   a. Penicillin
   b. Alcohol
   c. Aspirin
   d. Mushrooms

7. All of the following antibiotics have been used in the treatment of periodontal diseases except one. Which one is the exception? (pp. 110–111)
   a. Clindamycin
   b. Ciprofloxacin
   c. Erythromycin base
   d. Doxycycline hyclate

8 Which of the following antibiotics is contraindicated in children under 8 years old? (p. 115)
   a. Clindamycin
   b. Azithromycin
   c. Tetracycline
   d. Penicillin VK

9. Which of the following antibiotics cannot be taken concurrently with milk? (p. 115)
   a. Tetracycline
   b. Amoxicillin
   c. Metronidazole
   d. Penicillin

10. Which of the following antibiotics comprises Periostat? (p. 115)
    a. Tetracycline 250 mg caps
    b. Azithromycin 250 mg tabs
    c. Amoxicillin 500 mg cap
    d. Doxycycline 20 mg tab

11. Which of the following defines antimicrobial activity of an antibiotic that kills sensitive bacteria? (p. 101)
    a. Narrow-spectrum
    b. Broad-spectrum
    c. Bactericidal
    d. Bacteriostatic

12. All of the following are adverse reactions to antibiotics except one. Which one is the exception? (p. 101)
    a. Superinfections
    b. Gastrointestinal (nausea, vomiting, diarrhea)
    c. Allergic reactions
    d. Inhibits bacterial growth
    e. Photosensitivity

13. Antibiotics are effective against which of the following? (p. 101)
    a. Yeasts
    b. Bacteria
    c. Viruses
    d. Influenza

14. Which of the following symptoms occur in the oral cavity as a result of fungal overgrowth during antibiotic use? (p. 103)
    a. Stomatitis
    b. Hypersensitivity
    c. Caries
    d. Gingivitis

15. An overgrowth of which of the following organisms is responsible for antibiotic-associate diarrhea? (p. 103)
    a. *Streptococci mutans*
    b. *Mucobacterium tuberculosis*
    c. *Clostridium difficile*
    d. *Staphylococci aureus*

16. Which of the following active ingredients is found in Atridox? (p. 131)
    a. Chlorhexidine
    b. Tetracycline
    c. Doxycycline
    d. Minocycline

17. Which of the following active ingredients is found in Arestin? (p. 131)
    a. Chlorhexidine
    b. Tetracycline
    c. Doxycycline
    d. Minocycline

18. For which of the following patients is Atridox contraindicated? (p. 131)
    a. Alcoholics
    b. Diabetics
    c. Pregnant women
    d. Teenagers

19. Which of the following agents should not be taken immediately after using chlorhexidine oral rinse? (p. 128)
    a. Fluoride
    b. Alcohol
    c. Arestin
    d. Antacid

20. The percentage (%) of hydrogen peroxide found in antiseptic topical solutions is what? (p. 130)
    a. 1
    b. 2
    c. 3
    d. 4

SELECTED REFERENCES

American Academy of Periodontology position paper: Systemic antibiotics in periodontics. 2004. *J Periodontol* 75:1553–1565.

Dijani, A. S., K. A. Taubert, W. Wilson, A. F. Bolger, A. Bayer, et al. 1997. Prevention of bacterial endocarditis: Recommendations by the American Heart Association. *JAMA* 227:1794–1801.

Gums, J. G. Redefining appropriate use of antibiotics. *American Family Physician* 2004;69:35–36.

Hanes, P. J., and J. P. Purvis. Local anti-infective therapy: Pharmacological agents—A systematic review. *Ann Periodontol* 2003;8:79–98.

Hooton, R. M., and S. B. Levy. Antimicrobial resistance: A plan of action for community practice. *Am Fam Physician* 2001;63:1087–1098.

Newman, M. G. and A. J. van Winkelhoff. *Antibiotic and Antimicrobial Use in Dental Practice,* 2nd ed. Chicago: Quintessence Publishing Co., Inc. 2001.

Segelnick, S.L, Weinberg, M.A. Recognized doxycycline-induced esophagela ulcers in dental practice. *J Am Dent Assoc* 2008;139:581-585.

Vanden Eng, J., R. Marcus, J. L. Hadler, B. Imhoff, D. J. Vugia, P. R. Cieslak., et al. Consumer attitudes and use of antibiotics. *Emerg Infect Dis* 2003;9:1128-1135.

Wilson, W., K. A. Taubert, M. Gewitz, et al. Prevention of infective endocarditis. Guidelines from the American Heart Association Rheumatic Fever, Endocarditis and Kawasaki Disease Committee, Council on Cardiovascular Disease in the Young, and the Council on Clinical Cardiology, Council on Cardiovascular Surgery and Anesthesia, and the Quality of Care and Outcomes Research Interdisciplinary Working Group. *Circulation Journal of the American Heart Association.* 2007; Online and *JADA* 2007; 138(6):739–760.

WEB SITES

www.ncbi.nlm.nih.gov
www.fda.gov/bbs/topics
www.uspharmacist.com
www.ada.org
www.pharmacytimes.com
www.cdc.gov
www.perio.org

QUICK DRUG GUIDE

Bactericidal antibiotics

Penicillins

Natural penicillins: Narrow spectrum

- Penicillin V (Pen-vee K, V-cillin K, Veetids)
- Penicillin G (injectable)

Broad spectrum: Aminopenicillins

- Amoxicillin (Amoxil, Trimox)
- Ampicillin (Omnipen)

Beta-lactamase inhibitors

- Amoxicillin + clavulanate (Augmentin)
- Ampicillin + sulbactam (Unasyn)
- Piperacillin + tazobactam (injectable, Zosyn)

Penicillinase-resistant

- Dicloxacillin (Dycill)
- Nafcillin (injectable)
- Oxacillin (Bactocill)
- Cloxacillin (cloxacillin)

Anti-pseudomonal penicillins: Extended spectrum (All are injectables)

- Carbenicillin (Geocillin)
- Ticarcillin (Ticar)
- Mezlocillin (Mezlin)
- Piperacillin (Pipracil)

Cephalosporins

1st generation

- Cefadroxil (Duricef)
- Cephalexin (Keflex)

2nd generation

- Cefaclor (Ceclor)
- Cefprozil (Cefzil)
- Cefuroxime—axetil (Ceftin, Veftin)

3rd generation

- Omnicef (cefdinir)
- Cefixime (Suprax)
- Cefpodoxime (Vantin)
- Ceftibuten (Cedax)

4th generation: Only injectable

Nitroimadazoles

- Metronidazole (Flagyl)

Fluoroquinolones

1st generation

- Nalidixic acid (NegGram)

2nd generation

- Ciprofloxacin (Cipro)
- Ofloxacin (Floxin)

3rd generation

- Levofloxacin (Levaquin)
- Sparfloxacin (Zagam)
- Gatifloxacin (Tequin)
- Moxifloxacin (Avelox)

4th generation

- Trovafloxacin (Trovan)

Bacteriostatic antibiotics

Tetracyclines

- Tetracycline HCl (Sumycin, achromycin)
- Doxycycline hyclate (Vibramyin, Doryx)
- Doxycycline hyclate 20 mg (Periostat)
- Minocycline HCl (Minocin)

Erythromycins (macrolides)

- Erythromycin base (E-Mycin, Eryc, PCE, Ery-tab)
- Erythromycin estolate (Ilosone)
- Erythromycin ethylsuccinate (E.E.S., Eryped)

2nd generation macrolides (Azalides)

- Azithomycin (Zithromax)
- clarithromycin (Biaxin)

3rd generation (Ketolides)

- Telithromycin (Ketek)

Lincomycins

- Clindamycin (Cleocin)

Other Antimicrobials

Sulfonamides

- Sulfamethoxazole + trimethoprim (Bactrim)
- Sulfadiazine (Silvadene)
- Sulfamethoxazole (Gantanol)
- Sulfisoxazole (Gantrisin)
- Trimethoprim (Proloprim)

Glycopeptide antibiotic

- Vancomycin (Vancocin)

Aminoglycosides

- Neomycin (Bacitracin zinc-neomycin-polymyxin B sulfate)
- Gentamicin (Garamycin)
- Tobramycin (Nebcin)
- Amikacin (Amikin)

Chapter 7

Antiviral and Antifungal Agents

GOAL: To gain knowledge of the various treatments for herpes simplex virus infection and oral and systemic fungal infections.

EDUCATIONAL OBJECTIVES

After reading this chapter, the reader should be able to:

1. Illustrate the pathophysiology of herpes simplex viruses.
2. List various antiherpetic drugs.
3. Describe the appropriate dental management of patients with herpes labialis.
4. List the patients that are higher risk for fungal infections.
5. List common antifungal agents used to treat oral infections.
6. List common drug interactions of systemic antifungal agents.

KEY TERMS

Herpes simplex virus
Cold sore
Antiviral agents
Oral candidiasis
Antifungal agents

INTRODUCTION

Although dental hygienists do not treat and prescribe medications for oral conditions, they are probably the first to see changes of the patient's oral mucosa during an intraoral examination. Thus, the dental hygienist should be aware of the various common herpetic oral lesions and the medications used to manage them.

ANTIVIRALS FOR HERPES SIMPLEX

Antiviral drugs are used in the treatment of viral infections. There are mainly two serotypes of **herpes simplex virus (HSV):** Herpes virus type 1 (HSV-1) primarily causes oropharygeal disease (including eyes, vermillion border of the lips, mouth, face); herpes virus type 2 (HSV-2) primarily causes genital disease, which is considered a sexually transmitted disease. Herpes simplex virus infections occur in healthy as well as in immuno-compromised patients. There is transmission of HSV-1 to the genitals, and HSV-2 can cause oral herpes.

Herpes simplex type 1 (HSV-1) can occur either as a primary or recurrent infection. *Primary herpes simplex virus* or *primary herpetic gingivostomatitis* infections occur with the first exposure to HSV-1 or HSV-2. It can occur in infants, children (between 2 and 3 years of age), or adults, and is characterized by high fever, malaise, fatigue, nausea and vomiting and oral vesicles. Adults may have less typical clinical features, making a diagnosis more difficult. After primary exposure, herpes simplex virus may persist in a latent state in the trigeminal ganglion until it is disturbed and then reactivated in adulthood. Herpes infection is transmissible from human to human. An important part of the transmission is intimate contact between an infected shedding person (the host) and another susceptible person. Common stimuli that disturb the host's immune system include fever, menstruation, prolonged illness, exposure to sunlight, prolong use of steroids or surgery. By adulthood, up to 90 percent of individuals will have antibodies to HSV-1.

Painful intraoral vesicles on the oral mucosa rapidly rupture to form small ulcers with erythematous (red) haloes. HSV-1 is transmitted by contact with in-

Rapid Dental Hint

Patients with oral viral lesions should not use alcohol-containing mouthrinses.

fected saliva. Lesions appear 12 to 36 hours after the first symptoms. Lesions are self-limiting and will resolve within 10–14 days. There is also a generalized severe gingivitis present and cervical lymphadenopathy.

Treatment is palliative, including fluids and analgesics/antipyretics such as acetaminophen (Tylenol). Early treatment with acyclovir (Zovirax) or famciclovir (Famvir) may significantly shorten the duration of all clinical manifestations and infectivity of affected children. Antibiotics are not used in the treatment of primary herpes because they are used in bacterial infections, not viral; however, they may be helpful in preventing secondary infection.

Rapid Dental Hint

Patients should discard their toothbrush during periods of viral infection.

Recurrent herpes simplex virus infection is also caused by HSV-1 and occurs in individuals who previously had primary herpes. This infection occurs in and around the mouth and is referred to as herpes labialis, a **"cold sore"** or "fever blister" when it occurs on the vermillion border of the lip. (Figure 7–1) Recurrences of these lesions are thought to be due to stress, sunlight, fever, immunocompromised patients (HIV infection/AIDS), trauma (e.g., after a dental procedure), or other irritants (Figure 7–2). Usually there is a prodromal burning and itching at the site 12–35 hours preceding eruption of the vesicles (raised blisters). Clinically, a small well localized cluster of small vesicles appears on heavily keratinized oral mucosa (gingiva, palate, tongue, alveolar

Did You Know?

About 45 million Americans are infected with genital herpes (HSV-2).

Did You Know?

Incidence of ocular (eye) herpes infection is approximately 0.15%.

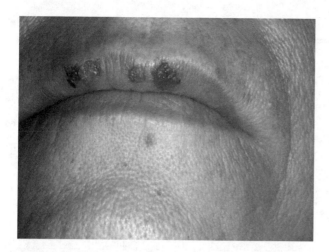

FIGURE 7–1 Herpes labialis on the vermillion border of the lip. (Courtesy of Dr. James B. Fine, Columbia College of Dental Medicine; U.S. Pharmacist)

ridges, and vermillion border of lips). The vesicles subsequently rupture, ulcerate, and crust within 24–48 hours. Lesions have the potential to last more than 14 days if left untreated.

Antibiotics should not be used, which will further suppress the immune system and prolong the infection.

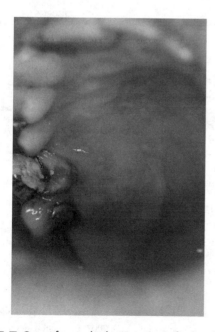

FIGURE 7–2 After multiple injections of a local anesthetic the patient developed herpetic lesions. (Courtesy of Dr. David Lefkowitz; U.S. Pharmacist)

Topical corticosteroids may be recommended in addition to oral antiviral agents to help reduce the pain and inflammation in herpes zoster, but their effectiveness in the treatment of recurrent herpes labialis infection is unknown. A 50:50 suspension of diphenydramine and Kaopectate and/or lidocaine viscous will help with the pain.

Table 7–1 lists the commonly used **antiviral agents** in the treatment of recurrent oral herpes simplex infection. Antiviral drugs inhibit viral DNA synthesis. These antiviral agents do not cure the condition but may reduce healing time, reduce viral shedding, and reduce frequency of recurrences.

Acyclovir is almost completely restricted to the herpes viruses (HSV-1, HSV-2, varicella zoster and Epstein Barr). Acyclovir (Zovirax) 5% cream/ointment is used in adults and adolescents 12 years old or more with recurrent herpes labialis. It is applied five times a day for 4 days.

Penciclovir 1% (Devavir) cream is highly recommended in immunocompetent (immune system is not compromised and the patient is healthy) patients. The cream should be applied during the prodromal (feeling before active disease) stage.

 Rapid Dental Hint

Patients should apply topical acyclovir and penciclovir with a finger cot.

Oral acyclovir is recommended in immunocompromised (HIV +) individuals with HSV-1 and in HSV-2 infection in immunocompetent (normal immune systems) patients. It has not been approved by the FDA for treatment of HSV-1 infections in immunocompetent patients, although many clinicians prescribe it.

Other products available OTC for the symptomatic treatment of herpes labialis include petroleum and cocoa butter to keep lesions moist and prevent cracking, which would make them more susceptible to secondary infection. Docosanol (Abreva), a 10% cream, is applied five times a day until the infection heals. It works by inhibiting the fusion of the virus with the human cell membrane, thereby blocking entry and subsequent viral replication.

If it is too late after the first symptoms appear to apply an antiviral agent, a topical anesthetic such as

Table 7-1 Antiherpetic Drugs

Drug Name	Indications and Adverse Effects	Drug Interactions	Dental Notes
Acyclovir sodium (Zovirax) 200 mg caps, 400, 800 mg tabs, suspension, topical ointment cream 5%, injectable; generic available	Topical: Recurrent herpes labialis Oral: herpes labialis, genital herpes (HSV-2) Side effects: Renal (kidney) impairment, changes in blood count, nausea, vomiting, rash, headache	Increased CNS effects when taken with zidovudine	Apply ointment every 3 hours up to six times a day for 7 days
Docosanol (Abreva) cream 10%	Over-the-counter for herpes labialis	No interactions	Apply five times a day at first sign of cold sore. Use until lesion is healed
Penciclovir (Denavir) cream 1%	FDA-approved for recurrent oral HSV. Side effects: Headache	No clinically significant interactions	Apply every 2 hours while awake for 4 days
Valacyclovir (Valtrex) tabs 500 mg, 1gram	For herpes labialis; genital herpes; well tolerated, Side effects: May cause anemia in immunocompromised patients	No clinically significant interactions	For cold sores: take 2 grams orally twice a day at a 12-hour interval for only one day
Famciclovir (Famvir) tabs 125, 250, 500 mg	For primary and recurrent genital herpes; headache, nausea, and diarrhea	No clinically significant interactions	250 mg tid × 7–10 days (primary infection) 125 mg bid × 5 days (recurrent infection)
Ganciclovir (Cytovene) injectable	Neutropenia (low white blood cells); treatment of HSV in immunocompromised patients	No clinically significant interactions	Not significant

20% benzocaine (Orabase-B) may reduce the pain, burning, and itching. Patients who are allergic to para-aminobenzoic acid (PABA) or sulfonamides may also be allergic to benzocaine and tetracaine. Products containing camphor (not greater than 3%) and menthol (not greater than 1%) act as an analgesic to relieve the pain and itching (Table 7–2). Natural products such as bioflavonoids or acidophilus are not FDA approved. Examples of prescriptions are shown in Figure 7–3.

Rapid Dental Hint

Patients should use a finger cot when applying Orabase products and remember to dab it, not rub it, on the lesion.

Table 7-2 Over-the-Counter (OTC) Analgesic Medications for Treatment of Herpes Labialis

Analgesic (chemical name)	Product Name
Allantoin	Herpecin-L
Benzocaine	Anbesol, Orabase with benzocaine 20%
Benzyl alcohol	Zilactin
Camphor and phenol	Campho-Phenique Cold Sore Gel, Blistex, Carmex, ChapStick Medicated
Dyclonine	Tanac Medicated Gel, Orajel CoverMed
Lidocaine	Zilactin L

(Adapted from Mackowiak, E. D. 2003. Prevention and treatment of cold sores. *U.S. Pharmacist* 28:77–84.)

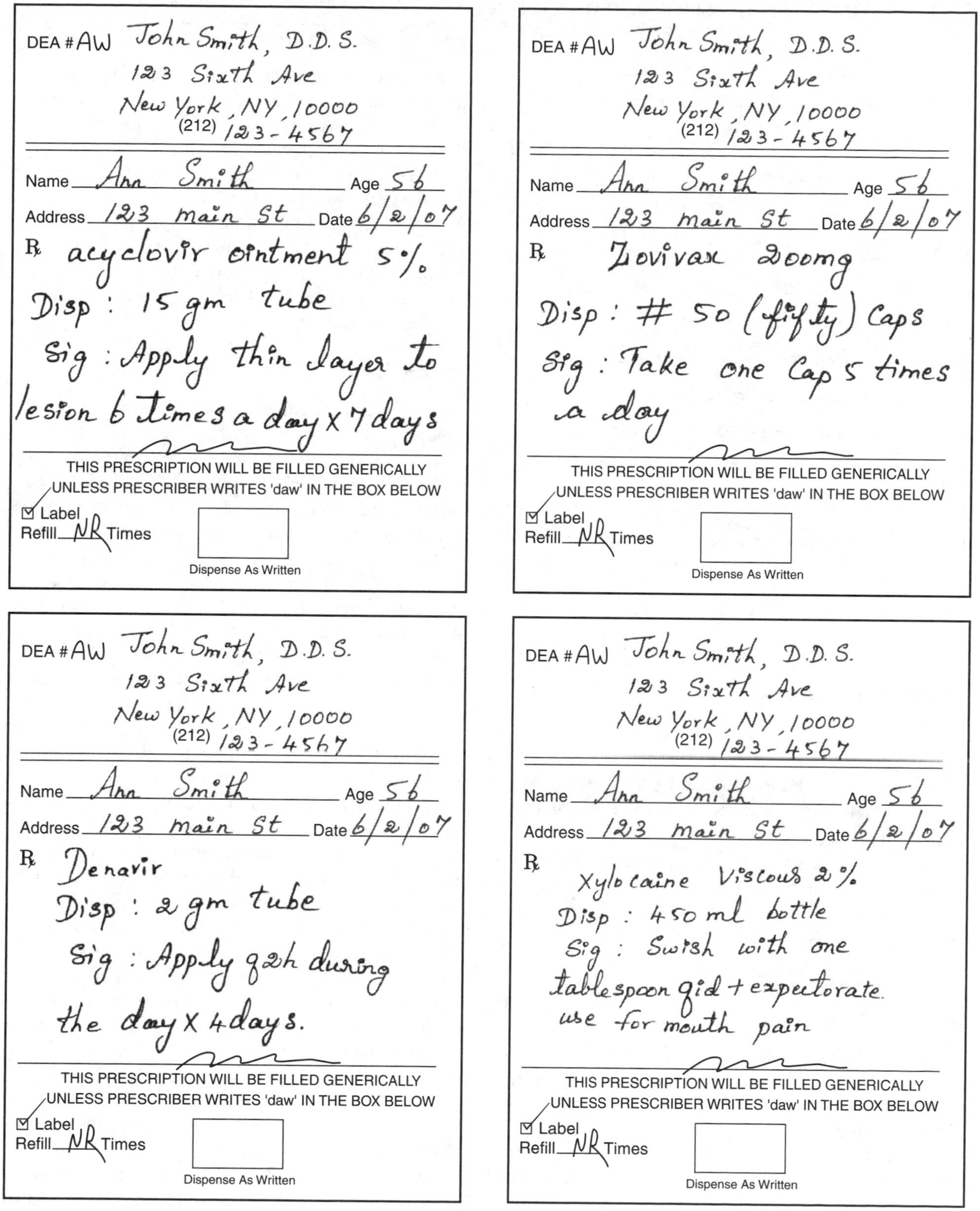

Prescription 1:

DEA #AW
John Smith, D.D.S.
123 Sixth Ave
New York, NY, 10000
(212) 123-4567

Name: Ann Smith   Age: 56
Address: 123 main St   Date: 6/2/07

Rx: acyclovir ointment 5%
Disp: 15 gm tube
Sig: Apply thin layer to lesion 6 times a day X 7 days

THIS PRESCRIPTION WILL BE FILLED GENERICALLY UNLESS PRESCRIBER WRITES 'daw' IN THE BOX BELOW
☑ Label
Refill NR Times
Dispense As Written

Prescription 2:

DEA #AW
John Smith, D.D.S.
123 Sixth Ave
New York, NY, 10000
(212) 123-4567

Name: Ann Smith   Age: 56
Address: 123 main St   Date: 6/2/07

Rx: Zovirax 200mg
Disp: # 50 (fifty) Caps
Sig: Take one Cap 5 times a day

THIS PRESCRIPTION WILL BE FILLED GENERICALLY UNLESS PRESCRIBER WRITES 'daw' IN THE BOX BELOW
☑ Label
Refill NR Times
Dispense As Written

Prescription 3:

DEA #AW
John Smith, D.D.S.
123 Sixth Ave
New York, NY, 10000
(212) 123-4567

Name: Ann Smith   Age: 56
Address: 123 main St   Date: 6/2/07

Rx: Denavir
Disp: 2 gm tube
Sig: Apply q2h during the day X 4days.

THIS PRESCRIPTION WILL BE FILLED GENERICALLY UNLESS PRESCRIBER WRITES 'daw' IN THE BOX BELOW
☑ Label
Refill NR Times
Dispense As Written

Prescription 4:

DEA #AW
John Smith, D.D.S.
123 Sixth Ave
New York, NY, 10000
(212) 123-4567

Name: Ann Smith   Age: 56
Address: 123 main St   Date: 6/2/07

Rx: Xylocaine Viscous 2%
Disp: 450 ml bottle
Sig: Swish with one tablespoon qid + expectorate. use for mouth pain

THIS PRESCRIPTION WILL BE FILLED GENERICALLY UNLESS PRESCRIBER WRITES 'daw' IN THE BOX BELOW
☑ Label
Refill NR Times
Dispense As Written

FIGURE 7–3 Sample prescriptions of drugs for oral herpes infection.

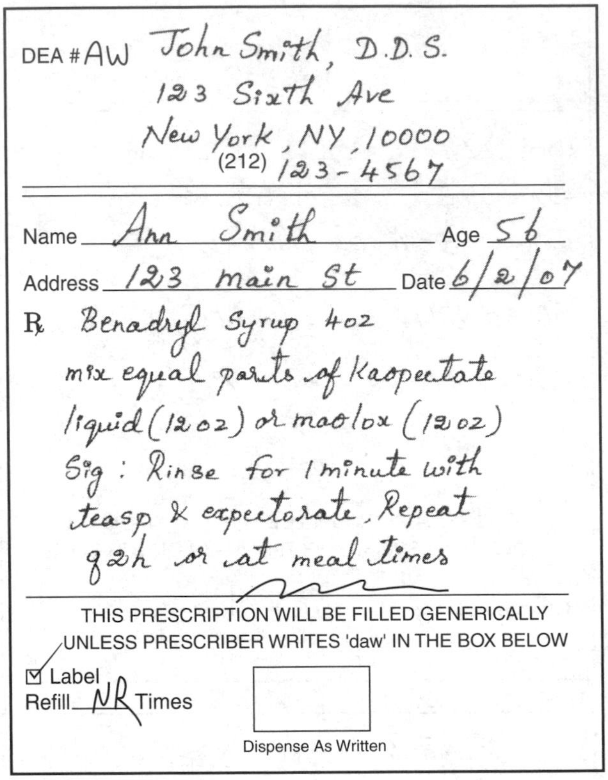

DEA # AW   John Smith, D.D.S.
123 Sixth Ave
New York, NY 10000
(212) 123-4567

Name _Ann Smith_   Age _56_

Address _123 main St_   Date _6/2/07_

R Benadryl Syrup 4oz
mix equal parts of Kaopectate
liquid (12oz) or maalox (12oz)
Sig: Rinse for 1 minute with
teasp & expectorate, Repeat
q2h or at meal times

THIS PRESCRIPTION WILL BE FILLED GENERICALLY
UNLESS PRESCRIBER WRITES 'daw' IN THE BOX BELOW

☑ Label
Refill _NR_ Times

Dispense As Written

FIGURE 7–3   (continued)

Rapid Dental Hint

There are no clinically significant dental implications with these drugs. To prevent reinfection or spread of infection, patients should not touch the lesion and should discard toothbrushes used during the infection.

ANTIFUNGAL AGENTS

Introduction

Fungal infections are caused by molds or yeasts. Some molds convert into yeasts once they infect the host. There are many types of fungal infections caused by different species of fungi.

The majority of healthy individuals have *Candida* species in the oropharyngeal (mouth) area. There are eight species of *Candida* that are regarded as clinically important pathogens in human disease. *Candida* is part of the normal flora in the gastrointestinal and vaginal tracts. Usually, *Candida* causes a localized superficial infection that is kept in check by the body; however, in certain circumstances such as immunocompromised hosts, the infection spreads.

The incidence of *Candida* infections has escalated over the years, with more immunocompromised individuals with AIDS. Histoplasmosis, a specific type of fungal infection caused by inhalation of dust-borne micro-organisms, is commonly found in the AIDS patient. These patients are also more prone to developing oral fungal infections.

Mycosis

Fungal infections (mycosis) are classified into three groups:

(1) systemic mycosis (e.g., soft tissue, meningitis, urinary tract infection); (2) superficial or mucocutaneous mycoses (e.g., nails, skin and mucous membranes); and (3) subcutaneous mycoses (e.g., infections from contaminated soil).

Dental clinicians are usually most concerned and are involved in the treatment of mucocutaneous mycoses of the mouth. Candidiasis may also present as vaginal candidiasis (vulvovaginitis, usually after antibiotic therapy) or as a diaper rash in infants. Other categories of mucocutaneous candidiasis include esophageal candidiasis and gastrointestinal candidiasis. The diagnosis of oral candidiasis is based on the clinical appearance of the lesions and by scraping of lesions.

Oral candidiasis usually responds to topical therapy if there are no systemic complications. Systemic antifungal agents are used primarily for fungal infections *not* involving the oropharyngeal area, but can be used for severe mucocutaneous candidiasis infections. Many fungal infections tend to recur after discontinuing drug treatment. Thus, antifungal drugs should be used for about 2 days after oral lesions disappear. Topical antifungal agents that can be applied to the oral mucosa include the oral suspension, vaginal cream, or ointment. Other formulations used in treating oral candidiasis include troches/pastilles or vaginal suppositories which are "sticky" and adhere to the oral mucosa so that they remain in the mouth for an extended period. Suppositories are less costly and have no sugar content, but may require psychological adjustment. Nystatin (Mycostatin) is usually given as an oral suspension that is swished around in the mouth and then swallowed, or as a lozenge (pastille) that dissolves slowly in the mouth. Nystatin functions to cause fungal cell lysis (break apart). Clotrimazole (Mycelex) is given as a 10 mg troche that is slowly dissolved in the mouth. Patients with a high caries index should not be given troches or nystatin oral suspension because of their high sugar content. An alternative choice is a systemic tablet. Severe and extensive oropharyngeal candidiasis can be treated with fluconazole (Diflucan), 100–200 mg orally twice a day. Prophylactic fluconazole is recommended for *Candida* suppression in HIV disease. Table 7–3 reviews common antifungal agents used to treat oral candidiasis. Figure 7–4 shows sample prescriptions for **antifungal agents** used in the management of oral fungal infections.

Table 7–3   Antifungal Agents: Mucocutaneous Candidiasis

Drug Name	Indications and Adverse Effects	Drug Interactions	Dental Notes
Topical	Indication: For mucocutaneous (superfical) mycoses; oral candidiasis (thrush) and skin/nail lesions	No significant drug interactions when using topical formulations.	No significant notes. Dentures should be soaked at night. Replace toothbrush after infection is cleared up.
Clotrimazole (Mycelex) Troche 10 mg (Lotrimin) cream	Troche: for oral (oropharyngeal candidiasis) lesions; to prevent oropharyngeal candidiasis in immunocompromised conditions (e.g., chemotherapy, radiotherapy). Cream/lotion: for severe skin and athlete's foot (tinea pedis); apply inside denture Nausea and vomiting (with oral troche) Rash, stinging, peeling with skin application	See above	Dissolve slowly (over 15–30 minutes) one troche (lozenge) five times a day (every 3 hours) for 14 days. The troche contains carbohydrates and should not be used on a long-term basis in patients with xerostomia because of increased incidence of caries.
Miconazole (Monistat) cream, lotion, vanginal suppositories, solution, powder, spray	If necessary can use for oral lesions (cream), but other products such as troches are better Vaginal infections; For vaginal candidiasis and tinea pedis (althlete's foot) Burning	See above	No significant notes
Nystatin (Mycostatin) oral suspension, pastilles (lozenge), vaginal tabs cream, ointment, powder	Oral suspension and pastille are effective for oral candidiasis, nausea, vomiting, diarrhea, abdominal pain, bad taste in mouth with lozenge and oral suspension. Vaginal tablets can be used orally since they are "sticky" to the oral mucosa. Cream, or powder are used for skin infections such as tinea pedis (althlete's foot).	See above	The oral suspension should be swished around in mouth for a few minutes and then swallowed. Use after meals and before bedtime. Do not eat or drink for 30 minutes after; Suck on the vaginal tablet or troche until it dissolves. Store in refrigerator. Dentures should be removed before using the oral suspension, lozenge or vaginal tablets. Remove dentures at night; the cream can be used orally by rubbing on to the affected area.

(continued)

Table 7–3   Continued

Drug Name	Indications and Adverse Effects	Drug Interactions	Dental Notes
			The lozenge contains carbohydrates and should not be used on a long-term basis in patients with xerostomia because of increased incidence of caries.
Systemic	Indication: Severe, chronic extensive subcutaneous and systemic mycosis. Oral and vaginal candidiasis caused by *Candida* sp.	See below	See below
Fluconazole (Diflucan) tab	For *severe oral lesions* or esophageal candidiasis. Systemic fungal infections (vaginal candidiasis, coccidioidal meningitis). Elevation of liver enzymes, nausea, vomiting, diarrhea	Metabolized by the P450 cytochromes in the liver. Several drug interactions, because ketoconazole inhibits the metabolism of several drugs by inhibiting the CYP3A4 isoenzyme, including: Benzodiazepines Calcium channel blockers Erythromycin Protease inhibitors (HIV). Slight increase in cyclosporine levels; Increases in phenytoin (Dilantin) blood levels Fluconazole is an inhibitor of CYP2C9 and warfarin is a substrate that is metabolized by CYP2C9: thus there is increased anticoagulant effect of warfarin. Decrease clearance of calcium channel blockers (e.g., diltiazem, verapamil).	Review medical history for medications. Make sure there are no interfering medications if the patient is prescribed fluconazole. Liver function tests need to be done monthly. Oropharyngeal candidiasis: 200 mg on day one followed by 100 mg every day for a minimum of 3 weeks and 2 weeks after symptoms resolve
Itraconazole (Sporanox) tab	For severe lesions (e.g., nail, vulvovaginal candidiasis) other than oral. Do not give to patients with heart failure or liver failure. Well tolerated. Some nausea, vomiting, headache, dizziness, hypertension	Decreased absorption when taken with antacids, anticholinergics, histamine H_2-antagonist, omeprazole sucralfate. Inhibits the CYP3A4 isoenzyme and inhibits metabolism of: Warfarin Benzodiazepines Calcium channel blockers Erythromycin Protease inhibitors (HIV). Cyclosporine levels are increased.	No significant dental notes. Do not take with antacids to reduce GI distress. Monitor liver function tests in patients with liver dysfunction.

Drug Name	Indications and Adverse Effects	Drug Interactions	Dental Notes
Ketoconazole (Nizoral) tab	For severe lesions other than oral. Well tolerated. Some side effects are nausea, vomiting, stomach discomfort	Decreased absorption when taken with antacids, anticholinergics, Histamine H_2-antagonist, omeprazole sucralfate. Metabolized by the P450 cytochromes in the liver and inhibits the CYP3A4 enzyme, causing increased blood levels of the above-mentioned drugs.	No significant dental notes. Monitor liver function tests.
Nystatin (Mycostatin) tab	Oral tablets are indicated for gastrointestinal candidiasis. Diarrhea, nausea, vomiting, GI upset, rash	No interactions	
Griseofulvin (Fluvicin, Grisactin, Grifulvin) tab	For severe lesions other than oral; not effective against *Candida.* For scalp and hair ringworm. High rate of hepatitis. Photosensitivity (increased incidence of burning when exposed to sun). Other drugs are more effective.	Induces liver metabolism of warfarin.	Not significant
Terbinafine (Lamisil) tab	For skin (Athlete's foot) and nail infections	Does not affect cyto-chrome P450 isoenzymes significantly. Clearance decreased with cimetidine (Tagamet).	Not significant
Amphotericin B (Fungizone) Parenteral	For severe skin fungal infection; (oral suspension for oral candidiasis); parenteral and topical administration; Hypertension, fever, chills, hypo-kalemia (low potassium levels), hypomagnesimia, GI discomfort, anemia, nephrotoxicity (kidney damage).	Additive nephrotoxicity with cyclosporine. Glucocorticosteroid may increase potassium loss.	Not significant

Did You Know?

Cryptococcus neoformas, a fungus discovered in the nineteenth century, can lead to brain infection and death in people with compromised immune systems (e.g., HIV).

Candidiasis: Acute Pseudomembranous Candidiasis (Thrush)

Acute pseudomembranous candidiasis or oral *thrush* appears on the oral mucous membranes as a white plaque that wipes off easily with gauze, leaving a raw, red, bleed-ing connective tissue surface. It is caused by an over-growth of *Candidia albicans,* which may be caused by factors that reduce the natural resistance, including:

- Systemic disease (uncontrolled diabetes mellitus)
- Immune-compromised patients (e.g., HIV/AIDS, chemotherapy, organ transplants)
- Use of broad-spectrum antibiotics
- Patients with poorly fitting dentures and who do not take it out at night (and are not immunocom-promised)

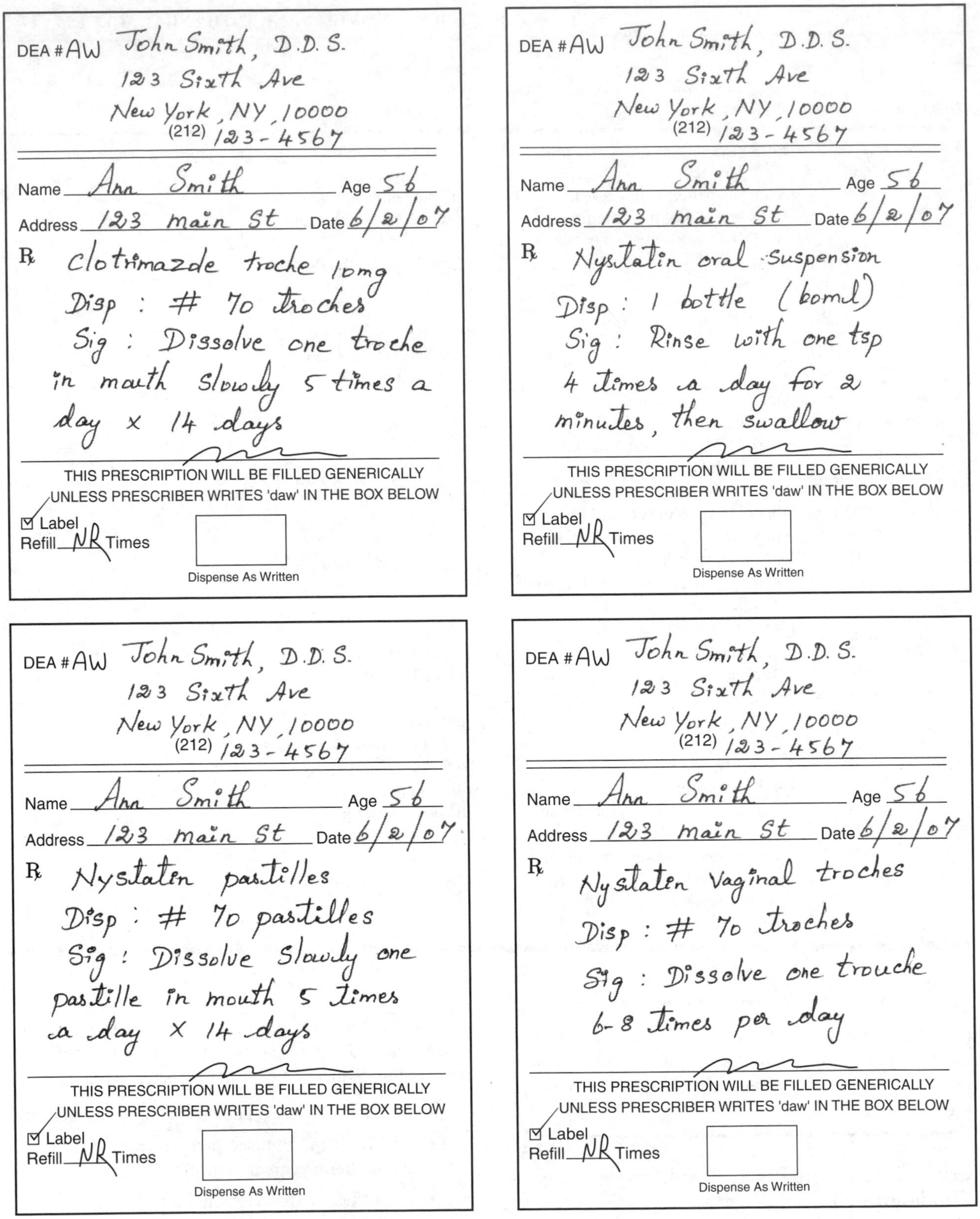

DEA #AW   John Smith, D.D.S.
           123 Sixth Ave
           New York, NY, 10000
              (212) 123-4567

Name   Ann Smith   Age 56
Address 123 main St   Date 6/2/07
℞   clotrimazde troche 10mg
    Disp : # 70 troches
    Sig : Dissolve one troche
    in mouth slowly 5 times a
    day x 14 days

THIS PRESCRIPTION WILL BE FILLED GENERICALLY
UNLESS PRESCRIBER WRITES 'daw' IN THE BOX BELOW
☑ Label
Refill NR Times   Dispense As Written

DEA #AW   John Smith, D.D.S.
           123 Sixth Ave
           New York, NY, 10000
              (212) 123-4567

Name   Ann Smith   Age 56
Address 123 main St   Date 6/2/07
℞   Nystatin oral suspension
    Disp : 1 bottle (60ml)
    Sig : Rinse with one tsp
    4 times a day for 2
    minutes, then swallow

THIS PRESCRIPTION WILL BE FILLED GENERICALLY
UNLESS PRESCRIBER WRITES 'daw' IN THE BOX BELOW
☑ Label
Refill NR Times   Dispense As Written

DEA #AW   John Smith, D.D.S.
           123 Sixth Ave
           New York, NY, 10000
              (212) 123-4567

Name   Ann Smith   Age 56
Address 123 main St   Date 6/2/07
℞   Nystaten pastilles
    Disp : # 70 pastilles
    Sig : Dissolve slowly one
    pastille in mouth 5 times
    a day x 14 days

THIS PRESCRIPTION WILL BE FILLED GENERICALLY
UNLESS PRESCRIBER WRITES 'daw' IN THE BOX BELOW
☑ Label
Refill NR Times   Dispense As Written

DEA #AW   John Smith, D.D.S.
           123 Sixth Ave
           New York, NY, 10000
              (212) 123-4567

Name   Ann Smith   Age 56
Address 123 main St   Date 6/2/07
℞   Nystaten vaginal troches
    Disp : # 70 troches
    Sig : Dissolve one trouche
    6-8 times per day

THIS PRESCRIPTION WILL BE FILLED GENERICALLY
UNLESS PRESCRIBER WRITES 'daw' IN THE BOX BELOW
☑ Label
Refill NR Times   Dispense As Written

FIGURE 7–4 Sample prescriptions of drugs for oral fungal infections.

DEA #AW John Smith, D.D.S.
123 Sixth Ave
New York, NY, 10000
(212) 123-4567

Name Ann Smith Age 56
Address 123 main St Date 6/2/07

℞ Mycolog II cream
Disp : 15 gm tube
Sig : Apply to affected area after meals and hs

THIS PRESCRIPTION WILL BE FILLED GENERICALLY
UNLESS PRESCRIBER WRITES 'daw' IN THE BOX BELOW
☑ Label
Refill NR Times

Dispense As Written

DEA #AW John Smith, D.D.S.
123 Sixth Ave
New York, NY, 10000
(212) 123-4567

Name Ann Smith Age 56
Address 123 main St Date 6/2/07

℞ Nystatin ointment
Disp : 15 g tube
Sig : Apply to infected area 4 times a day

THIS PRESCRIPTION WILL BE FILLED GENERICALLY
UNLESS PRESCRIBER WRITES 'daw' IN THE BOX BELOW
☑ Label
Refill NR Times

Dispense As Written

DEA #AW John Smith, D.D.S.
123 Sixth Ave
New York, NY, 10000
(212) 123-4567

Name Ann Smith Age 56
Address 123 main St Date 6/2/07

℞ Clotrimazole cream 1%
Disp : 15 g tube
Sig : Apply to affected area 4 times a day

THIS PRESCRIPTION WILL BE FILLED GENERICALLY
UNLESS PRESCRIBER WRITES 'daw' IN THE BOX BELOW
☑ Label
Refill NR Times

Dispense As Written

DEA #AW John Smith, D.D.S.
123 Sixth Ave
New York, NY, 10000
(212) 123-4567

Name Ann Smith Age 56
Address 123 main St Date 6/2/07

℞ Ketoconazole cream 2%
Disp : 15 g tube
Sig : Apply to affected area 4 times a day

THIS PRESCRIPTION WILL BE FILLED GENERICALLY
UNLESS PRESCRIBER WRITES 'daw' IN THE BOX BELOW
☑ Label
Refill NR Times

Dispense As Written

- elderly and pregnant women
- newborns are especially susceptible to an overgrowth of *Candida albicans* because they do not have an established oral flora or fully developed immune system

Treatment depends on the age of the patient. Nystatin oral suspension is recommended for infants. For adults, treatment is with topical or systemic antifungal agents such as fluconazole (Diflucan) or ketoconazole (Nizoral).

Chronic Atrophic Candidiasis (Denture Sore Mouth)

This condition is seen in patients with maxillary dentures. When the denture is removed the palatal tissue appears as either small, localized asymptomatic (not painful) red spots (in the mild form) and (in a more severe form) the entire tissue is red (outlining the shape of the denture) (Figure 7–5). This usually appears in patients who wear the denture continuously without removing it to clean it. It is a fungal infection caused by *Candida albicans.*

Since it is a fungal infection, topical antifungal agents are generally used. Nystatin (Mycostatin) pastilles/oral suspension/ointment, miconazole cream 2%, ketoconazole cream 2%, and clotrimazole (Mycelex) cream 2%/troches are some antifungal agents. The cream should be applied to the inner surface of the denture, a reline of the denture may be indicated. Patients with a high caries rate should not be given a suspension, trouches,

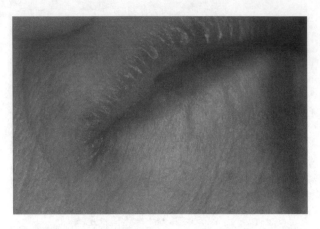

or pastilles because of the sugar content. The patient should be instructed not to wear the denture at night.

Angular Cheilosis

Angular cheilosis (or angular cheilitis) appears at the commissures of the lips (Figure 7–6). It is thought that this is a fungal infection caused by *Candida albicans* or a B-vitamin complex deficiency. Moist skin fold due to drooling and overclosure are added factors in the development of these lesions.

Since it is a fungal infection, topical antifungal creams/ointments are the drug of choice (Table 7–3).

Drug Interactions

There are many drug–drug interactions that are important with systemic agents and must be recognized. Drug interactions are reviewed in Table 7–3. Since systemic antifungal drugs are metabolized by the P450 cytochrome liver enzymes, many other drugs that also are involved in this system will interfere. Topically applied antifungal agents are not involved in this metabolism.

Subcutaneous and Systemic Mycosis

These fungal infections are not related to dentistry, and thus will not be discussed in depth. Sportrichosis is an example of subcutaneous mycoses seen especially in diabetics, and occurs usually after a splinter or a thorn from a plant that enters the skin.

Systemic or deep mycoses usually occur commonly after inhalation of the offending organism includ-

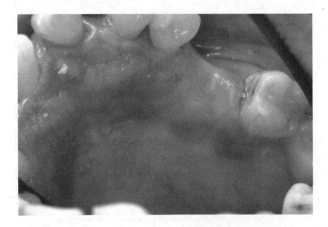

FIGURE 7–5   Denture sore mouth in a patient who never removed their partial denture at night. (Courtesy of U.S. Pharmacist).

ing *Aspergillus, Cryptoccocus* (from bird feces), *Blastomyces,* and *Candida.* Treatment of cryptococcosis is with amphotericin B, which is injectable and which can cause serious adverse effects.

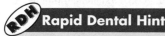

Rapid Dental Hint

Be aware of fungal infections in patients who wear dentures and do not practice good oral hygiene. Know their management.

DENTAL HYGIENE NOTES

In dentistry, mucocutaneous mycoses commonly present as infections of the oral mucous membranes. Thus, these infections will be managed by the dentist. Various causes of oral candidiasis (thrush), which is caused by the yeast *Candida albicans,* include broad-spectrum antibiotics, diabetes, inhalation corticosteroids, newborns, and in immunocompromised patients receiving immunosuppressive drugs that suppress the immune system and encourage fungi to overgrow.

Patients taking a broad-spectrum antibiotic (e.g., tetracycline, doxycycline, minocycline, amoxicillin) should be instructed to take supplemental acidophilus (found in the vitamin section of the pharmacy) or yogurt (not in combination with tetracycline) to help reduce the chances of developing a superinfection. Patients using a corticosteroid inhaler for asthma should be instructed to brush the teeth and rinse the mouth with water after each use to prevent development of oral candidiasis. Patients presenting with an oral infection (thrush) are best treated with a topical antifungal agent, which may be in the form of a troche, vaginal suppository, or oral suspension. Topical therapy has fewer side effects and a lower cost to the patient than systemic agents. If the oral infection is severe (oral and esophageal) such as in HIV disease, systemic antifungal agents may be used such as fluconazole (Diflucan).

Rapid Dental Hint

Remember to recommend to patients taking an antibiotic (e.g., tetraycycline, amoxicillin) to also take yogurt (except with tetracycline), or acidophilus to avoid developing a fungal infection.

KEY POINTS

- Herpes labialis is a herpes simplex type 1 viral infection.
- Antiviral drugs should be applied at the first sign of a cold sore.
- Antiviral drugs are noncurative, and only palliative.
- Acyclovir, famciclovir, and valacyclovir are systemic drugs used for herpes infections.
- Topical acyclovir and penciclovir are indicated for the management of herpes labialis.
- Docosanol (Abreva) is a cream that is available OTC.
- Oral candidiasis or thrush is caused by *Candida albicans.*
- Treatment of oral candidiasis is usually adequate with topical antifungal agents.
- Topical therapy for oral candidiasis is with nystatin oral suspension or clotrimazole troches.
- Many drug–drug interactions occur with systemic antifungal agents because these drugs are metabolized by the P450 cytochrome liver enzymes.

BOARD REVIEW QUESTIONS

1. Which of the following antiherptic drugs is recommended for herpes liabialis? (p. 140)
   a. Ganciclovir
   b. Famciclovir
   c. Valacyclovir
   d. Penciclovir

2. Which of the following drugs is contraindicated for treating herpes labialis? (p. 139)
   a. Hydrocortisone
   b. Docosanol
   c. Penciclovir
   d. Acyclovir

3. Herpes simplex virus 1 causes oral herpes. There is cross infection where both HSV-1 and HSV-2 are transmitted by intimate contact. (p. 138)
   a. Both statements are true.
   b. First statement is true and second is false.
   c. First statement is false and second is true.
   d. Both statements are false.

4. Which of the following antiviral agents is available over the counter for treating herpes labialis? (p. 140)
   a. Valacyclovir
   b. Docosanol

c. Penciclovir
d. Acyclovir

5. The major ingredient in Anbesol is? (p. 140)
   a. Lidocaine
   b. Camphor
   c. Benzocaine
   d. Benzyl alcohol

6. Which of the following terms is used for acute pseudomembranous candidiasis? (p. 145)
   a. Esophagitis
   b. Thrush
   c. Vaginitis
   d. Cryptococcosis

7. Which of the following drugs interacts with systemic fluconazole (Diflucan)? (p. 144)
   a. Erythromycin
   b. Penicillin
   c. Propranolol
   d. Digoxin

8. Which of the following is the treatment of choice in the prophylaxis and therapy of oral candidiasis? (p. 142)
   a. Nystatin suspension
   b. Ketoconazole tablets
   c. Fluconazole tablets
   d. Miconazole ointment

9. Which of the following clinical features is classic for oral candidiasis? (p. 142)
   a. Nonremovable creamy, white plaque
   b. Nonremovable creamy, white macule
   c. Removable creamy, white plaque
   d. Removable creamy, white macule

10. Which of the following agents is best for severe oropharyngeal candidiasis when topical therapy is inadequate? (p. 143)
    a. Griseovulvin
    b. Fluconazole
    c. Clotrimazole
    d. Nystatin

SELECTED REFERENCES

Abu-Elteen, K. H. and R. M. Abu-Elteen. 1998. The prevalence of *Candida albicans* populations in the mouths of complete denture wearers. *New Microbiol* 21:41–48.

Canker sores and cold sores 2005. *J Am Dent Assoc* 136(*3*):415.

Akpan, A. and R. Morgan. 2002. Oral candidiasis. *Postgraduate Medical Journal* 78:455-459.

Amir, J. 2002. Primary herpetic gingivostomatitis: Clinical aspects and antiviral treatment. *Harefusah* 141:81–84, 124.

Arduino, P. G. and S. R. Porter. 2006. Oral and perioral herpes simplex virus type 1 (HSV-1) infection: Review of its management. *Oral Dis* 12:254-370.

Birek, C. and G. Ficarra. 2006. The diagnosis and management of oral herpes simplex infection. *Curr Infect Dis Rep* 8:181–188.

Choi, S. Y. and H. Kahyo. 1991. Effect of cigarette smoking and alcohol consumption in the aetiology of cancer of the oral cavity, pharynx and larynx. *Int J Epidemiol* 20:878–885.

Engle, J. P. 2002. Oral pain and discomfort. In *APhA Handbook of Nonprescription Drugs: An Interactive Approach to Self-Care,* 13th ed. Washington, DC: American Pharmaceutical Association.

Fotos, P. G., S. D. Vincent, and J. W. Hellstein. 1992. Oral candidosis. Clinical, historical and therapeutic features of 100 cases. *Oral Sug Oral Med Oral Pathol* 74:41–49.

Heaton, M. L., I. Al-Hashimi, J. Plemons, T. Rees. 2006. Experimental chairside test for the rapid diagnosis of oropharyngeal candidiasis. *Compendium* 27:364–370.

Golecka, M., U. Oldakowska-Jedynak, E. Mierzwinska-Nastalska, A. Adamczyk-Kanli, F. Demirel, and Y. Sezgin. Oral candidosis, denture cleanliness and hygiene habits in an elderly population. *Aging Clin Exp Res* 2005;17:502–507.

Kolokotronis, A. and S. Doumas. 2006. Herpes simplex virus infection, with particular reference to the progression and complications of primary herpetic gingivostomatitis. *Clin Microbiol Infect* 12:202–211.

Mackowiak, Ed. Prevention and treatment of cold sores. *U.S. Pharmacist* 2003;28:77–84.

Ohman, S. C., G. Dahlen, A. Moller, and A. Ohman. Angular cheilitis: A clinical and microbial study. *J Oral Pathol* 1986;15:213–217.

Raborn, G. W., A. Y. Martel, M. Lassonde, M. A. O. Lewis, et al. Effective treatment of herpes simplex labialis with penciclovir cream: Combined results of two trials. *J Am Dent Assoc* 2002;133:303–309.

Reznik, D. A. Oral manifestastions of HIV disease. *Top HIV Med* 2005;13:143–148.

Rooney, J. F., S. E. Straus, M. L. Mannix, and C. R. Wohlenberg. Oral acyclovir to suppress frequently recurrent herpes labialis: A double-blind, placebo-controlled trial. *Ann Intern Med* 1993;118:268–272.

Seelig, M. S. Mechanism by which antibiotics increase the incidence and severity of candidiasis and later the immunological defenses. *Bacteriol Rev* 1966;30:442–459.

Sosinska, E. Candida-associated denture stomatitis in patients after immunosuppression therapy. *Transplant Proc* 2006;38:155–156.

Wong-Beringer, A. and J. Kriengkauykiat. Systemic antifungal therapy: New options, new challenges. *Pharmacotherapy* 2003;23(*11*):1441–1462.

Worrall, G. Herpes labialis. *Clin Evid* 2004;12:2312–2320.

WEB SITES

www.medscape.com
www.outlineMed.com
www.emedicine.com
www.jada.ada.org/cg/reprint/134/7/853.pdf

QUICK DRUG GUIDE

Antiherpetic Drugs

- Acyclovir sodium (Zovirax)
- Famciclovir (Famvir) tabs
- Valacyclovir (Valtrex) tabs
- Penciclovir (Denavir) Cream
- Docosanol (Abreva)
- Ganciclovir (Cytovene)

Antifungal Drugs

Topical

- Clotrimazole (Mycelex Lotrimen)
- Miconazole (Monistat)
- Nystatin (Mycostatin)

Systemic

- Fluconazole (Diflucan)
- Itraconazole (Sporanox)
- Ketoconazole (Nizoral)
- Griseofulvin (Fluvicin, Grisactin, Grifulvin)
- Terbinafine (Lamisil) tabs
- Amphotericin B (Fungizone)

Chapter 8

Local Anesthetics

GOAL: To gain knowledge of local anesthetics used in dentistry and their use in medically compromised patients.

EDUCATIONAL OBJECTIVES

After reading this chapter, the reader should be able to:

1. Discuss the mechanism of action of local anesthetics.
2. Classify local anesthetics used in dentistry.
3. Describe adverse effects of local anesthetics.
4. Describe the signs and symptoms of anesthetic toxicity.
5. Discuss the use of vasoconstrictors in medically compromised patients.

KEY WORDS

Local anesthetics
Nerve membrane
Vasoconstrictors
Epinephrine

INTRODUCTION

Local anesthetics are drugs used to prevent pain by inhibiting the conduction of nerve impulses along a nerve fiber. The degree of local anesthesia obtained is dependent on the method of administration, for example surface (applied directly to the surface that is to be anesthetized, such as the cornea), topical (drug is applied to the skin in the form of a cream/gel), infiltration (drug is injected below the skin), nerve block (injection close to a major nerve bundle), epidural (injection into the outer part of the spinal cord) or spinal (injection into the spinal canal).

HISTORY

The first local anesthetic agent to be used in dentistry was cocaine. In 1859, Albert Niemann discovered the intraoral anesthetic (numbing effect) of cocaine. Coca leaves were purified into coca extract and finally into cocaine. In 1884, Dr. Carl Koller, an Austrian ophthalmologist, performed the first surgery using topical cocaine on the cornea. In the same year, Dr. William Halsted used cocaine as an anesthetic agent for the first dental procedure. Due to the high incidence for addiction and a short

Did You Know?

Sigmund Freud, a famous psychiatrist, used cocaine on his patients as well as experimenting on himself, and became addicted.

duration of action, cocaine was no longer used for injections during dental procedures. Then in 1905 procaine, a synthetic substitute, was developed.

PROPERTIES OF LOCAL ANESTHETICS

Chemical Properties

The chemical aspects of local anesthesia are composed of an aromatic segment with either an amide bond or an ester bond to a basic side chain (Figure 8–1). Benzocaine is an exception to this, possessing no basic group. A bond links the lipophilic (fat-soluble) portion of the molecule with the hydrophilic (water-soluble) component. Local anesthetics without a hydrophilic portion are used only for topical administration. Local anesthetics of intermediate potency and duration of action, such as lidocaine, mepivacaine, and prilocaine are mainly used in dentistry.

The active ingredient in an anesthetic is called the anesthetic *base,* which is a weak base. A weak base does not ionize fully in an aqueous (body fluids) solution, resulting in a low pH level, which makes them poorly soluble in water and unstable in solution. Thus most anesthetics are combined with an acid such as hydrochloride (HCl) to form a salt, because it is more stable and soluble than the base.

Mechanism of Action

The **nerve membrane** or sheath is the site of action of local anesthetics. The pH (concentration of hydrogen H+ ion) of local anesthetics is generally about 4–5. Once the

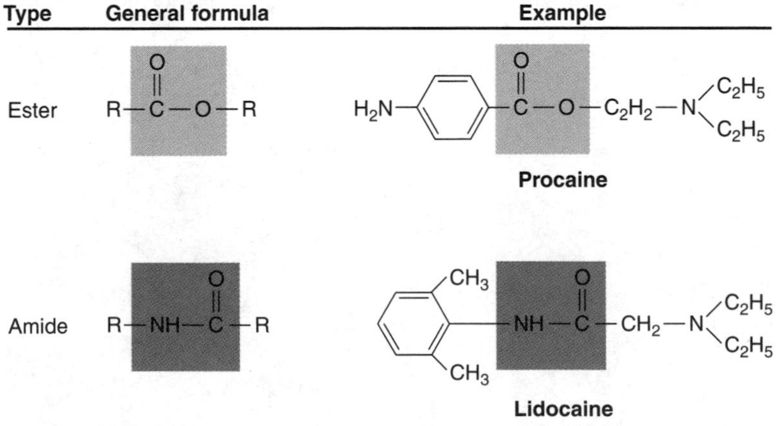

FIGURE 8–1   Chemical structures of ester and amide local anesthetics.

anesthetic solution is injected into the tissue, it changes rapidly to the more basic pH of the tissue, close to 7.4. In an aqueous solution such as body fluids, a local anesthetic will dissociate (dissolve and break down) into a nonionized (uncharged; neutral nonelectrolyte) form and an ionized (charged; electrolyte) form. When injected, the anesthetic is not in an active form. To be active, the nonionized or uncharged portion of the local anesthetic acts like a nonpolar (not water soluble), lipid-soluble compound that will readily transverse the lipid nerve cell membrane. Once inside the nerve, the ionized molecules block the sodium channels in the membrane, thus decreasing the permeability (passage) of the nerve membrane to sodium ions. This prevents the generation of action potentials (a stimulus applied to a nerve allowing sodium to move into the neuron) (Figure 8–2). The duration of action depends on the length of time that the drug can stay in the nerve to block the sodium channels.

Effects of pH

Local anesthetics are weak bases. pK_a has a direct effect on the onset of local anesthetics. pK_a determines the amount of base present in a solution, which also depends on the pH of the solution. When the pH is equal to the pK_a of a local anesthetic, then equal amounts of base and ionized species of the local anesthetic exist in solution. Thus, the lower the pKa value of the anesthetic, the more rapid the onset of action.

For instance:

Tissue pH = 7.4   Carbocaine pK_a = 7.6
Lidocaine pK_a = 7.9

There would be more molecules of carbocaine existing in the diffusible nonionized form because its pK_a is closer to tissue pH.

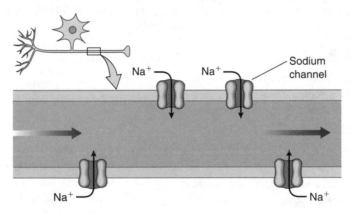

(a) Normal nerve conduction

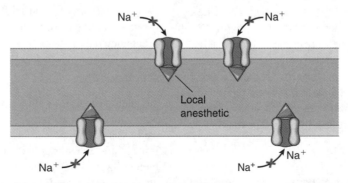

(b) Local anesthetic blocking sodium channels

FIGURE 8–2   How a local anesthetic blocks nerve conduction. (a) Normal nerve conduction; (b) local anesthetic blocking sodium channels.

Tissue Inflammation

At sites of tissue inflammation (e.g., abscesses) where the pH of the tissues is acidic (below a pH of around 6 or lower), the hydrogen ion concentration is increased, which increases the ionization of the local anesthetic and thus decreases the penetrability through the nerve sheath and its effectiveness.

Metabolism and Excretion

Metabolism of local anesthetic depends upon if it is an ester or amide. The ester local anesthetics are hydrolyzed (broken down) by plasma cholinesterase into para-aminobenzoic ACID (PABA). Amide local anesthetics are metabolized mainly in the liver by microsomal enzymes. Prilocaine has the lowest toxicity because it is metabolized the fastest. Active metabolites are excreted by the kidneys in the urine. Patients with severe kidney disease must have the dose reduced. Cocaine is the only local anesthetic that is excreted unchanged in the urine.

LOCAL ANESTHETIC AGENTS

Table 8–1 lists the various ester and amide agents. Today, amide agents (Table 8–2) have replaced the use of esters because lower incidence of allergies. Some amide agents include:

Lidocaine

First introduced in 1943, it is the most widely used amide anesthetic. It is available in an injectable form as 2% plain (without a vasoconstrictor; rarely used) and 2% with a vasoconstrictor (epinephrine) [1:100,000 (0.017–0.018 mg) and 1:50,000 (0.036 mg) epinephrine]. The amount of lidocaine per cartridge is 36 mg (20 mg/ml). As a topical anesthetic (ointment, cream, jelly, solution) it is available as a 10% concentration. Lidocaine is used in medicine as an antiarrhythmic to control cardiac (heart) excitability. Lidocaine has a pregnancy category of B. The maximum safe dose of lidocaine in a healthy adult should not exceed 500 mg. The maximum

> **Rapid Dental Hint**
>
> Remember to review the medical history before deciding on the appropriate local anesthetic.

dose in a child should not exceed 7 mg/kg of body weight in a single sitting.

Mepivicaine

First used in 1960. The brand name is Carbocaine. It has less vasodilation activity and low toxicity. The amount of mepivicaine per cartridge is 54 mg (of 3%) and 36 mg (of 2%). It is available in an injectable form as 2% solution with a vasoconstrictor [1:20,000 levonordefrin; 0.054 mg] and 3% plain. Levonordefrin is a less potent vasoconstrictor than epinephrine but is more likely to cause an increase in blood pressure. It has a rapid onset of action and is best used for dental procedures that require no more than 30 minutes of anesthesia.

The maximum dose should be calculated according to the patient's body weight. At any single dental sitting the total dose for all injected sites should not exceed 400 mg in adults. Mepivicaine has a pregnancy category of C.

Prilocaine

First introduced in 1960. The brand name is Citanest. It causes less tissue vasodilation than lidocaine. The advantage of using this agent is that it provides prolonged anesthesia with the least concentration of epinephrine. It is metabolized (converted) to *O*-toluidine, which is toxic and may cause methemoglobinemia if allowed to accumulate (see blood disorders).

Prilocaine is available in an injectable form as 4% with 1:200,000 epinephrine and 4% without a vasoconstrictor. There is less cardiac effect and it is especially useful in patients who are difficult to anesthetize. Anesthesia is adequate for up to 90 minutes. Prilocaine has a pregnancy category of B.

Articaine

An analogue of prilocaine. It was first used in the United States. Brand names are Septocaine, Zorcaine, and Ultracaine. It has a unique structure, containing both an amide linkage and as ester side chain. Since the ester does not metabolize to PABA, individuals allergic to ester are not allergic to articaine. It has a slightly faster onset of action and better diffusion than the other agents and long and profound anesthesia. The 4% solution has a higher incidence of paresthesia on mandibular blocks. Articaine has a pregnancy category of C.

Table 8-1 Local Anesthetic Agents

Drug	Onset	Vasoconstrictor	Duration of Action (with VC) (Infiltration) (Pulpal Anesthesia)	Duration of Soft Tissue Anesthesia (min)
Esters				
Benzocaine 20%, topical	Slow	None	Fast	N/A
Tetracaine (Pontocaine) topical, injectable	Slow	None	Fast	N/A
Amides				
Lidocaine 2% (Xylocaine) topical, injectable	Fast	EPI 1:100,000 1:50,000	60–90 min Moderate	180–240 min
Mepivacaine 2% (with vasoconstrictor), 3% (without vasoconstrictor) (Carbocaine; Polocaine)	Fast	Levonordefrin 1:20,000	2%: 50–75 min 3%: 25–40 min	2%: 120–240 min 3%: 120–180 min
Prilocaine 4% (Citanest) 4% without vasoconstrictor	Fast	EPI 1:200,000	45–90 min 20–60 min Plain	With VC:120–240 min Plain: 105 min
Bupivacaine 0.5% (Marcaine),	Intermediate	EPI 1:200,000	40–240 min	240–540 min
Etidocaine (Duranest)	Fast	EPI 1:200,000	40–240 min	240–540 min
Articaine 4% (Zorcaine, Septocaine, Ultracaine D-S, Ultracaine D-S Forte)	fast	EPI 1:100,000 1:200,000	60–95 min 45–60 min	120–360 min 120–360 min
Topicals, others				
Oraqix Periodontal Gel (Lidocaine/ prilocaine)	Slow	None	Fast	N/A
DentiPatch (Lidocaine Transoral Delivery)				

Adapted from: Haas, D. A. 2002. An update on local anesthetics in dentistry. *J Can Dent Assoc* 68(*9*): 546–551.

Bupivicaine

First made in 1956 as an epidural agent. The brand name is Marcaine. It was first used in dentistry in 1983 and is available in an injectable form 0.54% solution with epinephrine 1:200,000. It has a slow onset (up to 30 minutes, and may last two or three times longer than lidocaine and mepivacaine, up to 7 hours. Bupivicaine is usually used for lengthy dental procedures such as full mouth reconstruction and extensive and long periodontal or implant procedures. Bupivicaine can cause cardiotoxicity (e.g., ventricular arrhythmias) and has a pregnancy category of C.

Table 8–2   Recommended Maximum Doses of Local Anesthetics with Vasoconstrictor

Anesthetic	Maximum Dose	No. Cartridges
Articaine	Adult: 7 mg/kg (up to 500 mg)	7
	Child: 5 mg/kg	
Bupivicaine	Adult: 2 mg/kg (up to 200 mg)	10
	Child: 2 mg/kg	
Lidocaine	Adult: 7 mg/kg (up to 500 mg)	13
	Child: 7 mg/kg (3.2 mg/lb)	
Mepivicaine	Adult: 6.6 mg/kg (up to 400 mg)	11 (7 if plain)
	Child: 6.6 mg/kg	
Prilocaine	Adult: 8 mg/kg (up to 500 mg)	8
	Child: 8 mg/kg	

Example of calculation:

The maximum amount (number of cartridges) of lidocaine for a 40 lb child:

1. First convert lbs into kg
   Since 2.2 lbs = 1 kg, 2.2 × 18 = 40
   Thus, 40 lbs = 18 kg
2. Since the maximum dose is presented mg/kg, it is necessary to convert kg's into mg's.
   It is known that the maximum dose is 7 mg/kg (see above), which equals 7 mg per 1 kg of body weight.
   Thus, 7 × 18 kg = 126 mg
3. 2% lidocaine = 20 mg/ml (lidocaine: 20 mg of lidocaine/ml of solution) and each cartridge has 1.8 ml of solution, so there is 36 mg lidocaine/cartridge (20 × 1.8).
4. 126 mg divided by 20 mg/ml = 6 ml.
5. So, if there is 1.8 ml per cartridge, the maximum number of cartridges is 3.3 (6 divided by 1.8).

*Most U.S. manufacturers of local anesthetics made a labeling change in 2005. Each cartridge contains a minimum of 1.7 ml and a maximum of 1.8 ml. Calculations in this chapter used 1.8ml.
(Adapted from: Haas, D. A. An update on local anesthetics in dentistry. J Can Dent Assoc 2002;68(9): 546–551)

Etidocaine

A newer amide anesthetic that is similar to bupivicaine except it has a faster onset of action (3 minutes versus 6–10 minutes). The brand name is Duranest. It has a pregnancy category of B.

Lidocaine 2.5%/Prilocaine 2.5%

This is an anesthetic disc marketed under the name EMLA that is intended to reduce the pain of needle puncture. It is cream that is applied 1 hour before the shot or needle procedure and lasts for 1–2 hours after removal.

Topical Anesthetics

A topical anesthetic may be used before an injection of a local anesthetic to reduce discomfort associated with needle penetration. Systemic absorption of the topical anesthetic (e.g., lidocaine, benzocaine) must be considered when calculating the total amount of anesthetic ad-

ministered. Benzocaine has a pregnancy category of C and tetracaine B. Both anesthetics are contraindicated in patients taking a sulfa drug. Benzocaine is not administered by injection because of its tissue-irritating properties. If the patient is allergic to ester, topical benzocaine is contraindicated. Lidocaine and tetracaine produce effective local anesthesia whether they are injected into the tissue or used topically.

Oraqix, a gel that contains lidocaine 2.5%/prilocaine 2.5%, is administered into the gingival crevice for periodontal debridement. It has a pregnancy category of B.

VASOCONSTRICTORS IN LOCAL ANESTHETICS

Local anesthetics cause vasodilation, which increase the rate of absorption into the bloodstream (systemic circulation). This decreases the effectiveness of the local anesthetic and increases the anesthetic blood level, which may result in overdose. Essentially, there are two **vaso-**

constrictors used in local anesthetic solutions: epinephrine, or levonordefrin (Neo-Cobefrin). The addition of a vasoconstrictor counteracts the vasodilating effects of the anesthetic. Thus, the vasoconstrictor will:

- Constrict the blood vessels in the tissue, resulting in a decrease blood flow to the site of injection
- Slow the absorption of the agent into the bloodstream
- Lower blood levels that would decrease the risk of an overdose
- Decrease or prevent bleeding (hemostasis) at the site of injection
- Allow higher concentrations of the local anesthetic remaining in the nerve for a longer time (increase the duration of anesthetic effect). For example, 2% lidocaine lasts for about 10 minutes. With the addition of epinephrine, the duration of action is prolonged to about 60 minutes.

Epinephrine

Epinephrine is a more potent vasoconstrictor than levonordefrin. Epinephrine has no cardiac effect on the healthy individual. Epinephrine stimulates both α- and β-adrenergic (sympathetic) receptors at the same time; however, β_2-stimulation predominates at low doses and α-stimulation predominates at moderate to high doses.

Subcutaneous injection of epinephrine in *low doses* as used in dentistry will stimulate predominately β_2-receptors because these receptors have a higher affinity for epinephrine. Thus, epinephrine can selectively stimulate β_2-receptors, resulting in vasodilation of skeletal and smooth muscle. At high doses, the α_1-receptors will be occupied. Because there are more of these receptors, the primary effect at high doses is vascular smooth muscle contraction.

Epinephrine is available in many concentrations: 1:50,000, 1:100,000, and 1:200,000. *The maximum safe dose for epinephrine in healthy individuals is 0.2 mg and in cardiac patients is 0.04 mg.*

Levonordefrin

Levonordefrin (Neo-Cobefrin) is half as potent a vasoconstrictor as epinephrine. It primarily stimulates α-adrenergic (sympathetic) receptors, with little to no effect on the β-adrenergic receptors. Stimulation of α_1 receptors on tissues/organs causes vasoconstriction of blood vessels, resulting in hypertension (increased systolic and diastolic blood pressure). Epinephrine produces a greater stimulation of β_2-receptors than α_1 receptors, causing vasodilation and decreasing diastolic blood pressure. Higher doses produce more vasoconstriction and increased blood pressure. Since it is less effective/potent than epinephrine, it is used in higher concentrations (e.g., 1:20,000).

CLINICAL CALCULATIONS

Calculations of the recommended doses and maximum doses of anesthetics, the amount of the drug, and vasoconstrictor should be documented (Table 8–3).

SPECIAL PATIENT POPULATIONS
Children

The primary concern in children is the ease of overdose. Before administering a local anesthetic to a child, the child's weight must be used to calculate the appropriate dose (Table 8–2). In children under 10 years of age it is rarely necessary to administer more than 1/2 cartridge of lidocaine 2% with epinephrine per procedure.

It is best to administer a low-concentration solution such as lidocaine 2% with epinephrine 1:100,000. Bupivacaine should not be used because it has a long duration of action.

Pregnant and Nursing Women

Local anesthetics with vasconstrictors can be used safely in pregnant and nursing women. Because of its low concentration, lidocaine is preferred. The concentration of vascoconstrictors is low so that there is unlikely to be any affect on uterine blood flow.

Lidocaine	B
Mepivacine	C
Articaine	C
Bupivacaine	C

Elderly

There have been no documented differences in the response to local anesthetics with vasoconstrictors in the elderly versus younger adults; however, it is best to

Table 8–3   Calculation of the Amount of Local Anesthetic and Vasoconstrictor

Calculate the amount of lidocaine and EPI in 2 cartridges of 2% lidocaine/1:100,000 EPI:
1. Each cartridge contains 1.8 ml (average of 1.7–1.8 ml) of drug.* 2% lidocaine is equivalent to 36 mg lidocaine
2. Amount of epinephrine in 1:100,000 solution is 0.018 mg.
3. Thus, If you use 2 cartridges you have used 0.036 mg EPI and 72 mg of lidocaine.

Amount (in mg's) of Anesthetic (1.8 ml cartridge)

Percentage Concentration	Equivalent mg/ml (e.g., 2% = 20mg/ml)	Amount in a Cartridge (e.g., multiply by 1.8)
0.5%	5 mg/ml	9 mg
1%	10 mg/ml	18 mg
2%	20 mg/ml	36 mg
3%	30 mg/ml	54 mg
4%	40 mg/ml	72 mg

Amount of Vasoconstrictor (1.8 ml cartridge)

Vasoconstrictor	Dilution	Amount (mg) per Cartridge
Levonordefrin (in mepivicaine)	1:20,000	0.054
Epinephrine (in lidocaine)	1:50,000	0.036
Epinephrine (in lidocaine)	1:100,000	0.018

administer below the maximum recommended doses because the elderly may have slower metabolism.

ADVERSE EFFECTS OF LOCAL ANESTHETICS

Allergic Reactions

One of the most common adverse effects of local anesthetics that are reported by patients is allergy. However, in most cases it usually is not a true allergy and may be more of a reaction toward the epinephrine (e.g., the patient may experience palpitations and feel like their heart is racing). Predominately, there are allergies to ester because of para-aminobenzoic acid (PABA; used in some sunscreen products), its breakdown product. Antioxidants (e.g., sodium bisulfite and metabisulfite) are added to local anesthetics that contain vasoconstrictors to prevent biodegradation by oxygen. These antioxidants may cause an allergic potential.

At the end of the cartridge is the diaphragm, where the needle penetrates. This diaphragm is composed of latex and there is concern about patients with latex allergy because the latex allergen may leach from the diaphragm.

Central Nervous System

Toxicity of local anesthetics is a function of systemic absorption. High blood levels of the drug may be due to inadvertent intravascular injection or absorption (too much anesthetic injected).

Although the main systemic effect of local anesthetics is on the central nervous system (crosses the blood–brain barrier), in high blood concentrations there are cardiovascular effects, including hypotension and cardiac depression. At toxic levels they may cause seizures and cardiac arrhythmias. *Death from local anesthetic overdose is usually due to respiratory failure.* Local anesthetics may initially cause CNS stimulation (e.g., tremor, restlessness) followed by sedation and depressed CNS function. Patients may also experience headache and nausea. The danger to the systemic effects of epinephrine arise when the local anesthetic solution is injected into the blood vessels. Thus, it is imperative to use an aspirating syringe to ensure that no blood is found in the dental cartridge.

The use of cocaine (an ester) as a local anesthetic was first reported in 1884. Its potential to become addictive and its toxicity precludes its use as a dental anesthetic; however it is used for surface anesthesia (e.g., nose, ophthalmology) to obtain vasoconstriction. Cocaine, a very potent vasoconstrictor, works by inhibiting the reuptake of norepinephrine (NE), allowing for the accumulation of NE, which potentiates sympathetic nervous system activity (e.g., increased blood pressure and heart rate). It initially produces vasodilation, which is followed by an intense vasoconstriction of long duration.

Adverse reactions involving epinephrine include palpitations, tachycardia (rapid heart rate), anxiety, headache, tremor, and hypertension.

Blood Disorders

Methemoglobinemia

This is a rare and uncommon adverse reaction usually with high doses of prilocaine, but it may also occur with articaine and topical benzocaine. Normally, hemoglobin transports oxygen when the iron is in the ferrous form. When hemoglobin becomes oxidized, it is converted into methemoglobin, which does not bind to and transport oxygen. Normally, red blood cells are exposed to various oxidant stresses so that blood normally contains about 1% methemoglobin. Excessive methemoglobin levels (methemoglobinemia) reduce the amount of hemoglobin that is available for oxygen transport to the tissues. Clinical signs include blood that is dark in color, headache, weakness, confusion, chest pain and grayness/cyanosis of lips, mucous membranes, and nail beds. When methemoglobin levels are above 70 percent, death may result if not treated immediately. Treatment of

---

Did You Know?

In 1888, John S. Pemberton, a pharmacist, invented a beverage which contained caffeine and cocaine. Today, this beverage is known as Coca-Cola.

---

methemoglobinemia is with methylene blue administered with an IV over a 5-minute period. Results are typically seen within 20 minutes. Administration of methylene blue reduces methemoglobin back to hemoglobin.

Liver Disease

Since there is a decreased metabolism of local anesthetics in patients with severe liver disease (e.g., hepatitis, cirrhosis of the liver) a medical consultation with the patient's physician is required. A patient with severe liver disease still requires the standard amount of anesthetic, but the total dose must be reduced or minimized.

TREATMENT OF TOXICITY

Acute emergencies from local anesthetics are first managed by constant monitoring of cardiovascular and respiratory vital signs and the patient's state of consciousness. If there are changes in the patient's condition, oxygen should be administered. Convulsions may also occur. Emergency operation should be employed.

SELECTION OF THE LOCAL ANESTHETIC

Selection of the appropriate local anesthetic for the dental patient depends upon:

1. Duration of the dental procedure; amount of time pain control is required
   a. Short procedure (especially involving mandibular block): solutions without vasoconstrictor such as mepivicaine or prilocaine plain
   b. Longer procedure: bupivacaine has a long duration of action
2. Anticipation of postoperative pain; choose a longer duration anesthetic to cover postoperative pain
   a. Bupivicaine
3. Contraindications (e.g., drug interaction; disease) for a specific anesthetic
   a. If epinephrine is contraindicated, use mepivicaine or prilocaine plain
4. Routine procedures
   a. Use of EPI is justified for most dental procedures
   b. Lidocaine, articaine, prilocaine, or mepivicaine
5. Children and pregnant patients
   a. Lidocaine

DENTAL MANAGEMENT OF MEDICALLY COMPROMISED PATIENTS

Diseases and Disorders

Hypertension

Using vasoconstrictors in hypertensive patients is only contraindicated if it is severely uncontrolled; however, precautions using lower concentrations of vasoconstrictors and cardiac monitoring are taken in patients with controlled hypertension. Blood pressure should be monitored before and during dental treatment for any changes in blood pressure.

Patients taking a nonselective β_1/β_2- blocker such as propranolol (Inderal), metoprolol (Toprol), nadolol (Corgard), or timolol (Blocardren) may have an increased pressor response to epinephrine, but this effect is unlikely with low doses of epinephrine. Blocking vasodilating β_2-receptors in the blood vessels of skeletal and smooth muscle and the β_1-receptors, which lowers heart rate, causes epinephrine to act vascularly as a pure α_1-adrenergic stimulant. The initial dose should be minimal (1/2 cartridge), which should be injected slowly using aspiration to avoid intravascular injection. After waiting and monitoring for toxicity for a few minutes, more of the anesthetic may be injected. The maximum dose of epinephrine to be used in a patient taking nonselective β-blockers is 0.04 mg of epinephrine, equivalent to 2 cartridges (0.018 mg per cartridge 1:100,000) and 0.2 mg of levonordefrin (0.05 mg/cartridge 1:20,000). The benefits for maintaining adequate anesthesia (reducing the pain) outweigh the risks for toxicity. Careful monitoring for toxicity (e.g., increased blood pressure, cardiac arrhythmias including tachycardia) should be done. Epinephrine 1:50,000 should be avoided, as well as gingival retraction cord containing epinephrine used in restorative dentistry.

ⓇⒹⒽ Rapid Dental Hint

Remember: To reduce the incidence of toxicity, you should administer the local anesthetic slowly and aspirate or use an aspirating syringe.

Thus epinephrine or levodordefrin may be used in patients taking nonselective β-blockers, but the initial dose should be kept to a minimum (e.g., ½ cartridge of lidocaine with epinephrine 1:100,000).

There are no major concerns in patient taking cardioselective $\beta1$-blockers such as atenolol (Tenormin), metoprolol (Lopressor), acebutolol (Sectral), or betaxolol (Kerlone) because these drugs act only on $\beta1$-receptors.

Heart Failure/Angina/Stroke/Myocardial Infarction

In patients with heart failure and angina pectoris, the amount of vasoconstrictor should be minimized with prudent cardiac monitoring before and during anesthesia administration. Epinephrine is contraindicated in patients that have had a stroke or heart attack within the last 6 months. Epinephrine is also contraindicated in patients that had a coronary bypass or unstable angina within the last 3 months.

Diabetes Mellitus

Patients with controlled type 1 or type 2 diabetes mellitus can generally be given vasoconstrictors without special precautions. Patients who are not well controlled with fluctuating blood glucose (sugar) levels or taking high doses of insulin should have the amount of epinephrine limited. Epinephrine is able to counteract the hypoglycemic effects of insulin by elevating blood glucose. Epinephrine mobilizes liver carbohydrate stores and stimulates the production of lactic acid from glycogen in muscle (glycogenolysis). The lactic acid may be used by the liver to manufacture new carbohydrate (glucose), elevating blood glucose. Thus in these patients the amount of vasoconstrictor should be minimized.

Adrenal Disease

Vasoconstrictors are contraindicated in patients with pheochromocytoma. Pheochromocytoma is a tumor of the adrenal medulla characterized by increased secretion of epinephrine, which leads to hypertension and cardiac arrhythmias.

Thyroid Disease

Vasoconstrictors (e.g., epinephrine) should be avoided in patients with thyrotoxicosis (hyperthyroidism). Patients with excessive thyroid hormone levels develop hypertension and arrhythmias. However, in patients taking thyroid hormone replacement (Synthroid) and who are well controlled, no special precautions are needed.

Blood Dyscrasias

The use of prilocaine is contraindicated in patients with methemaglobinemia.

Asthma

Vasoconstrictor use should be minimized in asthmatic patients taking corticosteroids because the anesthetic solution contains sulfites, which may cause an allergic reaction in asthmatics.

Bronchitis

Bronchitis and emphysema are the most common forms of chronic obstructive pulmonary disease. No special precautions are needed with administration of local anesthetics.

Drugs

Cocaine User

Many times a patient may not willfully report the use of recreational cocaine. Vasoconstrictors should not be used in the patient for at least 24 hours after the last use of cocaine to allow for metabolism and elimination of the drug: Patients enter into irreversible cardiac arrhythmia, which is the primary cause of death.

Tricyclic Antidepressants and Monoamine Oxidase Inhibitors

The administration of local anesthetics with vasoconstrictors to patients receiving tricyclic antidepressants (e.g., Elavil) may produce severe, prolonged hypertension. There is no evidence of a significant interaction with monoamine oxidase inhibitors (MAOIs).

Tricycylic antidepressants block the reuptake of norepinephrine and serotonin back into the nerve. This causes an increase in the amounts of norepinephrine, which is deficit in patients with depression and obsessive-compulsive disorders. Epinephrine is also eliminated by the reuptake into the nerve endings. Norepinephrine (NE) differs from epinephrine in that it has a greater affinity for $\beta 1$-adrenergic receptors than for β_2-receptors. NE constricts all blood vessels; pinephrine constricts only some blood vessels and dilates others. Thus extreme precaution should be used in patients taking tricyclic antidepressants, because severe and prolonged hypertension may result. According to the drug insert from the manufacturer, the combination of a vasoconstrictor and a tricyclic antidepressant should be avoided. Other sources state that these patients should be treated similarly to cardiac patients receiving local anesthetics with vasoconstrictors. The amount of epinephrine used in the local anesthetic should be limited to two cartridges of lidocaine with 1:100,000 epinephrine, equivalent to 0.036–0.54

mg epinephrine; any additional injections should be given 30 minutes apart. Levonordefrin (contained in mepivacaine) should be avoided because of a greater chance of developing hypertension due to receptor stimulation. Gingival retraction cord containing epinephrine for tooth impressions should be avoided. The patient's cardiac condition should be monitored by taking blood pressure. If an adverse reaction occurs, this can be controlled by the use of an alpha-receptor blocker drug such as phentolamine.

Selective Serotonin Reuptake Inhibitors (SSRIs)

There are no vasoconstrictor interactions with SSRI such as paroxetine (Paxil), fluoxetine (Prozac), and sertraline (Zoloft). Blocking serotonin reuptake has no affect on epinephrine.

Antipsychotics

Antipsychotics such as aripiprazole (Abilify), clozapine (Clozaril), and olanzapine (Zyprexa) can block α-adrenergic receptors. Thus the use of epinephrine may cause hypotension and tachycardia (increased heart rate). Minimal amount of EPI may be used and the patient's vital signs should be monitored.

DENTAL HYGIENE NOTES

The use of local anesthetics with vasoconstrictors in medically compromised patients generally can be given safely. The anesthetic solution should be aspirated before injecting to avoid intravascular introduction of the solution, which would result in systemic involvement. The solution should then be administered slowly.

Selection of the type of anesthetic and whether to use a vasoconstrictor is based on patient history, and type and duration of the procedure (extraction, periodontal debridement, periodontal surgery). It is ideal to use a local anesthetic without a vasoconstrictor for short procedures using a mandibular block. On the other hand, bupivacaine is best for long procedures because it has a long duration of action. Lidocaine is preferred in children and pregnant patients. For conventional dental procedures, articaine, lidocaine, mepivicaine, or prilocaine can be considered. Prilocaine, and maybe articaine and topical benzocaine, should be avoided in patients with congenital methemoglobinemia. The goal is to use the minimal amount of anesthetic/vasoconstrictor that is needed to obtain profound anesthesia.

Documentation in the treatment record must include the type and dosage of local anesthetic in milligrams. Vasoconstrictor, if any, must be noted whether in milligrams or concentration (for example, 36 mg lidocaine 2% with 0.018 mg 1:100,000 epinephrine). Documentation must also include the type of injection given (e.g., infiltration, block).

KEY POINTS

- Anesthetics block sodium channels in the nerve cell membrane.
- anesthetic is less effective in inflamed, acidic tissue
- Levonordefrin (Neo-Cobefrin) is half as potent a vasoconstrictor as epinephrine
- levonordefrin stimulates α-adrenergic (sympathetic) receptors with little to no effect on the β-adrenergic receptors, causing hypertension
- precautions are needed when using vasconstrictors in certain medically compromised patients
- use no more than 0.04 mg of epinephrine for patients with cardiovascular disease
- Prilocaine, topical benzocaine, and topical lidocaine may cause methemoglobinemia clinically characterized by cyanosis (low oxygen).

BOARD REVIEW QUESTIONS

1. Which of the following agents primarily stimulates α$_1$-receptors, causing increased blood pressure? (p. 159)
   a. Lidocaine
   b. Mepivicaine
   c. Epinephrine
   d. Levonordefrin

2. Which of the following agents is available as a topical formulation? (p. 157)
   a. Mepivicaine
   b. Lidocaine
   c. Articaine
   d. Bupivicaine

3. The concentration (in mg's) of epinephrine in one cartridge of lidocaine 2% and 1:100,000 epinephrine is: (p. 160)
   a. 0.018
   b. 0.18
   c. 0.036
   d. 0.36
   e. 0.54

4. The concentration (in mg's) of levonordefrin in carbocaine 2% is: (p. 160)
   a. 0.018
   b. 0.18
   c. 0.036
   d. 0.36
   e. 0.09

5. Death from an overdose of a local anesthetic is usually due to: (p. 160)
   a. Cardiac stimulation
   b. Respiratory failure
   c. Bradycardia
   d. Tachycardia

6. Which of the follow anesthetics is an ester? (p. 157)
   a. Benzocaine
   b. Lidocaine
   c. Mepivicaine
   d. Etidocaine

7. Which of the following anesthetics is a potent vasoconstrictor? (p. 161)
   a. Cocaine
   b. Mepiviance
   c. Lidocaine
   d. Bupivicaine

8. Which of the following anesthetics contains levonordefrin as a vasoconstrictor? (p. 160)
   a. Lidocaine
   b. Procaine
   c. Bupvicaine
   d. Mepivicaine

9. The volume of an anesthetic cartridge is (p. 160)
   a. 1.8–1.9 ml
   b. 1.7–1.8 ml
   c. 2.0–2.4 ml
   d. 3.0–3.1 ml

10. Which of the following local anesthetics can cause methemaglobinemia? (p. 161)
    a. Prilocaine
    b. Lidocaine
    c. Articaine
    d. Bupivicaine

SELECTED REFERENCES

Bader, J. D., A. J. Bonito, and D. A. Shugars. 2002. A systematic review of cardiovascular effects of epinephrine on hypertensive dental patients. *Oral Surgery, Oral Medicine, Oral Radiology and Endodontics* 93:647–653.

Budenz, A. W. Local anesthetics in dentistry: Then and now. *J California Dental Association* 2003;31:388–396.

Budenz, A. W. Local anesthetics and medically complex patients. *J California Dental Association* 2000;28:611–619.

Carroll, A. and G. P. Sesin. A case study of benzocaine-induced methemoglobinemia. *U.S. Pharmacist* 2002;27(*12*):HS-44-HS-46.

Haas, D. A. 2002. An update on local anesthetics in dentistry. *J Can Dent Assoc* 68(*9*): 546–551.

Hersh, E. V., H. Giannakopoulos, L. M. Levin, P. A. Moore, M. Hutcheson, A. Mosenkis, and R. R. Townsend. The pharmacokinetics and cardiovascular effects of high-dose articaine with 1:100,00 and 1:200,000 epinephrine. *JADA* 2006;137(*11*):1562–1571.

Horlocker, T. T., and D. J. Wedel. Local anesthetic toxicity—Does product labeling reflect actual risk? *Regional Anesthesia and Pain Medicine* 2002;27:562–567.

Neal, J. M. Effects of epinephrine in local anesthetics on the central and peripheral nervous systems: Neurotoxicity and neural blood flow. *Regional Anesthesia and Pain Medicine* 2003;28:124–134.

Yagiela, J. A. Adverse drug interactions in dental practice: Interactions associated with vasoconstrictors. Part V of a series. *JADA* 1999;130:701–709.

WEB SITES

www.adha.org/governmental_affairs/downloads/local
anesthesia.pdf

www.guideline.gov

www.ada.org/prof/resources/topics/color.asp

www.ncbi.nlm.nih/gov/entrez/query.fcgi?cmd=Retrieve&db=
PubMed&list_uids=12636129&dopt=Abstract

QUICK DRUG GUIDE

Esters

- Benzocaine 20% (Hurricaine), topical
- Tetracaine (Pontocaine), topical, injectable
- Tetracaine + benzocaine (Cetacaine), topical
- Cocaine, topical

Amides

- Lidocaine (Xylocaine, Octocaine 50, 100)
  topical, injectable
- Mepivacaine (Carbocaine), injectable
- Prilocaine (Citanest), injectable
- Bupivacaine (Marcaine), injectable
- Etidocaine (Duranest), injectable
- Articaine (Septocaine; Zorcaine; Ultracaine D-S
  Forte, Ultracaine D-S), injectable

Other

- Lidocaine and prilocaine gel (Oraqix), topical
- Lidocaine (DentiPatch), transoral

Chapter 9

Sedation and General Anesthetics

GOAL: To gain knowledge about pharmacologic agents used for minimal-moderate sedation, anxiety control, and general anesthesia in the dental patient.

EDUCATIONAL OBJECTIVES

After reading this chapter, the reader should be able to:

1. Summarize the concepts of minimal, moderate and deep sedation.
2. List various pharmacologic agents used for moderate sedation.
3. List the objectives in using sedation to manage dental patients.
4. Discuss the role of nitrous oxide in the dental office.

KEY TERMS

Moderate sedation
Minimal sedation
General anesthesia
Nitrous oxide

INTRODUCTION

The management of fear and anxiety is an integral part of patient care in the dental office. Today a wide variety of equipment and medications are available to the dental clinician to help deal with patient apprehension of dental treatment.

Many types of drugs are used in anesthesia during minor and major surgery in hospitals and dental offices. These drugs produced CNS depression and analgesia, with a reversible loss of consciousness and the absence of response to painful stimuli. Dentists must be trained to use moderate sedation and general anesthesia. Dental hygienists may administer nitrous oxide.

TERMINOLOGY

Moderate sedation (previously known as conscious sedation) refers to the administration of drugs for the purpose of sedation (sleepiness), lack of awareness of surroundings (narcosis), amnesia (loss of memory), or analgesia (increased pain threshold without loss of consciousness so the patient still responds to verbal (arousable) and physical stimuli during stressful dental/medical procedures. Moderate sedation is not expected to induce depths of sedation that would impair the paitent's own ability to maintain the integrity of the airway. Thus intubation is usually not required, but may be in order to manage the airway and support vital signs. This procedure can be performed in the hospital or dental office by qualified dentists. General anesthesia is not routinely used for dental procedures because skeletal muscle relaxation and unconsciousness is not the goal. Thus, in dentistry minimal/moderate sedation/analgesia is used.

Minimal sedation (anxiolysis) is a drug-induced state during which patients respond normally to verbal commands. Although cognitive function and coordination may be impaired, ventilatory and cardiovascular functions are unaffected.

Deep sedation/analgesia is a drug-induced depression of consciousness during which patients cannot be easily aroused, but respond purposefully following repeated or painful stimulation. The patient breathes spontaneously but maintenance of a free airway may be impaired. Optimal sedation in these circumstances would include quick onset, low cardiopulmonary depression, and rapid recovery. It is possible to move from moderate sedation to deep sedation without recognition, and the varying levels of deep sedation may overlap with general anesthesia. Patients under deep sedation require more cardiac, blood pressure, and respiratory monitoring than under conscious sedation. Deep sedation is done in a hospital setting.

General anesthesia is an induced state of unconsciousness together with a *partial* or *complete* loss of protective reflexes, including the inability to maintain an airway independently and respond to physical stimulation or verbal command. A ventilator (endotracheal intubation is performed to put a tube into the trachea) breathes for the patient during the surgical procedure. General anesthesia is primarily used for lengthy surgical procedures. Balanced anesthesia is used where low doses of several drugs, rather than one drug, with different actions are given to minimize adverse events and provide recovery of the protective reflexes within a few minutes of the end of the surgical procedure.

ROUTES OF ADMINISTRATION

Different routes of administration of pharmacologic agents used to induce and maintain general anesthesia/conscious sedation are available and include:

- Enteral: Absorption is through the G.I. tract (e.g., oral, rectal, sublingual), the most common route for conscious sedation.
- Parenteral: absorption bypasses the G.I. tract, e.g., intravenous (IV) and subcutaneous (SC). The subcutaneous route of drug administration is usually used in pediatric dentistry because of a more rapid onset of action and more profound clinical effects.
- Inhalational: Gaseous or volatile drug is introduced into the lungs.
- Transdermal: Drug is administered by a patch or iontophoresis.

TYPES OF ANESTHESIA

- *Oral Moderate Sedation* is obtained via the enteral route. A disadvantage of this route is that a large initial dose must be given and absorption is not predictable, nor easily reversible.
- *Inhalation moderate sedation* is obtained via inhalation via the lungs. Nitrous oxide/oxygen is administered through this route only for anxiolysis, and not for anesthesia. Advantages of this route include easy adjustment of depth of sedation and rapid recovery.

- *Combined moderate sedation* is obtained via enteral and/or combination inhalation (e.g., nitrous oxide/oxygen)/enteral conscious sedation. The combined route is more effective than either route used alone.
- *Intravenous moderate sedation* is the most effective method of obtaining adequate and predictable sedation. A generalized misconception is that intravenous sedation is synonymous with general anesthesia. It is not, because the patient has a minimally depressed level of consciousness and can maintain an airway.
- *General anesthesia* is obtained via intravenous and inhalation of drugs.

THERAPEUTIC USES

General anesthesia is administered to patients undergoing major general surgery in the hospital in the treatment of injury, deformity, and disease. Areas of the body treated by general surgery include the stomach, liver, intestines, heart, and eyes.

Moderate sedation is administered to patients undergoing minor surgical procedures. It is used in the dental office or hospital to make the patients unaware of their surroundings and to provide analgesia (relieve pain). The same agents used for general anesthesia are used to induce conscious sedation.

PATIENT PHYSICAL STATUS CLASSIFICATION

Every patient seen in the medical/dental office or hospital is given a physical status classification according to the American Society of Anesthesiologists. This classification is used to determine the medical status of the patient and should be done before treatment is started. Patients receiving anesthesia should be medically stable with an ASA I or II. A medical consultation from the patient's physician may be required, especially for ASA III or IV. Table 9–1 reviews the classification of a patient's physical status.

MODERATE SEDATION IN THE DENTAL OFFICE

The goal of moderate sedation is to achieve anxiety reduction, pain control, and amnesia in the dental patient. The patient's mood must be altered so that dental treatment will be tolerated. The patient remains responsive

Table 9–1 Patient Physical Status Classification

ASA I	Normal, healthy patient
ASA II	Patient with mild systemic disease: type 2 diabetes, hypertension
ASA III	Patient with severe systemic disease: stable angina, type 1 diabetes, chronic obstructive pulmonary disease
ASA IV	Patient with severe systemic disease that is a constant threat to life: heart attack within 6 months, unstable angina, uncontrolled diabetes or uncontrolled epilepsy
ASA V	Moribund patient who is not expected to survive without the operation: patient is not expected to survive 24 hours with or without medical intervention
ASA VI	A declared brain-dead patient whose organs are being removed for donor purposes
E	Emergency operation used to modify any of the above classifications

ASA: the American Society of Anesthesiologists.
E: emergency.

and cooperative during the dental procedure. Additionally, the patient's airway remains open. Although dental hygienists cannot administer conscious sedation, they will be performing dental procedures on these patients and must be familiar with specific agents and their safe and effective use.

The objectives for moderate sedation differ depending upon the dental case. For instance, a long periodontal surgical procedure such as dental implants or grafting in an anxious and fearful patient may require a regimen that includes analgesic and amnesic properties, whereas managing an uncooperative patient during a minor restorative or periodontal procedure may just require orally administered mood alteration drugs or nitrous oxide.

Dentists providing moderate sedation must be qualified to recognize deep sedation, manage its consequences, and adjust the level of sedation to a moderate or minimal level.

Intravenous moderate sedation in the dental office can be administered with a combination of just a few drugs. Today, intravenous sedation is the most effective way to achieve adequate and predictable sedation in most dental patients. The most common method for achieving anxiety control in dental patients is with a combination of the following:

- Benzodiazepines such as diazepam (Valium, generics); midazolam (Versed) for its amnesia effect and reducing apprehension and fear
- Narcotic analgesics such as fentanyl (Sublimaze, generics), morphine, meperidine (Demerol, generics) for analgesia and euphoria
- Sedative /hypnotics: Nonbarbiturates such as propfol (Diprivan)
- Sedatives: Barbiturates such as pentobarbital may also be used if the patient cannot take benzodiazepines.

IV/ORAL/INHALATIONAL AGENTS FOR MODERATE SEDATION

Intravenous anesthetics are mainly used for the rapid *induction* of general anesthesia or moderate sedation, which is then maintained with an appropriated inhalational drug such as nitrous oxide-oxygen, or by intermittent or continuous infusion. Intravenous anesthetics are administered first to decrease anxiety and fear. These drugs may also be used alone to produce a light level of narcosis (unaware of the surroundings) for short surgical procedures, especially those performed with the aid of local anesthetics, which is used for an analgesic effect.

There is great individual variation in response to intravenous anesthetics. Some, but not all, of this is explained by lower tolerance of poor-risk patients or the increased requirements of those who have become tolerant to other CNS depressants such as alcohol or sleeping pills. Thus, assessment of individual requirements is necessary.

Intravenous anesthetics are administered directly into the blood and distribute to the lipid regions of the body so the onset of action is within seconds. The higher the lipid solubility of the agent, the more readily it is redistributed to other fatty regions. The drug is then slowly metabolized and excreted over several hours. Benzodiazepines take a few minutes to distribute to the brain, whereas barbiturates take about 20 seconds. Nonbarbiturates such as propofol and etomidate are highly lipid soluble and are rapid in onset, but shorter in duration of action. These agents are metabolized rapidly, with less accumulation in fatty deposits.

Sedation of children is different from sedation of adults. Generally, sedation is restricted to uncooperative children. According to the American Academy of Pediatrics, sedative and anxiolytic medications should only be administered by or in the presence of individuals skilled in airway management and cardiopulmonary resuscitation. The Academy (the American Academy of Pediatric Dentistry; reference manual, 2006) recognizes nitrous oxide/oxygen inhalation as a safe and effective technique to reduce anxiety, and produce analgesia.

Table 9–2 lists intravenous anesthetic agents used for the induction of general anesthesia or moderate sedation.

ANTIANXIETY AGENTS: BENZODIAZEPINES

Benzodiazepines are used to treat anxious dental patients. These drugs are sedating, reduce anxiety, induce relaxation, and produce amnesia. Some benzodiazepines used for IV sedation dentistry are diazepam (Valium) and midazolam (Versed). Diazepam, a long-acting benzodiazepine, can be irritating when administered IV and may cause pain at the injection site. On the other hand, midazolam, a short-acting benzodiazepine, causes less pain at the site of injection and is primarily used for preoperative sedation and for procedures that do not require a high level of analgesia. It has greater potential for respiratory depression in the elderly than in children, and has a pregnancy category of D (warning for use in pregnant women). For an adult the dosage is IV 1–1.5 mg, which may be repeated in 2 minutes prn or IM 0.07–0.08 mg/kg 30–60 minutes before the dental procedure (Table 9–2). Diazepam oral solution is recommended for children over 6 years. Another benzodiazepine, triazolam (Halcion), has a pregnancy category of X so it is contraindicated in pregnant women.

Respiratory status should be monitored in the dental patient taking a benzodiazepine. The effects can be reversed with flumazenil (Romazicon). Additionally, the dental hygienist should observe the patient for possible abuse and dependency on the drug.

Benzodiazepines are also used for oral minimal/moderate sedation of apprehensive and fearful dental patients. Orally administered benzodiazepines include lorazepam (Ativan), chlorazepate (Tranxene), alprazolam (Xanax), and triazolam (Halcion). The medication can be taken either the night before or one hour before the dental procedure. Oral benzodiazepines have the same drug interactions as injectable benzodiazepines.

Flumazenil (Mazicon, Romazicon) is a benzodiazepine antagonist and is given to patients to reverse the action of a benzodiazepine in cases of overdose.

Table 9–2 Classification of Intravenous Anesthetics Used for Moderate Sedation/Analgesia

Drug Name	Drug Interaction of Dental Significance
Benzodiazepines with Diazepam (Valium) Lorazepam (Ativan) Midazolam (Versed) Triazolam (Halcion)	• Benzodiazepines are metabolized by the CYP-3A4 liver enzymes. When taken alcohol, there is an increased CNS depression and sedation. • The depressant/sedation effect of the benzodiazepine is increased when taken with: cimetidine (Tagamet), a drug for ulcers; erythromycin or clarithromycin (Blaxin); ciprofloxacin (Cipro); grapefruit juice; fluvoxamine (Luvox; antidepressant); and fluconazole (Diflucan; antifungal). • Carbamazepine (Tegretol) and Phenytoin increases metabolism, decreasing serum levels and decreasing the benzodiazepine effect.
Opioids (Narcotics) Fentanyl (Sublimaze) Alfentanil (Alfenta) Sufentanil (Sufenta) Meperidine (Demerol)	• When taken with a benzodiazepine, there is increased respiratory depression. • When taken with cimetidine (Tagamet) there are increased levels of the narcotic analgesic, resulting in toxicity. • When taken with diuretics (water pill to lower blood pressure) there is an increased hypotensive (low blood pressure) effect.
Sedative/hypnotics Thiopental (Pentothal) Etomidate (Amidate) Methohexital (Brevital)	• When taken with alcohol there is increased sedation. • When taken with acetaminophen (Tylenol) there may be increased liver toxicity. • When taken with an oral contraceptive, the effects of the contraceptive are reduced.
Non-barbiturate Sedative Hypnotics Propofol (Diprivan) Ketamine (Ketalar) Chloral hydrate (Noctec)	• When chloral hydrate is taken with catecholamie (epinephrine), it may sensitize the heart to the actions of the epinephrine (vasoconstriction).
Reversal Drugs Naloxone (Narcan) Flumazenil (Mazicon, Romazicon)	• No significant interactions.

SEDATIVE/HYPNOTICS: BARBITURATES

Barbiturates are used for anxiety reduction, light sedation, and general anesthesia. Barbiturates used for moderate sedation are classified as sedative hypnotics. Barbiturates produce sleep by depression of central nervous system activity with minimal cardiovascular effects at sedative doses. Their popularity over the years has been reduced by the benzodiazepines, however, they still are being used because of the ease of multiple routes of administration.

Several disadvantages include respiratory depression, irritation of rectal mucosa with rectal administration, and slow onset with oral administration. Paradoxical excitement can occur when the barbiturate instead of causing depression causes excitement, especially when used for painful procedures. Barbiturates have primarily been replaced by other drugs that cause fewer adverse effects.

For dental situations, it is recommended to use a short-acting barbiturate such as pentobarbital or secobarbital. The duration of action is about 3 to 4 hours. Longer acting barbiturates such as phenobarbital are used as anticonvulsant drugs.

SEDATIVE/HYPNOTICS: NONBARBITURATES

Propofol

Nonbarbiturates are preferred over barbiturates because they have fewer side effects, including less cardiac depression. Propofol (Diprivan) is widely used for conscious sedation because it is associated with rapid recovery without hangover and nausea and vomiting. It has a rapid induction (40 seconds) and short duration of action (5–10 minutes) with a quick recovery. It can be

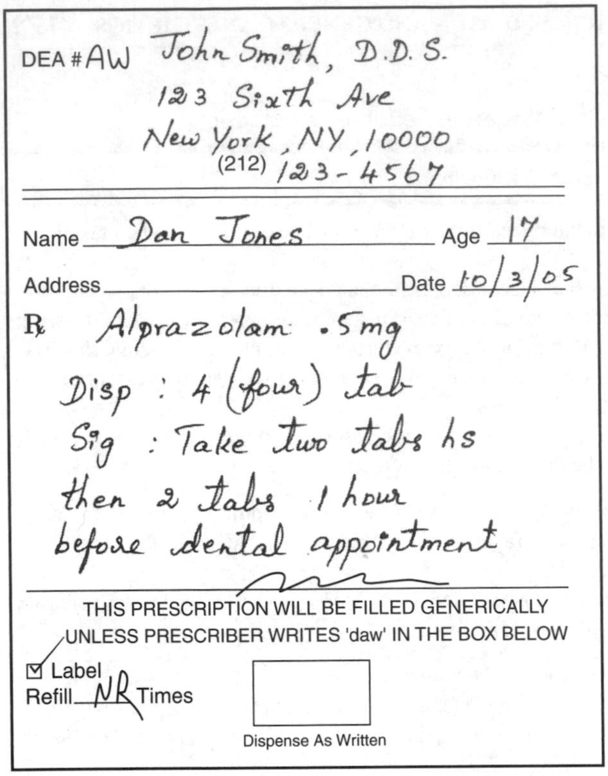

Prescription 1 (top left):

DEA #AW John Smith, D.D.S.
123 Sixth Ave
New York, NY, 10000
(212) 123-4567

Name Dan Jones   Age 17

Address _____ Date 10/3/05

℞ Alprazolam .5mg

Disp : 4 (four) tab

Sig : Take two tabs hs
then 2 tabs 1 hour
before dental appointment

THIS PRESCRIPTION WILL BE FILLED GENERICALLY
UNLESS PRESCRIBER WRITES 'daw' IN THE BOX BELOW

☑ Label
Refill NR Times

Dispense As Written

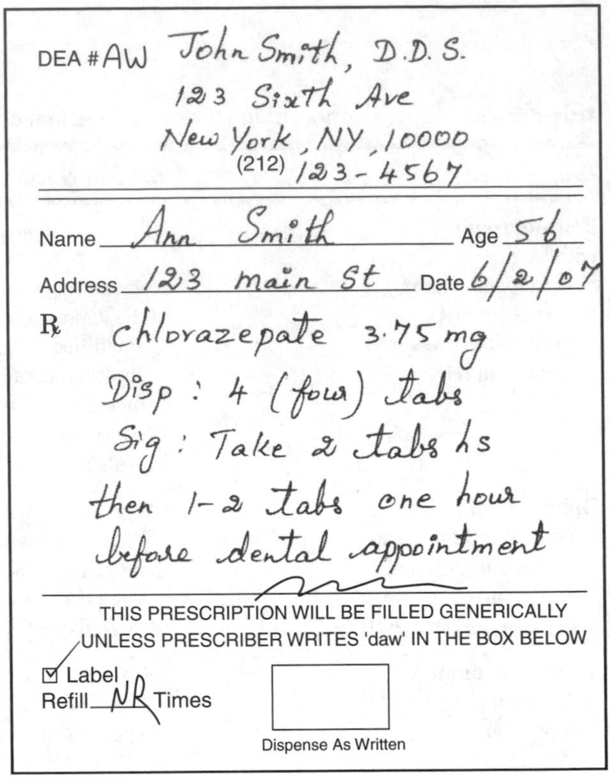

Prescription 2 (top right):

DEA #AW John Smith, D.D.S.
123 Sixth Ave
New York, NY, 10000
(212) 123-4567

Name Ann Smith   Age 56

Address 123 main St Date 6/2/07

℞ Chlorazepate 3.75 mg

Disp : 4 (four) tabs

Sig : Take 2 tabs hs
then 1-2 tabs one hour
before dental appointment

THIS PRESCRIPTION WILL BE FILLED GENERICALLY
UNLESS PRESCRIBER WRITES 'daw' IN THE BOX BELOW

☑ Label
Refill NR Times

Dispense As Written

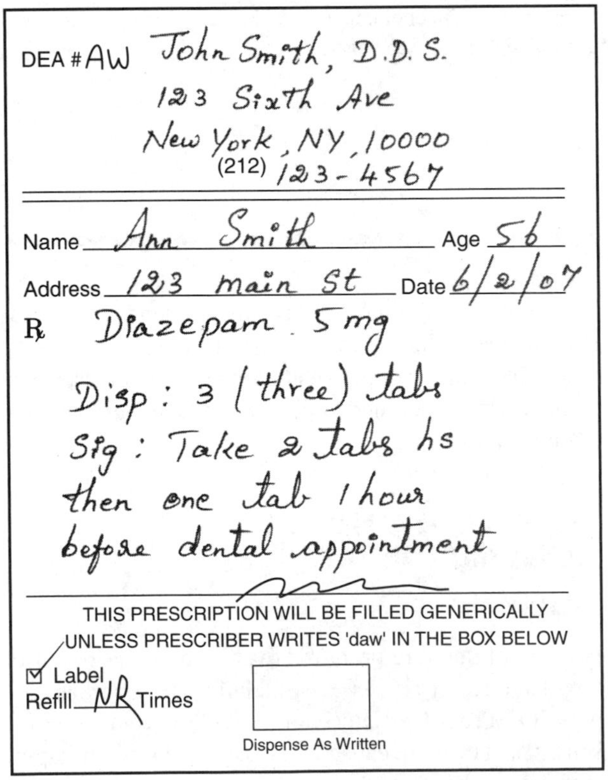

Prescription 3 (bottom left):

DEA #AW John Smith, D.D.S.
123 Sixth Ave
New York, NY, 10000
(212) 123-4567

Name Ann Smith   Age 56

Address 123 main St Date 6/2/07

℞ Diazepam .5mg

Disp : 3 (three) tabs

Sig : Take 2 tabs hs
then one tab 1 hour
before dental appointment

THIS PRESCRIPTION WILL BE FILLED GENERICALLY
UNLESS PRESCRIBER WRITES 'daw' IN THE BOX BELOW

☑ Label
Refill NR Times

Dispense As Written

FIGURE 9-1 Prescriptions of select benzodiazepines used in the dental office for dental anxiety.

used for lengthy surgical procedures, unlike thiopental, because is it rapidly metabolized by the liver and excreted in the urine. Propofol is usually combined with an analgesic agent or local anesthetic because by itself it provides no analgesia. Adverse effects include twitching, jerking, coughing and vasodilation, which can result in a marked hypotension.

It is available as an emulsion, which contains soybean oil and egg phosphatide. Adverse effects include twitching, jerking, coughing, and vasodilation, which can result in marked hypotension.

NARCOTICS

Opioids are used to produce mood changes, provide analgesia, and elevate the pain threshold. Narcotics are also used to reduce the dose of intravenous anesthetic and are usually used with benzodiazepines and as supplements to nitrous oxide. Narcotics commonly used for conscious sedation include fentanyl (Sublimaze) and meperidine (Demerol). For children, intranasal or oral transmucosal routes ("lollipop") for fentanyl (Sublimaze) and sufentanyl (Sufenta) are available and achieve both analgesia and sedation.

Narcotics have a direct effect on the gastrointestinal tract, causing constipation. Other side effects include respiratory difficulties, headache, itching, and nausea and vomiting.

 Rapid Dental Hint

Remember to monitor your patients. Watch for respiratory status, state of consciousness, heart rate, and blood pressure.

OTHERS

Chloral hydrate (Noctec) is a sedative/hypnotic with little to no analgesic properties. It is a useful and safe drug when properly administered orally (not very palatable) or rectally for anxious children, especially under 2 years, before a dental/medical procedure or for sedation before and after surgery. Particular care must be taken in calculating and admistering the proper dose. It is only given for conscious sedation and not for general anesthesia. It is readily absorbed, with an onset of action of 30–60 minutes and duration of action of 4–8 hours. It is metabolized in the liver to the active metabolite trichloroethanol. Chloral hydrate is not indicated as an analgesic for pain control and may actually cause excitement and delirium. Sudden death can occur due to cardiac arrest. Tachycardia can occur if alcohol is taken with chloral hydrate. At therapeutic doses, chloral hydrate has little effect on respiration and blood pressure.

MONITORING

The dental hygienist must be trained in monitoring the safety of patients and in the recognition and management of adverse reactions and emergencies that are associated with the use of these pharmacologic agents.

Did You Know

Chloral hydrate is the oldest hypnotic depressant (sleep pill); first synthesized in 1832, but not used in medicine until 1869.

Did You Know

The expression "knockout drops" or "Mickey Finn" is a drink consisting of a mixture of chloral hydrate and alcohol that is used on an unsuspecting victim to incapacitate them.

The patient should be assessed for adequate airway and gas exchange and cardiovascular response. The patient's vital signs, including pulse rate, blood pressure, and respiration rate, must be monitored and documented. Vital signs reflect changes in depth of anesthesia or physical status. A pulse oximeter is used to monitor the pulse rate and level of oxygen in the blood. An electrocardiogram (EKG) monitor can also be used to assist in monitoring the patient. The dental hygienist must also be aware of drug antagonists that are used to reverse the actions of some of these drugs. However, once some of these drugs are injected into the blood, it is not possible to reverse the actions.

NITROUS OXIDE

Properties and Indications: Nitrous Oxide

First discovered in 1783 by Joseph Priestley, **nitrous oxide** (referred to as "laughing gas" because of the euphoria that it produces) is the only anesthetic gas used today, and is the least soluble in blood of all inhalational anesthetics. Dr. Horace Wells was the first dentist to use nitrous oxide for tooth extractions (on himself!). Nitrous oxide (N_2O) is a colorless, sweet-smelling gas used for induction (if used alone for moderate sedation) or maintenance (if used after intravenous general anesthetic) of anesthesia. *It is a weak general anesthetic and is generally not used alone in anesthesia; however it has marked analgesic and amnesia properties,* is relatively nontoxic, and does not produce respiratory depression (slow breathing), bronchodilation, hypotension (low blood pressure), or heart arrhythmias. This makes it an ideal, safe sedative agent in the dental office (Tables 9–3 and 9–4).

The following are indications for nitrous oxide:

• Fearful, anxious patient (child/adult)
• Cognitively, physically, or medically compromised child, adult
• Gag reflex interfering with oral health care
• Profound local anesthesia cannot be obtained or tolerated.

Table 9–3   Features of Nitrous Oxide

	Adverse Effects	*Contraindications*	*Notes*
Nitrous oxide	Nausea and vomiting with very high concentrations, or on an empty or full stomach	Coronary heart disease; chronic obstructive pulmonary disease (COPD-bronchitis, emphysema); upper respiratory obstruction (e.g., cold, stuffy nose, blocked Eustachian tubes)	Does not cause respiratory depression, bronchodilation, or low blood pressure. Patients should avoid a large meal within 3 hours of dental visit to prevent vomiting.

When used alone, nitrous oxide has a rapid action (2 to 3 minutes) and a rapid recovery without loss of consciousness. It is easy to administer and can be self-delivered by the patient using the demand-valve positive

Table 9–4   Nitrous Oxide: Patient Response to Nitrous Oxide/Oxygen Mixtures

Nitrous Oxide Concentration (percentage)	*Patient Response*
10–20	Body warmth Tingling of hands and feet
20–30	Circumoral numbness Numbness of thighs
20–40%	Numbness of hands and feet Droning sounds present Hearing distinct but distant Dissociation begins and reaches peak Mild sleepiness Some analgesia Euphoria Feeling of heaviness or lightness of body
30–50%	Sweating Nausea Amnesia Increased sleepiness
40–60%	Dreaming, laughing, giddiness Further increased sleepiness, tending toward unconsciousness Increased nausea and possible vomiting
Greater than 50%	Unconsciousness and light general anesthesia

Reprinted from Bennett, C. R.: *Conscious-Sedation in Dental Practice.* Copyright (1974) with permission from Elsevier.

pressure method. Using this method, analgesia is obtained in less than 20 seconds and the patient is relaxed in 30–60 seconds. It is also acceptable for use in children. Besides its use in the dental office, nitrous oxide is used for many medical procedures, including minor painful orthopedic injuries or changing burn dressings.

Because of its analgesic properties and lack of major cardiovascular or respiratory depression, nitrous oxide is often used as a part of balanced anesthesia in combination with other anesthetic agents or drugs in low doses to reduce the requirements (MAC) of other, more potent agents. It cannot be used alone for surgical anesthesia because of its low potency.

Pharmacokinetics

Nitrous oxide is rapidly absorbed from the pulmonary alveoli into the bloodstream. The higher the concentration of nitrous oxide in the mask, the more rapidly the same concentration will develop in the lungs. When the high concentration of nitrous oxide at the mask is removed, the concentration falls and the nitrous oxide unchanged is removed from the body in the expired air at the same rate.

Method of Administration

Nitrous oxide is administered with oxygen by adjusting the concentration of nitrous oxide to titrate the patient to the desired level of sedation. There are two tanks: Oxygen is the green tank and nitrous oxide (N_2O) is the blue tank. Pure oxygen (100 percent) is administered with a mask for the first 2 to 3 minutes, and then nitrous oxide is added to the oxygen in 5 to 10 percent (up to about 20–30 percent) concentrations until the desired level of sedation is reached. The average patient requires 35 percent of nitrous oxide in oxygen, with a range of 10–50 percent. A 50/50 mixture of nitrous oxide and oxygen is commonly used during dental procedures. Table 9–4 shows the patient's response to different nitrous oxide/oxygen mixtures. Onset of sedation is usually within 3 to 5 minutes. When the dental procedure is finished the patient must be administered only 100 percent oxygen for at least 5 minutes. Diffusion hypoxia (low oxygen levels to the tissue; headaches can develop) may result when there is not enough oxygen delivered. To prevent hypoxia, the mask should not be removed until the patient receives enough oxygen.

Adverse Effects

The most common adverse effects include nausea and vomiting, which can be minimized by having the patient eat a light amount of food before the appointment. Chronic abuse of nitrous oxide is associated with a fall in the white-cell count, and neuropathy (nerve damage including numbness of limbs). Exposure of anesthetists or other operating room personnel to nitrous oxide should be minimized.

Drug Interactions, Contraindications

Nitrous oxide interacts with vitamin B_{12}, resulting in megaloblastic anemia. There may be an added sedative effect when a patient is also taking sedative drugs or St. John's wort.

Nitrous oxide should not be used in patients with coronary heart disease (because there may be diminished cardiac output), chronic obstructive pulmonary disease (e.g., bronchitis or emphysema), or respiratory obstructions (e.g., stuffy nose, blocked eustachian tubes) because the patient needs to breathe in the nitrous oxide/oxygen mixture, bowel obstructions and certain eye problems. Use of nitrous oxide during pregnancy is contraindicated. Chronic exposure to pregnant women increases the incidence of miscarriages.

Occupational Exposure

The National Institute of Occupational Safety and Health (NIOSH) reported nitrous oxide levels of approximately 50 ppm were achievable in the dental office. To keep occupational exposure to a minimum, the procedure time should be short and there should be ventilation and monitoring devices. Faulty equipment can pose hazards for dental/medical clinicians in the room, especially spontaneous abortion and genetic effects.

GENERAL ANESTHESIA
History

The first time general anesthesia was used for major surgery was in 1846 by William Morton at the Massachusetts General Hospital. He used only one agent, diethyl ether, which is no longer used in developed countries because of a slow rate of induction, with many postoperative adverse effects such as nausea and vomiting. General anesthesia allowed for longer and more sophisticated procedures to be done, not just quick procedures. Modern anesthesia uses a combination of many drugs to achieve surgical anesthesia rather than only one agent as William Morton did in the 1800s.

Indications

General anesthesia is not commonly used in dentistry except for patients who are very fearful of having dental procedures performed, mentally or physically challenged, or having very stressful and traumatic procedures done, such as multiple tooth extractions. General anesthesia is administered via inhalation and intravenous routes. General anesthetics are drugs that rapidly produce unconsciousness and total analgesia.

Stages

General anesthesia is a progressive process that occurs in distinct stages or levels (Guedel's signs). The most potent anesthetic agent can quickly induce all four stages, while others such as nitrous oxide are only able to induce Stage

Most surgery requires the patient to be in Stage III, called surgical anesthesia. Pupil dilation, tachycardia (increased heart rate), hypotension, and skeletal muscle relaxation are the four signs that indicate a patient is in Stage III surgical anesthesia. These stages of general anesthesia are listed in Table 9–5.

General anesthesia involves the administration of different drugs. To achieve balanced anesthesia the following regimens are used:

1. **Premedication** is administered to reduce anxiety and obtain analgesia (for short surgical procedures premedication is not necessary). Premedication is performed before the patient goes into the operat-

ing room. The patient may be premedicated with an antibiotic, anxiolytics (e.g., midazolam), or antiemetic (e.g., droperidol; to help prevent nausea and vomiting after the procedure; sometimes antiemetics are administered intravenously during anesthesia rather than as premedication)

2. **Induction** is most commonly obtained with intravenous agents. Induction refers to initiating anesthesia and is performed when the patient is in the operating room.
3. **Maintenance** of induction with inhalational agents. Maintenance occurs when the surgery is being performed and more anesthetic is required to finish the surgical procedure.
4. **Recovery** from anesthesia. Recovery begins when maintenance agent is discontinued up to the time when the patient is fully responsive and able to be dismissed. Medications may be given at this time to control pain or for nausea and vomiting.

Table 9–5   Stage of Surgical Anesthesia: Guedel's Classification

Stage	*Features*
Stage I	Amnesia and analgesia • Moderate sedation • nitrous oxide produces Stage 1 • loss of pain, loss of general sensation but still awake, even though the patient does not know anything is happening; semiconscious • reflexes intact
Stage II	Excitement/delirium • Patient may resist treatment; involuntary muscle movements • increase in blood pressure • irregular respirations • IV agents may be used to calm the patient; loss of consciousness to onset of anesthesia • Patient may become incontinent
Stage III	Surgical anesthesia • Required stage for major surgical procedures • loss of consciousness • dilation of pupils • tachycardia (increased heart rate) • hypotension • reflexes absent • skeletal muscles relaxed
Stage IV	Medullary paralysis: anesthetic overdose • Paralysis of the medulla region of the brain, which controls respiratory and cardiovascular activity • Death can occur if heart stops • Stop anesthetics and administer 100 percent oxygen

Classification and Chemistry

A variety of drugs can be used to provide sedation and analgesia. The classification of agents is listed in Table 9–6 and Table 9–7. The drugs used depend on whether the outcome is sedation, analgesia, and/or amnesia.

There are two main methods of inducing general anesthesia:

1. Intravenous agents are usually administered first to induce anesthesia quickly.
2. After the patient loses consciousness, inhaled agents are used to maintain the anesthesia.

Inhalational Anesthetics

Mechanism of Action: Inhalational Agents

Although the exact mechanism of action of *inhalational agents* is unknown, several theories have been postulated. The *lipid theory* states that inhaled anesthetics interact with hydrophobic parts of proteins in the lipid bilayer of membranes. These agents then dissolve in the membrane lipids, increasing chloride influx into the neurons on the CNS. Also, they may prevent the flow of sodium and calcium ions into neurons of the CNS. Thus there is a relationship between potency and lipid solubility of the agent, represented by the oil : gas partition coefficient.

The *protein theory* states that the inhalation agent binds to protein receptors located in or on the lipid bilayer

Table 9–6 Classification of Inhalational Anesthetics Used for General Anesthesia

Volatile Liquid General Anesthetics	Adverse Effects	Contraindications	Notes
Desflurane (Suprane) Enflurane (Ethrane) Halothane (Fluothane) Isoflurane (Forane) Methoxyflurane (Penthrane) Sevoflurane (Ultane)	• Nausea and vomiting • Halothane and sevoflurane have low respiratory depression. The others are moderate. • Sevoflurane has no bronchodilation effect. • All cause hypotension. • All have low arrhythmia effects except halothane, which is moderate.	Halothane is contraindicated in patients with cardiovascular conditions; sensitizes the heart to epinephrine (limit epinephrine use).	• Patient should be assessed for the use of alcohol or other CNS depressants before anesthetic use. • Postoperative monitoring for nausea and vomiting. • Halothane has a MAC of 0.75 (very potent). • Halothane is metabolized in the liver (20 percent).

of the neuronal cell membrane, which inhibits the activity of some excitatory neurotransmitter and enhances the activity of receptors for inhibitory transmitters such as gamma-aminobutyric acid (GABA).

Classification

Inhalational anesthetic agents are divided into two classifications (Table 9–6): nonhalongenated drugs and halogenated drugs. These agents are either gases or volatile liquids, and are used mainly for maintenance of anesthesia after induction with an intravenous induction agent.

Gaseous agents require suitable equipment for storage under pressure in metal cylinders, reduction to operating pressure, and monitoring of gas flow-rate. Most volatile agents are metered by calibrated vaporizers, using air or oxygen as carriers, though some can be given by direct drip onto a pad and vaporized by the patient's breath.

Table 9–7 Injectable General Anesthetics

Alfentanil	Narcotic
Droperidol	Narcotic
Etomidate	Sedative/hypnotic
Ketamine	Dissociative anesthetic
Methohexital	Barbiturate
Propofol	Nonbarbiturate sedative/hypnotic
Succinylcholine	Neuromuscular blocking drug
Sufentanil	Narcotic
Thiopental	Barbiturate

Chemistry and Pharmacokinetics

Unlike orally administered drugs, the dose of an inhalational agent is not expressed in terms of milligrams or grams of the drug, but in terms of partial pressure or percentage of inspired air. The potency of an inhalational anesthetic is expressed as the inspired concentration of the inhaled anesthetic required to induce surgical anesthesia in 50 percent of patients. This is referred to as the minimal alveolar concentration (MAC). MAC is used to measure and compare the potency of inhalational anesthetic agents. For example, agents with MACs greater than 1 are less potent than agents with an MAC of less than 1. Agents with low MACs are used in combination with nitrous oxide to reduce the concentration of each, resulting in less adverse side effects.

An individual gas in a mixture exerts a partial pressure according to its percentage concentration in the mixture that contributes to the total pressure exerted by the mixture. Each gas contributes partially to the total gas. For example, oxygen, which makes up about 21 percent of the atmospheric mixture of gases, contributes about 21 percent of the total pressure. Thus the partial pressure of oxygen is 21 percent, or 160 mm Hg.

Solubility of the gas in the blood is also important and is related to two barriers: lung tissue and blood. After inhalation gases will enter the blood and dissolve in it in proportion to their individual gas pressures. The absolute number of molecules of a gas that enters the blood depends on the pressure of the gas that surrounds it and also on the solubility of the gas. The more the pressure of a gas that is in contact, the more molecules of the gas will dissolve in it. Once a gas dissolves in the blood, the gas molecules may diffuse from regions of high pressure to regions of lower pressure. The speed at which induction of anesthesia occurs depends primarily on the solubility of the agent in the blood and the inspired concentration of gas. This is referred to as the blood/gas coefficient.

Metabolism is of little importance since general anesthesia is not maintained for prolonged periods of time. Recovery occurs because of redistribution of the drug away from the brain back into the lungs, where expiration occurs. Partial pressure in the lungs decreases as the administration of the gas stops, allowing for more drug diffusion from the lipid regions of the body to the blood. Recovery time for obese patients is longer because of greater distribution of the anesthetic to fat stores.

Adverse Effects

The inhalational anesthetics used in general anesthesia can cause severe reactions, including (Table 9–6):

- Airway irritation
- Bronchodilation
- Respiratory depression
- Low blood pressure (hypotension)
- Cardiac arrhythmia
- Nausea is common for a few hours after the procedure (avoid a heavy meal 3 hours before appointment to minimize vomiting)

Volatile Liquid General Anesthetics/Halogenated Drugs

Volatile liquids have replaced the older anesthetics such as diethyl ether, which was highly explosive, because these drugs have a more rapid rate of induction and recovery with less postoperative adverse effects such as nausea and vomiting. However, these drugs cause more respiratory and cardiovascular relaxation/depression, which is dose related (e.g., the more agent given, the increased incidence of side effects). It is liquid at room temperature and is converted to a vapor and inhaled. Carefully monitoring of vital signs is very important with these agents. Balanced anesthesia is usually achieved when these agents are administered with nitrous oxide (often in a 2 : 1 ratio with oxygen), opioids or skeletal muscle relaxants because by themselves they produce little analgesia or muscle relaxation. All of these anesthetics are volatile liquids at room temperature but are converted into a vapor and inhaled to produce their anesthetic effects. These agents are only used by dentists/anesthesiologists in a hospital setting.

Halothane

Halothane (Fluothane) is the prototype volatile liquid inhalational anesthetic. It is potent (MAC 0.75) and can be easy to overdose. It has a high blood : gas solubility (2.3) so that the rate of induction and recovery is slower than the other halogenated agents. Halothane is contraindicated in pregnancy and in patients with diminished hepatic (liver) function since it can be hepatoxic. It is extensively metabolized in the liver to toxic metabolites. Halothane decreases blood pressure and sensitizes the heart to epinephrine, which can cause heart dysrhythmias; thus caution should be used in patients with cardiac conditions. Since halothane does not cause as much muscle relaxation or analgesia as the other volatile anesthetics, it is used with other anesthetic drugs such as muscle relaxants and analgesics. It is used for the maintenance of anesthesia in major surgery and to supplement the action of nitrous oxide and oxygen in balanced anesthesia. Halothane has poor analgesic effects but is more potent and induces deep anesthesia (unconsciousness).

Drug Interactions and Contraindications   Levodopa (anti-Parkinson drug) should not be taken at the same time as administration of halothane because it causes elevated dopamine blood levels. Epinephrine (used for hemostatis or the control of bleeding) is limited with halothane.

Halothane is contraindicated in patients who previously were exposed to halothane within 4–6 weeks because of severe disturbances in liver function (toxic metabolites), including hepatitis and death.

Isoflurane

The most commonly used halogenated agent is isoflurane (Forane), which has moderate potency with a moderate onset of action and is inexpensive. It causes more muscle relaxation so additional muscle relaxants during surgery are not needed. However, isoflurane causes more respiratory depression (slow breathing), hypotension, and can induce heart rhythm abnormalities. Since a small amount of the drug undergoes liver metabolism, liver toxicity is not of concern. When used with nitrous oxide/oxygen, the MAC is reduced considerably.

Sevoflurane/Desflurane

Compared to the other halogenated agents, the newer agents sevoflurane (Ultane) and desflurane (Suprane) have a more rapid onset and shorter duration of action due to a low blood : gas solubility, which makes it easier to titrate the dose. They cause little cardiac toxicity. Desflurane is less potent and requires higher concentrations to be inhaled, which may be irritating to the respiratory tract causing coughing and breath-holding.

Injectable Anesthetics for General Anesthesia

Some drugs that were used in lower doses to produce moderate sedation are also used in general anesthesia, but in higher doses. Table 9–7 lists intravenous anesthetic agents used for the induction of general anesthesia.

Sedative/Hypnotics: Barbiturates

As an induction agent, thiopental has a rapid onset of 20 seconds but a long elimination time, resulting in a hangover effect and nausea and vomiting. It should not be continuously infused for long periods of time because it is slowly metabolized by the liver and can accumulate in the body. It is usually combined with nitrous oxide/oxygen to produce surgical anesthesia. Additionally, thiopental may cause bronchospasm, and was the primary agent until propofol was introduced.

Methohexital (Brevital) is an ultra–short acting barbiturate with an onset of 20–40 seconds and duration of action of 5–10 minutes. There is a high incidence of postoperative nausea and vomiting.

Propofol

Propofol is used for induction of general anesthesia or for maintenance of a balanced anesthesia technique. It provides complete anesthesia in and outside the operating room without having to transport an anesthesia machine.

Narcotics

Intravenous narcotics are not considered to be true anesthetics because they do not usually produce total unconsciousness, which is needed for general anesthesia. However, they have superior analgesic and sedative properties, which allow for easier endotracheal intubation and surgical incision. Sufentanil, alfentanil, and remifentanil are used most often in dentistry for deep sedation and general anesthesia. Fentanyl is combined with droperidol (premixed vial is marketed as Innovar), an antipsychotic drug, to produce an analgesia where the patient is conscious but insensitive to pain and unaware of the surroundings.

Dissociatives

Ketamine (Ketalar) affects the senses, and produces a dissociative/hallucinatory anesthesia where the patient may appear to be awake and receptive but does not respond to sensory stimulation. It has potent analgesic properties, and mild respiratory depression. Ketamine is recreationally abused for intoxicating and hallucinatory effects. It is used in pediatric patients because it can be administered by intramuscular injection.

Muscle Relaxants

Neuromuscular-blocking drugs are used for the induction and maintenance of skeletal relaxation during general anesthesia. These drugs are also used during premedication to facilitate endotracheal intubation by relaxing the muscles of the trachea. Some examples include succinylcholine (Ancetine) and pipecuronium (Arduan).

Typical Sequence of Events for Intravenous Sedation

A typical sequence is to induce loss of consciousness for 2–3 minutes with propofol or other intravenous anesthetic and maintain anesthesia with nitrous oxide/oxygen (50/50) mixtures supplemented, when necessary, with halothane or other potent inhalational anesthetic, or with a narcotic analgesic. The action of the anesthetic is enhanced by the narcotic analgesic, and overall anesthetic requirements are reduced. (This is balanced anesthesia.) Adequate muscle relaxation, if needed, is given.

Postoperative Problems: General Anesthesia

Many postoperative adverse events can occur in patients after general anesthesia. These include:

1. Respiratory
   - Airway obstruction
   - Sore throat
   - Difficulty breathing
   - Hypoxia (low oxygen)
2. CNS/Neurologic
   - Pain

• Muscle weakness
• Sleepiness
3. Cardiovascular
  • Hypotension (low blood pressure)
  • Hypertension (high blood pressure)
  • Arrhythmias
4. Gastrointestinal
  • Constipation (with narcotics)
  • Nausea and vomiting

DENTAL HYGIENE NOTES

Nitrous oxide is used in dental offices for its anti-anxiety effects rather than its anesthetic effects. The dental hygienist should have a general knowledge of the medical status of patients who are candidates for nitrous oxide and IV sedation, as well as knowledge of the pharmacology of these agents. The patient should be instructed to eat a small amount of food before coming to the dental appointment to minimize nausea that can occur after nitrous oxide use. The dental hygienist should question the patient about medications they are taking to avoid any drug–drug interactions.

KEY POINTS

• The goal of general anesthesia is to provide a rapid and complete loss of sensation; general anesthesia is not used in the dental office but is used in dentistry (in a hospital setting) for a certain group of patients, for example, patients who are fearful and apprehensive about having multiple tooth extractions at one time.
• General anesthesia is administered by anesthesiologists or certified registered nurse anesthetists (CRNA).
• Intravenous moderate sedation is not synonymous with general anesthesia.
• Intravenous sedation is performed by well trained, qualified dentists in the dental office.
• The goal of minimal sedation or moderate sedation/analgesia in the dental office is to relieve patient anxiety, and produce some amnesia and pain control.
• Usually a benzodiazepine and a narcotic are used for intravenous (IV) sedation in the dental office.
• Benzodiazepines are used for oral minimal sedation or moderate sedation/analgesia.
• Nitrous oxide is the only gas used for inhalational anesthesia.

• Nitrous oxide is the least potent of inhalational anesthetics and does not reduce consciousness: It has strong analgesic and amnesia properties, and is good as a sole agent in the dental office.
• Nitrous oxide cannot be used in patients who have nasal obstruction and fear losing consciousness, and who are mentally unstable.
• Sedation is obtained with nitrous oxide.
• The most serious danger of anesthesia is overdosage, which results in death.
• Intravenous anesthetics are primarily used for rapid induction of general anesthesia with inhalational anesthetics for maintenance.

BOARD REVIEW QUESTIONS

1. Which of the following agents is considered to be a gas? (p. 173)
   a. Nitrous oxide
   b. Fentanyl
   c. Propofol
   d. Diazepam

2. Which of the following inhalational anesthetics does not cause respiratory depression and hypotension? (pp. 173–175)
   a. Nitrous oxide
   b. Enflurane
   c. Isoflurane
   d. Halothane

3. All of the following statements are true about moderate sedation except one. Which one is the exception? (p. 168)
   a. Complete loss of protective reflexes
   b. Total unconsciousness
   c. Patent airway
   d. Responds to physical stimulation

4. Propofol is preferred over thiopental as an intravenous anesthetic because of its: (pp. 171–172)
   a. Recovery characteristics
   b. Can be taken orally
   c. Long onset of action
   d. Prolonged duration of action

5. Which of the following side effects is common after general anesthesia? (p. 178)
   a. Diarrhea
   b. Esophageal reflux

c. Nausea and vomiting

d. Muscle weakness

6. Which of the following ratios of nitrous oxide/oxygen is usually used in dentistry? (p. 174)
   a. 25/25
   b. 25/50
   c. 50/50
   d. 50/75

7. Use of nitrous oxide/oxygen is contraindicated in patients with: (p. 175)
   a. Allergies to pollen
   b. Upper respiratory infection
   c. Bacterial infections
   d. Hepatitis

8. Which of the following ASA classification describes a patient with mild hypertension? (p. 169)
   a. I
   b. II
   c. III
   d. IV
   e. V

9. Which of the following agents is used in sedation of children who are anxious in the dental chair? (p. 173)
   a. Halothane
   b. Diazepam
   c. Chloral hydrate
   d. Ketamine

10. At which of the following stages of anesthesia is surgical anesthesia attained? (p. 176)
    a. 1
    b. 2
    c. 3
    d. 4

SELECTED REFERENCES

ADA Guide to Dental Therapeutics, 3rd ed. 2003.

American Academy of Pediatric Dentistry. 2004. Clinical guideline on use of anesthesia-trained personnel in the provision of general anesthesia/deep sedation to the pediatric dental patient. *Pediatr Dent* 26:104–105.

American Dental Association. 2003. *Guidelines for Teaching the Comprehensive Control of Anxiety and Pain in Dentistry.* Chicago: American Dental Association.

American Dental Association House of Delegates, October 2003.

American Association of Oral and Maxillofacial Surgeons. Spring 1997. Anesthesia in the dental office.

Bell, C. Z., N. Kain. 1997. Anesthesia and Sedation away from the operating room. In: *The Pedeatric Anesthesia Handbook,* p. 433–452. Mosby: St. Louis.

Byrne, B. E., and L. S. Tibbetts. Conscious sedation and agents for the control of anxiety. In: *ADA Guide to Dental Therapeutics.* 3rd ed. Chicago: ADA Publishing, pp. 17–53.

Nick, D., L. Thompson, D. Anderson, and L. Trapp 2003. The use of general anesthesia to facilitate dental treatment. *Gen Dent* 51:464–468.

Shampaine, G. S. 1999. Patient assessment and preventive measures for medical emergencies in the dental office. Dental Clinics of North America 43:383–400.

Standards for Sedation and Anesthesia Care from the Joint Commission. *Moderate/deep Sedation Stands Comprehensive Accreditation Manual for Hospitals.* February 1, 2003 update.

WEB SITES

www.ada.org/prof/resources/positions/statements/anxiety_guidelines.pdf.

www.chclibrary.org

www.mescape.com

www.aapd.org/media/policies_guidelines/g_sedation.pdf.

Q U I C K   D R U G   G U I D E

Oral Anti-Anxiety Agents for Minimal to Moderate Sedation

Benzodiazepines

- Alprazolam (Xanax)
- Clorazepate (Tranxene)

- Diazepam (Valium)
- Lorazepam (Ativan)
- Triazolam (Halcion)

Minimal/Moderate Sedation/Deep Sedation/General Anesthesia

Intravenous Agents

Benzodiazepines

- Diazepam (Valium)
- Lorazepam (Ativan)
- Midazolam (Versed)
- Triazolam (Halcion)

Opioids

- Fentanyl (Sublimaze)
- Alfentanil (Alfenta)
- Sufentanil (Sufenta)
- Meperidine (Demerol)

Sedative/hypnotics

- Pentobarbital
- Secobarbital

Nonbarbiturate Sedative Hypnotics

- Propofol (Diprivan)
- Ketamine (Ketalar)
- Chloral hydrate (Noctec)

Reversal Drugs

- Naloxone (Narcan)
- Flumazenil (Mazicon)

Inhalational Agents

- Nitrous Oxide-Oxygen

General Anesthesia/ Inhalation Agents

Halogenated (volatile liquids)

- Desflurane (Suprane)
- Enflurane (Ethrane)
- Halothane (Fluothane)
- Isoflurane (Forane)
- Methoxyflurane (Penthrane)
- Sevoflurane (Ultane)

IV Agents

- Methohexital (Brevital)
- Thiopental

Chapter 10

Fluorides in Dental Practice

GOAL: To provide an overview of the pharmacology of fluorides and their benefits in community and dental office fluoride use.

EDUCATIONAL OBJECTIVES

After reading this chapter, the reader should be able to:

1. Describe the chemical composition, metabolism, and systemic intake of fluoride.
2. Describe the various types of fluoride available in dentistry.
3. Explain acute and chronic fluoride toxicity and how it relates to systemic and topical use.

KEY TERMS

Fluoride
Hydroxyapatite
Safely tolerated dose (STD)
Certainly lethal dose (CLD)

CHEMICAL COMPOSITION

Fluorine is a natural occurring element found in living and nonliving things. Its atomic number is 9, and it is found in the halogen group (VIIa) of the periodic table. In its standard state, fluorine is a pale yellow corrosive gas. It is the most electronegative and reactive of all elements. When a fluoride ion combines with a sodium ion, the compound sodium fluoride (NaF) is formed. The chemical formula NaF represents the salt of hydrofluoric acid. The compounds of potassium **fluoride** (KF) and hydrogen fluoride (HF) are also commonly found in dentistry.

Bone consists primarily of two compounds. About 70 percent of bone is an inorganic ionic compound of **hydroxyapatite,** [Ca10 (PO4)6(OH)2], while the other 30 percent is organic, consisting of protein collagen fibers. Fluoride ions can react with hydroxyapatite to create fluorapatite. A chemical reaction takes place where the negative hydroxide ion (OH^-) is replaced by the highly negative fluoride ion (F^-). The fluroride ions have a stronger chemical bond to the apatite matrix, making it more difficult chemically to change the matrix again. This confers increased strength and density to bone.

$$Ca_{10}(PO_4)_6(OH)_2 + 2F^- \longrightarrow Ca_{10}(PO_4)_6F_2$$
Hydroxyapatite   Fluorapatite

Fluoride can be added in ratios or parts per million (ppm) to water, dentifrices, mouth washes, gels, or to tablets as supplements for ingestion. One ppm is one part in 1,000,000, 1 milligram (mg) per kilogram (kg) of weight, or 1 cent in $10,000. Depending upon the sources, time of use or ingestion, fluoride can chemically react with and be incorporated into the enamel and dentinal structures. This makes the tooth harder, denser, and structurally sounder.

PHARMACOKINETICS

Fluoride in its mineral compound state is considered a nonessential nutrient for daily consumption because there are no known essential metabolic reactions it functions in. There are no recommended daily intake values. However many studies have indicated its effectiveness when retained in teeth and bones. When taken orally, fluoride is adsorbed and taken up into the plasma of the blood stream. The plasma then circulates throughout the body to bathe bone. Fluoride in the saliva can remain chemically active for up to 3 hours, effectively bathing the teeth.

Fluoride is retained by the body in hard, calcified tissue such as bone and teeth, and is excreted through the kidneys in the form of urine. The timing of ingestion, age, and tooth or bone formation at the time determine the concentrations of the fluoride stored. Fluoride is not appreciably found in breast or cow's milk; the concentrations are 0.01 ppm and 0.05 ppm respectively.

SOURCES

Fluoride is found naturally in tea, seafood, chicken, and in some water sources. Raw tea leaves can have up to 400 parts per million (ppm) of fluoride, while brewed tea would have 3 ppm. Often fluoride is added to water supplies, dentifrices, and school water systems. This can be of concern when foods are commercially prepared in areas that fluoridate their water because the fluoride ions will remain in these foods. This is important when considering fluoride content in processed foods such as baby foods, seafood products, fruit juices or other beverages, and—most important—infant formulas reconstituted with fluoridated water, which can often be forgotten. Ready-to-eat formula may contain 0.1 to 0.2 mg/L of fluoride. Grape juice, especially white grape juice, and baby food with processed chicken have higher levels of fluoride. Unless the manufacturing location or the amount of fluoride in the water used to reconstitute the product is known, this can make it very difficult for the consumer to evaluate the amount of fluoride in a product. Moreover, some countries such as France, the United States, Switzerland, and Jamaica add fluoride to table salt.

If water is naturally fluoridated it may contain greater than the acceptable concentration of fluoride. When potable water sources are found to have over the acceptable level of 0.07–1.2 ppm of fluoride content, the water source is defluoridated to ensure fluorosis does not occur. Another potable water source, bottled water, generally contains less than 0.3 ppm fluoride. It is usually distributed as spring or natural water, distilled, drinking, or mineral water; this labeling is regulated by the Food and Drug Administration (FDA). Any bottled water with fluoride added, such as bottled water for children, is required to state: with

---

Did You Know?

Fluorine, from which fluoride is derived, is the 13th most abundant element.

or added fluoride. There are water purification systems available to make it possible for consumers to purify home water sources. These systems may work by reverse osmosis, activated charcoal, or ozonation. Most purification systems are done by filtration, which does not appreciably remove fluoride; however, distillation and reverse osmosis do remove fluoride. Due to the perception that municipal water sources are not palatable or healthy, the use of water purification devices along with the growing trend to drink bottled water have become a great concern in caries prevention, and undermine the health benefits of community water fluoridation. In order to project someone's total fluoride intake, one must consider the amount of processed foods ingested, especially reconstituted foods, use of bottled water, and water purification devices.

USES

Diseases that affect oral health are not localized, but can affect individuals systemically. With many people living longer due to advances in medicine, they are looking at quality of life. Poor dentition can cause decreased mastication, leading to malnutrition. Poor gingival health can cause oral infections, which may spread systemically through the blood supply and cause bacteremia or endocarditis. In *Healthy People 2010,* the national goal is stated to "prevent and control oral and craniofacial diseases, conditions, and injuries and to improve access to related services." The oral health objectives in *Oral Health in America,* a report of the Surgeon General, are intended to prevent, decrease, or eliminate oral health disparities in the U.S. population. In the United States, reports indicate that by age 6 only 5.6 percent of schoolchildren have tooth decay in their permanent teeth but by age 17, 84 percent of individuals have an average of eight permanent tooth surfaces affected. This indicates that despite the great strides the United States has made in the decline of dental caries, it is still the most common dental disease affecting its children and adults.

Caries are an infectious bacterial-based disease caused by *Streptococcus mutans* and *Lactobacilli* that colonize in the biofilms which line the oral cavity. These bacteria produce organic acids as byproducts of their metabolism. These acids can diffuse across the biofilm and into the tooth structure. The acids will erode the enamel and dentin and cause weakening of the hydroxyapatite matrix structure of the tooth, thereby causing caries. Fluoride can help in disease modification and prevention. When fluoride is exposed during or after enamel formation, fluoride ions will displace the hydroxide ions in hydroxyapatite, creating fluoroapatite. This new matrix is much more stable, less soluble, and more resistant to the acid attack of the bacterial metabolic byproducts.

Fluoride has antimicrobial properties. It can inhibit enolase and ATPases, enzymes found in the bacteria's metabolic pathway. When found in saliva, fluoride can diffuse out and through dental plaque to depress the metabolic activity of bacteria. Decreased saliva production causes dry mouth, or xerostomia. This can occur in patients who have been irradiated for head and neck cancer or individuals with Sjögren's autoimmune disease. With decreased saliva, bacteria will grow exponentially. Fluoride, when used in mouthrinses, pastes or when ingested, decreases the bacterial count very effectively in individuals who are at increased risk of caries.

Osteoporosis is a clinical condition of age related to decline in bone mass whereby the bones can become brittle and porous. This condition is important for the mandible and maxillae, bones that support the teeth. Treatment for this condition may include bisphophonates, calcium supplements, and weight-bearing exercise. In addition, treatment with sodium fluoride is under investigation. Sustained-release sodium fluoride has been shown to augment spinal bone mass and reduce spinal fractures in older women with osteoporosis. Greater fluoride absorption occurs as the bones are forming and plateaus at about 50–60 years of age. In later years, more fluoride is excreted in urine than stored in bones.

DELIVERIES

Fluoride can be delivered to the teeth through systemic or topical measures or a combination of both means. If fluoride is ingested during tooth development stages from birth to adulthood third molars, it can be incorporated into the tooth structure in the form of fluorapatite. This delivery of fluoride is systemic, meaning that the fluoride absorbed from the gut, then transferred to plasma, is exposed to all parts of the body where blood plasma will flow. Any method of ingested fluoride such as fluoridated water, fluoride tablets, or drops or vitamins with fluoride, natural foods, and ingested toothpaste are considered systemic delivery of fluoride.

Topical delivery of fluoride means the surface of the tooth is bathed with fluoride-containing solutions. It may be from saliva (a systemic source) or applied to the teeth but after eruption. The fluoride is incorporated into the tooth surface by replacing the hydroxyl ion. The concentration of the delivered fluoride will vary depending upon the methods used; the amount of fluoride incorporated to the tooth will vary. The more fluoride incorporated, the longer the teeth will withstand an acid attack and therefore greater caries resistance.

SYSTEMICS

Sources of naturally occurring fluoride are water and food. Fluoride can be added to water, referred to as water fluoridation. The amount of fluoride added is 0.7–1.2 ppm in order to have the maximum reduction in dental decay, without causing fluoroisis or altered enamel formation. Fluorosis can have an effect on the tooth structure and also cause tooth staining. Water concentrations in moderate climates are at 1 ppm, in colder climates at 1.2 ppm. As climate warmth increases, individuals are more likely to drink increased amounts of water; in warmer climates the water is fluoridated between a 0.6 and 0.8 ppm ratio.

Approximately 65 percent of the population on public systems in the United States has fluoridated water; this comprises about 57 percent of the total U.S. population. As of 2003, 42 of the largest cities in the United States had fluoridated water.

Community Water Fluoridation

Fluoride is added to the water source in such compounds as hydrofluorosilic acid, sodium fluoride, or sodium silicofluoride. The fluoride must be soluble in order to be released in the ionized form and become available for uptake into the blood stream. The compound must also be relatively inexpensive, safe, and easily regulated in distribution. The results of community water fluoridation may result in 40–65 percent fewer caries in children exposed to water fluoridation. There is also a 50 percent reduction of root caries in populations who have been exposed to water fluoridation over a lifetime. One cup (8 oz) provides approximately .2 mg of fluoride.

School Fluoridation

By adjusting the fluoride content in a school water source, the amount can be raised to over 4.5 times the

┌─ **Did You Know?** ──────────────────
│ Grand Rapids, Michigan was the first city in the
│ United States to put fluoride in its drinking water.
└──────────────────────────────────────

amount of fluoride in natural water. This has and can be done to compensate for the limited hours per day the child is in school and the amount of water consumed. The results show a 20–30 percent reduction in caries over the 12 years in school. The cost and practicality of added fluoride in this manner is weighed against the more effective community water fluoridation.

Prescriptions and Supplements

Supplements given orally can come as liquid drops, tablets, or in a combination form with vitamins. The clinician must consider the age of the child and the amount of active fluoride in drinking water when prescribing the dosage of fluoride to be taken in supplement form. The clinician should do a 3-day intake diary of the child's food and drinks to get a more accurate fluoride intake history. The clinician should also factor in other sources of fluoride such as natural foods or teas, prepared foods, beverages, or formulas prepared with fluoridated water, and deficiency, if there is too little fluoride such as in well water or bottled water use. The chart by the ADA (Table 10–1) gives the usual amount of concentration and age. The method of fluoride delivery must also be considered when prescribing for children. The child's ability to chew a tablet needs to be assessed or, if unable, liquid may be added to the formula or other beverages as an alternative method of supplementation. Milk or other calcium products should not be consumed within an hour, as the calcium will bind with the newly released fluoride ion, making it insoluble and not bioavailable.

Naturally Fluoridated Water

Water can naturally contain trace amounts of fluoride. About 10 million people in the United States live in communities where water is fluoridated naturally at 0.7 ppm or higher. In communities where natural fluoridination occurs at high levels, people are at an increased risk of dental fluorosis, a hypomineralization of the enamel. Partial defluoridation can be accomplished to reduce the level to the acceptable 0.7–1.2 ppm by diluting the water with nonfluoridated water or by chemically removing enough fluoride to bring it to the recommended level.

Fluorosis

Dental fluorosis or mottled enamel can only occur with systemically ingested fluoride. This is different from fluoride toxicity, when there has been a one-time lethal dose of fluoride ingestion. Fluorosis has its effect on the

Table 10-1 Fluoride Supplement Dosage Schedule

Age	Fluoride Ion Level in Drinking Water (ppm)*		
	< 0.3 ppm	0.3−0.6 ppm	>0.6 ppm
Birth–6 months	None	None	None
6 months–3 years	0.25 mg/day**	None	None
3–6 years	0.50 mg/day	0.25mg/day	None
6–16 years	1.0 mg/day	0.50 mg/day	None

This schedule has been approved by the American Dental Association, American Academy of Pediatrics, and American Academy of Pediatric Dentistry.
* 1.0 ppm = 1 mg/liter.
** 2.2 mg sodium fluoride contains 1 mg fluoride ion.

ameloblasts which occur in tooth architecture during development. Most tooth development occurs from 6 months to 6 years; fluoride ingestion must be actively monitored during this time. Studies indicate that the maxillary centrals are at the greatest risk in males from 15 to 24 months, and in females from 21 to 30 months. Any combination of systemic fluoride over the total acceptable level of 0.7–1.2 ppm can cause fluorosis. Therefore it is very important for the dental clinician to evaluate all sources of fluoride in order to prevent this unwanted effect. Once the crown is formed, no amount of ingested fluoride can cause additional fluorosis damage to teeth.

Clinically, mild fluorosis will appear as chalky, with striations barely visible. It may be seen just at the incisal edge, involving less than one-third of the crown, this is referred to as "snow capping." A score of 0–7 is used to quantify the amount of tooth involvement from excess fluoride.

Teeth with fluorosis are less susceptible to caries; however, as the effect increases, the enamel becomes more pitted and irregular, making teeth not aesthetically pleasing. Staining can occur if the intact enamel or the dentin are visible. This is like a floor tile with a crack in it; the stain becomes more visible in the crack than the rest of the tile. Large areas of enamel may be missing.

Dental hygienists must be aware of patients' systemic fluoride intake to reduce the risk of fluorosis in formulating teeth.

Rapid Dental Hint

For esthetic purposes, prosthetics such as veneers or crowns are commonly used for severe fluorosis.

TOPICALS

Topical fluoride can be applied to erupted teeth. The fluoride delivered in this method is absorbed into the tooth surface from the topically applied solution. The fluoride found in saliva that bathes the tooth acts in this method. Topical sources of fluoride may appear to overlap systemic, affecting the erupted teeth and ideally not the developing teeth. Many sources of topical fluoride are self-applied by the patient, or can be applied in an office setting by the dental clinician. The home or self-applied fluorides are less concentrated and are to be used over a longer time period compared to office treatments, which are a more concentrated form and are applied once or twice a year.

In May 2006, evidence-based clinical recommendations were developed by the American Dental Association Council on Scientific Affairs (CSA) that evaluated the effectiveness of professionally applied topical fluoride for caries prevention. The complete article and table, "Professionally Applied Topical Fluoride: Evidence-Based Clinical Recommendations," is available online at www.ada.org/goto/ebd.

The most common active forms of fluoride found in topical fluoride delivery systems are sodium fluoride and acidulated phosphate fluoride; stannous fluoride is also available. Many of these products can be found over the counter. A prescription may be needed if the percentage of fluoride indicated is greater than over-the-counter FDA regulations. Stannous fluoride (GelKam 0.4%) is used primarily in the management of dentinal hypersensitivity, not for caries prevention, and can be purchased over the counter without a prescription. Table 10–2 reviews the more commonly used fluoride products.

Table 10–2   Common Fluoride Products

	Preparation	Generic/brand names	Notes
Systemic Fluorides			
	Community water fluoridation		Estimated daily consumption of water is 0.7 to 1.2 ppm
	Dietary Supplements		
	Chewable tablets with/without vitamins	Poly-Vi-Flor, Tri-Vi-Flor; Vi-Daylin/F, Luride Lozi-Tabs; generics	0.25, 0.5, and 1 mg sodium fluoride (NaF); recommended up to age 16 in areas where drinking water is less than the recommended levels
	Drops with vitamins	Generics; Luride, Thera-Flur, Pediaflor drops, Poly-Vi-Flor	NaF; recommended up to age 16 in areas where drinking water is less than the recommended levels
Topical Fluorides	**Self-Applied**		
	Rinse	Phos-Flur (OTC)	4.4 mg acidulated phosphate fluoride (APF); sodium fluoride (NaF)
		Fluorigard (OTC)	0.05% (5 mg) NaF
		ACT (OTC)	0.05% (5 mg) NaF
		Gel-Kam Oral Care Rinse (Rx)	0.63% stannous fluoride
	Gel	PreviDent Rinse (Rx)	0.2% neutral NaF
		PreviDent 5000 Plus (Rx)	1.1% NaF
		PreviDent Gel (Rx)	1.1% NaF
		Oral-B NeutraCare (Rx)	1.1% neutral NaF
		Phos-Flur Gel (Rx)	1.1% NaF/APF
		PreviDent 500 Sensitive (Rx)	5% potassium nitrate; for dentinal hypersensitivity
		PreviDent 5000 Booster (Rx)	1.1% NaF
Topical Fluorides	**Office-Applied**		
	Gel, foam	Oral-B Minute Foam	1.23% Fluoride ion
		Oral-B Neutra-Foam	2.0% Neutral NaF
		Oral-B Minute-Gel	1.23% APF
		Fluoro-Foam	1.2% APF88
	Varnish	Duraphat (Rx)	5% NaF (for dentinal sensitivity)
		Duraflor (Rx)	5% NaF (for dentinal hypersensitivity)
		PreviDent Varnish (Rx)	5% NaF (for dentinal hypersensitivity)

Self-Applied Dentifrices

Dentifrice (toothpastes/gels and powders) are the most commonly used method of self-applied topical fluoride. A 30 percent decrease in dental caries can be achieved from the twice daily use of fluoridated dentifrice. Sodium fluoride at 0.22% (1,100 ppm) or sodium monofluorophosphate at 0.76% (1,100 ppm) are the common active forms of fluoride seen in dentifrices. This would indicate that a single ribbon of toothpaste on the brush will yield about 1 mg of fluoride when released. Therefore, it is extremely important for young children to limit the amount of fluoride on the brush to no more than a pea and to expectorate (spit out) the paste. A child can ingest up to 0.3 mg of fluoride in a single brushing session. Even more can be ingested if the child continues to refill the brush and swallow the paste, or has not formed the ability to properly spit out upon request. This extra ingestion of fluoride could lead to fluorosis.

Extra strength toothpaste at 1,500 ppm will release increased amounts of bioavailable fluoride ion for remineralization. As with toothpaste, this should be kept out of the reach of children and if used by a child should only be done so under adult supervision paying close attention to the amount used.

Toothpastes are given an ADA seal of approval for therapeutic caries preventative action based on the amount of bioavailable fluoride and the toothpaste's degree of caries reduction. The other components found in toothpaste may be assessed for varying amounts of abrasivity, calculus reduction, gingivitis reduction, desensitizing action, or whitening, or combined effects. These separate effects should be understood when recommending a toothpaste.

Mouthrinses

Mouthrinses may be cosmetic or therapeutic. Mouthrinses that contain fluoride must be studied for their effectiveness. If they have been proven in caries prevention, they may then be included in the home care regime. The most common fluoride used in mouthrinses is sodium fluoride (NaF) at concentrations of 0.05% for daily use. This delivers 264 mg of NaF or 120 mg free fluoride. A 500 mL bottle of 0.05% NaF contains 100 mg of fluoride; therefore the bottle must be kept out of the reach of children and packaged with a child-proof cap. Children over 6 years of age who can rinse and spit the solution out properly may be instructed on how to use the mouthrinse. Several of these low-potency mouthrinses are available over the counter, such as Act, Fluorigard, and Reach.

Higher concentrations and less frequency solutions of fluoride are available at 0.2% sodium fluoride solution (1,000 ppm). These prescription products can be found under product label names such as Fluorinse, Phos-Flur or Point Two. These may be used in a pediatric population under supervision, such as in a school rinse program or at home use with parents. When used appropriately, both prescription and nonprescription concentrations have been shown to result in a 35 percent caries reduction.

Brush-On Gels

Home use brush-on gels may be over the counter or prescription depending upon the concentration and the use. Daily gels such as Stop, Gel-Kam, or Omni-Gel may contain 0.4% stannous fluoride (1,000 ppm). Prescription fluoride gels such as Prevident or Karigel may contain 1.1% sodium fluoride (5,000 ppm) or 0.05% acidulated phosphate fluoride 5,000 ppm prescription gel to be used once daily. These gels may be applied with a custom tray or brush-on technique after using conventional toothpaste. Consideration of the dentition and

 Rapid Dental Hint

The dental hygienist should consider the staining effect of stannous fluoride or the etching effect of an acidulated phosphate fluoride for veneers or laminates.

restorations should be given when determining if stannous, neutral, or acidulated phosphate fluoride is selected.

Professionally Applied Fluoride

Professionally applied fluorides decrease caries by 30–40 percent when applied during the eruptive stages of the tooth. They are delivered in solutions, gels, or foams and vary in the percentage of fluoride they contain. They can be applied in trays or painted on and are in one-minute or four-minute application delivery systems.

Neutral sodium fluoride at 2% delivers 9,000 ppm of fluoride in concentration and is applied twice a year or as the caries risk assessment indicates. Four applications are given one week apart during the ages of 3, 7, 10, and 13. It does not discolor teeth, or cause gingival irritation. Also, a basic pH of 9.2 makes this type of fluoride treatment recommended for adults who have anterior restorations or laminates.

A 1.23% acidulated phosphate fluoride in 12,300–12,500 ppm concentration is another treatment option for those with a high risk of caries formation. It is applied twice yearly or as indicated. This combination or 2.0% NaF and 0.34% hydrofluoric acid can be delivered as a gel or aqueous solution. Since this treatment is at 3.0–3.5 pH, a side effect may be pitting or etching of porcelain or composite restorations. A full dental history should be taken when deciding to use these methods.

Stannous fluoride at 8% contains 20,000–25,000ppm of bioavailable fluoride. It is rarely used now due to the bitter taste it has and its propensity to cause extrinsic brown staining. Its pH is 2.4 to 2.8, making it very acidic and it may cause gingival irritations.

CHOOSING TREATMENT METHODS

Determining which fluoride delivery system and frequency depends upon client risks, age, natural intake of fluoride, eruption of teeth, presence of exposed cementum, types of restorations, and overall dietary issues. Children and adults should be considered for fluoride if the risk factors assessment indicates that there is a need. Children who do not receive the recommended levels of fluoride from common sources should be considered for systemic and topical deliveries. Adults at risk of caries from dietary changes, recessions, cancer therapies, xerostomia or medications that can affect salivary flow should be considered for fluoride treatments.

The age of the child must be considered when determining which delivery method to recommend, such as, the tray, paint-on, or rinse. The ability not to swallow the solutions and spit the excess or rinse without swallowing must be considered when planning an intervention. Mainly children by the age of 6 will have the capacity fully to understand what it means not to swallow. Moreover, consideration of the child's inadvertent swallowing of toothpaste as a source of fluoride must be included when tabulating the daily fluoride intake of the patient.

TOXICOLOGY

Acute toxicity refers to the rapid intake of an excess dose of fluoride over a short time. Depending on the dose ingested, this can result in mild nausea or upset stomach, to death. Upon ingestion of the fluoride compound a chemical reaction takes place where the atoms dissociate into hydrogen and fluoride, making hydrofluric acid (HF). This is one of the strongest acids that can be made and is highly irritating to the stomach mucosa. Pain and vomiting will result even if the quantities ingested are small. A dose of on average of 4 to 5 grams is such a lethal level that there will be systemic symptoms. These symptoms include muscular weakness, spasms, paresthesia, central nervous system depression, bronchospasm, ventricular fibrillation, and cardiac arrest. Death can occur within 4 hours after the lethal dose is ingested if emergency actions are not taken. The blood toxicity can reach its maximum level within 30 minutes, meaning symptoms can begin soon after ingestion.

Rapid Dental Hint

While formulating the care plan, the dental hygienist considers all benefits for fluoride for all age groups and all systemic conditions, not just children during tooth eruption years.

If under 2.3 mg fluoride/lbs body weight have been ingested, give calcium (milk). If more than 2.3 mg fluoride/lbs body weight have been ingested, induce vomiting and give orally soluble calcium (e.g., a mild 5% calcium gluconate or calcium lactate solution) and seek immediate assistance.

The lethal dose of fluoride is the amount of fluoride which is likely to cause death if not intercepted with emergency treatment. When computing this amount, the person's weight must be considered. The **safely tolerated dose (STD)** is the amount of fluoride that can be ingested without causing any serious reaction for the client. This can be about one-quarter of the **certainly lethal dose (CLD)**. The CLD will result in death for the client if emergency care is not rendered. In order to calculate the STD or the CLD, the practitioner must know the percentage of fluoride in the compound, the amount ingested, and the weight of the client.

The CLD of a 70 kg (154 lb) adult is about 5–10 grams of NaF or 32–64 mg of fluoride per kilogram (kg). The CLD for a child depending upon weight is 0.5 to 1.0 grams of sodium fluoride taken at once. The STD for an adult of 70 kg is about 1.25 to 2.5 grams of NaF or 8–16 mg of fluoride per kilogram (f/kg). For a child the STD is 0.5 grams of sodium fluoride taken at once. In order to compute the amount of fluoride released from a solution, gel, or paste, the following formula is to be used. It has been calculated that less than 1 gram (1,000 mg) of fluoride, if ingested in one huge dose, can be fatal for a child 12 years or younger depending upon weight and for a child 6 years or younger, it may be as little as 500 mg of fluoride in order to be lethal.

As an example, if a 2% NaF solution is used, a conversion ratio of the fluoride compound is to be multiplied. To calculate this ratio of a compound such as NaF, the combined molecular weight should be assessed, e.g., Na 23 + F 19 = 42. Then the ratio of fluoride to the compound is 19 to 42 = 19/42, or 0.452. Similarly, the ratio of stannous fluoride is 1 divided by 4.1 and APF (Na_2PO_3) is 1 divided by 7.6. It follows that if a 2% solution of NaF is used and 5 ml of solution were ingested, the amount of available fluoride would be 45.5 mg F. It would require about 105 ml of 2% solution to yield a CDL (1,000 mg, or 1 gram) of fluoride for a child.

DENTAL HYGIENE NOTES

With any use of fluoride it is suggested that the clinician be aware of the full amount of fluoride used systemically and topically. Also, the amount of topical fluoride should be considered if the child inadvertently ingests during tooth brushing. Certain people and cultures may eat more shellfish or drink more tea than others, and this needs to be considered in determining fluoride applications.

Consuming products containing calcium (dairy) or magnesium may decrease the absorption of fluorides.

The current risk of caries and in the future depends upon given lifestyle changes and drug therapies. These risks impact upon the recommendations made when fluoride is used as a systemic or topical additive. It is the responsibility of the clinician to determine completely the amount of fluoride and the risk of caries for the patient before prescribing fluoride treatments. Here the dental hygienist plays a primary role in documentation and assessment before the delivery of fluoride treatment to the patient.

KEY POINTS

- Fluoride supplement is primarily used for caries prevention.
- Dental fluorosis is seen when there is excessive ingestion of fluoride.
- Before prescribing or advising on a fluoride supplementation, many factors must be assessed, including the age of the child and the amount of fluoride ingested in the diet.
- Once in the saliva, fluoride can remain chemically active for up to 3 hours.

BOARD REVIEW QUESTIONS

1. A condition related to hypomineralization due to excessive ingestion of fluoride is known as: (pp. 186–187)
   a. Fluorosis
   b. Caries
   c. Hypercalcification
   d. Demineralization

2. The teeth can acquire fluoride during (p. 184)
   a. Pre-eruptive mineralization stage
   b. Pre-eruptive maturation stage

   c. Post-eruptive stage
   d. a and b
   e. All of the above

3. Which is not an effect of fluoride? (pp. 185, 188)
   a. Prevents demineralization
   b. Enhances remineralization if incipient lesion
   c. Alters plaque bacteria
   d. Increases enamel solubility and decreases enamel resistance

4. Soduim fluoride is available in (pp. 188, 190)
   a. 2% solution
   b. 2% gel
   c. 2% foam
   d. all of the above

5. Which is *not* an indication for acidulated fluoride application? (p. 189)
   a. Primary teeth
   b. Active caries
   c. Teeth supporting an overdenture
   d. Porcelain restorations

SELECTED REFERENCES

Bowen, W. H. Fluorosis: Is it really a problem? 2002. *JADA* 133:1405–1407.

Hays, D. R. and C. Westphal. 2006. Fluorides' balancing act. *Dimensions of Dental Hygiene* May: 20–21.

Healthy People 2010. Office of Disease Prevention and Health Promotion, U.S. Department of Health and Human Services.

Oral Health in America: A Report of the Surgeon General. May 2000.

Weinberg, M. A. Guide to fluoride use. 2005. *U.S. Pharmacist* 30:48–58.

WEB SITES

www.ada.org/public/topics/fluoride/fluoride_article01.asp
www.dentistry.com/oralhygienecenter003.asp
www.atsdr.cdc.gov/tfacts11.html
www.healthypeople.gov
www.oralhealthamerica.org

QUICK DRUG GUIDE

SYSTEMIC FLUORIDES

- Community water fluoridation

Dietary Supplements

- Chewable tablets with/without vitamins
- Drops with vitamins

- Poly-Vi-Flor, Tri-Vi-Flor; Vi-Daylin/F, Luride Lozi-Tabs; generics
- Generics; Luride, Thera-Flur, Pediaflor drops, Poly-Vi-Flor

TOPICAL FLUORIDES

Self-applied

- Phos-Flur Rinse
- Fluorigard
- ACT
- PreviDent 5000 Plus
- PreviDent 5000 Booster
- PreviDent Brush on Gel
- PreviDent Dental Rinse
- Oral-B NeutraCare Rinse

- Gel-Kam Oral Care Rinse
- Gel-Kam Treatment Gel   } for dentinal hypersensitivity
- PreviDent 5000 Sensitive

Office-applied

- Oral-B Minute Foam, Gel
- Oral-B Neutra Foam
- Fluoro-Foam
- Duraphat varnish } for dentinal hypersensitivity
- Duraflor varnish

Chapter 11

Management of Common Oral Lesions and Conditions

GOAL: To introduce basic treatment regimens for common oral lesions seen in the dental office.

EDUCATIONAL OBJECTIVES

After reading this chapter, the reader should be able to:

1. Review common oral mucous membrane lesions including signs, symptoms and treatments.
2. Choose the appropriate treatment for xerostomia.

KEY TERMS

Oral lesion

Recurrent minor aphthous ulcers

Xerostomia

INTRODUCTION

Since dental hygienists are probably the first to see changes in the patient's oral cavity, they must be proficient in recognizing oral lesions. When an **oral lesion** is noted during an intraoral examination, the dental hygienist should note the size, shape, and color of the lesion. The patient should be questioned as to whether they are aware it is present in the mouth, and how long it has been there. This chapter will review common oral conditions/lesions and appropriate therapy; herpetic and fungal infections were discussed in Chapter 7. After a brief explanation of the oral lesion, sample prescriptions of drugs used in the treatment of these lesions are presented (Table 11–1). It should be noted that there are many OTC products, and only some are mentioned in this chapter.

RECURRENT MINOR APHTHOUS ULCERS (RAU)

The etiology of **recurrent minor aphthous ulcers** (canker sores) is essentially unknown; however, an immune response has been proposed involving immune cells. Toothpaste ingredients (e.g., sodium lauryl sulfate) can increase aphthous ulcerations. Clinically, aphthous ulcers appear on movable mucosa only (e.g., inner lower lip, soft palate). The ulcerations are usually round with

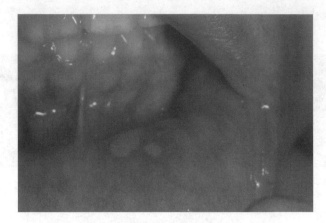

FIGURE 11–1 Recurrent aphthous ulcers. (Courtesy Dr. James B. Fine, Columbia College of Dental Medicine.)

a depressed center and a red margin and do not fuse (Figure 11–1). They are very painful, especially when speaking and eating.

Treatment

Though painful, these lesions will heal in about 7–10 days. Most patients with mild aphthae require no treatment or only periodic topical analgesic therapy such as viscous lidocaine 2% rinse, which is a prescription product. Besides analgesics, anti-inflammatories (steroids), and antibiotics have been used. Orabase with benzo-

Table 11–1 Medications Used in Treatment of Common Oral Lesions

Disease	Prescription Products	Common OTC Products
Aphthous Ulcers (Canker Sores)	Lidocaine 2% viscous, Timamcinolone (Kenalog) in Orabase, Orabase HCT Amlexanox (Aphthasol) 5% paste Tetracycline Chlorhexidine gluconate Severe: • Flucinonide gel 0.05% mixed with equal parts of Orabase • Dexamethasone elxir	• Orajel • Orabase • Gly-Oxide • Peroxyl
Xerostomia	Pilocarpine (Salagen) Initial dose is one 5 mg tablet tid or qid increasing to 3-6 tabs (15 to 30 mg) a day. At least 6 to 12 weeks of uninterrupted therapy may be needed before improvement is seen Cevimeline (Evoxac) 30 mg tid	• Oasis mouthrinse • Biotène (mouthrinse, spray, toothpaste, gum) • Oralbalance Long-lasting moisturizing gel • Saliva substitutes: Xero-Lube Salivart Optimoist • Moi-Stir Salix MouthKote Saliva stimulants: • Natrol Dry Mouth Relief

caine (Orabase-B) is dabbed on the ulcer using a finger cot.

Anti-inflammatory (corticosteroid) agents may be the most helpful in increasing healing time and relieving pain. Triamcinolone 0.1% (Kenalog in Orabase) or hydrocortisone in Orabase is dabbed on to ulcers 2–4 times daily. If Orabase products are rubbed on the mucosa, the paste will not stay on the tissue. Orabase products also provide a protective coating for the ulcer. For more severe and extensive ulcers, dexamethasone elixir may be used as a rinse and expectorated.

Amlexanox (Aphthasol) 5% paste is a topical preparation that should not be applied more than four times daily. It may increase healing and decrease pain, but not reduce the frequency of RAU episodes. It is a potent inhibitor of the formation and release of inflammatory mediators from mast cells and neutrophils.

Randomized, controlled studies have supported the use of tetracycline: one 250 mg capsule opened and dissolved in 180 mL of water to be used as a rinse four times daily for 5 days. A tetracycline syrup (20 mg/5 mL) has also been used four times daily for 5 days.

There are numerous OTC agents that are available, including Kank-A, Orabase-B (benzocaine), and Gly-Oxide or Peroxyl mouthrinse (carbamide peroxide) (Table 12–1). Alternative therapies include zinc lozenges (suck one lozenge 4–6 times daily), vitamin C (500 mg, four times daily), and vitamin B complex (one tablet, four times daily).

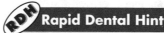

Rapid Dental Hint

Be able to make a differential diagnosis of aphthous ulcers and herpetic ulcers. The difference is location!

Orabase plain (Colgate Oral Pharm) and Orabase-B are available OTC.

LICHEN PLANUS

Lichen planus (LP) is a benign, chronic inflammatory mucosal condition of unknown etiology affecting the skin, oral mucosa, or both. Current theory suggests an immune-mediated mechanism. It affects all ages, but female adults over 40 years of age predominate.

Two major forms exist: reticular and erosive. Reticular LP is usually asymptomatic and classically presents

as reticular, lacy white lines on the buccal mucosa called Wicham striae. Lichen planus also occurs on other intraoral sites including the tongue, lips, floor of the mouth and gingival tissue. Erosive LP presents with generalized erythema and ulceration of the gingival tissue known as desquamative gingivitis.

Treatment

Asymptomatic lesions do not need treatment. Patients that are symptomatic may require topical corticosteroid gels, such as flucoinonide and/or corticosteroid mouthrinses. Meticulous oral hygiene may improve gingival lesions.

BURNING MOUTH SYNDROME

Burning mouth syndrome is defined as burning pain in the tongue or oral mucosa, usually without accompanying clinical and laboratory findings. Patients usually visit many healthcare providers for effective management. It is most prevalent in postmenopausal women. Other causes include nutritional/vitamin deficiency, xerostomia, and cranial nerve damage. Onset of symptoms may occur after a dental procedure, recent illness, or antibiotic therapy. Other symptoms include xerostomia and alterations in taste. There is a strong psychologic component where there may be mood and personality changes.

Treatment

Treatment of burning mouth usually deals with its symptoms. Medications include tricyclic antidepressants and benzodiazepines (anti-anxiety), and anticonvulsants.

Rapid Dental Hint

Burning mouth syndrome is very difficult to diagnose and treat. Listen carefully to the patient's symptoms.

PERICORONITIS

Pericoronitis refers to inflammation in the gingival tissue around the crown of a partially erupted tooth, usually the mandibular 3rd molar. There is a gingival flap (referred to as an operculum) surrounding the crown which is usually inflamed and is continuously bitten on, causing more pain. Pericoronitis is caused by a bacterial infection that can spread to other areas of the mouth, including the oropharyngeal area. Patients may experience difficulty and pain on swallowing and opening, fever, and malaise.

Treatment

Includes irrigation under the operculum to flush the area, and systemic antibiotics; however, recurrence is high. The most definitive treatment of a pericoronal abscess is extraction of the offending partially erupted tooth.

NECROTIZING ULCERATIVE GINGIVITIS

Necrotizing ulcerative gingivitis (NUG) is an infectious periodontal condition caused by fusiform-spirochete (*Borrelia vincentii*) bacteria. NUG is confined to the gingival tissue and characterized by pain of rapid onset, interdental necrosis, and bleeding. The onset of NUG is usually associated with increased psychological stress, immunosupression, tobacco use, and decreased nutritional intake. Usually, the patient is in extreme pain so that periodontal debridement is impossible until the pain is relieved.

Treatment

First the pain must be relieved with analgesics. The infection can be treated with antibiotics such as doxycycline, penicillin or metronidazole. Mouthrinses with hydrogen peroxide or chlorhexidine are helpful. Then plaque control is reviewed and periodontal debridement is performed.

XEROSTOMIA

Xerostomia or dry mouth can either be due to medications, illness (e.g., Sjøgren's syndrome, HIV, cancer) or aging. Some medications that cause xerostomia include psychotropics, antidiarrheals, decongestants, antihistamines, and antihypertensives. Salivary glands receive sympathetic innervation in addition to cholinergic innervation. Activation of either autonomic system will increase secretions; however, cholinergic activation is the more important system. Anticholinergic drugs bind to the cholinergic (muscarinic) receptors thus inhibiting salivary secretions from the salivary glands, resulting in dry mouth. Examples of drugs that cause anticholinergic side effects include antihistamines, antianxiety drugs, and antidepressants. Other drugs will decrease norepinephrine release and hence decrease salivation, resulting in dry mouth.

In patients with xerostomia, there is an increased risk for caries and periodontal disease.

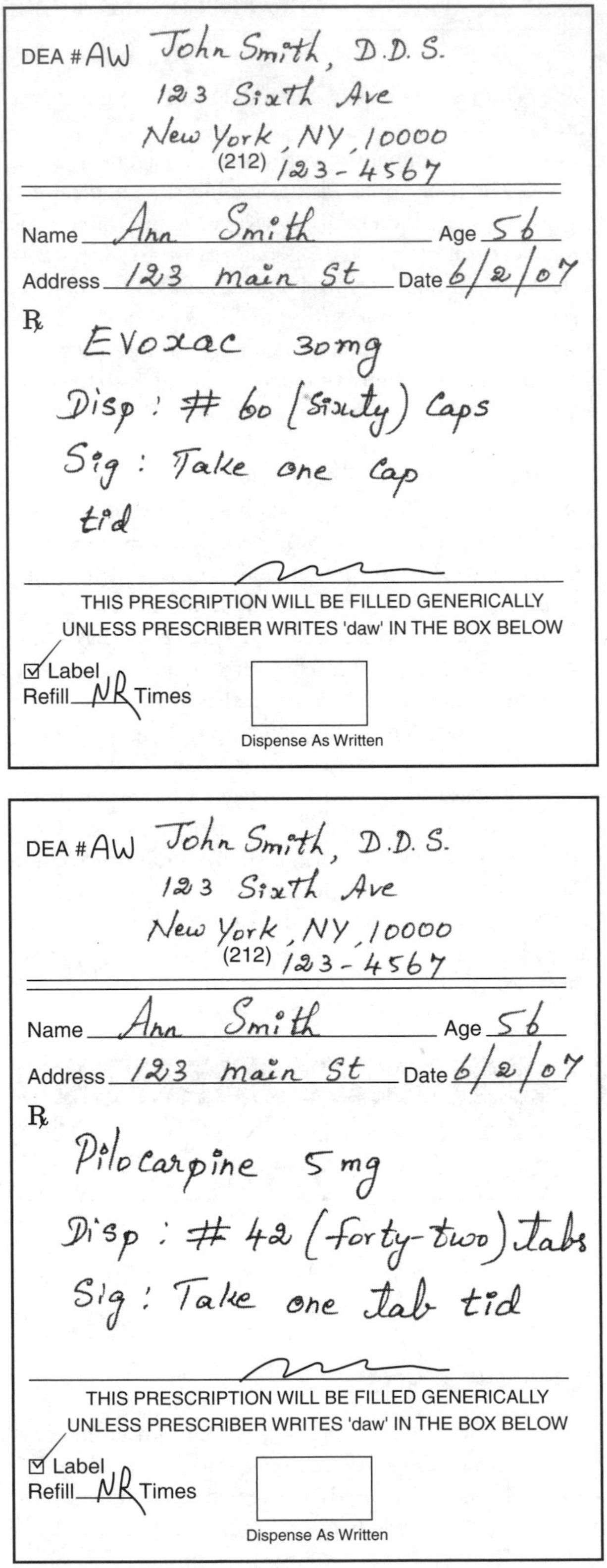

DEA #AW John Smith, D.D.S.
123 Sixth Ave
New York, NY, 10000
(212) 123-4567

Name Ann Smith Age 56
Address 123 main St Date 6/2/07
℞
Evoxac 30mg
Disp: # 60 (Sixty) Caps
Sig: Take one cap tid

THIS PRESCRIPTION WILL BE FILLED GENERICALLY UNLESS PRESCRIBER WRITES 'daw' IN THE BOX BELOW
☑ Label
Refill NR Times
Dispense As Written

DEA #AW John Smith, D.D.S.
123 Sixth Ave
New York, NY, 10000
(212) 123-4567

Name Ann Smith Age 56
Address 123 main St Date 6/2/07
℞
Pilocarpine 5 mg
Disp: # 42 (forty-two) tabs
Sig: Take one tab tid

THIS PRESCRIPTION WILL BE FILLED GENERICALLY UNLESS PRESCRIBER WRITES 'daw' IN THE BOX BELOW
☑ Label
Refill NR Times
Dispense As Written

FIGURE 11–2 Prescriptions for drugs used in the management of xerostomia

Treatment

Treatment is aimed at increasing secretions. Many saliva substitutes are available OTC, but patient adherence is poor. These products come in a variety of formulations, including solutions, sprays, gels, and lozenges (Table 11–1). Generally, they contain an agent to increase viscosity, such as carboxymethylcelluose or hydroxyethylcellulose, minerals such as calcium phosphate and fluoride, preservative such as propylparaben, and flavoring.

There are also many OTC mouthrinses such as Biotène and Oasis. Sample prescriptions are shown in Figure 11–2.

For patients with some salivary function, a sialagogue may be beneficial; pilocarpine HCl (Salagen) and cevimeline (Evoxac) are cholinergic drugs that act directly on cholinergic muscarinic receptor sites, mimicking acetylcholine and increasing salivary secretions. These drugs are contraindicated in patients with uncontrolled asthma, narrow-angle glaucoma, and have a pregnancy category C. Excessive sweating, urinary urgency, GI upset and nausea are the most common adverse effects with these drugs.

In addition to medications, the patient can chew or suck on sugar-free gum or candy and increase intake of water.

KEY POINTS

- Aphthous ulcers (canker sores) are self-limiting and are treated by alleviating the pain.
- Monitor susceptible patients for xerostomia and when indicated, use appropriate prescription or OTC drugs

BOARD REVIEW QUESTIONS

1. Which of the following medications is used to treat canker sores? (p. 194–195)
   a. Systemic steroids
   b. Hydrogen peroxide
   c. Lidocaine, viscous
   d. Steroid gel

2. Which of the following patients is cevimeline contraindicated? (p. 197)
   a. Uncontrolled asthma.
   b. Hypertension
   c. Cardiac arrhythmias
   d. Prostate hypertrophy

3. Which of the following lesions occurs on movable mucosa? (p. 194)
   a. Aphthous ulcers
   b. Herpetic labialis
   c. Cold sores
   d. Angular cheilosis

4. Which of the following medications is used for the management of burning mouth syndrome? (p. 195–196)
   a. Antidepressants
   b. Chlortimazole troche
   c. Nystatin tablets
   d. Mycostatin pastilles

5. Which of the following is a prescription drug used in the management of xerostomia? (p. 196)
   a. Salivart
   b. Optimoist
   c. Pilocarpine
   d. Mycelex

REFERENCES

ADA Division of Communications. 2005. For the dental patient: Canker sores and cold sores. *J Am Dent Assoc* 136(*3*):415.

Akintoye, S. O., and M. S. Greenberg. 2005. Recurrent aphthous stomatitis. *Dent Clin North Am* 49:31–47, vii–viii.

Grushka, M., J. B. Epstein, M. Gorsky. 2002. Burning mouth syndrome. *Am Fam Physicians* 65:615–620, 622.

Huan Xin Meng. Periodontal Abscess. 1999. *Ann Periodontol* 4:79–82.

Jurge, S., R. Kuffer, C. Scully, Porter S. R. 2006. Mucosal disease series. Number VI. Recurrent aphthous stomatitis. *Oral Dis* 12:1–21.

Neville, B. W., D. D. Damm, C. M. Allen, J. E. Bouqout. 2002. Recurrent aphthous stomatitis (recurrent aphthous ulcerations; canker sores). In: *Oral and Maxillofacial Pathology*. Philadelphia: W.B. Saunders Company, pp. 285–290.

Porter, S., C. Scully. Aphthous ulcers (recurrent). 2005. *Clin Evid* 13:1687–1697.

Sugarman, B., N.W. Savage, X. Zhou, L. J. Walsh, M. Bigby. 2000. Oral lichen planus. *Clin Dermatol* 18:533–539.

Volkov, I., I. Rudoy, U. Abu-Rabia, T. Masalha, R. Masalha. 2005. Case report: Recurrent aphthous stomatitis responds to vitamin B_{12} treatment. *Can Fam Physician* 51:844–845.

Chapter **12**

Vitamins and Minerals

GOAL: To introduce the dental clinician to the essentials of vitamins and minerals and oral symptoms resulting from deficiency states.

EDUCATIONAL OBJECTIVES

After reading this chapter, the reader should be able to:

1. Evaluate the role of vitamins in the health of an individual.
2. Describe oral signs and symptoms in deficiency states.
3. List the various types of water-soluble and fat-soluble vitamins.
4. Explain the importance of drug–drug interactions with selected vitamins.
5. Discuss how select vitamins affect dental treatment.

KEY TERMS
Vitamins
Recommended daily allowances
Antioxidants
Minerals

INTRODUCTION

Maintaining Health

Vitamins are organic compounds required for normal growth, development, and maintenance, but are not synthesized by the human body. Therefore, vitamins must get into the body from outside sources, including food and water, or by orally or intravenously administered formulations. Vitamins and minerals are used for the prevention and treatment of specific deficiency conditions or where the diet is known to be inadequate to maintain plasma levels. Some vitamins may actually be harmful to individuals, especially if taken in more than the prescribed dose.

According to the Food and Nutrition Board, the **recommended dietary allowances** or RDAs of vitamins and minerals are stated requirements that are essential for the needs of an individual. IU stands for International Units, and is used for the measurement of vitamins. It is defined as the quantity of a vitamin that produces a biological effect agreed upon as an international standard, and is dependent on the potency of the vitamin.

Daily values (DVs) represent two sets of reference values for nutrients: daily reference values (DRVs) and reference daily values (RDVs). Only the DVs are listed on product labels as a reference point to help individuals understand their overall daily dietary needs.

If an individual's diet contains a combination of fresh vegetables, fruits, dairy products and meat, a vitamin or mineral supplement is probably not needed. However, when an individual cannot get an adequate diet, or in diseases of intestinal malabsorption, pregnancy, lactation or other conditions with increased tissue requirements, then vitamin/mineral supplementation is recommended by a physician. Fortunately, today most vitamin deficiencies are rarely seen in the United States.

┌ Did You Know? ───

In 1929, Sir Frederick Gowland Hopkins won the Nobel Prize for his discovery of vitamins (actually, growth-stimulating vitamins). Vitamin was named after "vita" meaning life and "amine" from compounds found in the thiamine that was isolated from rice husks.

CLASSIFICATION OF VITAMINS

Vitamins are classified as either fat soluble or water soluble (Table 12–1). Vitamins A, D, E, and K are fat soluble because they are extracted with fat solvents and are found in the fat parts of animal tissue. These vitamins are absorbed from the small intestine most effectively when ingested with dietary fat. Fat-soluble vitamins are stored in the liver and used by the body when the body is not getting enough of them in the diet. Thus, deficiencies in vitamins A, D, E, and K are uncommon. However, toxicity (referred to as hypervitaminosis) may occur if supplements are taken when there are adequate levels in the plasma.

Vitamins B and C are water soluble and not stored in the body; these vitamins must be obtained daily through food or supplements. Toxicity is uncommon because these vitamins are water soluble and easily excreted in the urine and feces. The effects of many vitamin deficiencies are seen in the mouth (Table 12–1).

Two types of multivitamin preparations are available over the counter: supplemental and therapeutic. Supplemental multivitamins contain ½ to 1½ times the RDA requirements. Therapeutic multivitamins are available with a prescription and are used for the nutritional support of severe disease states.

 Rapid Dental Hint

Deficiency in many vitamins cause oral lesions/conditions. When oral conditions such as glossitis, angular cheilitis, or xerostomia are recognized in your patients, a vitamin deficiency must be ruled out.

WATER-SOLUBLE VITAMINS

- Vitamin B_1 (thiamine)
- Vitamin B_2 (riboflavin)
- Vitamin B_3 (niacin, nicotinic acid)
- Vitamin B_5 (pantothenic acid)
- Vitamin B_6 (pyridoxine)
- Vitamin B_{12} (cobalamin)
- Folic acid
- Biotin
- Vitamin C (ascorbic acid)

Table 12–1 Vitamins

Vitamin	RDA	Sources	Oral Deficiency/Notes
Water-Soluble			
Vitamin B_1 (thiamine)	Men: 1.2 mg Women: 1.1 mg	Liver, grains, dried yeast, whole grains, meat	Glossitis (burning tongue, red, raw, fissured), loss of taste, stomatitis, angular cheilosis
Vitamin B_2 (riboflavin)	Men: 1.4–1.8 mg Women: 1.2–1.3 mg	Milk, cheese, liver, eggs, enriched cereals	Angular cheilosis (painful, dry cracked corners of the mouth), atrophy of villiform papillae, glossitis, magenta tongue
Vitamin B_3 (niacin)	Men: 15–20 mg Women: 13–15 mg	Dried yeast, meats, fish, whole grains, green vegetables, beans	Angular cheilosis, glossitis, swollen red fungiform papillae, loss of filliform papillae (smooth, red appearance)
Vitamin B_6 (pyridoxine)	Men: 2 mg Women:1.5–1.6 mg	Dried yeast, liver, organ meats, beans, whole-grain cereals	Angular cheilosis, glossitis, mucosal ulcerations and erosions
Vitamin B_{12} (cobalamin)	Men: 2.0 mcg Women: 2.0–2.2 mcg	Liver, meats, milk, eggs, yeast	Xerostomia, angular cheilosis, stomatitis, glossitis, smooth and shiny tongue
Vitamin C	Men and women: 60 mg	Citrus fruits, green and red peppers, spinach, tomatoes, strawberries	Gingival bleeding, abnormal redness, poor wound healing
Folic acid	Men: 200 mcg Women: 160–180 mcg (pregnant women: 400 mcg)	Liver, yeast, leafy vegetables, beans	Stomatitis, glossitis
Fat-Soluble			
Vitamin A (retinol)	Men: 1,000 RE Women: 800 RE	Preformed Vitamin A: Fish, liver, butter, milk, cream Carotenoids: dark green, leafy vegetables and yellow-orange vegetables (carrots)	Xerostomia, abnormal size and shape of teeth
Vitamin D (cholecalciferol)	Men and women 5 to 10 mcg (cholecalciferol = 400 IU of vitamin D	Sunlight, milk, cheese, yogurt, fish, eggs	Enamel hypoplasia, loss of bone
Vitamin E (tocopherol)	Men: 10 mg/day Women: 8 mg/day	Vegetable oils, green vegetables, nuts, wheat germ	None
Vitamin K	Men: 70–80 mcg Women: 60–65 mcg	Phylloquinone (green leafy vegetables); Menadione (liver)	increased risk of bleeding and candidiasis

Data obtained from: Food and Nutrition Board. *Recommended Dietary Allowances.* Washington, DC: National Academy Press. www.iom.edu.
Vitamin A: 1 retinol equivalent (RE) = 1 mcg retinol or 6 mcg beta-carotene.
Vitamin E: 1 mg alpha tocopherol = 1 TE alpha-tocopherol = 1.5 IU.
Niacin: 1 niacin equivalent is equal to 1 mg of niacin or 60 mg of dietary tryptophan.
Vitamin D: 10 mcg cholecalciferol = 400 IU vitamin D.

B Vitamins

The B vitamins, also referred to as the B complex of vitamins, consist of:

- Thiamine (B_1)
- Riboflavin (B_2)
- Niacin (B_3)
- Pantothenic acid (B_5)
- Pyridoxine (B_6)
- Cobalamin (B_{12})
- Folic acid
- Biotin.

Dietary sources and the RDA for the B complex vitamins are listed in Table 12–1.

Thiamine

Actions   Thiamine (B_1) is important for carbohydrate metabolism, nerve cell function, and heart function.

Sources   Sources of thiamin include dried yeast, whole grains, liver and pork, enriched cereal, nuts, legumes, and potatoes.

Deficiency   Signs of thiamine deficiency, also known as beriberi, include peripheral neuritis (paralysis of the sensory and motor parts of the extremities), impaired memory, loss of appetite (anorexia), muscle weakness, and feeling tired. Dental signs and symptoms include glossitis (inflammation of the tongue), glossodynia (burning tongue), stomatitis (sores of the mouth and lips), and loss of taste. Thiamine deficiency is primarily seen in individuals with liver damage, chronic diarrhea, pregnancy, "junk food" diets, and in people with alcoholism (alcohol interferes with thiamine absorption). Deficiency of thiamine is managed by administering thiamine. It is used in patients with liver disease.

Riboflavin

Actions   Vitamin B_2 (riboflavin) is essential for cell growth, red blood cell production, and protein metabolism. It is involved in the cytochrome P450 isoenzyme system in the liver, which metabolizes drugs. Epidemiological studies link riboflavin supplementation to prevention of cardiovascular diseases, cancer, and development of corneal cataracts.

Sources   Riboflavin is found in milk, liver, eggs, broccoli, cheese, green vegetables, and fish. A decline in

consumption of milk and milk products in Western countries may contribute to poor riboflavin status.

Deficiency   Signs of riboflavin deficiency include appearance of magenta-colored mucosa, glossitis, angular cheilosis, and seborrheic dermatitis. A deficiency of riboflavin rarely occurs alone but most likely will occur with the other B vitamins. Riboflavin deficiency is most common in individuals with chronic diarrhea, liver disease, and alcoholism.

Use   There are no known therapeutic uses for vitamin B_2 except that it is used in combination with other B vitamins to treat vitamin B deficiency, or in multivitamins.

Niacin

Actions   Vitamin B_3 (niacin) exists in two forms: nicotinic acid and nicotinamide. It is necessary for cellular respiration and for carbohydrate metabolism. Niacin improves circulation and, in high doses, is used to treat hyperlipidemia (lower blood triglycerides and LDL cholesterol, and raise HDL cholesterol). Patients seen in the dental office may be taking niacin without approval from their physician.

Deficiency   A severe deficiency in niacin results in a condition called pellagra, which consists of dermatitis, diarrhea, dementia, neuropathy, increased salivation, enlarged salivary glands, loss of papillae on tongue, glossitis, and stomatitis.

Adverse effects   Adverse effects/toxicity can result in facial flushing, hypertension, diarrhea and skin lesions. Niacin sustained-release formulation or aspirin can be used 30 minutes prior to niacin to minimize facial flushing. Chronic use can cause dry skin, xerostomia, peptic ulcer disease, and hyperglycemia.

Pantothenic Acid

Actions   Vitamin B_5 is an essential component of coenzyme A, a cofactor for protein metabolism. Pantothenic acid is usually nontoxic, even in high doses.

Guidelines for Patients With Vitamin B Deficiency and Patients Taking Vitamin B

- Monitor patients for signs of deficiency: angular cheilosis, glossitis, glossodynia, smooth tongue (atrophy of filiform papillae), and stomatitis.
- No special dental care needed.

Guidelines for Patients with Niacin Deficiency and Patients Taking Niacin

- Oral sign/symptoms of niacin deficiency are glossitis and stomatitis.
- As a supplement, niacin can cause flushing and dry mouth.
- Monitor your patient's vital signs.
- No drug interactions of dental concern.

Sources Food sources include chicken, beef, potatoes, oats, tomatoes, liver, yeast, egg yolk, grains, and green leafy vegetables.

Deficiency Pantothenic acid deficiency usually is accompanied with deficiency of other B vitamins. Symptoms of vitamin B_5 deficiency include numbness and burning of the feet, abdominal upset, fatigue, and muscle cramping.

Pyridoxine

Actions Vitamin B_6 is the generic term for three forms of the vitamin: pyridoxal, pyridoxine, and pyridoxamine. It is important in the metabolism of amino acids.

Sources Sources include meat, whole-grain cereals, dark green, leafy vegetables, and potatoes.

Deficiency Deficiency states can be the result of alcoholism, hypothyroidism, or heart failure. Isoniazid (INH), a drug used to treat tuberculosis, can cause a deficiency of the vitamin.

Signs and symptoms of deficiency consist of oral changes, skin lesions on the face, increased irritability, seizures (especially in children), and neuritis (degeneration of peripheral nerves). Pyridoxine is usually nontoxic even in large doses. It is used to prevent and to treat vitamin B_6 deficiency.

Cobalamin

Actions Vitamin B_{12} is essential for hematopoiesis (production of red blood cells), DNA synthesis, and nerve function. Since humans cannot make vitamin B_{12} in the body, it must be obtained from the ingestion of animal protein (meat). Then it is absorbed in the stomach by intrinsic factor (IF) (Figure 12–1).

Sources Natural sources of these vitamins are liver, yeast, and animal products. Otherwise, to obtain these vitamins a supplemental source must be taken.

Did You Know?

Brown rice is high in vitamin B_6, niacin, magnesium, and selenium.

Deficiency Individuals with pernicious anemia (the inability to make red blood cells) do not produce enough IF to absorb vitamin B_{12}, resulting in a deficiency of the vitamin, causing megaloblastic anemia. Dietary vitamin B_{12} deficiency can occur in strict vegetarians. It takes many years for megaloblastic anemia to develop because very little of the vitamin B_{12} is used up. Signs and symptoms of pernicious anemia are weakness, sore tongue (glossitis), anorexia, and pallor. Treatment of vitamin B_{12} deficiency is cyanocobalamin. Other clinical manifestations for vitamin B_{12} deficiency include paresthesia (nerve numbness) and psychiatric problems such as irritability, depression, dementia and psychosis. Long-term use of histamine H_2-receptor blockers and proton pump inhibitors for the treatment of ulcers may cause impaired breakdown of vitamin B_{12} from food, causing malabsorption and eventual depletion of vitamin B_{12} stores in the body.

Folic Acid

Actions Folic acid is a B-complex vitamin (vitamin B_9). Together with vitamin B_{12} it is involved in protein, lipid, and carbohydrate metabolism. It is also important in red blood cell development and neural-tube development in the fetus.

Sources Dietary sources include orange juice, lentils, beans, whole-grain breads and cereals, liver, and green, leafy vegetables.

Deficiency The prevalence of folic acid deficiency has decreased since the United States introduced a mandatory folic acid fortification program in 1998. People with excessive alcohol intake and malnutrition are still at high risk of folic acid deficiency.

Use A healthy individual has about 500–20,000 mcg of folate in body stores. Humans need to absorb approximately 50–100 mcg per day in order to replenish daily degradation and loss through urine and bile. Folic acid is used to treat anemia caused by folate deficiency, and the prevention of neural-tube defects in the developing fetus. Studies have shown that folic acid may reduce elevated levels of homocysteine, which may be associated with atherosclerotic vascular disease. It may counteract damage to the liver from certain medications.

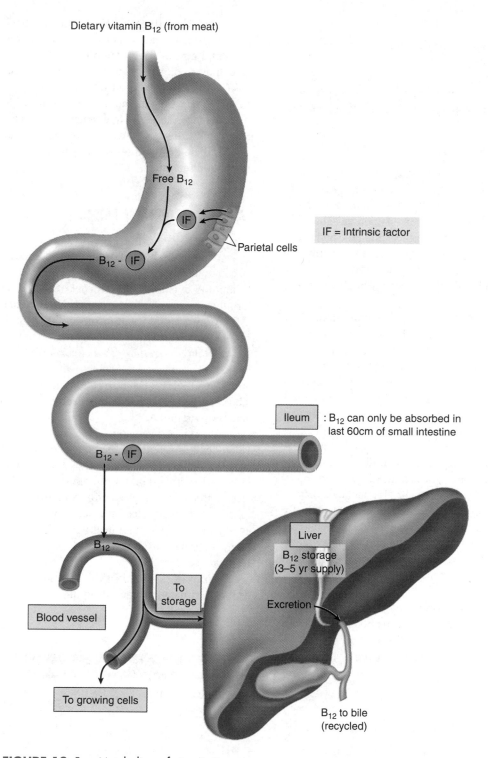

Dietary vitamin B_{12} (from meat)

Free B_{12}

IF

IF = Intrinsic factor

Parietal cells

B_{12} - IF

Ileum : B_{12} can only be absorbed in last 60cm of small intestine

B_{12} - IF

B_{12}

Liver

B_{12} storage (3–5 yr supply)

To storage

Excretion

Blood vessel

To growing cells

B_{12} to bile (recycled)

FIGURE 12-1   Metabolism of vitamin B_{12}.

Biotin

Biotin functions as a co-enzyme in gas exchange and in fat and carbohydrate metabolism.

Chronic consumption of raw egg whites, which contain a biotin antagonist, results in dermatitis and tongue swelling that responds to administration of biotin.

Ascorbic Acid

Actions Vitamin C is required for synthesis and maintenance of collagen and intercellular ground substance of body cells, blood vessels, cartilage, bones, teeth, skin, ligaments, and tendons. It is also required for tissue repair (wound healing). Unlike most mammals, humans cannot synthesize or store ascorbic acid in the body so it must be consumed daily. Ascorbic acid is reversibly oxidized to dehydroascorbic acid in the body.

Sources Vitamin C is plentiful in all fruits and vegetables.

Deficiency Although an adequate amount of ascorbic acid is usually obtained from dietary sources, in patients with G.I. absorption problems vitamin C may not be absorbed completely. A severe form of vitamin C deficiency called scurvy is usually not seen in the general population today because of obtaining it from food sources. Scurvy was first documented in sailors who had an inadequate diet, without fruits and vegetables.

Years ago periodontal literature found an association between scurvy and periodontal diseases, particularly gingival bleeding. An article in the *Journal of Periodontology* (2000;71:1215–1223) concluded that dietary intake of vitamin C showed a weak, but statistically significant, relationship to periodontal disease in current and former smokers as measured by clinical attachment. Patients taking the lowest levels of vitamin C and who also smoke are likely to show the greatest clinical effect on periodontal tissues.

Adverse effects Although vitamin C is a water-soluble vitamin and is excreted by the body, when taken in large doses kidney stones may form. Other adverse effects include diarrhea, nausea, headache, abdominal cramps, and insomnia.

Did You Know?

Vitamin C was the first vitamin to be artificially synthesized, in 1955.

Use Ascorbic acid is used therapeutically for the prophylaxis and treatment of scurvy and as a dietary supplement. Large doses of vitamin C for the prevention of the common cold are not well documented. This concept was originally introduced by Linus Pauling.

Vitamin C is an antioxidant that may block some of the damage caused by free radicals, which are byproducts from the body's conversion of food into energy.

Individuals who smoke may require an additional amount of vitamin C.

FAT-SOLUBLE VITAMINS

Vitamin A (Retinol)

Actions The term vitamin A includes a number of compounds referred to as retinoids and carotenoids. Vitamin A exists in many forms: retinol (the alcohol form/the most active form/vitamin A_1); retinal (the aldehyde form); retinoic acid (a metabolite of retinol); and beta-carotene (provitamin A). *Beta-carotene is a precursor of vitamin A (retinol) that is converted to vitamin A* in the wall of the small intestines, which is then absorbed in the small intestine and stored in the liver. During metabolism, each molecule of beta-carotene yields two molecules of vitamin A.

Vitamin A is essential for general growth and development, especially of the bones, teeth, and epithelial tissues, including surface tissues (e.g., mucous membranes). It is important for protein synthesis and cell differentiation during reproduction and growth. The health of the skin is influenced by vitamin A. Vitamin A is necessary for proper wound healing and is one of the pigments required for night vision. It is also considered to be an antioxidant.

Sources Vitamin A is found in two forms: retinol and beta-carotene. Vitamin A is obtained from

Guidelines for Patients Taking Vitamin C

- Today, vitamin C deficiency is very rare.
- Excessive use of chewable ascorbic acid (vitamin C) tablets may lead to tooth caries.
- There in an increased excretion in the urine if taking aspirin.

foods containing beta-carotenes. Retinol is present in eggs, whole milk, butter, meat, and oily salt-water fish (cod liver oil). Provitamin A pigments (beta-carotene) are found in green, yellow, and orange vegetables and fruits, and are converted to retinol in humans.

Deficiency Vitamin A deficiency can result from intestinal disease such as celiac disease, cystic fibrosis, resection of the small intestine, excessive mineral oil ingestion, massive intestinal infections, and hepatic (liver) cirrhosis. An inadequate dietary intake may be the cause in malnourished children and the elderly.

Deficiency symptoms include dry or rough skin, night blindness, poor growth (bone growth), weak tooth enamel (hypoplasia), xerophthalmia (dry eye disorder leading to blindness), and digestive problems.

Toxicity Since vitamin A is a fat-soluble vitamin and is stored in the body, overdosing is a possibility. Massive overdose can cause drowsiness, irritability, severe headache, vomiting, liver damage, hair loss and aching bones.

Products Many pharmaceutical preparations are used for the treatment of acne, psoriasis, and other skin disorders.

Tretinoin (Retin-A, Renova) is a retinoic acid derivative that improves the appearance of the skin by decreasing the cohesiveness of follicular cells, causing a superficial peeling of the top layer of the skin (epidermis). The epithelial cells multiply and turn over more rapidly, which prevent skin pores from becoming clogged. This topically applied product may cause dry, peeling skin. It is contraindicated in patients also taking photosensitive drugs such as tetracyclines.

Isotretinoin (Accutane) is an oral product that is a highly toxic metabolite of retinol (vitamin A) with a pregnancy category X, and is contraindicated in women who are or may become pregnant. It regulates epithelial cell differentiation and proliferation, and is indicated for severe recalcitrant cystic or nodular acne unresponsive to conventional therapy, including systemic antibiotics. A dentally related side effect is xerostomia.

Etretinate (Tegison) is an oral product that is a second generation retinoid related to retinoic acid and retinol (vitamin A). Its mechanism of action is unknown. It reduces redness, scaling, and thickness of psoriasis lesion by normalizing epidermal differentiation and decreases skin thickness. Indications are for the treatment of severe recalcitrant psoriasis in patients unresponsive to or intolerant of standard therapies. It has a pregnancy category X and is teratogenic.

Vitamin E (Alpha-Tocopherol)

Vitamin E exists in many forms: α (alpha), β (beta) γ (gamma), and δ (delta) tocopherols and tocotrienols. The most biologically active natural form of the vitamin is α-tocopherol, which is converted by the body to vitamin E and is the only one of pharmacologic importance.

Actions Vitamin E is stored in muscle, fat, and liver tissue. Acting as an antioxidant it protects cells of organs from the effects of free radicals, potentially damaging byproducts of energy metabolism. Free radicals can damage cells and may contribute to the development of cardiovascular disease and cancer. A 2005 study published in the Journal of the American Medical Association (Lee LM, Cook NR, Gazrano JM et al.) Vitamin E in the primary prevention of cardio vascular disease and cancer, 294:56–65) concluded that 600 IU of natural-source vitamin E taken every other day provided no overall benefit for major cardiovascular events or cancer, did not affect total mortality, and decreased cardiovascular mortality in healthy women. These data did not support recommending vitamin E supplementation for cardiovascular disease or cancer prevention among healthy women (Lee et al., 2005). Vitamin E also protects polyunsaturated fatty acids, which make up the cell membrane, and other oxygen-sensitive substances such as vitamin A and C from oxidation in the cells of the body and prevents breakdown of body tissues.

RDH ► **Rapid Dental Hint**

Remember to ask patients if they are taking vitamin E. Vitamin E may act like a blood thinner, which increases the risk of bleeding. Recommend discontinuing vitamin E at least 24 hours before dental surgery.

Sources and RDA: The RDA for vitamin E is 10 mg for men and 8 mg for women (1 mg = TE, tocopherol equivalents) per day. RDAs for vitamin E are listed as TE to account for the different biological activities of the various forms of vitamin E. The conversion of TE is: 1 mg alpha-tocopherol = 1 TE alpha-tocopheral = 1.5 IU. Eating a variety of foods containing vitamin E is the best way to get an adequate amount. The daily value (amount per day of the vitamin that is recommended to keep within normal range) is 10 to 30 mg. Requirement for vitamin E increases as the intake of polyunsaturated fats increases. Thus, individuals on a high carbohydrate/low fat diet may require more vitamin E supplementation.

Deficiency Vitamin E deficiency may lead to red blood cell hemolysis (anemia) and nerve damage, and is usually seen in premature babies and malabsorption diseases. There are no documented oral changes. To prevent vitamin E deficiency in premature, low-birth-weight babies, oral vitamin E is administered.

Products For drug use, vitamin E is available as a dietary supplement as *d* or *dl*-alpha-tocopheryl acetate, *d* or *dl*-alpha-tocopheryl acid succinate or *d* or *dl*-alphatocopherol. The natural form of vitamin E is labeled *d* while the synthetic form, which is only half as active as the natural form, is labeled *dl*.

Topical preparations are available to treat dry, cracked skin.

Interactions High-dose of vitamin E may increase the risk of bleeding and potentiates the anticoagulant effect of warfarin (coumadin). Concurrent use of vitamin E and warfarin cause an increase in protrombin time (PT) due to a depletion of vitamin K–dependent clotting factors. Increased gingival bleeding may occur in patients taking vitamin E and aspirin. Bleeding effects are seen in quantities of vitamin E over 300 IU/day. Some dental clinicians may ask the patient to discontinue vitamin E during periodontal or oral surgery.

Vitamin D (Cholecalciferol; Ergocalciferol)

Actions and Sources Vitamin D consists of a group of chemicals with similar activities. Chlolecalciferol (vitamin D_3) is the natural form of vitamin D that is formed in the skin when exposed to sunlight.

Sources Approximately 10 to 15 minutes of sunlight during the day is sufficient for most individuals to produce the vitamin. Vitamin D_2 (ergocalciferol) is found in fortified milk, fish liver oils, butter, liver, and egg yolk. Vitamin D is unique among the vitamins in that it is considered to be a prohormone because it is converted in the liver and kidneys to its active form. In the

skin, the inactive form of vitamin D, called cholecalciferol, is synthesized from cholesterol. Cholecalciferol is obtained from exposure of the skin to sunlight and from dietary products such as milk or other foods fortified with vitamin D. Cholescalciferol is further metabolized in the kidneys to calcitriol, the most active form of vitamin D. This form is responsible for the absorption of calcium and phosphates, with subsequent deposition in and mineralization of bone and enamel of teeth.

Deficiency and Toxicity A deficiency of vitamin D can result in rickets (bone mineralization is decreased in a growing person) and osteomalacia (softening of the bones due to insufficient levels of vitamin D). Causes of deficiency include dietary deficiency, gastrointestinal conditions such as malabsorption or chronic pancreatitis, or renal disease. An overdose can lead to anorexia, renal (kidney) failure and metastatic calcification.

Products Calcitriol (Calcijex, Rocaltrol) is a synthetic form of an active metabolite of ergocalciferol (vitamin D_2). Patients with nonfunctioning kidneys are unable to make enough calcitriol, and thus must get it exogenously. This product is used in the management of hypocalcemia in patients undergoing chronic renal dialysis.

Dihydrotachysterol (DHT) is a product of ergocalciferol and is used in patients with hypocalcemia associated with hypoparathyroidism.

Vitamin D is used as an adjunct with calcium for the treatment and prevention of osteoporosis.

Vitamin K

Actions and Sources Vitamin K is essential for the formation of prothrombin and other blood clotting factors. There are two forms: vitamin K_1 (phytonadione), present in foods, and vitamin K_2 (menaquinone), synthesized by bacteria in the intestine. Menadione (vitamin K_3) is the synthetic form of vitamin K.

Deficiency Deficiencies in adults are rarely seen because enough is obtained from the diet and from bacteria. However, only small stores are in the body so deficiency can occur within 1 to 2 weeks. Newborns are especially prone to vitamin K deficiency. Breast milk is low in vitamin K and the newborn does not have any vitamin K–producing bacteria in the intestine. This form of vitamin K deficiency in newborns is called hemorrhagic disease of the newborn.

Interactions Anticoagulants (e.g., warfarin) and the long-term use of broad-spectrum antibiotics (e.g.,

---

Guidelines for Patients Taking Vitamin E

- Question patients about vitamin E intake.
- Since it causes bleeding, patients should discontinue use for invasive oral/periodontal surgical procedures.

CHAPTER 12 VITAMINS AND MINERALS **207**

tetracyclines, amoxicillin, and ampicillin) interfere with the function and absorption of vitamin K, leading to bleeding. These antibiotics eradicate normal gastrointestinal bacteria that synthesize vitamin K, resulting in a deficiency. Patients with normal vitamin K intake who take these antibiotics concurrently with oral anticoagulants are not implicated in this interaction. Taking probiotic supplements such as acidophilus or eating yogurt with active cultures replaces beneficial intestinal bacteria, and they should be taken with all broad-spectrum antibiotics.

Products Phytonadione (vitamin K_1) is used as an antidote for overdosage of warfarin (Coumadin), an anticoagulant. Vitamin K is also used in the treatment of patients with clotting factor deficiency.

Phenytoin (Dilantin) interferes with the body's ability to use vitamin K. Taking phenytoin during pregnancy may deplete vitamin K in the newborn. Aspirin may decrease vitamin K absorption, resulting in reduced blood levels.

ANTIOXIDANTS

Antioxidants are compounds that inhibit chemical reactions with oxygen. They protect cells in the body against damage by free radicals, which are reactive by-products of normal cell activity. They work to protect membranes in the nerves, muscles and cardiovascular system. Naturally occurring antioxidants include vitamin A (retinoids), vitamin C (ascorbic acid) and vitamin E (tocopherols). Natural antioxidants are added to food to prevent deterioration. There are claims that antioxidants can lower the risk of heart disease, some forms of cancer, and macular degeneration of the eyes. The Food and Nutrition Board (FNB) states that it cannot be certain that there is a direct link between antioxidants and the lower incidence of chronic diseases. As was mentioned earlier in the chapter, a 2005 article in *JAMA* concluded from a large clinical trial that taking 600 IV of vitamin E provided no overall benefit for major cardiovascular events or cancer in women.

COMMON MINERALS

Minerals are inorganic substances that must be obtained daily from dietary sources in amounts of 100 mg or higher. Only selected elements will be discussed, including iron, zinc, and calcium.

Macrominerals

Macrominerals are minerals or inorganic substances required by humans in amounts of 100 mg/day or more.

Calcium

Actions Calcium is obtained from the diet. About 90 percent is stored in bone where there is a constant exchange between blood, tissues, and bone. Calcium is important in blood clotting, muscle contraction, nerve transmission, and bone and tooth formation (almost 99 percent of total body calcium is found in teeth and bones). Calcium is absorbed in the intestine and excreted in urine and feces. The absorption and deposition of calcium is controlled by vitamin D, parathyroid hormone, and calcitonin. *Vitamin D is required for proper calcium absorption.*

Sources and RDA Calcium is found in milk, cheese, yogurt, Chinese cabbage, beans, cereal products, fish, kale, and broccoli. The recommended daily intake of calcium is 800 to 1,200 mg (1.2 g) in men and women and 1,200 mg in pregnant women.

Deficiency and Toxicity Since calcium is critical for physiologic function, the body will take calcium from the bones when there is insufficient dietary intake. Calcium deficiency can cause osteoporsis, osteomalacia, muscle spasms, and muscle cramps. Excessive consumption of calcium (12 gm of a calcium product) may result in kidney stones, hypercalcemia (high blood calcium levels) and renal insufficiency.

Supplements Calcium supplements are used to prevent and treat osteoporosis, calcium-deficient states, and to prevent and treat hyperphosphatemia (excessive phosphate blood levels seen in patient with renal failure). For absorption of calcium to occur in the duodenum (intestine) and then into the blood it must be in a soluble, ionized form.

Various calcium salt forms are available that contain different milligrams of elemental calcium. Calcium carbonate is the most efficient and inexpensive calcium salt for replacement because it contains 40 percent of elemental calcium, the highest amount available. However, calcium carbonate and calcium phosphate are insoluble and must be taken with meals to lower the pH for absorption. Calcium carbonate is the active ingredient in Tums, an antacid for the relief of acid indigestion and a calcium supplement. Calcium citrate (Citracal), calcium lactate, and calcium gluconate (Kalcinate) are soluble and allow for better absorption.

Guidelines for Patients Taking Calcium Supplements

If the patients are prescribed tetracycline (doxycycline, minocycline) for a dental infection, tell them to take the calcium 1 hour before or 2 hours after the tetracycline.

Calcium supplements should not be taken concurrently with tetracyclines, due to formation of a complex which is not readily absorbed.

Phosphorous

Actions Phosphorous is used to lower urinary calcium concentration and to correct phosphate deficiency. It is contraindicated in patients on a sodium- or potassium-restricted diet. It is an essential mineral that is often bound to calcium in the form of calcium phosphate in bones.

Sources Meat, poultry, fish, eggs, milk, and dairy products.

Deficiency Symptoms include weakness, muscle tremor, anorexia, weak pulse, and bleeding abnormalities.

Supplements Sodium phosphate and potassium phosphate are available for phosphorous deficiencies.

Magnesium Sulfate

Actions Cofactor for many enzymes in the breakdown of carbohydrates and proteins, and necessary for normal nerve conduction and muscle contraction.

Sources Whole grain, nuts, seeds, legumes, green leafy vegetables.

Deficiency Hypomagnesemia is generally asymptomatic until serum magnesium falls below 1.0 mEq/L.

Supplements When given orally, magnesium salts are a laxative or antacid (magnesium citrate, magnesium hydroxide) and are used to treat hypomagnesemia.

Microminerals

Microminerals, also referred to as trace elements, are required by humans in amounts under 100 mg/day.

Zinc

Actions Zinc is a part of many enzymes and is important to insulin function, reproduction, skin integrity, growth, and wound healing.

Sources Zinc is obtained in the diet and is found in animal products, oysters, liver, peanuts, and whole grain cereals.

Deficiency A deficiency in zinc can cause growth retardation, skin changes, altered immune function, and loss of hair.

Supplements Zinc is used to treat deficiencies and improve wound healing. It is available in a lozenge for the management of the common cold.

Iron

Actions As a component of hemoglobin (the oxygen-transporting component of red blood cells composed of heme and globin) in the body, iron is important in oxygen transport. Iron is also a component of myoglobin (muscle hemoglobin). Iron exists in the body as essential and nonessential. Approximately 60 to 70 percent of iron is found as hemoglobin in red blood cells (essential iron); some is associated with myoblobin and iron-containing enzymes; and the remainder (nonessential) is stored in the liver in the form of ferritin and hemosiderin.

Sources Iron is obtained primarily from the diet from the ferrous form of iron rather than the ferric form. It is absorbed most efficiently.

Sources and RDA The average diet contains 10 to 15 mg a day, which is adequate for most individuals. Foods high in iron (heme) include meat (liver and heart), egg yolks, wheat germ, and most green vegetables. Heme sources of iron, found in animal products, are absorbed better than nonheme sources. RDAs are expressed as elemental iron. Amounts greater than the RDA are needed to rebuild normal stores of iron. Iron is also recommended for vegetarians.

Deficiency Although iron is present in most foods, only about 10 percent is actually absorbed into the blood. Iron-deficiency anemia occurs secondary to menstruation and pregnancy. Anemia secondary to low dietary intake takes years to develop. Anemia can also occur secondary to blood loss due to a bleeding peptic ulcer, diverticulitis, ulcerative colitis, and colon cancer. In cases of iron-deficiency anemia, hemoglobin levels will decrease. Signs and symptoms of iron-deficiency anemia include fatigue, skin pallor and a pale, atrophic, smooth/slick tongue.

Toxicity Iron toxicity rarely occurs in adults, but is frequently seen in children. Signs of iron poisoning include vomiting and diarrhea. Treatment starts with inducing vomiting and lavage.

Supplements Iron is used therapeutically to correct iron-deficiency anemia or as a supplement to the diet in certain individuals (e.g., vegetarians, pregnancy, during a growth period or excessive menstruation).

Various forms of ferrous salts are available, including ferrous sulfate, ferrous gluconate, and ferrous fumarate, which contain different percentages of elemental iron. Ferrous calcium citrate is used in pregnant women to provide iron and calcium. Ferrous sulfate is usually used for the treatment of anemia and contains 20 percent elemental iron. When treating iron-deficiency anemia, it is suggested for the patient to take three to four tablets of ferrous sulfate daily for 3 months. Constipation is an adverse side effect of iron preparations.

Iron should not be taken concurrently with tetracyclines because a complex is formed that decreases the absorption of the tetracycline.

Iodine

Actions Iodine is a micromineral and a component of thyroid hormones.

Sources Iodized salt.

Deficiency Deficiency of iodine causes goiter; excess suppresses thyroid function.

MULTIVITAMINS

Many multivitamin preparations are on the market, with little standardization of the formulas. Individuals having a well balanced diet will find no additional benefits from a multivitamin. Once the body has obtained the amounts of vitamins and minerals needed to carry on metabolism, the excess is excreted or stored.

Products containing more than 100 percent of the daily value may be beneficial for individuals with severely restricted food intake, alcoholics, pregnant or nursing women, those with chronic kidney or liver disease, or the elderly. Although a product may have some vitamins that are more than the 100 percent DV, only about 10 percent may actually be absorbed. Multivitamin formulations should contain only essential vitamins that have a recommended RDA. Some products contain iron and calcium which may be useful for certain individuals such as pregnant women, but other essential minerals are usually obtained from the diet. A multivitamin not contain-

ing iron is best for men and menopausal women. If the product contains the letters USP, that means that it meets the standards of the U.S. Pharmacopeia. Most brand-name vitamins are not labeled USP. The labels on these products list the amount of each nutrient and the percentage of the "daily value."

The Food and Nutrition Board (FNB) has expressed concern regarding this claim as many people will consume vitamin *megadoses*. Megavitamin therapy uses large amounts of vitamins, often greater than the RDA, to treat diseases. The efficacy of various megavitamin therapies is controversial. Megavitamin therapies are not entirely recognized, although they are increasingly used as adjuncts to conventional medicine. Administration of large doses of fat-soluble vitamins may have adverse side effects. In the healthy individual, megadoses of any vitamin are not necessary and not recommended.

DRUG-INDUCED VITAMIN DEFICIENCY

Some medications that patients take can cause vitamin deficiencies. Excessive alcohol intake can cause a vitamin B_1 deficiency. Phenytoin, phenothiazines, oral contraceptives and barbiturates may cause decreased folic acid levels. Oral contraceptives and alcohol interfere with vitamin B_{12} absorption.

DENTAL HYGIENE NOTES

The dental hygienist can help to identify vitamin deficiencies and overdoses in patients, and to consult them in vitamin supplementation.

Interviewing the patient about vitamins is very important. The general public does not understand that vitamins are drugs and there are adverse effects and interactions. Vitamin E causes increased bleeding, thus caution should be used when performing periodontal surgery. The patient may be told to discontinue use until after surgery.

Many vitamin deficiencies have oral manifestations of which the dental clinician should be aware. Vitamin B deficiencies have oral manifestations including glossititis, stomatitis, pale, smooth tongue and angular cheilosis. A careful intraoral examination can detect these vitamin deficiencies. Additionally, the dental clinician can educate the patient on recognizing vitamin deficiencies and toxicities and recommend a proper diet and/or supplements that best fits the patient's profile.

KEY POINTS

- Water-soluble vitamins do not accumulate in the body.
- Vitamins E, C, and A are antioxidants: They protect cells in body against damage by free radicals, reactive byproducts of normal cell activity. It has not yet been proven that there is a direct link between antioxidants and a lower incidence of chronic diseases such as heart disease and cancer.
- Vitamin E is an anticoagulant and increases bleeding; caution for use during periodontal/oral surgery procedures.
- Deficiencies of vitamin C and B_2, B_3, and B_6 have oral manifestations, including gingival bleeding (vitamin C) and angular cheilosis, stomatitis, glossitis, and denuded tongue.

BOARD REVIEW QUESTIONS

1. Which of the following signs/symptoms is found in vitamin B_2 deficiency? (p. 201)
   a. Glossitis
   b. Bleeding
   c. Hepatitis
   d. Blindness

2. Which of the following situations occurs if a patient is taking high doses of vitamin E and having periodontal surgery? (pp. 205–206)
   a. Increased salivation
   b. Increased probing depths
   c. Increased bleeding tendency
   d. Decreased salivation
   e. Decreased bleeding

3. Which of the following vitamins are considered to be antioxidants? (p. 207)
   a. A, E
   b. A, D
   c. C, B
   d. C, D

4. Which of the following abbreviations indicates the measurement of a vitamin? (p. 199)
   a. RDA
   b. IU
   c. mg
   d. ml

5. Which of the following vitamins must be consumed daily because humans are unable to synthesize it? (p. 199)
   a. C
   b. D
   c. K
   d. A

SELECTED REFERENCES

Brody, T. *Nutritional Biochemistry.* 1998. San Diego: Academic Press, Inc.

Donjon, R. P. and B. J. Goeckner. 1999. *Mosby's OTC Drugs.* St. Louis: Mosby.

Food and Nutrition Board. 1989. *Recommended Dietary Allowances.* Washington, DC: National Academy Press. 10th Ed.

Lee, I. M., N. R. Cook, J. M. Gaziano, D. Gordon, P. M. Ridker, et al. 2005. Vitamin E in the primary prevention of cardiovascular disease and cancer. *JAMA* 294:56–65.

Wishida, M., S. G. Grossi, R. G. Dunford, et al., 2000. Dietary Vitamin C and the risk for Periodental disease of Periodontol; 71(8): 1215–1223.

Oh, R. C. and D. L. Brown. 2003. Vitamin B_{12} deficiency. *American Family Physician* 67:979–986,993–994.

WEB SITES

www.iom.edu/board
www.fda.gov/fdac/special/foodlabel/dvs.html
(U.S. Food and Drug Administration)

QUICK DRUG GUIDE

Water-Soluble Vitamins

- Vitamin B_1 (thiamine)
- Vitamin B_2 (riboflavin)
- Vitamin B_3 (niacin)
- Vitamin B_5 (pathothenic acid)
- Vitamin B_6 (pyridoxine)
- Vitamin B_{12} (cobalamin)
- Vitamin C
- Folic acid

Fat-Soluble Vitamins

- Vitamin A (retinol)
- Vitamin D (cholecalciferol)
- Vitamin E (tocopherol)

Minerals

- Calcium
- Zinc
- Iron
- Phosphate
- Magnesium
- Iodine

Chapter **13**

Autonomic Drugs

GOALS:

- To gain knowledge of the fundamentals of the sympathetic and parasympathetic nervous system; this is essential for understanding the mechanism of action of many drugs used in dentistry and medicine.
- To provide knowledge about the fundamentals of the autonomic nervous system drugs used to treat various medical conditions and how these drugs affect dental treatment.

EDUCATIONAL OBJECTIVES

After reading this chapter, the reader should be able to:

1. Understand the differences between the sympathetic and parasympathetic divisions of the autonomic nervous system.
2. Illustrate the different types of receptors and neurotransmitters in the autonomic nervous system.
3. Identify drugs affecting the autonomic nervous system (sympathetic and parasympathetic divisions).
4. Understand the differences between adrenergic and cholingeric drugs.
5. Describe the role of autonomic nervous system drugs in dentistry.
6. Explain the use of vasoconstrictors (in local anesthetics) in dental patients.

KEY TERMS

Autonomic nervous system
Neuron
Neurotransmitters
Sympathomimetics
Sympatholytics
Cholinergic
Anticholinergic

INTRODUCTION

Some medications used by dental clinicians and many drugs taken by dental patients act upon the autonomic nervous system. Thus, it is essential that the dental hygienist be familiar with these medications.

THE NERVOUS SYSTEM

Structurally, the human nervous system is divided into the central nervous system (CNS) and the peripheral nervous system (PNS). The *central nervous system* is com-

posed of the brain and spinal cord, which receive sensory input from the peripheral nervous system. The *peripheral nervous system* is functionally divided into the **autonomic nervous system (ANS)** and the *somatic nervous system*. The somatic nervous system, also called the *voluntary* nervous system, innervates the skeletal muscles, causing contractions. The autonomic nervous system, or the *involuntary* (digestion, circulation) nervous system, is composed of motor nerve cells that transmit impulses to smooth muscles (e.g., intestinal, urinary bladder, uterus, eyes, lungs, and small arteries and veins), cardiac muscle and glands (Figure 13–1). These impulses

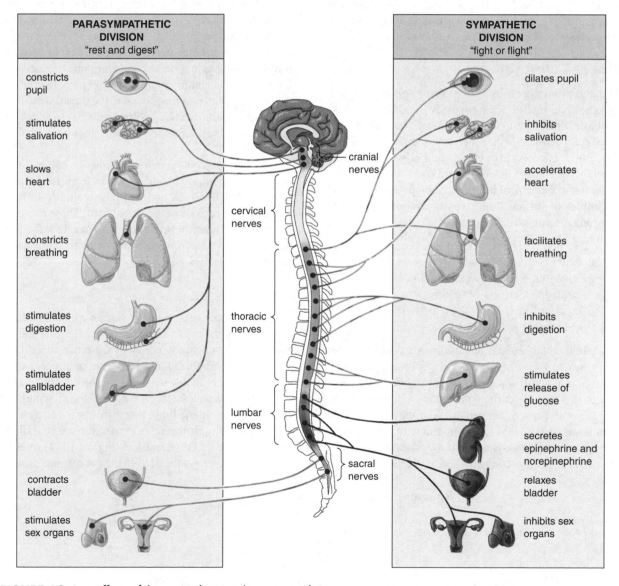

FIGURE 13–1 Effects of the sympathetic and parasympathetic nervous systems.

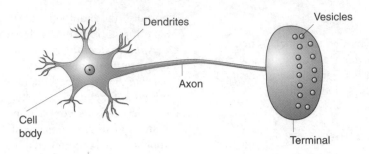

FIGURE 13–2   Diagram of a neuron.

are involuntary, and cannot be consciously controlled. The autonomic nervous system is further subdivided into *sympathetic* and *parasympathetic divisions.*

Nerve Cell Anatomy

The autonomic nervous system is a two-neuron chain. So what is a neuron? A **neuron** is the unit of cellular structure of the central nervous system. In the brain there are about 10 billion neurons. Neurons are nerve cells that transmit messages throughout the body. The neurons communicate with each other and transmit information in the form of electrical influx or action potential in which a stimulus of sufficient intensity is applied to a neuron. Neurons are composed of four parts (Figure 13–2):

- *Cell body* or soma, where normal cellular processes occur
- *Dendrites,* where receptors are located
- Axon, an extension or sending part
- Axon terminal, where the axon terminates; within the terminal are vesicles

Individual neurons do not directly contact one another. Instead, one neuron closely approaches another neuron, but is still separated from the other by a small space. This type of neuronal junction is called the *synapse* and the actual space is called the *synaptic cleft.* Neurons communicate with other neurons and with the target (effector) organ at these synapses. If the connection between the two neurons is outside the CNS, it is called a ganglion.

The neurons of the *sympathetic division* originate in the thoracolumbar portion of the spinal cord as *preganglionic* (or *presynaptic*) *nerve fibers (neurons).* The axons of these motor nerves leave the spinal cord and travel with the spinal nerves and enter one of a series of interconnected chain ganglia. The long, *postganglionic (or postsynaptic) neurons* extend to the organs they innervate (e.g., heart, eye, lung, blood vessels, stomach and intestines, kidney, secretory glands, and urinary bladder) (Figure 13–1).

In the *parasympathetic division,* the cell bodies of the *preganglionic neurons* originate from four cranial nerves (CN III, VII, IX and X) in the brain and from the sacral (S2–5) regions of the spinal cord. These nerves do not travel through the spinal nerves but rather the short *postganglionic neurons* synapse at or near the target organ.

Neurotransmitters

So how does one neuron communicate with another neuron and with the organ they innervate? Because the two neurons do not actually contact each other, a nerve impulse from the brain cannot cross from one neuron to the next. Instead, in the synapse region the electrical signal that has been transmitted the length of the preganglionic neuron located in the brain is transformed into a chemical signal through the release of a substance called a neurotransmitter (Figure 13–3, Figure 13–4). **Neurotransmitters** are synthesized in the neuron and stored in

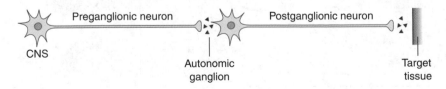

FIGURE 13–3   Basic structure of the autonomic nervous system.

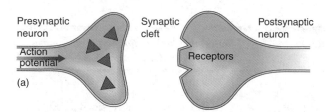

FIGURE 13-4a   Synaptic transmission.(a) Action potential reaches synapse;

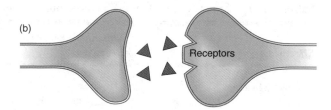

FIGURE 13-4b   (b) neurotransmitter released synaptic cleft;

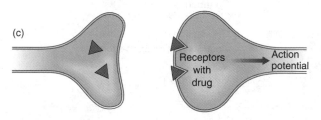

FIGURE 13-4c   (c) neurotransmitter reaches receptors to regenerate action potential.

vesicles or boutons located in the axon terminal of one neuron. In response to a nerve action potential (nerve impulse) the neurotransmitter is released from the vesicles into the synaptic space and binds to receptors on the postsynaptic or postganglionic neuron. This interaction of a neurotransmitter with a postsynaptic receptor results in the creation of a new action potential with the release of more neurotransmitter, which crosses the synapse and binds to receptors on the target organ. This results in either an inhibitory or excitatory action of the organ (e.g., increased heart rate or decreased intestinal movement). Thus, *the purpose of the neurotransmitter is to carry nerve impulses across the synapse.* Once the neurotransmitter has reacted with the receptor, it is rapidly removed to allow the arrival of a second signal. The neurotransmitter is removed by enzymes which degrade it into an inactive metabolite or by a process of "reuptake" whereby the specific neurotransmitter is taken back up into the axon terminal, where it is inactivated by enzymes.

There are many types of neurotransmitters. The primary neurotransmitters found in the ANS are acetylcholine (ACh) and norepinephrine (NE; released from adrenal glands). Other neurotransmitters include epinephrine (EPI), dopamine, serotonin, and GABA (gamma aminobuteric acid).

Receptors

Receptors are structures, usually proteins, that receive neurotransmitters released from the axonal terminals of the neuron. Receptors are located on the dendrites of postganglionic neurons and on/in smooth muscle, cardiac muscle, and glands (Figure 13–2).

FUNCTIONS OF THE AUTONOMIC NERVOUS SYSTEM: NEUROTRANSMITTERS AND RECEPTORS

Most organs of the body are innervated by neurons of both the sympathetic and parasympathetic divisions of the ANS. The only organs not innervated by both are the sweat glands, smooth muscles of the hair follicles, the adrenal medulla, and blood vessels of the skin.

Generally, stimulation of the sympathetic (adrenergic) and parasympathetic (cholinergic) nerves cause opposite responses (Table 13–1; Figure 13–3). If one division increases the activity of an organ, the other generally decreases it. The sympathetic nervous system is sometimes called the "fight or flight response" and the parasympathetic system as the "resting and digestive response." The sympathetic division prepares the individual for emergency/stressful situations, such as those responses required during aggressive or defensive behavior. These reactions include increased heart rate, increased blood flow to the skeletal muscles, and dilation of the bronchi. In contrast, the parasympathetic division maintains the body organs at activity levels that are most efficient in maintaining normal homeostasis of the body. It slows the heart rate, lowers the blood pressure, and stimulates the gastrointestinal tract.

Table 13-1 Effects of the Autonomic Nervous System

Effector Organ	Sympathetic (Adrenergic) Response (Receptor)	Parasympathetic (Cholinergic) Response (Receptor—All Muscarinic)
Cardiac Muscle		
Heart	↑ Heart rate, contractility (β_1) ↑ BP	↓ Heart rate, contractility, blood pressure
Smooth Muscle		
Lung (bronchioles)	Dilation (relaxation) (β_2)	Constriction (contraction)
Digestive tract (stomach; small intestines) (G.I.)	Increased acid secretion (α_1, β_2) Decreased motility (constipation)	Increased motility
Urinary bladder	Relaxation (urinary retention) (α_1)	Contraction (urine flow)
Eye		
Iris	Dilation of pupil (mydriasis) (α_1)	Contraction of pupil (miosis)
Ciliary muscle	Relaxation for far vision (β_2)	Contraction for near vision
Skin		
Arrector pili muscles	Contraction ("goose bumps") (α_1)	No innervation
Liver	Breakdown of glycogen (β_2)	—
Blood Vessels		
Coronary (heart)	Constriction (α_1) Dilation (β_2)	Dilation; decreased heart rate
Mucosal linings	Constriction (α_1)	No innervation
Skin	Constriction (α_1)	No innervation
Skeletal muscles	Constriction (α_1); dilation (β_2)	No innervation
Sex organs		
Uterus	Relaxation (β_2); contraction (α_1)	No innervation
Penile	Ejaculation (α_1)	Erection
Glands		
Lacrimal (tear)	No innervation	Secretion of tears
Sweat	Sweat (muscarinic)	No innervation
Adrenal medulla	Secretion of EPI	No innervation
Salivary	Secretion of thick, mucous saliva (α_1)	Secretion of thin, watery saliva

Sympathetic Nervous System (Adrenergic): Neurotransmitters

The neurotransmitter released from *every* preganglionic nerve terminal in the sympathetic division is acetylcholine, which causes excitation of the adrenergic postganglionic nerve and initiates the synthesis and release of norepinephrine from *most* postganglionic nerve terminals into the neuroeffector junction (Figure 13–5). Norepinephrine then diffuses across the neuroeffector junction and exerts its effects on the effector tissue [smooth muscle (e.g., intestines, uterus, and small arteries and veins), gland or cardiac muscle]. Catecholamines, also known as adrenergic neurotransmitters, are derived from the amino acid tyrosine. The principal catcholamines are EPI, NE, and dopamine.

Nerve fibers that synthesize and release ACh are called *cholinergic fibers* and cause cholinergic effects. Neurons that secrete NE are called *adrenergic neurons* and causes adrenergic effects.

There are a few exceptions to this general rule:

1. Sweat glands are innervated only by sympathetic cholinergic pathway, which releases ACh to cause sweating. Thus, these postganglionic fibers are cholinergeric, not adrenergic.
2. The adrenal medulla. The central part of the adrenal glands located superior to the kidneys consists of the adrenal medulla. Each adrenal medulla is innervated by a sympathetic *preganglionic* nerve, which releases ACh. The ACh then causes the release of two hormones, EPI (85 percent) and NE

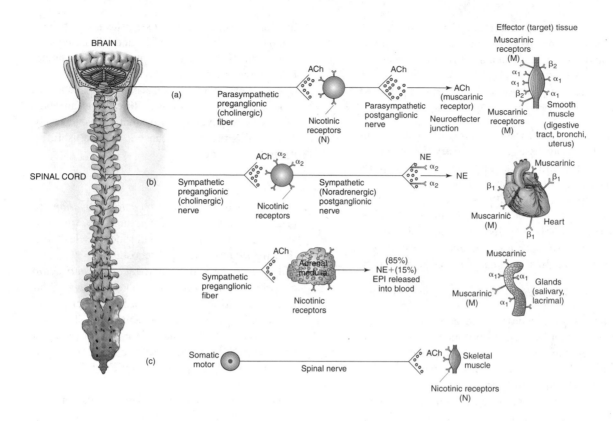

FIGURE 13–5   (a) Parasympathetic pathway. ACh is released from the preganlionic neuron over the synapse and stimulates cholinergic (nicotine) receptors. Then ACh is released from the postganglionic neuron, which activates the cholinergic (muscarinic) receptors on the target tissue. (b) Sympathetic pathway: Acetylcholine (ACh) is released from the preganglionic neuron and stimulates cholinergic (nicotine) receptors on the postganglionic neuron. Then, norepinephrine (NE) is released from the end of the postganlionic neuron, which is then transmitted to the target tissue, where it activates receptors on the surface. These adrenergic (sympathetic) receptors are either alpha (α) or beta (β). (c) Somatic motor pathway: nicotinic receptors on skeletal muscle.

(15 percent). Thus, there are no postganglionic fibers innervating the adrenal medulla.

3. Blood vessels to skeletal muscles, skin, brain, and nose. A different type of nerve transmission occurs when an axon terminates on a skeletal muscle fiber, skin, brain, and nose. From an anatomical point of view these structures are innervated only by the sympathetic nervous system and not by the parasympathetic nervous system. The sympathetic preganglionic nerves originate in either the thoracic or lumbar segments of the spinal cord. The majority of these sympathetic postganglionic fibers release NE to produce vasconstriction of the blood vessels which carry blood to skeletal muscle, skin, brain, and the nose.

Sympathetic Nervous System: Receptors

Different effector tissues (smooth muscle, cardiac muscle, and glands) contain different types of receptors with which the sympathetic neurotransmitters, NE and EPI, may interact. The two types of *adrenergic receptors* are referred to

---

Did You Know?

Did you know that when you are scared of an insect or a snake your sympathetic nervous system gets activated to help you deal with this frightening episode?

as alpha- (α)- and beta (β)-receptors. Certain effector tissue contains only α-receptors, other tissues contain only β-receptors, and other tissues contain both α and β-receptors (Figure 13–5; Tables 13–1, 13–2, 13–3).

There are two *subtypes* of α-adrenergic receptors; α_1 and α_2-receptors:

- α-1 receptors are located on preganglionic smooth muscle (blood vessels, genitourinary system, sweat glands, eye, intestine). Activation of α_1-receptors causes contraction of smooth muscles.
- α_2-receptors are typically located on the preganglionic neurons and are called autoreceptors because activation of α_2-receptors causes inhibition of NE release, decreases secretion of insulin, decreases blood pressure, and decreases eye secretion.

There are three *subtypes* of β-adrenergic receptors:

- β_1-adrenergic receptors are located on cardiac tissue and when stimulated produce heart stimulation, leading to a positive chronotropic effect (increased heart rate) and a positive inotropic effect (increased contractility or strength).
- β_2-adrenergic receptors are located on bronchial, uterine, and vascular (arteries, veins) smooth muscle. Ac-

tivation of β_2-receptors causes relaxation of these smooth muscles. Whereas EPI and NE are equally potent and effective at β_1-receptors on cardiac tissue, EPI is more potent than NE on β_2-receptors.

- β_3-receptors are found on fat cells (adipocytes) and produce breakdown of lipids. Research is currently underway to develop a drug that will selectively activate this receptor because it may be useful in the treatment of obesity.

General Rules

1. Those responses due to α-*receptor activation* are primarily *excitatory* or stimulating (e.g., vasoconstriction, contraction of the uterine muscles) with the *exception* of intestinal relaxation.
2. Those responses due to β-*receptor activation* are primarily *inhibitory* or relaxing (e.g., vasodilation, relaxation of the uterine muscles and bronchial tree) with the *exception* of stimulant effects on the heart. The β-receptors of the heart are referred to as β_1 receptors. All other β-receptors (lungs, eye, uterus) are referred to as β_2-receptors.
3. *Epinephrine* released (in response to some forms of stress) by the adrenal medulla acts on both α and

Table 13–2 Neurotransmitters of the Autonomic Nervous System

Pathway	Neuron/Neurotransmitter
Sympathetic	**Smooth Muscle; Cardiac Muscle; Glands** Preganglionic neuron (cell body located within the CNS): Releases acetylcholine (ACh) into the synapse Postganglionic neuron (cell body located outside CNS): Releases norepinephrine (NE) into the neuroeffector junction (NE will then have a pharmacologic effect on the effector tissue, including smooth muscles, cardiac muscles and glands) **Adrenal Medulla** Adrenal medulla (located on top of each kidney): Only preganglionic neurons, which release ACh. This stimulates the secretion of EPI (85%) and NE (15%). **Sweat Glands** Innervated by only sympathetic cholingeric neurons which release ACh
Parasympathetic	**Neurons** Preganglionic neuron: Releases acetylcholine (ACh) into the synapse Postganglionic neuron: Releases acetylcholine (ACh) into the neuroeffector junction (ACh will then have a pharmacologic effect on the effector tissue)

Table 13-3   Classification of Autonomic Receptors

Nervous System Division/Neurotransmitter	Receptor	Location of Receptor (found on the surface of effector tissue/organ and/or axonal terminal of neurons)	Therapeutic Objective
Sympathetic Norepinephrine (NE) (postganglionic/adrenergic receptors)	α_1	Located in/on most sympathetic effector tissues, including the blood vessels of smooth muscle of most organs (e.g., heart, skin, eye, bladder, intestine, salivary glands, mucous membranes) except the heart muscle. (Note: α_1-receptors are located in blood vessels of the heart but not heart muscle, causing vasocon-striction and increased blood pressure)	Vasoconstriction (constrict blood vessels) Dilates pupil (mydriasis) Urinary retention Decrease gastrointestinal motility Ejaculation Inhibits insulin release
	α_2	Located on neurons that release NE (presynaptic); termed auto-receptors because they inhibit the amount of NE released when levels get too high; also found in eye, intestinal, hepatic, plate-lets, renal, and endocrine tissues	Lowers blood pressure by inhibiting release of NE at the neuroeffector junction
	β_1	Primarily on heart muscle and blood vessels of the heart	Heart stimulation; renin secretion
	β_2	All organs except the heart muscle vasodilation; (e.g., smooth muscle of the bronchioles, smooth muscle of the blood vessels in skeletal muscle)	Relaxation of smooth muscle: bronchodilation; uterine relaxation; relaxation for distant vision
	β_3	Adipose (fat) tissue	Lipolysis (breakdown of fat)
Cholinergic/ ACh (preganglionic/cholinergic receptors)	Muscarinic	Sweat glands	Increased sweating
Parasympathetic Acetylcholine (cholinergic) (pre- and postganglionic/ cholinergic receptors)	Nicotinic	Postganglionic nerves and neuro-muscular junction of skeletal muscle	Muscle contraction
	Muscarinic	Smooth muscle, heart and glands	Smooth muscle contraction: (bronchoconstriction), increased G.I. motility (diarrhea), erection Gland secretion (mucous secretion, salivation, lacrimation—tears) Decrease heart rate
Somatic Acetylcholine	Nicotinic	Skeletal muscle	—

Table 13–4 Affinity of Neurotransmitters for Receptors

Receptor/Neurotransmitter	Affinity To
α_1	NE > EPI
α_2	NE > EPI
β_1 (cardiac tissue)	NE = EPI
β_2 (smooth muscle)	EPI > NE

β-receptors, but its effects are more potent on β_2-receptors (because it stays on these receptors longer; higher affinity).

4. *Norepinephrine (NE)* (released from the adrenal medulla or sympathetic postganglionic nerves) acts on *all* α-receptors and *some* β-receptors and is thus chiefly a *vasoconstrictor*. NE does not act on the β-receptors of smooth muscles of the liver, lungs, stomach, urinary bladder, and ciliary muscle of the eye.

5. β_1- receptors predominate (95 percent) in the heart (coronary) blood vessels and blood vessels to skeletal muscle. EPI produces vasodilation of these blood vessels since the β-receptors outnumber the α-receptors. NE produces vasodilation of the coronary blood vessels of the heart (Beta effect), but produces vasoconstriction of blood vessels to skeletal smooth muscle due to a greater effect of norepinephrine on the α-receptors.

6. Certain tissues contain an equal amount of α- and β-receptors. Two such tissues are the pulmonary (lung) blood vessels and the cerebral blood vessels. Epinephrine and NE *constrict* pulmonary blood vessels to relieve congestion related to asthma. Epinephrine produces only *mild* vasodilation, if any, of cerebral blood vessels; however, NE does produce vasoconstriction of cerebral blood vessels.

Parasympathetic Neurotransmitters and Receptors

Parasympathetic innervation predominates over sympathetic innervation of salivary glands, lacrimal glands, and erectile (penile) tissue. Stimulation of the parasympa-thetic division causes secretion of saliva and tearing, bronchiole contraction, and gut relaxation.

Acetylcholine is the neurotransmitter released from the parasympathetic preganglionic and postganglionic nerves. In each instance, the released ACh binds to and acts on cholinergic receptors contained in the postgan-glionic nerve and the effector tissue. The cholinergic re-ceptors do not appear to be identical; thus there are two types of cholinergic receptors:

- *Muscarinic cholinergic receptors* are located in tis-sue innervated by parasympathetic postganlionic nerves (and by sympathetic cholinergic nerves) which innervate sweat glands and blood vessels to skeletal muscle. Activation of muscarinic recep-tors resembles those produced when a person in-gests the poisonous mushroom *Amanita muscaria*.
- *Nicotinic cholinergic receptors* are located in auto-nomic ganglia (sympathetic and parasympathetic) and motor end plate of skeletal muscle. When ac-tivated, muscarinic receptors mediate smooth mus-cle contraction, and slow cardiac function and gland secretions. Activation of nicotinic receptors on skeletal muscle causes muscle contraction. There are not many pharmacologic applications of stimulating nicotinic receptors.

Acetylcholine that does not bind to the receptors is either destroyed by enzymes, taken up into the presyn-patic neuron to be recycled, or diffused away from the synaptic cleft.

Other Types of Neurotransmitters and Receptors

Dopamine Dopamine receptors are activated by dopamine, but not by other adrenergic receptor agonists. Currently, there are five classes of dopamine receptors (D_1, D_2, D_3, D_4, and D_5) which mediate muscle relax-ation in vascular smooth muscle and regulate neurotrans-mitter release. Dopamine plays an important role in the pathogenesis and treatment of certain brain disorders such as Parkinson's disease and schizophrenia. Antago-nism of the dopamine D_2 receptor, which prevents dopamine from attaching to the receptor, is a mechanism common to antipsychotic drugs.

Serotonin More than 15 subtypes of serotoner-gic receptors have been discovered. Pharmaceutical com-panies have been attempting to develop compounds that will act specifically at a single receptor subtype, hoping to obtain a profound therapeutic effect that is free from adverse effects.

Serotonin, or 5-hydroxytryptamine (5-HT) is a neurotransmitter that is produced primarily by platelets, cells in the gastrointestinal tract, and neurons. Serotonin is produced locally in peripheral tissues, and is also found in the brain. Its physiologic effects include platelet aggregation, stimulation of gastrointestinal motility, vasoconstriction, and controlling sleep, pain, behavior, and emotions such as depression. Certain drugs can act to affect the synthesis, storage, release or reuptake of serotonin.

AUTONOMIC DRUGS

Autonomic drugs work by acting as either agonists or antagonists at cholinergic and adrenergic receptors. Various autonomic drugs exert their effects at different steps in the neurotransmission process. Drugs that act as *agonists* bind to a receptor on the tissue and produce the maximal response, excitatory or inhibitory, obtainable in the tissue. *Antagonists* only produce a submaximal response in the tissue by blocking and reversing the effects of the neurotransmitter; an antagonist is opposite of an agonist.

SYMPATHOMIMETIC DRUGS: DRUGS AFFECTING SYMPATHETIC TRANSMISSION

Drugs that act as mediators of sympathetic transmission and cause a sympathetic response are called **sympathomimetics** or adrenergic agonists. Drugs that decrease sympathetic activity are called **sympatholytics** or **adrenergic antagonists.**

Many of the actions of sympathomimetic drugs (or the effects they produce) can be better understood in terms of specific drug–receptor interactions. The excitatory action of sympathomimetics (e.g., contraction of smooth muscle) is due to stimulation of α-receptors. This action is antagonized by an α-adrenergic blocking agent. The cardiac excitatory action of sympathomimetics is due to stimulation of the β_1-adrenergic receptors. This action is antagonized by β-blocking agents.

The most striking and characteristic actions of sympathomimetic drugs are exerted on the cardiovascular system. The changes in blood pressure caused by these drugs can be used as a model to understand how their actions on the adrenergic receptors contribute to the response. In this regard it is important to keep in mind the following points:

1. The effect of a sympathomimetic drug on blood pressure is sum of the stimulant or excitatory actions of the drug on both α- and β-receptors.
2. There are many more α-receptors in blood vessels than β-receptors. However, the affinity of a drug with the ability to stimulate both types of receptors will be greater for the β-receptor than for the α-receptor.

These two points are illustrated in the following example. Usually, following the injection of moderate to large doses of epinephrine there is an initial increase in blood pressure. This is due to α_1-receptor stimulation in the blood vessels supplying the heart because there are more α-receptors than β_2-receptors in blood vessels. But as the epinephrine concentration decreases, the epinephrine stays on the β_2-receptors longer because EPI has a higher affinity for β_2-receptors which are located in blood vessels in the heart. This causes a continued effect of vasodilation and a decrease in blood pressure. Beta$_2$-stimulation tends to dampen the increase in blood pressure from the α_1-receptor stimulation. Thus, epinephrine initially causes the blood pressure to increase via stimulation of α-receptors followed by β_2-stimulation, which tends to decrease the blood pressure. On the other hand, with lower doses of epinephrine, as is used in dentistry, there is no biphasic effect; there is simply an increase in systolic pressure due to α-stimulation and a β_1-stimulation which is a direct stimulation of heart muscle. There is not enough of the drug to give a β_2-stimulation.

ADRENERGIC (SYMPATHETIC) AGONISTS

Adrenergic agonists are divided into drugs that act *directly* binding to and activating the α or β receptors on the tissue, imitating the action of the neurotransmitter and drugs that act *indirectly* (that do not themselves bind or act on the receptor, but cause the release of norepinephrine from the nerve terminals). The effects of these drugs are actually the result of the released NE interacting with the receptor sites.

Adrenergic agonists are also classified according to *receptor site specificity* (α_1, α_2, β_1, β_2) (Table 13–5). It is best to select a drug that has selectivity for the receptor intended so as to minimize adverse effects.

Table 13–5 α and β-Adrenergic Agonists

	α-*Agonists*	*Clinical Use*	β-*Agonists*	*Clinical Use*
Direct acting	Phenylephrine (Neo-Synephrine) α_1	Nasal decongestant	Isoproterenol (Isuprel)—nonselective β_1 β_2 (better to use a selective β_2 drug)	Asthma
	Oxymetazoline (Afrin) α_1	Nasal decongestant		
	Tetrahydrozoline (Visine) α_1	Ocular decongestant	Albuterol (Ventolin, Proventil)—selective β_2	Asthma
	Norepinephrine (Levarterenol, Levophed) $\alpha_1 = \alpha_2$, β_1	Hypotension and shock	Terbutaline (Brethine)—selective β_2	Asthma
			Metaproterenol (Alupent, Metaprel)—selective β_2	Asthma
	Epinephrine $\alpha_1 = \alpha_2$, $\beta_1 = \beta_2$	Prolongs action of local anesthetics, reduction in bleeding	Epinephrine (Adrenalin)—α and nonselective β agonist	Anaphylactic shock (reverses hypotension-α_1) ; bronchodilator (asthma—β_2); stimulates heart in heart failure (vasoconstriction—β_1); in local anesthetics (β_2)
Central α_2 agonists	Clonidine (Catapres)—α_2 agonist	Hypertension; withdrawal from alcohol and cigarettes	Salmeterol (Serevent) β_2	asthma
	Methydopa (Aldomet)—α_2 agonist	Hypertension	Dobutamine (Dobutrex)—β_1, dopamine agonist	Drug of choice to stimulate heart (β_1)
			Isoetharine (Bronkosol)—nonselective	Asthma ($\beta_1\beta_2$)
Mixed	Ephedrine α_1/β	Nasal decongestion (vasoconstriction)	Ephedrine (preferable to use a β_2 selective bronchodilator)	Bronchodilation
	Pseudoephedrine (Sudafed and others) α_1/β	Nasal decongestion	Pseudoephedrine (preferable to use a β_2 selective bronchodilator)	Bronchodilation
Indirecting acting	Amphetamine	ADHD, narcolepsy		
	Cocaine	Topical anesthetic		

A review of the actions of adrenergic receptors:

1. *Alpha$_1$ (α_1)-receptors* are located on/in smooth muscle of the blood vessels supplying organs such as the heart, skin, heart, skin, and salivary glands, and smooth muscle of the eye, glands, G.I. tract, and urinary bladder; α_2-receptors are located on the on the axonal terminal of neurons releasing NE. The pharmacologic activation of the α_1-receptors leads to vasoconstriction, dilation of the pupils (to let more light in), and contraction of isolated smooth muscle. The exception to this rule is stimulation of α_1-receptors in the intestines, which leads to intestinal relaxation. Stimulation of α_2 receptors (autoreceptor) by released NE reduces further NE release, which is a negative feedback.

2. Beta (β_1)-receptors are located on cardiac muscle of the heart, stimulation leads to increase heart rate and force. Beta (β_2)-receptors are located on smooth muscle of the bronchioles (lungs) and intestine; stimulation of these receptors causes relaxation of smooth muscle. The effect of β-receptors can be blocked with β-blocking agents such as propranolol (Inderal).

Direct-Acting Adrenergic Receptor Agonists

α-adrenergic Agonists: *Vasoconstriction (Constriction of Blood Vessels): Ocular and Nasal Decongestants*

Many of the direct-acting agonists are catecholamines (e.g., epinephrine, norepinephrine, dopamine, isoproterenol, and dobutamine) and are used in the treatment of hypotension and shock by increasing blood pressure via constriction of blood vessels (vasoconstriction) (Tables 13–5 and 13–6).

Table 13–6   Common Adrenergic Blocking Drugs (Antagonists)

Drug Category	Drug Name	Drug Action	Clinical Use
α_1-blockers	Prazosin (Minipress)	Selective α_1 antagonist	Hypertension
	Doxazosin (Cardura)	Selective α_1 antagonist	Hypertension
	Terazosin HCl (Hytrin)	Selective α_1 antagonist	Hypertension, prostate hypertrophy, urinary retention
	Tamsulosin (Flomax)	Selective α_1 antagonist	Prostate hypertrophy
α_2-blockers	Yohimbine (Aphrodyne)	α_2-receptor blocker	Penile erectile dysfunction (impotency)
Nonselective β-blockers (blocks both β_1 and β_2-receptors)	Naldolol (Corgard)	β_1, β_2 blocking	Hypertension
	Propranolol (Inderal)	90% bound to plasma proteins and rapidly metabolized by liver	Hypertension, migraine headaches, mitral valve prolapse, tremors
	Timilol (Blocadren)	β_1, β_2 blocking	Hypertension, myocardial infarction, migraine headaches, glaucoma
Selective β_1-blockers	Metoprolol (Lopressor)	Selective β_1 blocking	Hypertension
	Atenolol (Tenormin)	Selective β_1 blocking	Hypertension
	Esmolol (Brevibloc)	Selective β_1 blocking	Hypertension
	Bisoprolol fumerate (Zebeta)	Selective β_1 blocking	Hypertension
α and β-blockers	Carvedilol (Coreg)	α and β blocking activity	Hypertension, atrial fibrillation,
	Labetalol (Normodyne)	α and β blocking activity	Hypertension

Drugs that bind to and activate α_1-receptors also stimulate vasoconstriction and increase blood pressure. These drugs, such as norepinephrine and dopamine, are used to treat shock and hypotension. Since they may cause an increase in blood pressure through arteriolar constriction, caution should be used in patients with a heart condition, since there is an increased risk of developing palpitations and tachycardia. Drugs used to treat hypotension and shock include dopamine and norepinephrine.

Epinephrine is unsuitable for oral administration because enzymes would destroy it, and thus can only be given in an injectable form. In dentistry, epinephrine is incorporated into local anesthetic solutions such as lidocaine to cause vasoconstriction, vasostimulation of α_1 receptors, of the blood vessels, which reduces bleeding and keeps the local anesthetic solution at the injection site longer.

The sympathomimetic effect on nasal mucous membranes (α_1-*adrenergic* receptors) is constriction of the blood vessels of the nasal mucosa, which reduces vascular congestion and mucus secretions, thus opening the nasal passages and increasing breathing. These drugs are administered topically as nose drops or nasal sprays to produce a *decongestant effect*. Examples are phenylephrine (Neo-Synephrine) and oxymetazoline (Afrin).

An adverse effect of using most short-acting nasal decongestants longer than 3–5 days is rebound congestion with mucosal swelling. The topical decongestant must be slowly discontinued and replaced with normal saline (e.g., Aryl, Ocean). Additionally, local irritation including burning, sneezing, and dryness are seen.

It is not selective for β_2-receptors acting on α_1-, β_1-, and β_2-receptors at the same time. Epinephrine is also used as a bronchodilator, by stimulating β_2-receptors, to counteract bronchoconstriction in anaphylactic shock, a severe, life-threatening drug reaction accompanied by hypotension. Additionally, epinephrine increases glycogenolysis (β-receptor) which increases glucose production and decreases the release of insulin, resulting in hyperglycemia. Being nonselective, epinephrine has adverse effects including tachycardia (increased heart rate due to β_1 stimulation), hypertension (due to α_1 stimulation), palpitations, cardiac arrhythmias (β_1), and dizziness. *Stimulation of β_2-receptors (in blood vessels of the heart) causes vasodilation which decreases blood pressure.* Excessive cardiac stimulation from high doses of EPI may result in angina or cardiac arrhythmias, which may lead to a stroke. Epinephrine causes the production of thick, viscous saliva.

When epinephrine has done its job, it is removed from the area via two methods:

1. Metabolized (breakdown) by monoamine oxidase (MAO) and catechol-O-methyl transferase (COMT), both enzymes present in the gastrointestinal tract
2. Reuptake back into the nerve terminal

Norepinephrine (Levophed) has a stronger affinity for α_1- and β_1-receptors and does not stimulate β_2-receptors. There is pure α_1-stimulation which is pure vasoconstriction with an enormous increase in blood pressure. This α_1-stimulation is so great that often the heart rate will slow down (bradycardia) as part of a physiologic adjustment to the high blood pressure. Norepinephrine is primarily used as a vasoconstrictor in shock (hypotensive) patients. It is removed by reuptake into the nerve terminals for by metabolism by MAO and COMT.

Levonordefrin (Neo-Cobefrin) is a vasoconstrictor found in dental local anesthetics. Levonordefrin is half as potent a vasoconstrictor as epinephrine. *It primarily stimulates α-adrenergic receptors with little to no effect on the β-adrenergic receptors.* Thus, stimulation of α_1-receptors on tissues/organs causes vasoconstriction of blood vessels, resulting in hypertension (increase systolic and diastolic blood pressure). Epinephrine produces a greater stimulation of β_2 receptors than α_1 receptors, thereby causing vasodilation and decreasing diastolic blood pressure. Higher doses produce more vasoconstriction and increased blood pressure.

Rapid Dental Hint

Remember to assess your patients before choosing a local anesthetic containing epinephrine.

Dopamine, a catecholamine, is often used for hypotensive shock (not anaphylactic shock). A person in shock has a high sympathetic output and kidney function stops. Dopamine increases renal blood flow.

Central α_2-Agonists
Centrally (central nervous system) active α_2- agonists stimulate α_2-receptors in the *brain,* and turn off the activity of sympathetic nerves due to an inhibition of NE re-

lease from the nerve terminals. Even though these drugs are agonists, they stimulate a receptor that turns off the sympathetic nervous system response and work like blockers. These drugs are used to treat hypertension by decreasing heart rate. Adverse effects include xerostomia and orthostatic hypotension. The prototype drug in this class is clonidine (Catapres). The xerostomia from clonidine is very severe and uncomfortable for the patient.

β_1/β_2-Adrenergic Agonists: Adrenergic Bronchodilation: Bronchial Asthma
Drugs used in the treatment of bronchial asthma affect the β_2-*adrenergic receptors,* causing dilation of the bronchial smooth muscle and vasoconstriction of the bronchial blood vessels. Drugs are administered through inhalation, orally or injected. The prototype drug is isoproterenol (Isuprel). Since isoproterenol is nonselective and acts on both β_1- and β_2-adrenergic receptors, besides affecting the bronchioles it also affects the heart by causing an increased heart rate (β_1). So, blood pressure can go up or down, because there is vasodilation and increased cardiac output which makes blood pressure increase.

Selective β_2-adrenergic agonists (albuterol, metaproterenol, terbutaline) selectively affect only the tissues with β_2 receptors and not cardiac muscle; thus there are less effects on the heart. These selective β_2 agonists, which are given via inhalation, were developed for asthma patients and are ideal for use in the treatment of asthma, bronchitis, or chronic obstructive pulmonary disease. Since these drugs are not catecholamines (as is epinephrine and isoproterenol), they are not digested by the same enzymes and therefore have a long duration of action. Ritodrine (Yutopar) is a selective β_2-adrenergic agonist used to stimulate uterine smooth muscle, which will prevent or delay preterm labor.

Indirect-Acting Agonists
Amphetamine releases stores of NE from the sympathetic neurons. The released NE activates adrenergic receptors and causes a powerful sympathomimetic effect with vasoconstriction, cardiac excitation, and increased blood pressure. A drug called Adderall, which is indicated in narcolepsy (individual falling asleep uncontrollably) and in attention deficit hyperactivity disorder (ADHD), contains mixed salts of a single-entity amphetamine product (dextroamphetamine sulfate, dextroamphetamine saccharate, amphetamine aspartate monohydrate, amphentamine sulfate).

Cocaine is a naturally occurring drug. It is the most potent vasoconstrictor and is used as a local anesthetic. Its mechanism of action is to block the reuptake of NE, thus increasing the concentration of NE in the synapse. The sympathomimetic effects include cardiac stimulation and elevation of blood pressure.

Mixed-Acting Adrenergic Receptor Agonists

Ephedrine and pseudoephedrine (Sudafed) activate both α_1- and β_2- adrenergic receptors by direct and indirect methods. These drugs are used as nasal decongestants due to stimulation of α_1-receptors, resulting in vasoconstriction. These drugs produce bronchodilation by stimulating β-receptors. However, since they are not selective for β_2-adrenergic receptors, other drugs are preferred such as albuterol sulfate. Side effects include increased blood pressure and increased heart rate (tachycardia).

Pseudoephedrine and ephedrine are used by drug traffickers to manufacture methamphetamine, a Schedule II controlled substance, for the illicit market. As of April 2006, federal law imposed a limit on the amount of pseudoephedrine products: Consumers can buy to 3.6 grams a day, 9 grams for an entire month.

Therapeutic Uses

- α_1-receptor agonists cause smooth muscle contraction, which leads to *vasoconstriction,* dilation of the pupils, and contraction of the bladder muscle. These drugs are used in the treatment of shock and hypotension and as a nasal/ocular decongestant.
- α_2-receptor agonists are used in the treatment of hypertension to *lower blood pressure.* These drugs will inhibit the release of NE, resulting in lower levels of NE.
- β_1-receptor agonists are used to increase the rate and force of heart contractions in patients with hypotension and shock. These drugs are given intravenously.
- β_2-receptor agonists are used to cause relaxation or dilation of smooth muscle in the lungs in patients with asthma. These long-acting drugs are given orally or inhaled. It is best to use a selective β_2 drug such as albuterol or terbutaline to keep adverse effects to a minimum.
- Dopamine-receptor agonists cause renal (kidney) vasodilation.

Adverse Effects

Adverse effects of sympathomimetic drugs primarily occur as a result of the drug's pharmacologic actions. Taking higher doses of direct-acting catecholamines (e.g., epinephrine, isoproterenol, norepinephrine) may cause severe hypertension due to excessive cardiac stimulation; arrhythmias, tachycardia, and ventricular fibrillation may occur. Other side effects include xerostomia, nausea, vomiting, headache, dizziness, and palpitations. Nonselective β-agonists may cause hyperglycemia, and should not be taken by diabetic patients.

Drug abuse may occur with amphetamines and cocaine. An overdose may result in excessive cardiac stimulation. Cocaine inhibits the reuptake of NE, and amphetamine increases the release of NE into the synapse.

Drug Interactions

Tricyclic antidepressants (e.g., amitriptyline, desipramine, nortirptyline, and imipramine) act by blocking the reuptake of catecholamines and thus may increase the hypertensive effects of EPI. Nonselective β_1, β_2 agonists may also cause a hypertensive crisis. Nonselective β-blockers block β_2 vasodilatory effects of EPI. Thus, the amount of epinephrine should be limited to 0.04 mg (2 cartridges of 1:100,000) in patients taking these drugs. A severe hypertensive reaction with death can occur when cocaine and epinephrine are taken together.

ADRENERGIC RECEPTOR ANTAGONISTS

Sympatholytics are drugs that directly block the α- and β-adrenergic receptors on tissues resulting in a decrease of sympathetic activity. These drugs are used in the treatment of cardiovascular conditions (hypertension), urinary retention, migraine headache, and glaucoma. Sympatholytics can be classified according to their effect on the receptors: α-blockers and β-blockers. Essentially the symptoms produced are similar to the resting

Did You Know?

In literature, Sherlock Holmes injected cocaine in his arm. The author Robert Louis Stevenson wrote *Dr. Jekyll and Mr. Hyde* while under the influence of cocaine.

and digesting symptoms seen in the cholinergic or parasympathetic nervous system response.

Most of the therapeutic effects are primarily due to the blocking of α_1- or β_1-adrenergic receptors, and any adverse effects are due to the blockade of α_2- or β_2-receptors. Because of this, drugs have been developed that selectively block either α_1- or β_1-adrenergic receptors and do not affect the other receptors, thus eliminating any adverse effects.

α_1-Adrenergic Receptor Antagonists (Blockers)

The α_1-adrenergic blockers are used in the treatment of hypertension by blocking the vasoconstrictive actions of NE and EPI on vascular smooth muscle. This causes arteriolar vasodilatation and lowers peripheral vascular resistance, which increases blood flow to the tissues so the heart does not have to work as hard. Taking an initial dose of these drugs can result in orthostatic hypotension, where a sudden drop in blood pressure occurs when the individual rises quickly from a sitting or reclining position, causing dizziness or fainting. Allow the individual to remain sitting for a while before getting up.

Alpha-blockers are classified as *nonselective α-adrenergic blockers* that bind both α_1 and α_2 receptors on smooth muscle of blood vessels. As a result alpha-receptor sites are unable to react to norepinephrine. The *selective α_1-adrenergic blockers* include prazosin (Minipress) and terazosin (Hytrin) and block only α_1-receptors. Yohimbine (Yocon) is a *selective α_2-adrenergic antagonist* that blocks α_2-receptors and is used in the treatment of impotency in men.

These drugs produce vasodilation and decrease blood pressure and they are used in the treatment of chronic essential hypertension. Because these drugs relax the smooth muscle of the bladder and prostate, they are used in the treatment of urinary retention due to benign hypertrophy of the prostate. When the prostate becomes enlarged the flow of urine is reduced. The α_1-adrenergic blockers relax the smooth muscle, increasing urinary flow. Adverse effects of selective α_1-adrenergic blockers are due primarily to excessive vasodilation, which may cause hypotension, dizziness, fainting, reflex tachycardia, and palpitations.

Prazosin is used in the treatment of chronic essential hypertension. Since it undergoes extension first-pass metabolism, most of the drug is metabolized before it is excreted. Severe syncope (fainting) is possible with the first dose.

β-Adrenergic Receptor Antagonists (β-blockers)

Drugs classified as β-blockers are either nonselective or selective in blocking the β-receptors. All of the β-blockers are competitive antagonists. Therapeutic uses of β-blockers include:

- Hypertension
- Angina
- Heart arrhythmias
- Panic attacks
- Migraine headaches
- Glaucoma

Nonselective β-Blockers (Treatment of Hypertension, Angina Pectoris, Glaucoma)

The nonselective β-blockers block both β_1 receptors on the heart tissue and β_2 receptors on smooth muscle, liver, lung, and other tissues, thus affecting all of these tissues and causing adverse effects such as a bronchospasm, bradycardia, and hypoglycemia.

Blocking β_1-receptors located on the heart reduce sympathetic stimulation of the heart, thus reducing cardiac output (cardiac work is decreased) and blood pressure. Blocking β_1-receptors on the kidneys reduce the secretion of a substance called renin, involved in the formation in the bloodstream of a vasoconstrictor substance called angiotensin II that causes hypertension. Blockade of β_1-receptors in the eye reduces secretions and intraocular pressure.

The prototype nonselective β-blocker is propranolol (Inderal). Its therapeutic effect is to decrease cardiac output and blood pressure and thus it is used in the treatment of hypertension. Since it decreases oxygen demand to the heart and produces peripheral vasoconstriction, it is used in the treatment of angina and tachycardia. Since it is a nonselective β_1-blocker it will also block β_2-receptors on the lungs, which may cause bronchoconstriction in asthmatics. By blocking β_2-receptors in the liver these drugs have a hypoglycemic effect, inhibiting EPI-stimulated glycogenolysis, the breakdown of glycogen into glucose. Precaution should be used in diabetics taking insulin. Propranolol is also used in the prevention of migraine headache and for essential tremors, involuntary trembling of the hands. Propranolol and other β-blockers may reduce the incidence of sudden death in patients with acute mycocardial infarction (heart attack). Elevated thyroid hormone levels (thyroid storm) tend to stimulate the heart, and propranolol is used to reduce the hormone levels.

Selective β₁-Blockers (Treatment of Hypertension)

Selective β₁-blockers have a greater affinity for β₁-receptors than for β₂-receptors. These drugs are referred to as *cardioselective β-blockers* because β₁-receptors are located primarily on heart tissue. The prototype selective β-blocker is atenolol (Tenormin).

Because these drugs are more selective toward the β1-receptors, there are fewer adverse effects than occur with the nonselective β-blockers. However, there still may be some affinity toward β₂-receptors, thus they should be used with caution in patients with asthma.

Indirect-Acting Adrenergic Antagonists

These drugs do not directly block α- or β-adrenergic receptors, but they block the release of NE from nerve endings. They antagonize the effects of the sympathetic system. The two drugs in this category are reserpine and guanethidine (Ismelin), used in the treatment of hypertension.

Adverse Effects of Adrenergic Blockers

- α-blockers can cause postural hypotension and bradycardia with initial doses. Taking the drug with food may reduce the incidence of dizziness. Food may delay absorption, but does not affect the extent of absorption.
- All β-blockers can cause heart failure or heart block. Caution should be used in diabetics, as these drugs increase insulin action resulting in hypoglycemia. Nonselective β₂-blockers may cause bronchoconstriction, and are contraindicated in asthmatics.

Drug Interactions

Additive hypotensive effects occur with α₁-blockers when used concurrently with other antihypertensive drugs and diuretics.

Concurrent administration of phenothiazines with the β-blockers has an additive hypotensive effect. Cimetidine (Tagamet) decreases elimination and increases

effects of propranolol. Diuretics and other antihyhpertensive agents will increase the hypotensive effects.

DRUGS AFFECTING CHOLINERGIC TRANSMISSION

Drugs that act as mediators of cholinergic/ACh transmission are called parasympathomimetics (or **cholinergic agents**) and parasympatholyics (or **anticholinergics**) are agents which block the effects acetylcholine on parasympathetic nervous activity.

Parasympathomimetic Drugs

Cholinergic Agonists

There are two types of cholinergic agonists: (1) directing-acting agents and (2) indirecting-acting cholinergic agonists (also referred to as cholinesterase inhibitors).

Directing-acting agents have affinity and activity at cholinergic receptors at either nicotinic or muscarinic receptors. Ideally, the drug should have a greater affinity for the muscarinic receptors, because these receptors are found at the organ site. The muscarinic effects act directly on the postsynaptic nerve endings. They can produce a slowing of the heart and increase smooth muscle tone of the G.I. and urinary tracts, which may result in nausea and evacuation of the bladder. They also may cause bronchial and pupil constriction (miosis). The nicotinic effect refers to the cholinergic action at the autonomic ganglia and at the neuromuscular junction (Table 13–7).

The prototype direct-acting cholinergic receptor agonists are acetylcholine and bethanechol (Urecholine). Acethycholine (ACh) has almost no clinical use because it is rapidly destroyed and causes a lot of adverse effects.

Natural plant alkaloids that are cholinergic agents include muscarine, nicotine, and pilocarpine. Pilocarpine, obtained from a plant shrub, is used to treat xerostomia by binding to and stimulating cholinergic muscarinic receptors. Muscarine, found in mushrooms, has no current medical use. Nicotine is obtained from plants and cigarettes and other tobacco products. It is contained in chewing gum and transdermal patches for smoking cessation.

One class of *indirect-acting cholinergic receptor agonists* are *cholinesterase inhibitors* (or anticholinesterase) (Table 13–8). These drugs have cholinergic action by inhibiting cholinesterase, the enzyme that breaks down acetylcholine, allowing for the accumulation of acetylcholine at the receptor site. These agents show a mixture

Table 13-7 Direct-Acting Cholinergic Agonists Agents

Drug Name	Mechanism of Action	Clinical Use
Acetylcholine	Muscarinic and nicotinic receptor activation	Rarely used because it produces widespread effects and is rapidly broken down
Carbachol (Miostat)	Muscarinic and nicotinic receptor activation	Intraocular administration, glaucoma, miosis for eye surgery
Bethanechol (urecholine)	Muscarinic receptor stimulation	Oral administration: prevents urinary retention and increases intestinal motility after surgery
Pilocarpine (Pilocar)	Greater affinity for muscarinic than for nicotinic	Intraocular administration: open-angle glaucoma. Oral administration: treatment of xerostomia
Methacholine	Muscarinic receptor stimulation	Diagnosis of asthma and bronchial hyperreactivity
Nicotine	Nicotine	Smoking cessation (oral, transdermal patch)

of muscarinic and nicotinic effects. They are divided into two classes, depending upon their duration of action: reversible inhibitors, which do not bind tightly to receptors, and irreversible inhibitors, which bind irreversibly to receptors. Examples of reversible inhibitors include neostigmine and pyridostigmine, used to treat symptoms of myasthenia gravis. Physostigmine is used in the treatment of glaucoma.

Donepezil (Aricept) and tacrine (Cognex) are newer, centrally acting, reversible cholinesterase in-

hibitors that concentrate in the brain and are used in the treatment of Alzheimer's disease.

Irreversible cholinesterase inhibitors are all organophosphates and are primarily used as pesticides. Some agents were developed as nerve gases (chemical warfare). These include tabun, sarin, and soman. Since these agents are highly lipid soluble they are absorbed through the skin and eye. Poisoning is a problem, and can occur through these routes as well as by oral ingestion. Some agents are used medically (such as echothio-

Table 13-8 Indirect Acting Cholinergic Agonists

Drug Name	Route of Administration	Clinical Uses
Reversible inhibitors		
Donepezil (Aricept)	Oral	Alzheimer's disease
Tacrine (Cognex)	Oral	Alzheimer's disease
Edrophonium	IV	Test for myasthenia gravis; antidote for curare
Neostigmine	Oral, IM, SC	Treatment for myasthenia gravis, postsurgery urine retention
Physostigmine	Topical (ocular)	Glaucoma
	IM, IV	Reverse anticholinergic overdose
Pyridostigmine	Oral, IM, IV	Myasthenia gravis
	IV	Reversal of muscle relaxants
Irreversible inhibitors		
Echothiophate	Ocular	Refractory glaucoma
Nerve gases (sarin, tabun, soman)	Absorbed through the skin, eyes	Poisoning

phate and isofluophate in the treatment of chronic glaucoma) that are refractory to other agents.

Anticholinergic Drugs

Cholinergic Receptor Antagonists (Anticholinergic Agents)

Cholinergic antagonists block both the muscarinic and nicotinic receptors. The muscarinic receptor antagonists compete with ACh for muscarinic receptors at the organ site, thereby inhibiting the effects of parasympathetic nerve stimulation (Tables 13–9 and 13–10).

There are two types of *muscarinic receptor antagonists:* belladonna alkaloids, and semisynthetic and synthetic muscarinic receptor antagonists. Belladonna alkaloids include atropine and scopolamine.

In low doses, atropine and scopolamine cause dry mouth and inhibit sweating. In higher doses they relax

Table 13–9 Muscarinic (Cholinergic) Blocking Agents

Organ System	Pharmacologic Effect	Drug Name
CNS	Antimotion sickness Sedation	Scopolomine Atropine
Eye (ocular)	Mydriasis (pupil dilation)	Atropine, homatropine
Lung (bronchi)	Bronchodilation	Ipratropium (Atrovent)
G.I. tract	Relaxation, slow motility (preoperative)	Dicyclomine (Bentyl), Propantheline (Pro-Banthine)
Heart	Bradycardia	Atropine
Salivary glands	Preoperative: Decrease salivation	Methantheline (Banthine)
Bronchial secretion	Preoperative: Decrease secretions	Atropine

smooth muscle, causing a decrease in G.I. and urinary tract contractions; decrease G.I. secretions (these drugs are used in the treatment of peptic ulcers); decrease respiratory secretions; and increase heart rate and cardiac conduction. Thus, with higher doses of atropine the severity of effects increases. Indications for using atropine include:

1. Ocular: To produce dilation (mydriasis) and facilitate an eye examination
2. Cardiac: Treat bradycardia after a mycocardial infarction
3. Gastrointestinal and urinary tract—treat gastrointestinal and bladder spasms;
4. Central nervous system—prevent motion sickness and treat excessive muscle movement, especially of the face and neck (acute dystonia) caused by antipsychotic medications;
5. Preoperative: dry up secretions
6. Organophosphate poisoning

Scopolamine is primarily used to prevent motion sickness, but has the same effects as atropine. Hyoscyamine is used primarily to treat intestinal spasms and other types of gastrointestinal disorders.

These agents are used to dilate the pupil to allow an examination of the eye. The most popular drug used for this is topicamine (Mydriacyl).

The pharmacologic effects of semisynthetic and synthetic muscarinic receptor antagonists are similar to atropine. Under certain conditions these agents are helpful. For instance, dicyclomine (Bentyl) and propantheline (Pro-Banthine) are synthetic agents with a strong affinity to muscarinic receptors in the G.I. tract, making them useful in decreasing gastrointestinal motility in irritable bowel syndrome. Tolterodine (Detrol) is used for the treatment of urinary incontinence.

Nicotinic receptor antagonists include ganglionic blocking agents and neuromuscular blocking agents.

The ganglionic nicotinic receptor blocking agents selectively block nicotinic receptors at the sympathetic and parasympathetic ganglia.

Adverse effects of anticholinergic drugs include xerostomia, blurred vision, constipation, and urinary retention.

Adverse Effects

There are many adverse effects with anticholinergic agents. Basically, the adverse effects are primarily sympathetic in nature. There is xerostomia, urinary retention,

Table 13–10 Selective Anticholinergic (Cholinergic Receptor Antagonists) Drugs

Drug Name	Route of Adminstration	Clinical Uses	Drug Interactions
Muscarinic Receptor Antagonists			Additive effects when taken with other drugs with anticholinergic activity (e.g., tricyclic antidepressants)
Atropine sulfate	IV/IM/SC IV/IM IV/IM Inhalation Drops/ointment	Produces a dry field before surgery Cardiac arrythmias/bradycardia Organophosphate (nerve gas) antidote Short-term COPD Mydriasis before eye exam	
Hyoscyamine sulfate	IV/IM/SC/PO/SL (sublingual)	Gastrointestinal (G.I.) spasms	
Scopolamine	PO/IV/IM/SC PO/topical patch Drops	Adjunct to anesthesia Motion sickness Mydriasis (pupil dilation) for eye exam	
Dicyclomine HCl (Bentyl)	PO	Irritable bowel syndrome	
Flavoxate HCl (Uripas)	PO	Nocturia (night urination), incontinence	
Ipratropium bromide (Atrovent)	Inhalation, nebulizer	COPD (bronchodilator for chronic bronchitis and emphysema), rhinitis/common cold	
Oxybutynin chloride (Ditropan)	PO	Pain/spasms in urinary incontinent patients	
Tolterodine tartrate (Detrol)	PO	Urinary incontinence (less incidence of dry mouth)	
Tropicamide (Mydriacyl)	drops	Mydriasis (pupil dilation) for eye exam	
Nicotinic Receptor Antagonists			General anesthesia; reduce dose of neuromuscular blocking drug
Atracurium besylate	IV	Skeletal muscle relaxation during surgery (for intubation)	
Doxacurium chloride	IV	Skeletal muscle relaxation during surgery	
Pancuronium bromide	IV	Skeletal muscle relaxation during surgery	
Pipecuronium	IV	Skeletal muscle relaxation during surgery	
Succinylcholine chloride	IV/IM	Presurgical muscle relaxation to facilitate intubation	
d-tubocurarine	IV/IM	Skeletal muscle relaxation during surgery (for intubation)	

blurred vision, constipation and tachycardia. Anticholinergic drugs are contraindicated in glaucoma and in urinary tract obstruction (e.g., benign prostatic hypertrophy—BPH). Atropine and other muscarinic receptor antagonists are contraindicated in heart disease because they may cause tachycardia.

Drug Interactions

Additive anticholinergic side effects are seen when these drugs are given concurrently with drugs that have anticholinergic effects, such as tricyclic antidepressants and antihistamines such as diphenhydramine (Benadryl).

DENTAL HYGIENE NOTES

Many patients in the dental office will be taking one or more drugs that act on the autonomic nervous system. Drug actions of the autonomic nervous system on various organs including the heart, eye, arterioles, glands (salivary and lacrimal or tear), skin, lung, G.I. tract, and urinary bladder result in either stimulation or relaxation of these organs.

A local dental anesthetic (e.g., lidocaine) containing a sympathomimetic vasoconstrictor (e.g., epinephrine) should be used with precaution if the patient is a cocaine abuser or taking amphetamines. A severe hypertensive crisis and cardiac damage—even death—can occur due to toxic levels of epinephrine, which is a sympathetic agonist. Epinephrine is a vasoconstrictor, and cocaine is the most potent vasoconstrictor. Thus, epinephrine should not be used for at least 24 hours after the last dose of cocaine.

The amount of epinephrine injected in dental anesthesia will produce an α_1 and β_2 response, with β_2 predominating. Small doses of epinephrine produce constriction of blood vessels in the skin and mucous membrances (α_1 response) and a decrease in diastolic blood pressure and increase blood flow to skeletal muscle (β_2 response).

It is not a contraindication to use lidocaine with epinephrine in patients with hypertension and patients taking a tricyclic antidepressant (e.g., Elavil), but the patient should be treated similar to a cardiac patient. Thus

the administration of two to three cartridges (0.036–0.054 mg epinephrine) of 2% lidocaine with 1:100,000 epinephrine is considered safe. The patient's blood pressure should be monitored during all dental procedures.

Levonordefrin (Neo-Cobefrin) is another type of vasoconstrictor used in the local anesthetic mepivacaine. It is half as potent a vasoconstrictor as epinephrine and it primarily stimulates α-adrenergic (sympathetic) receptors, with little to no effect on the β-adrenergic receptors. Stimulation of α_1-receptors on tissues/organs causes vasoconstriction of blood vessels, resulting in hypertension (increased systolic and diastolic blood pressure). Thus, levonordefrin should not be used in patients taking a tricyclic antidepressant. Levonordefrin and epinephrine may be used in patients taking nonselective β-blockers, but the amount should be reduced. When evaluating a patient's medical history it is important to know every drug the patient is taking, both over the counter (OTC) and prescription. It is interesting to note that most of the adrenergic agonists (namely, α_1-adrenergeric agonists) are nasal decongestants and are OTC drugs. These drugs cause a local (nasal mucosa) vasoconstiction. Patients may not realize that OTC drugs are chemical drugs and must be mentioned in the medical history.

β_1-adrenergic receptors are found predominately on the heart and, when stimulated, cause an increase in the rate and force of contraction. β_1-*adrenergic agonist drugs* acting selectively on β_1-receptors are used in the treatment of heart failure and are given IV. These patients will most likely not be seen in the dental office.

β_2-receptors are found on the lungs, uterus, and arterioles and veins. β_2-*adrenergic agonist* drugs acting on β_2-receptors are used in the treatment of asthma. These drugs are selective for β_2-receptors, avoiding cardiac adverse effects. The dental clinician should be aware of which drugs are selective β_2-agonists acting only on the bronchioles.

Patients taking α_1-blockers are being treated for hypertension. Orthostatic hypotension is an adverse effect of these drugs. To prevent syncope, allow the patient to sit in an upright position in the dental chair before getting up.

Blood pressure should be taken at every office visit on patients taking β_1-blockers, which are used primarily in patients with hypertension to decrease blood pressure. The patient should be asked if he/she took medication that day. Use of local anesthetics containing epinephrine

epinephrine is not contraindicated; however, caution should be used. Two or three cartridges of 2% lidocaine with 1:1,000,000 epinephrine can safely be administered to a patient taking these medications.

The primary adverse effect of anticholinergic drugs is xerostomia. The dental clinician plays an important role in teaching the patient to care for the mouth. To minimize the effects of dry mouth on the oral mucosa, the patient should be instructed to maintain good oral home care, drink plenty of water, avoid sugar candy, and avoid alcohol-containing mouthrinses. Numerous OTC salivary substitutes are available.

Additionally, the patient may experience tachycardia, or increased heart rate, while taking anticholinergic drugs. The patient's blood pressure should be monitored at every dental visit.

KEY POINTS

- Stimulation of the sympathetic (adrenergic) and parasympathetic (cholinergic) nerves cause opposite responses.
- Function of neurotransmitters is to carry nerve impulses (action potentials) across the synapse.
- Stimulation of the sympathetic pathway starts a "flight or fight" response, and activation of the parasympathetic pathway initiates a "resting and digestive" reaction.
- Sympathetic nervous division: Norepinephrine has a higher affinity and binding to all α-receptors and some β-receptors. Epinephrine has a higher affinity to β_2-receptors in blood vessels/smooth muscle.
- α_1-receptors are found in skin, coronary tissue, the kidney, mucosa, salivary glands, blood vessels, eye muscle, and sphincters of the gastrointestinal tract.
  - α_1-receptor agonist drugs: nasal decongestant and hypotension
- α_2-receptors are autoreceptors found at terminal endings of neurons that release norepinephrine. They function to inhibit release of norepinephrine and its effects.
  - α_2-receptor agonist drugs: treatment of hypertension
- All α-receptor mediated effects of sympathomimetic drugs are excitatory except in the intestines, where they cause an inhibitory type of response.
- β_1-receptors are found on heart muscle.

- All β-receptor mediated effects of sympathomimetic drugs are inhibitory.
  - β_1-receptor agonists drugs: treatment of heart conditions and shock
- β_2-receptors are found in certain blood vessels/smooth muscle (lung, liver, intestines, bladder)
  - β_2-agonist drugs: treatment of asthma
- The cardiac excitatory effects of sympathomimetic drugs are β_1-mediated and are inhibited by a β-blocking agent.
- Sympathomimetic drugs are used primarily for their effects on the heart, bronchial tree, and nasal passages.
- Adrenergic blockers are used primarily to treat hypertension and are the most widely prescribed class of autonomic drugs.
- The primary use of β-blockers is in the treatment of hypertension.
- Initial effect of epinephrine (in a local anesthetic) is an increase in blood pressure due to α_1-receptor stimulation (this causes blood vessel constriction). This is followed by a decrease in blood pressure due to epinephrine having a higher affinity for β_2-receptors, which causes a continued effect of vasodilation (opening of blood vessels) and a decrease in diastolic blood pressure.
- Parasympathomimetics (cholinergic drugs) have few therapeutic uses because of their numerous side effects.
- Cholinergic drugs are primarily used in the treatment of xerostomia (cevimeline, pilocarpine) and Alzheimer's disease (donepezil, tacrine, rivastigmine).
- Anticholinergic drugs are used to increase heart rate (atropine), urinary incontinence (oxybutynin), motion sickness (scopolamine), and irritable bowel syndrome (dicyclomine, propantheline, scopolamine).

BOARD REVIEW QUESTIONS

1. Which of the following neurotransmitters is released from sympathetic postganglionic neurons? (p. 217)
   a. Dopamine
   b. Serotonin
   c. Acetylcholine
   d. Norepinephrine

2. Which of the following receptors is classified as an autoreceptor? (p. 218)
   a. Nicotinic
   b. α_1
   c. α_2
   d. β_1
   e. β_2

3. Which of the following receptors is primarily found on heart tissue? (p. 218)
   a. Nicotinic
   b. α_1
   c. α_2
   d. β_1
   e. β_2

4. Which of the following organs is the origin of presynaptic (preganglionic) sympathetic neurons? (p. 217)
   a. Heart
   b. Brain
   c. Spinal cord
   d. Skeletal muscle
   e. Adrenal medulla

5. Which of the following organs is only innervated by sympathetic preganglionic neurons? (p. 217)
   a. Lacrimal glands
   b. Heart muscle
   c. Kidneys
   d. Bronchioles
   e. Adrenal medulla

6. Which of the following receptors does epinephrine primarily stimulate to cause vasoconstriction? (pp. 218–219)
   a. α_1
   b. α_2
   c. β_1
   d. β_2

7. A patient is taking propranolol (Inderal) for hypertension. Which of the following signs should be monitored? (p. 224–225)
   a. Kidney function
   b. Blood pressure
   c. Body temperature
   d. CNS function

8. Which of the following types of drugs is used in the treatment of nasal congestion? (pp. 222–223)
   a. β_1 agonists
   b. β_2 selective antagonists
   c. α_1 agonists
   d. α_2 agonists

9. All of the following drugs cause xerostomia as an adverse effect *except* one. Which is the exception? (pp. 225, 229–230)
   a. Atropine
   b. Scopolamine
   c. Pilocarpine
   d. Hyoscyamine

10. Which of the following drugs is used in the treatment of asthma? (p. 222)
    a. Timolol
    b. Reserpine
    c. Albuterol
    d. Dobutamine

11. Which of the following drugs may cause xerostomia? (pp. 229, 230)
    a. Epinephrine
    b. Dopamine
    c. Cevimeline
    d. Atropine

12. Which of the following drugs should be limited in patients taking Elavil (a tricyclic antidepressant)? (p. 225)
    a. Epinephrine
    b. Acetylcholine
    c. Dopamine
    d. Serotonin

13. Epinephrine is added to local anesthetics as a vasoconstrictor. Which of the following receptors are activated initially by epinephrine? (p. 231, 232)
    a. α_1
    b. α_2
    c. β_1
    d. β_2

14. Epinephrine goes through a biphasic response concerning blood pressure. After the initial increase in blood pressure, there is a decrease. This decrease in

blood pressure is due to stimulation of which of the following receptors? (p. 223)

a. α_1
b. α_2
c. β_1
d. β_2

15. Which of the following receptors is stimulated when pilocarpine is taken? (p. 228)

a. Cholinergic nicotinic
b. Cholinergic muscarinic
c. Adrenergic α
d. Adrenergic β

SELECTED REFERENCES

Bousquet, P., L. Monassier, J. Feldman. 1998. Autonomic nervous system as a target for cardiovascular drugs. *Clin Exp Pharmacol Physiol* 25:446–448.

Bylund, D. B. 1995. Pharmacologic characteristics of α_2-adrenergic receptor subtypes. *Ann NY Acad Sci* 763:1–7.

Herman, W. W., J. L. Konzelman Jr., M. Prisant. 2004. New national guidelines on hypertension: A summary for dentistry. *JADA* 135:576–584.

Hieble, J. P., R. R. Ruffolo. 1996. The use of α-adrenoceptor antagonists in the pharmacological management of benign prostatic hypertrophy: An overview. *Pharmacol Res* 33:145–160.

Jaradeh, S. S. and T. E. Prieto. 2003. Evaluation of the autonomic nervous system. *Phys Med Rehabil Clin N Am* 14:287–305.

Lepor, H. et al. 1997. Doxazosin for benign prostatic hyperplasia: Long-term efficacy and safety in hypertensive and normotensive patients. *J Urol* 157:525–530.

Wallingford, A. 2000. Beta blockers and heart disease. *Lancet* 35(4):1751–1756.

WEB SITES

www.medscape.com
www.uspharmacist.com

Q U I C K   D R U G   G U I D E

Sympathomimetics (Adrenergic Agonists)

Directing Acting α-agonists (vasoconstriction; ocular (eye) and nasal decongestants; treatment of hypotension and shock, antihypertensive)

- Phenylephrine (NeoSynephrine) (nasal decongestant; increases BP) α_1
- Oxymetazoline (Afrin) (nasal and ocular decongestant) α_1
- Tetrahydrozoline (Visine) (ocular decongestant) α_1
- Norepinephrine (hypotensive shock to increase blood pressure) $\alpha_1 = \alpha_2$, β_1
- Epinephrine (shock, cardiac arrest, prolong action of local anesthetics) $\alpha_1 = \alpha_2$, $\beta_1 = \beta_2$
- Clonidine (Catepres) (autoreceptor; antihypertensive drug) α_2

Direct Acting β-agonists (anti-asthmatic/bronchodilator; shock/heart failure)

- Isoproterenol (Isuprel) (β_1/β_2 nonselective; heart stimulation and asthma)
- Albuterol (Ventolin, Proventil) (asthma) selective β_2

- Terbutaline (Brethine) (asthma; uterus relaxation—premature labor) selective β_2
- Metaproterenol (Alupent) (asthma) selective β_2
- Epinephrine (Adrenalin) β_1/β_2 nonselective
- Dobutamine (Dobutrex) (shock/heart failure) β_1/β_2
- Isoetharine (Bronkosol) (asthma) selective β_2
- Salmeterol (Serevent) (asthma) selective β_2

Indirect-acting agonists

- Amphetamine (increase NE release) (ADHD)
- Cocaine (inhibits NE reuptake into nerve terminals) (topical anesthetic)

Mixed-acting agonists (nasal decongestants)

- Ephedrine α_1, β_2
- Pseudoephedrine (Sudafed and others) α_1, β

Centrally acting α2-agonists (hypertension)

- Clonidine (Catapres)
- Methyldopa (Aldomet)

Adrengergic antagonists (blockers)

α-blockers

Nonselective α_1/α_2-receptor blockers

- Phenoxybenzamine (Dibenzyline) (hypertensive episodes in pheochromocytoma)
- Phentolamine (hypertensive episodes in pheochromocytoma)

Selective α_1- blockers (antihypertensive drugs)

- Prazosin (Minipress)
- Doxazosin (Cardura)
- Terazosin (Hytrin) (also indicated in prostate hypertrophy)
- Tamsulosin (Flomax) (prostate hypertrophy)

Selective α_2- blockers (impotency in men)

- Yohimbine (Aphrodyne)

β-blockers

selective β₁- blockers (cardioselective; antihypertensive drugs)

- Metoprolol (Lopressor)
- Atenolol (Tenormin)
- Esmolol (Brevibloc)
- Bisoprolol (Zebeta)

Nonselective β₁,₂ blockers (affects both heart and other tissues with β-receptors; antihypertensive drugs; also has α-1 blocking action)

- Naldolol (Corgard) (hypertension)
- Propranolol (Inderal) (hypertension)
- Timolol (Blocadren) (for glaucoma)

α- and β-Blockers (antihypertensives)

- Carvedilol (Coreg)
- Labetalol (Normodyne)

Indirect acting adrenergic antagonists (do not directly block α or β adrenergic receptors. They block the release of NE from the nerve endings; treatment of hypertension)

- Reserpine
- Guanethidine

Parasympathomimetics

Direct-acting cholinergic receptor agonists (reduction in intraocular pressure, miosis; stimulate G.I. smooth muscle postoperative)

- Bethanechol (Urecholine)—Stimulates G.I. smooth muscle postoperative; prevents urine retention
- Carbachol (Miostat)—Glaucoma (openangle)
- Cevimeline (Evoxac)- Treatment of xerostomia
- Pilocarpine (Pilocar)—Glaucoma (open-angle), xerostomia

Indirect-acting cholinergic receptor agonists

- Donepezil (Aricept)—Alzheimer's disease
- Edrophonium—Diagnosis of myasthenia gravis
- Galantamine (Razadyne)—Alzheimer's disease
- Neostigmine—To diagnose myasthenia gravis
- Physostigmine—Concurrently used with pilocarpine for glaucoma; diagnosis myasthenia gravis
- Echothiophate and isoflurophate—Longer acting drugs for glaucoma
- Rivastigmine (Exelon)—Alzheimer's disease

Parasympatholytics (Anticholinergics)

Muscarinic-receptor antagonists

- Atropine—Prototype; preoperative medication to dry up secretions, prevents bradycardia during spinal anesthesia; cholinergic poisoning
- Dicyclomine (Bentyl)—Irritable bowel syndrome (decreases G.I. motility/antispasmodic)
- Flavoxate (Uripas)—Urinary incontinence
- Ipratropium (Atrovent)—Bronchodilator
- Oxybutynin (Ditropan)—Spasm in urinary incontinence
- Propantheline—Irritable bowel syndrome (decreases G.I. motility/antispasmodic)
- Scopolamine—Motion sickness

- Tolterodine (Detrol)—Urinary incontinence
- Tropicamide (Mydriacyl)—Mydriasis (pupil dilation) for eye exam

Ganglionic-blocking drugs

- Trimethaphan—Produces controlled hypotension during surgery

Neuromuscular blocking agents

- Succinylcholine—To induce skeletal muscle relaxant during surgery to help with intubation
- d-Tubocurarinre—To induce skeletal muscle relaxant during surgery to help with intubation

Chapter **14**

Cardiovascular Drugs

GOAL: To gain knowledge of common drug therapy and dental management of heart-related diseases.

EDUCATIONAL OBJECTIVES

After reading this chapter, the reader should be able to:

1. Describe the different types of heart diseases.
2. List the different categories of drugs used in the treatment of heart conditions.
3. Discuss the adverse effects of these drugs that are important in the dental office.
4. Describe steps used to monitor a cardiac patient who is being administered a local anesthetic with a vasoconstrictor in the dental office.

KEY TERMS
Cardiovascular system
Hypertension
Angina pectoris
Arrhythmia
Lipoproteins
Anticoagulant drugs
Anitplatelet drugs
Thrombosis

INTRODUCTION

The **cardiovascular system**, which comprises the heart and blood vessels, functions to supply blood and oxygen to the body through contractions of the heart and the vasculature. As the body's demand for oxygen increases, the vasculature contracts or dilates to direct blood flow to the areas of the body requiring more oxygen. The cardiovascular system can fail either when the heart does not contract sufficiently or there is blockage of a blood vessel, referred to as atherosclerosis. Cardiovascular disorders are classified as hypertension, angina pectoris, heart failure, and arrhythmias.

HYPERTENSION

Pathogenesis

Hypertension is defined as a sustained elevation in arterial pressure due to the amount of blood in the vessel being greater than the space available. In 2003, the Joint National Committee on Prevention, Detection, Evaluation, and Treatment of High Blood Pressure released its seventh report (*JNC-VII*). This most current classification of blood pressure is summarized in Table 14–1. According to *JNC-VII,* normal blood pressure is less than 120/80 mm Hg, whereas prehypertension indicates a patient is at risk of developing hypertension. Additionally, there is new emphasis on elevated systolic pressure (SBP) being an important risk factor for cardiovascular disease, rather than elevated diastolic blood pressure, which has been emphasized for many years.

Hypertension affects as many as 50 million Americans. It is listed as the principal cause of death in approximately 40,000 people per year and as a contributory cause of death in more than 200,000 others. Generally, hypertension is an asymptomatic condition in its initial stages.

Blood pressure is regulated by the sympathetic nervous system and the kidneys. Hypertension having no identifiable cause is termed primary or essential and accounts for 90 percent of all cases. It results in an increase in systolic and diastolic pressure due to alterations in the mechanisms regulating cardiac output and total peripheral vascular resistance. Secondary hypertension is the term given to elevated blood pressure due to a known physical abnormality.

Although the etiology of essential hypertension is relatively unknown, certain genetic and environmental risk factors are listed in Table 14–2. Risk factors for secondary hypertension include renal disease, hyperthyroidism, medication-induced (estrogen), Cushing's disease (glucocorticoid excess), diabetes mellitus, and pheochromocytoma (rare malignant neoplasm). Complications arising from hypertension include stroke and renal failure, which leads to congestive heart failure.

Three factors are responsible for creating blood pressure and controlling cardiac function: cardiac output, peripheral resistance, and blood volume (Figure 14–1).

- *Cardiac output* is the volume or amount of blood pumped out per minute by the ventricle of the heart and is determined by the heart rate and stroke volume, which is the amount of blood pumped by a ventricle in one contraction.
- *Peripheral resistance* (afterload) refers to the resistance of blood vessels to blood flow.
- *Blood volume* is the total amount of blood in the circulatory system, which is approximately 5 liters.

Table 14–1   JNC-VII Classification of Blood Pressure for Adults

Category	Systolic (mm Hg)		Diastolic (mm Hg)	Followup
Normal	< 120	*and*	< 80	Check again in 2 years
Prehypertension	120–139	*or*	80–89	Check again in 1 year
Hypertension				
Stage 1	140–159	*or*	90–99	Confirm within 2 months
Stage 2	≥160	*or*	≥ 100	Evaluate in < 1 week

When blood pressures fall into different categories, the higher category should be selected to classify the individual's blood pressure status.
(Adapted from Chobanian, A. V., H. R. Black, W. C. Cushman et al. 2003. The seventh report of the Joint National Committee on Prevention, Detection, Evaluation, and Treatment of High Blood Pressure. *JAMA* 289:2560–2571.)

Table 14–2   Major Risk Factors for Hypertension

- Smoking
- Obesity
- Sedentary lifestyle
- Alcohol
- Stress
- Male
- Family history of cardiovascular disease
- Postmenopausal woman
- Sodium intake

Other factors include:

- *Preload,* the volume of blood returned to the heart before it beats
- *Contractility,* the forcefulness with which the heart contracts

The main function of the heart is to receive blood from the body at low pressure and pump it back out to the body at a high enough pressure so that it will be pumped back to the heart. Systolic pressure is the pumping or contraction of the left ventricle, forcing blood out; the diastolic pressure is the relaxation of the left ventricle, allowing for refill with blood.

Treatment

Treatment of essential hypertension is aimed at restoration of the balance between cardiac output and total peripheral vascular resistance, so that the blood pressure

(cardiac output times total peripheral vascular resistance) falls to acceptable levels before irreversible damage occurs to organ systems such as the eyes, the kidneys, or the cardiovascular system. Secondary hypertension is treated by removing the causative agent, re-evaluating the cardiovascular system for damage, and initiating treatment, if necessary.

It is important to realize that treatment of hypertension not only involves pharmacotherapy, but major lifestyle modifications, including: weight reduction, limiting alcohol consumption, increasing aerobic physical activity, restricting sodium intake, and smoking cessation.

There are over 100 drugs that have been approved by the U.S. Food and Drug Administration (FDA) for the treatment of hypertension. Thus, it is important that a drug be selected that is most appropriate for the specific needs of the patient. Many patients with hypertension will have a cormorbidity (another coexisting disease) which makes choosing the correct medication more challenging to prevent any drug–drug or drug–disease interactions. For instance, patients with hypertension and arthritis may be taking a nonsteroidal anti-inflammatory drug (e.g., ibuprofen) that could lower the effects of some

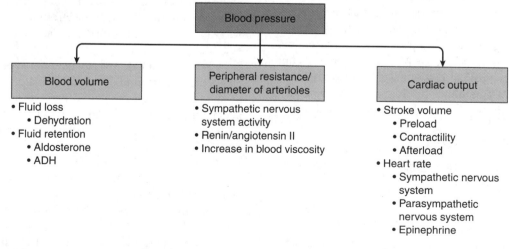

FIGURE 14–1   Major three factors creating blood pressure.

antihypertensive drugs. The desired target blood pressure goal is lower than 140/90 in patients without compelling indicators, and lower than 130/80 on patients with compelling indicators such as diabetes mellitus.

Recommendations of the *JNC-VII* give preference to thiazide diuretics for initial drug therapy of *uncomplicated stage 1 hypertension* because they have consistently been shown to reduce cardiovascular morbidity and mortality in controlled clinical trials. If this drug is not tolerated, is ineffective, or is contraindicated, then one of the other drug classes should be used instead or used in combination with thiazide. Other drugs that may be considered include:

Angiotensin-converting enzyme (ACE) inhibitors

angiotensin II receptor blocker (ARB)

α_1-blockers

α/β-blockers

calcium channel blockers

Patients with *uncomplicated stage 2 hypertension* will require two or more medications to achieve blood pressure goals. Several major classes of antihypertensive agents have been recommended; for use as initial therapy (Table 14–3). An outline for the treatment of hypertension is given in Figure 14–2. If a patient has concurrent diabetes mellitus (type 1), an ACE inhibitor is recommended; if the patient has concurrent congestive heart failure, an ACE inhibitor or diuretic is recommended; and in the elderly patient, a diuretic is preferred.

Pharmacotherapy

Figure 14–3 illustrates the sites of action of drugs that reduce blood pressure.

Diuretics

Diuretics were the first drugs used in the treatment of hypertension, in the 1950s. They are still considered to be the drug of choice because they produce few adverse

effects and are very effective for treating mild to moderate hypertension.

There are three classes of diuretics: thiazides, loop, and potassium-sparing, which act in different parts of the kidney (Figure 14–4). Diuretics act by increasing the volume of urine production by excretion of excess fluid in the body.

Because of increased loss of fluids, electrolyte disturbance with loss of sodium, potassium and magnesium, dehydration, orthostatic hypotension (due to reduced blood volume) and xerostomia are common adverse side effects.

Thiazide Diuretics Thiazide diuretics act in the distal tubule of the kidney to inhibit sodium chloride (NaCl) reabsorption back into the blood allowing an increased level of sodium in the tubule, which holds water, resulting in increased urination (Figure 14–4). Because of the increased sodium load in the tubule, excretion of potassium is usually increased, resulting in hypokalemia. Hydrochlorothiazide is the prototype thiazide.

Over months the diuretic effect of thiazides decreases, with kidney function returning to normal in regard to sodium (sodium reabsorbs back into the blood and is not excreted), but the antihypertensive effect remains. Thiazides are effective in lowering blood pressure 10–15 mm Hg in patients with *mild essential hypertension*. Thiazides may increase total cholesterol and loss of electrolytes, which may predispose the patient with heart disease to arrhythmias. Potassium supplements (e.g., food or drugs) may be necessary to replenish lost potassium. Thiazides are contraindicated in diabetics because they increase blood glucose and may decrease the effectiveness of antidiabetic drugs. Monitoring of blood electrolytes including K^+, N^+, Mg^+, Cl^-, and serum lipids and cholesterol, is essential.

An important drug–drug interaction occurs when an NSAID (nonsteroidal anti-inflammatory drug) such as naproxen sodium, or ibuprofen is taken with a thiazide diuretic for more than 5 days. This combination of drugs reduces the antihypertensive effect of the thiazide diuretic, which may result in elevated blood pressure.

Table 14–3 lists common diuretics with adverse reactions and drug interactions.

Loop Diuretics Loop diuretics are the most effective diuretics and are more potent than thiazides, resulting in greater and more rapid diuresis with loss of fluids through kidney excretion and severe potas-

Table 14-3 Classification of Antihypertensive Agents

Drug Name	Mechanism of Action	Adverse Effects; Precautions	Significant Dental Drug Interactions
Diuretics	Decreases blood volume and cardiac output		
Thiazides	Inhibits reabsorption of Na, Cl, and H_2O in the kidney tubule, resulting in elimination of water, Na, Cl, and potassium (K). Must replace potassium that is lost with either a potassium medication or foods (e.g., bananas)	Hypokalemia (low blood potassium), hyperglycemia (high blood glucose) xerostomia, orthostatic hypotension	Dental drug interaction: NSAIDs (nonsteroidal anti-inflammatory drugs)such as naproxen sodium and ibuprofen can decrease the effectiveness of the anti-hypertensive action of the thiazide diuretic, resulting in rapid elevation of blood pressure
Chlorothiazide (Diuril) Hydroclorothiazide (Hydrodiuril)			
Loop Diuretics	Inhibit reabsorption of sodium chloride in the Loop of Henle (a part of the kidney)	Postural hypotension, xerostomia, hypokalemia, hyperglycemia	No dental drug interactions; Colestipol and cholestyra-mine (cholesterol-lowering drugs) reduce the diuretic effects of furosemide
Furosemide (Lasix) Blumetanide (Bumex)			
Potassium–Sparing Diuretics	Inhibit sodium reabsorption with a reduction of potassium excretion	Hyperkalemia (elevated potassium serum, gynecomastia, (enlargement of breasts in both males and females), fatigue with rapid weight loss	No dental drug interactions; increase potassium blood levels if taken with ACE inhibitor (antihypertensive drugs) and digoxin
Amiloride (Midamor) Spironolactone (Aldactone) Triamterene (Dyrenium)			
Potassium–Sparing/ Thiazide Amiloride/ hydrochlorothiazide (HCTZ) (Moduretic) Spironolactone/HCTZ (Aldactazide) Triamterene/HCTZ (Dyazide)	Inhibit sodium reabsorption with a reduction of potassium excretion	Hyperkalemia, hyperglycemia, skin rash, xerostomia	Increase potassium blood levels if taken with ACE in-hibitor (antihypertensive drugs)
ACE inhibitors	Inhibiting the formation of angiotensin II	Angioedema (fluid leakage into dermis of skin), cough, dizziness, sudden drop in blood pressure after initial dose	NSAIDs (nonsteroidal anti-inflammatory drugs) such as naproxen sodium and ibuprofen can decrease the effectiveness of the antihypertensive action of the ACE inhibitor, resulting in rapid elevation of blood pressure.

(continued)

Drug Name	Mechanism of Action	Adverse Effects; Precautions	Significant Dental Drug Interactions
Captopril (Capoten) Lisinopril (Prinivil) Enalapril (Vasotec) Ramipril (Altase) Benazepril (Lotensin) Fosinopril (Monopril) Quinapril (Accupril) Moexipril (Univasc) Trandolapril (Mavik)			
Angiotensin II blockers (ARBs) Candesartan cilexetil (Atacand) Eprosartan (Teveten) Irbesartan (Avapro) Losartan (Cozar) Telmisartan (Micardis) Valsartan (Diovan)	Block angiotensin II receptor site	See above	NSAIDs (nonsteroidal anti-inflammatory drugs) such as naproxen sodium and ibuprofen can decrease the effectiveness of the antihypertensive action of the thiazide diuretic resulting in rapid elevation of blood pressure.
Central Presynaptic α_2-Adrenergic Release Inhibitors Clonidine (Catapres) Methyldopa (Aldomet)	Stimulates α_2-adrenergic receptors in the central nervous system	Depression, dizziness, significant xerostomia, sedation, orthostatic hypotension Liver problems	Tricyclic antidepressants (e.g., amitriptyline) may reduce the hypotensive effects. Increases effects of lithium
Peripheral Presynaptic Adrenergic Release Inhibitors Reserpine (Serpasil) Guanethidine	Deplete neurons of their catecholamine stores and prevent norepinephrine release from nerves that end in the heart	Drowsiness, gastrointestinal disturbances	No significant interactions
α_1-Adrenergic Blockers (also Vasodilators) Doxazosin (Cardura) Prazosin (Minipress) Terazosin (Hytrin)	Block the α_1-receptors on the heart Also used for prostate enlargement	First-dose syncope (sudden drop in blood pressure after initial dose), dizziness, headache	NSAIDs may decrease the hypotensive effect of prazosin; beta-blockers may enhance postural (fainting) effects of prazosin.

Drug Name	Mechanism of Action	Adverse Effects; Precautions	Significant Dental Drug Interactions
β-Adrenergic Blockers	Block beta-receptors on the heart and other tissues if it is not cardioselective	Cardioselective (β_1) blockers have fewer side effects than noncardioselective drugs: sedation, fatigue, depression, dizziness, bronchocontriction (in noncardioselective drugs), impotence (sexual dysfunction)	Epinephrine may produce hypertensive effects.
Atenolol (Tenormin)	Cardioselective β_1	Sedation, depression	No precautions regarding use of EPI in local anesthetic
Acebutolol (Sectral)	Cardioselective β_1	See above	No precautions regarding use of EPI in local anesthetic
Betaxolol (Kerlone)	Cardioselective β_1	See above	No precautions regarding use of EPI in local anesthetic
Bisoprolol (Zebeta)	Cardioselective β_1	See above	No precautions regarding use of EPI in local anesthetic
Carteolol (Cartrol)	Cardioselective β_1	See above	No precautions regarding use of EPI in local anesthetic
Metaprolol (Lopressor)	Cardioselective β_1	See above	No precautions regarding use of EPI in local anesthetic
Labetalol (Normodyne)	α and β blocker; treat chronic hypertension and hypertensive emergencies	Dizziness, sexual dysfunction, xerostomia, orthostatic hypotension	Use minimal amount of EPI (two cartridges 1:100,000)
Nadolol (Corgard)	Not cardioselective; blocks both β_1 and β_2	Dizziness, sexual dysfunction, xerostomia, orthostatic hypotension	Use minimal amount of EPI (two cartridges 1:100,000)
Propranolol (Inderal)	Not cardioselective; blocks both β_1 and β_2	Dizziness, sexual dysfunction, xerostomia, orthostatic hypotension	Use minimal amount of EPI (two cartridges 1 1:100,000)
Calcium Channel Blockers (CCBs)	Cause vasodilation (widening of coronary arteries) by blocking calcium ion channels	Orthostatic hypotension, gingival enlargement (especially with nifedipine), constipation, headache	Diltiazem inhibits the metabolism (breakdown) of cyclosporine (used to prevent organ rejection). Grapefruit juice increases the absorption of felodipine.
Nondihydropyridines Diltiazem (Cardizem) Verapamil (Calan, Isoptin)	See above	See above	See above
Dihydropyridines Amlodipine (Norvasc) Felodipine (Plendil) Isradipine (Dynacirc) Nicardipine (Cardene) Nifedipine (Adalat, Procardia) Nisoldipine (Sular)	See above	See above	See above
Direct Vasodilators	Direct vasodilator action on vascular (blood vessel) smooth muscle to reduce pressure	Too rapid drop in blood pressure; nausea, headache, sweating	No significant interactions
Hydralazine (Apresoline) Minoxidil (Loniten) Nitroprusside (Nitropress)		Hair growth (used topically as Rogaine)	

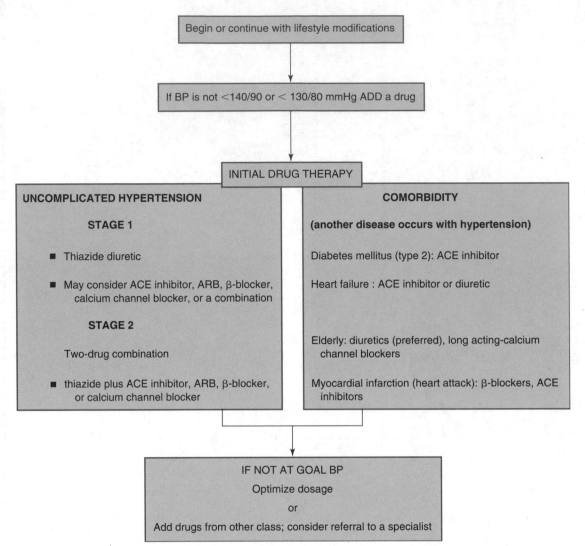

FIGURE 14–2 Algorithm for hypertension [Joint National Committee (JNC) VII Recommendations].
(Adapted from: The seventh report of the Joint National Committee on Prevention, Detection, Evaluation, and Treatment of High Blood Pressure. 2003. *JAMA* 289:2560–2571.

sium loss and orthostatic hypotension. These drugs inhibit reabsorption of sodium chloride in another part of the kidney called the Loop of Henle but also in the distal tubules (Figure 14–3). Furosemide (Laxis) is the prototype drug, has an onset of about 1 hour after oral administration, and causes significant electrolyte loss because it produces a more dilute urine and excretion of electrolytes. Potassium supplements are usually necessary. Loop diuretics may also increase glucose levels.

Potassium-sparing Diuretics Potassium-sparing diuretics act in the distal tubule, where inhibition of sodium reabsorption results in a corresponding *reduction* in potassium excretion (Figure 14–4) so potassium supplements are not necessary. In order to equalize the potassium effects, these drugs are usually prescribed with a potassium-wasting diuretic such as hydrochlorothiazide. Thus these diuretics work differently than thiazide and loop diuretics.

Spironolactone (Aldactone), a type of potassium-sparing diuretic, is an antagonist of a hormone called al-

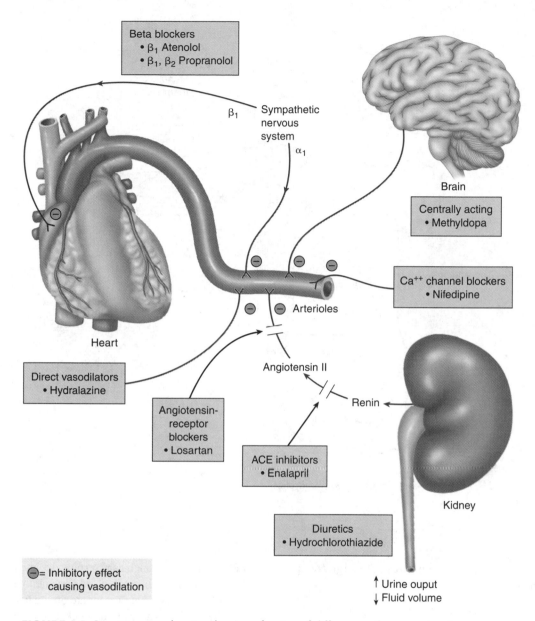

FIGURE 14-3   Diagram showing the sites of action of different antihypertensive drugs.

dosterone. Aldosterone prevents the reabsorption of sodium in exchange for potassium.

Triamterene (Dyrenium) promotes sodium excretion in the collecting tubules of the kidneys. Potassium is not exchanged for sodium; sodium is not reabsorbed and stays in the tubules along with water.

Since there is less potassium loss, hyperkalemia can occur, and monitoring of serum potassium levels is necessary.

Adrenergic Blockers (Antagonists) and Adrenergic Agonists

Elevated sympathetic nervous system activity may result in transient or sustained hypertension by:

1. Directly stimulating the heart via β_1-receptors
2. The release of NE and/or
3. Constricting peripheral blood vessels via stimulating α_1-receptors

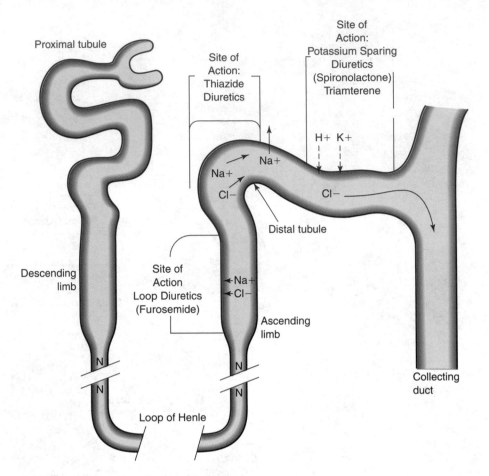

FIGURE 14–4 Site of action of diuretics.

Since hypertension stimulates adrenergic/sympathetic effects, drugs are selected to:

1. Block β_1-adrenergic postsynaptic receptors, preventing stimulation of the heart
2. Stimulate α_2-receptors, which inhibit the release of catecholamines, causing vasoconstriction or
3. Block α_1-receptors, which inhibits vasoconstriction

Adrenergic Agents Presynaptic α_2-adrenergic agonists are divided into *central and peripheral* antiadrenergics. Centrally acting drugs such as clonidine (Catapres) work in the central nervous system to reduce norepinephrine release by stimulating areas of the brain that inhibit sympathetic outflow. These drugs are not routinely used because of their adverse side effects. Periph-

erally acting drugs such as reserpine deplete the neurons of their catecholamine stores and prevent norepinephrine release from nerves that terminate on the heart.

Selective α_1-adrenergic blockers (vasodilators) decrease blood pressure by causing vasodilatation of peripheral blood vessels. Prototype drugs include prazosin (Minipress) and doxazosin (Cardura). Terazocin (Hytrin) is also used to treat benign prostatic hypertrophy (BPH).

Beta-blockers reduce the heart rate and contractility and decrease CNS sympathetic output. Binding to β-receptors results in decreased norepinephrine release, which is responsible for increased blood pressure.

When selecting a β-blocker for the treatment of hypertension, it is best to use a cardioselective β_1-blocker such as atenolol (Tenormin) so it can be given to patients with diabetes and asthma with fewer undesirable side effects.

Angiotensin-Converting Enzyme Inhibitors (ACE Inhibitors) and Angiotensin-Receptor Blockers (ARBS)

As mentioned earlier in the chapter, the kidney plays a major role in controlling blood pressure by regulating blood volume. When blood pressure increases in the blood vessels, the kidney can excrete more sodium, which will lower blood volume, resulting in a decrease in cardiac output and the blood pressure returning to normal.

Renin is produced and secreted in the kidney in response to a decrease in renal blood flow. Renin converts angiotensinogen, which is produced in the liver, into angiotensin I. Angiotensin-converting enzyme (ACE), made in the lung, cleaves angiotensin I into angiotensin II, which is a potent vasoconstrictor and causes an increase in blood pressure (Figure 14–5).

Drugs called angiotensin-converting enzyme (ACE) inhibitors act on the renin-angiotensin-aldosterone system, blocking the conversion of angiotensin I to the active angiotensin II by inhibiting the converting enzyme. These drugs do not have a substantial effect on cardiac output and heart rate (Table 14–3), but reduce peripheral vascular resistance, resulting in lower blood pressure. ACE inhibitors are ideal in hypertensive patients with diabetes.

While monotherapy with ACE inhibitors in mild-to-moderate hypertension will significantly lower blood pressure, it is usually combined with another antihypertensive agent, such as a diuretic or calcium channel blocker. Precautions must be taken, especially in elderly patients, because both drugs can cause excessive volume depletion. ACE inhibitors have not been shown to reduce associated cardiovascular outcomes, such as stroke, heart failure or coronary artery disease.

A common side effect of all ACE inhibitors is a nonproductive, persistent cough which can develop immediately or after months of therapy. It is not dose dependent, which means that it may develop no matter how much of the drug is taken. Other adverse effects include dizziness, headache, fatigue, angioedema (fluid leakage into the skin), orthostatic hypotension, and xerostomia.

An important drug–drug interaction occurs when an NSAID such as naproxen sodium or ibuprofen is taken with an ACE inhibitor. This combination of drugs reduces the antihypertensive effect of the ACE inhibitor, which may result in elevated blood pressure.

Angiotensin-II Receptor Blockers (ARBs)

Angiotensin-II receptors are found in a variety of tissues throughout the body. Angiotensin-II receptor blockers (ARBs) block the receptors from receiving angiotensin II,

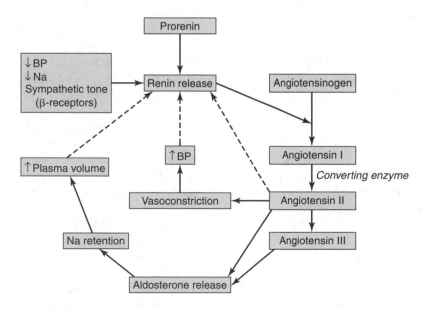

FIGURE 14–5   Renin-angiotensin system.

limiting angiotensin II–mediated vasoconstriction and reducing aldosterone secretion. Aldosterone is a mineralocorticoid that acts on kidney cells to increase reabsorption of sodium and water in exchange for the excretion of potassium. These drugs are well tolerated and have a low incidence of cough.

Combination of an ARB and NSAID reduces the antihypertensive effect of the ARBs, which results in elevated blood pressure.

Calcium Channel Blockers (CCBs)

Calcium channel blockers were first approved in the treatment of angina in the 1980s. A side effect was lowering of blood pressure in hypertensive patients. As previously discussed, peripheral blood vessels are constricted in hypertension, thus vasodilation is one of the goals of treatment.

Calcium channel blockers cause vasodilation by inhibiting the influx of calcium into cardiac and smooth muscle by blocking calcium channels. This reduces peripheral vascular resistance, with little effect on cardiac output. Verapamil (Nifedipine) has the most inhibitory effect on cardiac conduction and the greatest effect on decreasing blood pressure, while diltiazem (Cardizem) has a moderate effect on decreasing blood pressure and on cardiac conduction.

Common adverse effects include orthostatic hypotension, reflex tachycardia (increase heart rate due to a rapid fall in BP caused by the drug), hypotension, and gingival enlargement.

There are two classes of calcium channel blockers:

1. Dihydropyridines [e.g., amlodipine (Norvasc), nifedipine (Procardia), felodipine (Plendil)]
2. Nondihydropyridines [e.g., verapamil (Calan) and diltiazem (Cardizem)]. Of the entire class of calcium channel blockers, verapamil and diltiazem have the greatest effect on reducing blood pressure. Calcium channel blockers are the most frequently used because they are good for the treatment of all types of hypertension and can be used in asthmatics. Gingival enlargement is a common adverse side effect.

Other Vasodilators

Direct-acting vasodilators relax smooth muscle cells surrounding blood vessels by an unclear mechanism. These drugs include hydralazine (Apresoline), diazoxide (Hyperstat), minoxidil (Loniten), and nitroprusside (Nitropress). These drugs are usually used in combination with other antihypertensive agents for the treatment of moderate to severe hypertension. Used alone, they cause fluid retention and angina. Minoxidil is used in the management of refractory hypertension where the patient has not responded with other types of drugs. A side effect of minoxidil is hair growth, making it useful treatment for hair loss. This drug is topically applied and is sold under the trade name Rogaine. Nitroprusside and diazoxide are administered intravenously in hypertensive emergencies. These are usually not the drug of choice because of many adverse side effects.

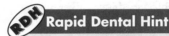

Rapid Dental Hint

Monitor vital signs when administering a local anesthetic to cardiac patients.

Dental Hygiene Notes

The patient should be asked what medications he/she is currently taking for blood pressure, and if these medications are being taken as prescribed. These medications are usually taken in the morning or at night. Vital signs should be monitored at every dental visit. Since some drugs are used to treat different types of cardiovascular disorders, the clinician should ask the patient for what condition the drug(s) is (are) being taken.

Any hypertensive drug has the ability to cause orthostatic hypotension, a fall in blood pressure of 20/10 mm Hg or more within 5 minutes of standing from a supine position, which can result in syncope. Care must be taken to allow the patient to remain sitting upright for a few minutes after being in a supine position to this.

Using vasoconstrictors in the hypertensive patient is not contraindicated. In the hypertensive patient, high doses of epinephrine may cause excessive cardiac stimulation, resulting in angina or cardiac arrhythmias which can lead to increased blood pressure and stroke. Patients taking a nonselective β-blocker such as propranolol (Inderal), nadolol (Corgard), or timolol (Blocardren) may have an increased vasopressor response to epinephrine. Blood pressure should be monitored before and during dental treatment for any changes. The initial dose should be minimal (1/2 cartridge), injected slowly using aspiration to avoid intravascular injection. After waiting and monitoring for toxicity for a few minutes, more of the anesthetic may be injected. The maximum dose of epinephrine to be used in a patient with controlled hypertension or cardiovascular disease is 0.04 mg which is equivalent to two cartridges (0.018 mg EPI per cartridge 1:100,000; note that the volume in a cartridge is now 1.7–1.8 ml). The benefits for maintaining adequate anesthesia outweigh the risks for toxicity. Careful monitoring for toxicity (e.g., increased blood pressure, cardiac arrhythmias including tachycardia) is important. Epinephrine 1:50,000 should be avoided, as well as retraction cord containing epinephrine.

There is no major concern for the use of EPI in patients taking cardioselective β_1 blockers.

Levonordefrin, a vasoconstrictor contained in mepivicaine, stimulates primarily α-adrenergic receptors. This will increase blood pressure, and the drug should not be used in the hypertensive patient.

A dry, sore mouth caused by diuretics and central-acting adrenergic inhibitors are dealt with by educating the patient to increase fluid intake, avoid alcohol and alcohol-containing mouthrinses, and use artificial salivary drugs.

Gingival enlargement is a common side effect of calcium channel blockers (e.g., nifedipine) (Figure 14–6). Discontinuation of the drug usually results in a disappearance of the enlargement. Treatment involves meticulous oral home care and possible surgical removal of excess gingiva.

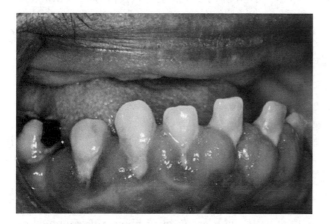

FIGURE 14–6   Gingival enlargement in a patient taking nifedipine.

 Rapid Dental Hint

In patients with drug-induced gingival enlargement, consultation with the patients' physician may be necessary to change the calcium channel blocker to another drug category.

ANGINA PECTORIS

Pathogenesis

Angina pectoris (AP) occurs when the metabolic demands of the heart exceed the ability of the coronary arteries to supply adequate blood flow and oxygen to the heart. Although the typical symptom of angina is severe chest pain upon exertion, angina may develop unexpectedly with minimal or no exertion.

The majority of myocardial ischemia (reduced blood flow) represents a manifestation of atherosclerosis (Figure 14–7). Other risk factors for AP include smoking, elevated serum lipids, family history, obesity, male gender, sedentary lifestyle, hypertension, and a type A personality.

Stable angina occurs when chest pain is intermittent on exertion but relieved by rest. Each attack generally resembles the previous attack, to such an extent that the patient can predict the attack and change his way of life to avoid the precipitating cause. The classical symptoms are squeezing chest pain that radiates to the left arm, right arm, or both, and to the jaw. There may be shortness of breath, nausea, vomiting, and sweating. Acute coronary syndromes (ACS) or myocardial ischemia include unstable angina and myocardial infarction. *Unstable angina* occurs when oxygen demand exceeds oxygen supply at rest and the frequency and severity of attacks increases. *Variant angina* (Prinzmetal's angina) is due to a heart vasospasm, often occurring during sleep. About 90 percent of patients present with stable angina and 10 percent have unstable angina that progresses to myocardial infarction and requires antiplatelet drugs and/or surgery.

Pharmacotherapy/Treatment

The goals of treatment are to reduce morbidity and mortality and to control the angina. Risk factors must be controlled, including smoking and alcohol cessation.

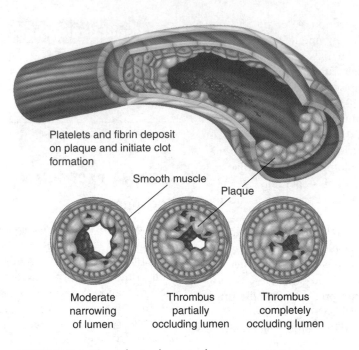

Platelets and fibrin deposit
on plaque and initiate clot
formation

Smooth muscle

Plaque

Moderate
narrowing
of lumen

Thrombus
partially
occluding lumen

Thrombus
completely
occluding lumen

FIGURE 14–7 Atheroscleosis in the coronary arteries.

The goal of drug therapy is to reduce angina by restoring the balance between heart oxygen supply and demand, either by increasing oxygen supply or decreasing oxygen demand.

The following are drugs/modifications used in the treatment of angina (Table 14–4) (Figure 14–8):

- Nitrates
- β₁-blockers
- calcium channel blockers
- Aspirin: platelet inhibition
- Lifestyle modifications
- Cholesterol reduction
- Homocysteine reduction

Nitrates

Nitrates work by relaxing vascular smooth muscle, resulting in vasodilation. This reduces ventricular filling and heart tension and thus oxygen requirements. In addition, nitrates dilate the large coronary arteries. It is recommended for long-term use to do interval dosing with a several-hour "nitrate-free" time, since tolerance can develop. The prototype drug is nitroglycerin, a short-acting nitrate available as a patch (transdermal), topical ointment, or oral formulation. Sublingual nitroglycerin should be given initially at the onset of acute chest pain and continue for prevention of attacks with the patch or ointment form (2%). The sublingual form is used initially because of its fast onset, within seconds. The patch releases 5 to 10 mg of nitroglycerin over 24 hours. Adverse side effects due to vasodilation include orthostatic hypotension, dizziness, hot flashes, and reflex tachycardia. Nitroglycerin given in sustained-release capsules is used to prevent angina attacks.

Due to the first-pass effect, orally administered nitrates such as isosorbide dinitrate are only effective when given in high doses (30–40 mg qid) but is effective sublingually in a 5 mg dose. Isosorbide dinitrate is used for acute angina attacks and for prophylactic management in situations likely to provoke angina attacks. It is given sublingually, with an onset of about five minutes, or orally with an onset of thirty minutes and duration of action of about five hours.

Table 14–4 Antianginal Drugs

Drug	Mechanism of Action	Adverse Effects	Drug Interactions
Nitrates Nitroglycerin (NitroBid, Nitrostat, Nitro-Dur) Isosorbide dinitrate (Isordil)	Dilates and relaxes coronary blood vessels	Headache, dizziness and/or flushing, orthostatic hypotension	Alcohol increases side effects. Sildenafil (Viagra): serious hypotension
Calcium Channel Blockers Amlodipine (Norvasc) Bedpridil (Vasocor) Diltiazem (Cardizem) Nifedipine (Procardia, Adalat) Verapamil (Calan, Isoptin)	Slows heart rate and dilates coronary arteries	Orthostatic hypotension, gingival enlargement (especially with nifedipine), constipation, headache	Diltiazem inhibits metabolism (break down) of cyclosporine (drug used to prevent organ rejection); Grapefruit juice increases the absorption of felodipine
Beta-Blockers Atenolol (Tenormin)-β_1 cardioselective Metoprolol (Lopressor)-β_1 cardioselective Nadolol (Corgard) Propranolol (Inderal)	Reduces cardiac load and thus oxygen demand	Cardioselective (β_1) blockers have fewer side effects than noncardioselective drugs: sedation, fatigue, depression, bronchocontriction (in non-cardioselective drugs), impotence	Epinephrine may produce hypertensive effects

Beta-blockers

Beta-blockers have been proven to reduce mortality and are used in patients with stable angina who require long-term treatment or in patients who also have hypertension. These drugs decrease myocardial oxygen demand by decreasing heart rate, contractility and tension. Cardioselective β-blockers such as atenolol (Tenormin), timolol (Blocardren), or metoprolol (Lopressor) are preferred so that only the β_{1-} receptors are stimulated. These drugs are *cardioselective* because they do not cause bronchoconstriction and the hypoglycemic effects of nonselective beta-blockers. The noncardioselective beta-blockers will block both β_1 and β_2 receptors, so these drugs should be used with extreme caution in patients with asthma and diabetes.

Calcium Channel Blockers

Calcium channel blockers (CCBS) reduce anginal symptoms but do not reduce mortality. Calcium channel blockers are the drug of choice in Prinzmetal's angina but can also be used in chronic stable angina, hypertension, and arrhythmias. CCBs reduce peripheral resistance, decrease in force of heart contraction, and decrease contractility.

Nonnitrates

Dipyridamole (Perstantine) is used only for prophylaxis and not for an acute attack, and may decrease platelet aggregation. This drug acts primarily on small resistance blood vessels in the heart.

Aspirin

Aspirin or acetylsalicylic acid is a type of antiplatelet drug and is effective in a wide range of atherosclerotic heart diseases, exerting its effect by inhibiting the production of thromboxane A_2 (platelet aggregation), thus preventing blood clot formation. It has been shown to reduce mortality in patient with unstable angina and prevention of strokes.

Dental Hygiene Notes

Upon review of the patient's medical history, it should be determined when the patient's last attack was and what was the precipitating factor. Patients taking any form of nitrates must be careful when sitting up and getting out of the dental chair. Orthostatic hypotension may develop whereby the patient will get dizzy. Have the patient remain in an upright position in the chair for a few minutes

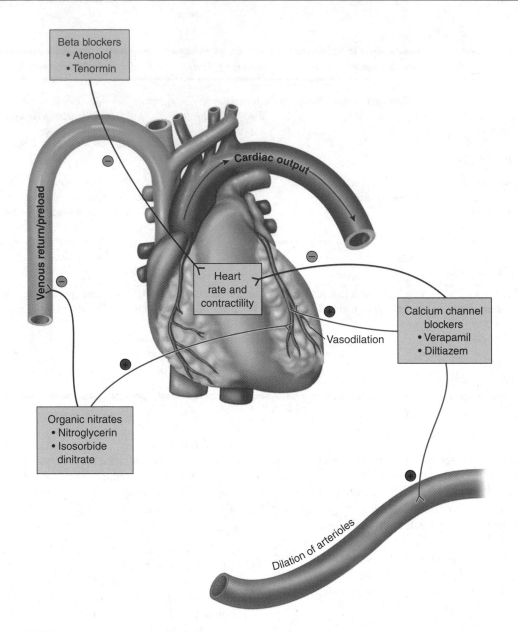

FIGURE 14–8 Mechanisms of action of drugs used to treat angina.

before attempting to get out. Sildenafil (Viagra) taken with a nitrate can cause a serious decrease in blood pressure. Otherwise, there are no contraindications or complications to dental treatment. No special precautions are needed with epinephrine.

If going to the dental office may provoke an attack, the patient should take a sublingual tablet or translingual spray prophylactically 5–10 minutes prior to the appointment.

It is usually not necessary to discontinue aspirin for routine periodontal debridement. For surgical procedures, aspirin should be discontinued for approximately 1 week, which is the time it takes to reform platelets. If in doubt, get a physician's consult.

The use of vasoconstrictors in local anesthetics in stable angina patients is recommended to reduce stress. However, it is suggested to use a maximum of two cartridges containing 1 : 100,000 epinephrine. Elective dentistry should be postponed in patients with unstable angina.

HEART FAILURE

Heart failure occurs when decreases in contractility prevent the heart from pumping forcefully enough to deliver blood to meet the body's demands. Decreases in cardiac output activate reflex responses in the sympathetic nervous system which attempt to compensate for the reduced cardiac output. These reflex responses include: increase in heart rate, increased preload, which causes edema, and increased afterload. Ultimately, the heart fails.

Heart failure can be classified into systolic dysfunction (left ventricular), which is referred to as congestive heart failure, and diastolic dysfunction (right ventricular). Causes of left ventricular heart failure (decreased emptying of the left ventricle) include hypertension, coronary artery disease, mitral regurgitation, anemia (decrease number of red blood cells or hemoglobin), and Paget's disease. These conditions impair the ability of the heart muscle to contract. Symptoms of left heart failure include cough, dyspnea (increased breathing) during exercise or when lying flat, and pulmonary edema (fluid in lung).

Right ventricular heart failure occurs with a decreased emptying of the right ventricle. Symptoms include pitting edema (fluid accumulation in the interstitial spaces is especially seen in the ankles), liver enlargement, nausea, vomiting, anorexia, and abdominal distention.

The goals of therapy are to relieve the symptoms of heart failure and to prolong the survival rate. Exercise, dietary restrictions and medications are part of the management guidelines (Table 14–5) (Figure 14–9).

Pharmacotherapy

The impaired function of the failing heart can be improved by:

1. Indirectly reducing cardiac work load (decrease preload) and reduction of edematous fluid (preload) with diuretics
2. Increasing heart contractions with cardiac glycosides
3. Using vasodilators to increase cardiac output and blood pressure (ACE inhibitors, angiotensin-II receptor blockers, calcium channel blockers, and direct vasodilators) and/or

4. reducing sympathetic stimulation to the heart with β_1-blockers (e.g., carvedilol)

Diuretics

Diuretics are the most commonly used drugs for the initial treatment of heart failure. Generally, furosemide or other loop diuretics are used, and a thiazide diuretic can be added if necessary. Loop diuretics are most effective in the treatment of severe heart failure because they are effective in reducing systemic, or peripheral or pulmonary, edema. Urinary loss of potassium and magnesium is a major problem and must be monitored, as well as dehydration and xerostomia. Although highly effective in the management of acute congestion, diuretics do not prevent disease progression. Once the patient is stabilized with a diuretic, an ACE inhibitor is added.

Cardiac Glycosides

Since the primary cause of heart failure is a weak myocardium, it is ideal to have a drug that causes the muscle to beat more forcefully (increase heart contractions). The ability to increase the strength of contraction is called a positive inotropic effect. Digitalis (cardiac) glycosides have a positive inotropic effect, negative chronotropic effect (decrease heart rate), and decrease heart size. They cause the heart to beat more forcefully and more slowly, improving cardiac output. The primary cardiac glycoside is digoxin (Lanoxin), which originates from the leaves of the purple foxglove plant (*Digitalis purpurea*). Until the discovery of ACE inhibitors, cardiac glycosides were the mainstay of heart failure treatment. Today, digoxin is a second line drug.

Cardiac glycosides have a narrow therapeutic index and can cause fatal adverse effects. At therapeutic doses, these drugs cause an increase in the force of contraction of the cardiac muscle due to an increase in calcium in the cells and decrease heart rate. At slightly higher doses, there is an increased excitability of the heart, seen as tachycardia and arrhythmias. One of the more common adverse effects is hypokalemia, which increases the risk of digitalis cardiotoxicity when combined with diuretics. Treatment with potassium may be indicated in digitalis-induced tachycardia. The most common visual disturbances of digitalis toxicity are blurring and change in color vision (yellow, green, red, and white). Digitalis toxicity is managed by discontinuing the drug, treating the electrolyte imbalance, and monitoring arrhythmias.

Table 14-5 Drugs in the Treatment of Congestive Heart Failure

Drug	Mechanism of Action	Adverse Effects	Drug Interactions
Diuretics Thiazides Loop diuretics furosemide (Lasix)	Increases fluid loss, which reduces cardiac load	Hypokalemia, xerostomia	NSAIDs (nonsteroidal anti-inflammatory drugs) such as naproxen sodium (Aleve) and ibuprofen Advil, Motrin) can decrease the effectiveness of the antihypertensive action of the thiazide diuretic, resulting in rapid elevation of blood pressure. Cholestyramine decreases furosemide absorption.
Positive Inotropics *Cardiac Glycosides* Digoxin (Lanoxin)	Cardiac glycosides: increase calcium concentration, which enhances heart contractility	Cardiac glycosides: digitalis toxicity (color vision changes) and hypokalemia (low potassium)	β-blockers may worsen CHF when taken with digoxin; oral antacids impair digoxin absorption.
Adrenergic Receptor Agonist Dobutamine (Dobutrex) dopamine	Adrenergic agonists: stimulates β-receptors, which increases cardiac contractility	Adrenergic receptor agonists: hypertension, increased heart rate	β-blockers may make dopamine ineffective
Vasodilators Hydralazine (Apresoline)	To increase cardiac output	Headache, tachycardia, fixed drug eruption	β-blockers and other antihypertensives increase hypotensive effect
ACE Inhibitors Captopril (Capoten) Enalapril (Vasotec) Lisinopril (Prinivil, Zestril) Quinapril (Accupril) Fosinopril (Monopril)	Reduces peripheral resistance by causing vasodilation	Angioedema (fluid leakage into dermis of skin), cough, dizziness, sudden drop in blood pressure after initial dose	NSAIDs (nonsteroidal anti-inflammatory drugs) such as naproxen sodium (Aleve) and ibuprofen (Advil, Motrin) can decrease the effectiveness of the antihypertensive action of the ACE inhibitor resulting in rapid elevation of blood pressure.
Calcium Channel Blockers Non-dihydropyridines Diltiazem (Cardizem) Verapamil (Calan, Isoptin) Dihydropyridines Amlodipine (Norvasc) Felodipine (Plendil) Isradipine (Dynacirc) Nicardipine (Cardene) Nifedipine (Adalat, Procardia) Nisoldipine (Sular)	Increases cardiac output	Orthostatic hypotension, gingival enlargement (especially with nifedipine), constipation, headache	Diltiazem inhibits metabolism (break down) of cyclosporine (used to prevent organ rejection). Grapefruit juice increases the absorption of felodipine.
Other Drugs Carvedilol (Coreg)	Nonselective β-blocker and selective α_1-blocker; reduces sympathetic stimulation to the heart		

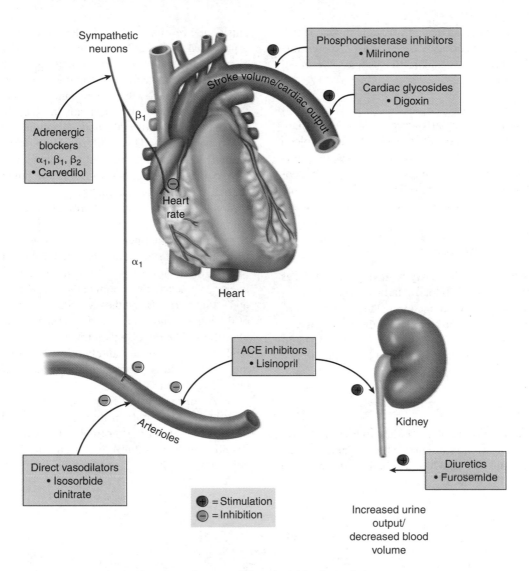

FIGURE 14–9 Mechanisms of action of drugs used for heart failure.

Vasodilators

Vasodilators are useful in the treatment of HF because of their ability to reduce blood pressure, which decreases edema, and dilate arteries, which increases cardiac output.

ACE Inhibitors

The primary function of ACE inhibitors is to lower peripheral resistance (reduces load on the heart/afterload) and reduce blood volume by increasing sodium and water excretion. The diminished afterload required of the heart allows for increased cardiac output. A reduction in vas-

cular tone decreases the work and oxygen demand of the failing heart.

In patients who cannot tolerate ACE inhibitors because of cough, either combination therapy with hydralzazine (Apresoline) or a nitrate, or with an angiotensin receptor antagonist such as losartan, valsartan or irbesartan is indicated.

β-blockers

β_1-blockers reduce excessive sympathetic stimulation of the heart and circulation in patients with heart failure. These drugs should only be used after standard treatment has been tried, never during acute heart failure. One of the newer drugs, carvedilol (Coreg), has considerable vasodilative properties and is the best to use of all β-blockers.

Sympathomimetics

Sympathomimetics drugs (β$_1$-receptor adrenergic agonist) increase contractility with a minimal effect on blood vessels. Dobutamine (Dobutrex) stimulates β$_1$ receptors on the heart, resulting in an increase in the force of contraction of the heart. Adverse effects include increasing heart rate and hypertension. This drug is also used in the treatment of shock.

Dental Hygiene Notes

Patients with heart failure may be taking similar drugs (e.g., duiretics, ACE inhibitors, beta-blockers) as a hypertensive patient. Thus, when recording the type of medication, it is also important to record the indication for usage.

Limitation of a vasoconstrictor (1 : 100,000 epinephrine) in a local anesthetic should be limited to two cartridges.

ARRHYTHMIAS

In an unstimulated neuron, potassium ions (K$^+$) are present in higher concentration inside the cell than outside, and sodium ions (Na$^+$) are found in higher concentration outside the cell than inside. In this situation the neuron is polarized. If the cell membrane becomes depolarized, allowing the rapid movement of K$^+$ ions outside the cell and Na$^+$ inside the cell, a stimulation or action potential results, which causes the cell to contract. This action potential is the stimulus that normally initiates the contraction of the heart. During the depolarization phase the cell cannot be reactivated by an electrical impulse, and is considered refractory to further stimulation. For the cell to return to a resting state, Na$^+$ ions must be pumped out of the cell and K$^+$ ions back into the cell, known as repolarization. This action potential process is spontaneous or automatic.

In the normal heart, an electrical impulse or contraction originates from the sinoatrial (SA) node, a small mass of tissue in the right atria, and travels through the internodal tracts in the atrium to the atrioventricular (AV) node (Figure 14–10). At the AV node, a momentary delay of the impulse allows for atrial contraction and ventricular filling. The impulse then travels through the bundle of His, bundle branches, and Purkinje fibers to stimulate the ventricles to contract and pump blood into the systemic circulation.

An **arrhythmia** occurs when either the impulse rhythm does not start in the SA node, or the rate of heartbeats is abnormal (normally the heart beats about 70–80 times per minute), or it is not under automatic control.

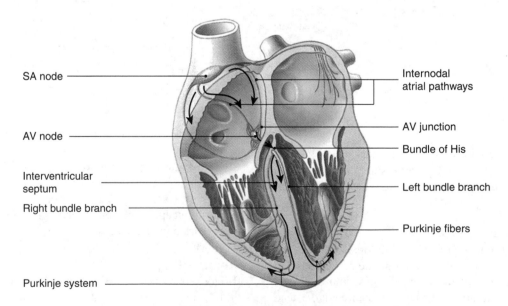

FIGURE 14–10 Diagram of the heart showing normal conduction pathway.

Classification of arrhythmias is based on the anatomical site of the abnormal rhythm:

Atrial (atrium)

Ventricular (ventricle) or

Supraventricular (atrium or above the ventricles)

When the heart is beating too slowly but at a regular rate, it is called sinus bradycardia. There is an increased parasympathetic stimulation which causes the heart to beat slowly. If the heart is beating too fast, it is called sinus or ventricular tachycardia or atrial flutter. Of the different arrhythmias seen in clinical practice, the most common is atrial fibrillation, where the heart is beating without regard for impulses originating from the SA node. Other types of arrhythmias are ventricular tachycardia, ventricular fibrillation, and premature ventricular contractions (PVCs).

Anti-arrhythmics (Table 14–6) suppress the arrhythmia by blocking either autonomic function or calcium, potassium or sodium channels, which slows conduction of the cardiac impulse. Anti-arrhythmics should only be used to treat symptomatic arrhythmias. Based upon these mechanisms, there are four Vaughan Williams classifications of antiarrhythmics:

* Class I drugs, the largest group of antiarrhythmics, have a mechanism of action similar to local anesthetics. These drugs block sodium entry into the cell, preventing transmission of the nerve impulse and reducing the rate of depolarization. Class I drugs are further divided into:
  Class I-A: Includes quinidine (Quinidine, Quinaglute), procainamide (Pronestyl, Procan SR), and disopyramide (Norpace). These drugs prolong

Table 14–6   Anti-Arrhythmic Drugs

Drug	Adverse Effects	Significant Drug Interactions
Class I: Sodium Channel Blockers *Class I-A* Quinidine (Quinidine) Procainamide (Pronestyl) Disopyramide (Norpace)	Diarrhea, nausea, vomiting Procainamide causes a lupus-like skin lesion (rash)	Quinidine increases plasma levels of digoxin and oral anticoagulants (e.g., warfarin)
Class I-B Lidocaine (Xylocaine) Tocainide (Tonocard) Mexiletine (Mexitil)	Drowsiness, numbness, slurred speech	not significant
Class I-C Flecainide (Tambocor) Propafenone (Rythmol)	Flecainide: blurred vision, headache	not significant
Class II β-Adrenergic Blockers Esmolol (Brevibloc) Metoprolol (Lopressor) Propranolol (Inderal)	Fatigue, depression, sexual dysfunction	Epinephrine may produce hypertensive effects
Class III Potassium Channel Blockers Amiodarone (Cordarone) Bretylium Sotalol (Betapace)	Photosensivity (exaggerated sunburn when exposed to the sun)	Amiodarone increases warfarin's anticoagulant effects
Class IV Calcium Channel Blockers Diltiazem (Cardizem) Nifedipine (Adalat, Procardia) Verapamil (Calan)	Dizziness, constipation, hypotension	Diltiazem inhibits metabolism (break down) of cyclosporine (drug used to prevent organ rejection)

the action potential in supraventricular and ventricular arrhythmias.

Class I-B: Includes Lidocaine (Xylocaine), tocainide (Tonocard), and mexiletine (Mexitil). These drugs shorten the action potential and are used in ventricular arrhythmias.

Class I-C: Includes flecainide (Tambocor) and propafenone (Rythmol). These drugs slow cardiac conduction without affecting the action potential; for supraventricular and ventricular arrhythmias.

- Class II anti-arrhythmics: Include esmolol (Brevibloc), metoprolol (Lopressor), and propranolol (Inderal). These drugs are beta-blockers used for the prevention and treatment of supraventricular arrhythmias. They function to slow the heart rate, decrease the AV node conduction rate, and increase the AV node refractory period.
- Class III drugs: Include amiodarone (Cordarone, Pacerone), bretylium, and sotalol (Betapace). These drugs are potassium channel blockers and prolong the action potential duration and refractory period. Indications for usage are to suppress ventricular arrhythmias.
- Class IV antiarrhythmics: Include diltiazem (Cardizem, Dilacor) and verapamil (Calan). These drugs are calcium channel blockers that have significant effects on cardiac tissue. They act to decrease the AV node conduction velocity and increase the AV node refractory period. They are used to treat supraventricular tachycardia and suppress AV node conduction.

Other antiarrhythmics include adenosine (Adenocard), digoxin (Lanoxin) for supraventricular arrhythmias, and magnesium sulfate.

Dental Hygiene Notes

Determine which drugs the patient is taking for a specific cardiovascular condition. There are no special precautions when treating a patient with controlled arrhythmias. The patient's pulse should be taken to determine normal rate and rhythm.

It is necessary for the patient's physician to determine the status of the patient. Local anesthetics with vasoconstrictors should be used to minimize stressful situations. It is reasonable, as is with most cardiovascular conditions, to limit the use of 1 : 100,000 epinephrine to two cartridges.

EPINEPHRINE IN CARDIAC PATIENTS

Epinephrine initially acts primarily on α_1-receptors on smaller arterioles. Although epinephrine stimulates both α- and β-receptors, at low doses used in dental anesthesia the β_2-receptors will be occupied because these receptors have a higher affinity for epinephrine. Thus, epinephrine can selectively stimulate α_1-receptors, resulting in vasoconstriction and an increase in systolic blood pressure. Stimulation of β_2-receptors produce vasodilation and a decrease in diastolic blood pressure and an increase blood flow to skeletal muscles. The primary effect at high doses is vascular smooth muscle contraction.

Low epinephrine concentrations used in dental anesthesia result in an:

- Increase in heart rate due to stimulation of β_1-receptors in the heart
- Increase in force of heart contraction (positive inotropic effect) and increase rate of contraction (positive chronotropic) due to stimulation of β_1-receptors in the heart
- Increase in blood pressure: Cardiac output will increase due to β-receptor effects on heart rate and stroke volume.

There is 0.018 mg of epinephrine in one cartridge (1.7–1.8 ml) of lidocaine 2% with 1 : 100,000 EPI. In normal healthy patients, the maximum amount of EPI is 0.2 mg per appointment and in patients with clinically significant cardiovascular impairment, 0.04 mg per appointment. If necessary, a physician's consultation may be appropriate. Many physicians will not allow the use of EPI in cardiac patients because in medicine EPI is used in emergency situations for anaphylaxis and cardiac arrest where the dosage is much higher, from 0.5 to 1 mg, than used in dentistry.

The table summarizes the types of cardiovascular diseases, goal of treatment, and medications used to treat the disease.

Disease	Goal of Treatment	Common Drugs
Hypertension	1. To reduce decrease blood volume (preload)	Diuretics (thiazides, loop, potassium sparing): increase Na and water excretion
	2. To reduce peripheral resistance	ACE inhibitors: inhibit angiotensin II
	3. To reduce sympthathetic stimulation causing vasodilation (afterload)	α_2-adrenergics (clondine): inhibit NE release
	4. Vasodilation (afterload)	α_1-blockers (Prazocin), calcium channel blockers (nifedipine)
	5. Block β_1-receptors on the heart (reduces cardiac output)	β-blockers (atenolol, metroprolol, etc.)
Angina Pectoris	1. To reduce cardiac output (workload of heart); dilates arteries (decrease afterload)	Nitroglycerin
	2. Smooth muscle relaxation and suppress cardiac activity (decrease afterload)	Calcium channel blockers (diltiazem)
	3. Reduce the frequency of angina; decrease heart rate and contractility	β_1-blockers (atenolol)
Heart Failure	1. Decrease workload (decreasing blood volume)	Diuretics (furosemide); in mild heart failure, use thiazide
	2. Increasing cardiac contractility	Digitalis
	3. Vasodilation	ACE inhibitors, angiotensin II receptor blockers, calcium channel blockers, and direct vasodilators
Arrhythmias	1. Restore heart rate and covert the rhythm	Class I–IV (sodium channel blockers, beta-blockers, potassium channel blockers, calcium channel blockers)

LIPID-LOWERING DRUGS

It is estimated that nearly 97 million American adults have total serum cholesterol levels of 200 mg/dL or higher. Almost half of deaths occurring from coronary heart disease are due to high cholesterol and lipid plasma levels.

The major plasma lipids include cholesterol and triglycerides. Cholesterol is an important part of cell membranes and is a precursor to steroid production in the body. Triglycerides are the main storage form of fuel to support the generation of high-energy compounds in the body.

Because lipids are insoluble in plasma, they must be transported in the circulation in the form of **lipoproteins** (Figure 14–11). These lipoproteins transport cholesterol esters and triglycerides from the sites of synthesis to either sites of utilization. There are different types of lipoproteins, including chylomicrons, very low-density lipoproteins (VLDL-C), low-density lipopro-

teins (LDL-C), intermediate-density lipoproteins (IDL-C), high-density lipoproteins (HDL-C) and lipoprotein; the C refers to cholesterol. Each lipoprotein contains various amounts of triglyceride, protein, cholesterol, and phospholipids.

The pharmacologic treatment of hyperlipidemia (high serum lipids) and hypercholesterolnemia (high cholersterol) is based on this sequence of events (Figure 14–12):

- *Triglycerides,* formed in the liver from fatty acids, are absorbed into the blood in the form of very low density lipoproteins (*VLDL*).
- *Cholesterol,* primarily from the diet and made in the liver, enters the liver and then is also absorbed into the blood in the form of very low density lipoproteins (*VLDL*).
- After delivering triglycerides to adipose (fat) and muscle tissue, VLDL becomes low density lipoproteins (*LDL*), which are removed from the plasma

by LDL receptors present on the liver. Lowering LDL levels has been shown to decrease the incidence of coronary artery disease.

- LDL transports the highest amount of cholesterol to various sites in the body. For this reason LDL, is considered the "bad" cholesterol. HDL also transports cholesterol from the tissues to the liver, where it is broken down and excreted in the feces (Figure 14–12) and is incorporated into atherosclerotic plaques. Because HDL transports cholesterol for destruction and removal from the body, it is considered "good" cholesterol. On the other hand, elevated levels of LDL cholesterol are somewhat responsible for the development of coronary artery disease and other disorders. The ratio of LDL to HDL is an important factor in predicting cardiovascular disease. A high cholesterol level (hypercholesterolemia) contributes to the development of atherosclerosis.

Hypercholesterolemia can result from overproduction of VLDL, increased clearance of VLDL to LDL, or defective clearance of LDL. LDL is the major cholesterol-carrying lipoprotein in humans and is responsible for about 70 percent of total cholesterol in plasma.

The high density of HDL is due to the larger concentration of proteins to lipids. HDL transports cholesterol from peripheral tissues to the liver, termed reverse cholesterol transport, and may be responsible for the inverse correlation between HDL cholesterol levels and the risk of coronary artery disease. Exercise increases serum concentrations of HDLs, which is associated with reduced risk of coronary artery disease.

When dietary cholesterol reaches the liver, elevated cholesterol concentrations suppress LDL-receptor synthesis, resulting in high levels of LDL and total cholesterol.

In 2001, the National Cholesterol Education Program (NCEP) Expert Panel on Detection, Evaluation, and Treatment of High Cholesterol in Adults (known as the Adult Treatment Panel III, ATP III) made recommendations for cholesterol management. *This panel agreed that elevated LDL cholesterol is the primary target of cholesterol-lowering therapy.* Drug therapy is generally reserved for patients who fail to respond to diet or other measures such as weight reduction, or treatment of an underlying disease. Cholesterol intake should be under 200 mg a day.

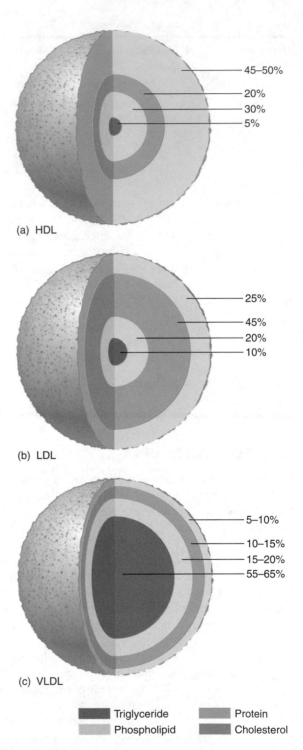

FIGURE 14–11   Composition of lipoproteins: (a) HDL; (b) LDL; (c) VLDL.

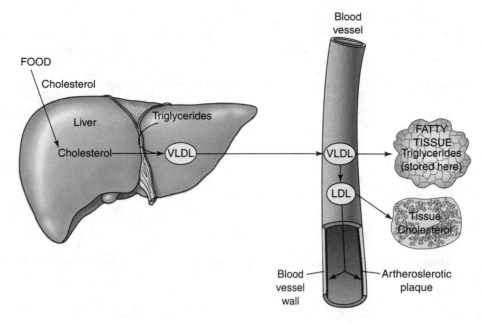

FIGURE 14–12 Lipid metabolism.

Treatment of hyperlipidemia may consist of implementing dietary restrictions with or without drug therapy. Blood levels of all types of lipids including triglycerides, total cholesterol, and the LDL : HDL ratio must be addressed. Drugs for hyperlipidemia are primarily used to treat hypercholesterolemia and hypertriglyceridemia or both. These drugs include (Table 14–7) (Figure 14–13):

- HMG-CoA reductase inhibitors (or "statin" drugs), primarily used to treat hypercholesterolemia (lowers LDL)
- Bile acid sequestrants and niacin, primarily used to treat hypertriglyceridemia or marked HDL deficiency
- Fibric acid drugs, used to lower triglycerides
- Combination drugs

HMG-CoA REDUCTASE INHIBITORS (STATIN DRUGS)

These drugs primarily reduce LDL-C and have been shown to slow the progression of coronary artery disease. The mechanism of action is inhibiting the enzyme 3-hydroxy-3-methyl-glutaryl-coenzyme A (HMG-CoA), which results in less cholesterol formation by the liver. The primary adverse effects of the statin drugs include liver toxicity (hepatotoxicity), as seen by elevated serum liver enzymes, and muscle weakness (myopathy). Atorvastatin (Lipitor) is the prototype drug. It has a pregnancy category of X. See Table 14–7 for drug–drug interactions.

Statin drugs are metabolized by CYP3A4. Erythromycin and clarithromycin inhibit this enzyme, resulting in elevated blood levels of the statin drugs; grapefruit juice has the same mechanism of action. Erythromycin or clarithromycin should not be given at the same time as the statin drugs.

Most of the statin drugs, except atorvastatin (Lipitor), should be taken at night because cholesterol synthesis is highest at this time of the day.

Did You Know?

Grapefruit juice inhibits the breakdown of statin drugs, increasing their blood levels.

Table 14–7 Drugs Used in the Treatment of Hyperlipidemia

Drug	Adverse Effects	Drug Interactions
HMG CoA Reductase Inhibitors ("Statin" Drugs) Lovastatin (Mevacor) Simvastatin (Zocor) Pravastatin (Pravachol) Fluvastatin (Lescol) Atorvastatin (Lipitor)	Increased liver enzymes, myopathy (muscle weakness)	Increased risk of myopathy when taken with: cyclosporine, niacin, erythromycin, clarithyromycin or grapefruit juice, which inhibits metabolism of statin drugs
Bile Acid–Binding Resin (Sequestrants) Cholestyramine (Quesytran) Colestipol (Colestid)	G.I. distress, constipation	Interferes with metabolism of digitalis and warfarin (anticoagulant)
Fibric Acid Derivatives Clofibrate (Atromid-S) Gemfibrozil (Lopid)	Gallstones, myopathy, dyspepsia (indigestion)	Caution with anticoagulants
Natural Products Niacin	Flushing, hyperglycemia (elevated blood sugar)	Anticoagulants (increased bleeding); adjust dose of diabetic medications; do not use with HMG-CoA drugs
Combination Drugs Amlodipine/atorvastatin (Caduet) Ezetimibe/simvastatin (Vytorin)	Back pain, abdominal pain (from the cholesterol absorption inhbitors amlodipine and ezetimibe)	Increased risk of myopathy when taken with: cyclosporine, niacin, erythromycin, clarithyromycin, or grapefruit juice, which inhibits metabolism of statin drugs
Other Drugs Ezetimibe (Zetia)	Fatigue, headache, coughing, back pain, myalgia	No significant dental interactions. Cyclosporine can significantly increase ezetimibe levels

BILE ACID SEQUESTRANTS

The bile acid sequestrants bind bile acids (a greenish liquid secreted by the liver, aiding in absorption and digestion) and prevent reabsorption. These drugs (e.g., cholestyramine) are especially valuable in patients with moderately elevated LDL-C, but there is either no change or an increase in triglyceride levels. These drugs may cause constipation and a rash, and interfere with the absorption of digitalis and warfarin.

FIBRIC ACID DRUGS

High triglyceride levels appear to be positively correlated with risk for coronary heart disease. Fibric acid derivatives primarily reduce triglyceride levels and are used

in combination with statins. There are many adverse side effects, including allergic reactions, blood disorders, and myopathy. The prototype drug is gemifibrozil (Lopid). Fibric acid analogs can displace other highly protein-bound drugs (e.g., warfarin) from their receptors, causing elevated plasma levels.

NATURAL PRODUCTS

Nicotinic Acid

Nicotinic acid (Niacin), a B-complex vitamin, reduces LDL cholesterol, increases HDL cholesterol, and is preferred for lowering triglyceride levels because bile acid sequestrants may raise triglyceride levels. Nicotinic acid is available with a prescription or as an over-the-counter

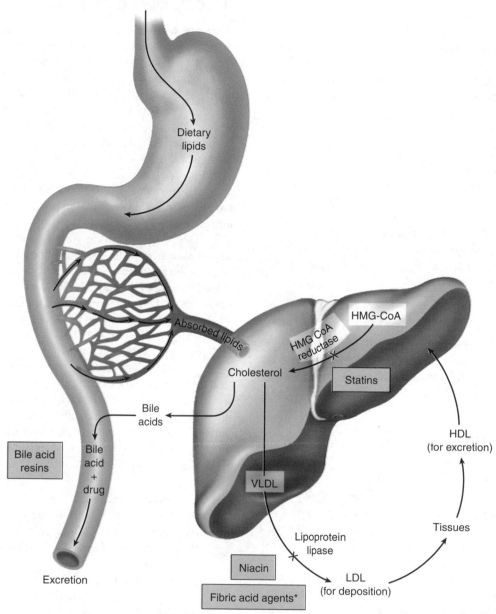

Dietary
lipids

Absorbed lipids

HMG-CoA

HMG CoA
reductase
X

Cholesterol

Statins

Bile
acids

HDL
(for excretion)

Bile acid
resins

Bile
acid
+
drug

VLDL

Excretion

Tissues

Lipoprotein
lipase
X

Niacin

LDL
(for deposition)

Fibric acid agents*

*Mechanism not completely understood

FIGURE 14–13   Mechanisms of action of lipid-lowering drugs.

dietary supplement which is not FDA approved. One form of OTC niacin called nicotinamide has no lipid-lowering effects; patients should be under medical supervision and not self-medicate.

Nicotinic acid causes flushing and an itching or burning feeling of the skin, which may reduce compli-

ance. To help prevent flushing, a nonsteroidal anti-inflammatory drug or aspirin can be taken 30 minutes before. Nicotinic acid also causes liver toxicity, gastrointestinal disturbances, glucose intolerance, and peptic ulcers. It is contraindicated in diabetics and people with peptic ulcer disease.

Vitamin E

Vitamin E, a naturally occurring antioxidant and fat-soluble vitamin, may have a protective role against atherosclerosis and coronary artery disease by preventing the oxidation of LDL cholesterol. Adverse effects include muscle weakness, blurred vision, and, in large doses, iron deficiency anemia.

Coenzyme Q10

Coenzyme Q10 (CoQ10) is a vitamin-like substance found in most animal cells, important in producing energy or ATP. Because the heart requires high levels of ATP, a sufficient level of CoQ10 is essential to that organ. Coenzyme Q10 and cholesterol share the same metabolic pathways. Although clinical studies show positive results, CoQ10 has not been widely accepted in the conventional medical community.

OTHER DRUGS

Ezetimibe (Zetia) inhibits absorption of cholesterol by the small intestine. It is usually administered alone or with HMG-CoA reductase inhibitors as an adjunctive therapy to diet for reduction of elevated total cholesterol and LDL.

Combination Drugs

The newest drugs for LDL reduction are combination drugs, which have less adverse effects and may be more superior to the statins. *These new drugs not only block absorption of cholesterol (cholesterol-absorption inhibitors) from food but reduce the cholesterol that the body makes in the liver.* All of the other drugs, including the statins, affect only dietary cholesterol. Examples of these drugs include amlodipine/atorvastatin (Caduet) and ezetimibe/simvastatin (Vytorin). Ezetimibe and amlodipine are cholesterol absorption inhibitors; atorvastatin and simvastatin are statin drugs. Combination therapy achieves a greater LDL-C reduction than statin monotherapy.

Dental Hygiene Notes

There are no contraindications or precautions to follow for patients on hypolipidemia drugs. Erythromycin should not be prescribed to a patient taking statin drugs. There are no special precautions to follow for these patients regarding the administration of local anesthetics/vasoconstrictors.

THROMBOLYTIC DRUGS

Normally, when a blood vessel is injured, a constriction occurs in the vessel which prevents hemorrhage (bleeding). The constriction brings the inner walls of the vessel together and the internal cells become "sticky" and adhere to one another. Normally, within an undamaged vessel, platelets circulate freely and do not stick to the vessel walls; in an injured blood vessel, platelets adhere to the underlying tissues and a platelet plug or clump forms and, finally, a fibrin clot. The clot is then removed by the process of fibrinolysis. Platelets or thrombocytes are small fragments found in the blood which promote blood clotting. This coagulation process prevents blood loss after injury or damage to a blood vessel.

This process occurs as part of the normal hemostasis mechanism. In pathologic conditions (e.g., atherosclerosis) of the blood vessels, increased clotting may occur in the presence of thrombus (a fibrinous clot formed in a blood vessel). Formation occurs where a clot forms within a blood vessel which can completely occlude the vessel. Thus, the inhibition of thrombin is essential in preventing and treating thromboemoblic disorders.

Anticoagulant drugs retard coagulation and extend the time taken for blood to clot, preventing the occurrence or enlargement of a thrombus (Figure 14–14). These drugs include heparin sodium, given intravenously/subcutaneously, and warfarin sodium (Coumadin) in an oral and injectable form. Warfarin is an antagonist of vitamin K. Warfarin is involved in inhibiting:

1. The pathological formation of blood clots within blood vessels by inhibiting the synthesis of clotting factors II, VII, IX, and X, which are made in the liver. It takes about 3 days for an anticoagulant effect to occur.
2. The synthesis of proteins C and S, which are endogenous anticoagulants that inactivate factors V and VII. It takes about 2 days for this to occur.

A period of several days is also required for coagulation factor levels to return to normal after oral anticoagulants are discontinued.

Dicumarol is a coumarin derivative. It is not commonly used because it is not completely absorbed in the G.I. tract, causing much gastrointestinal upset.

Heparin, one of the oldest drugs currently used, is a naturally occurring anticoagulant produced by basophils and mast cells in the body. Heparin can only be give parenterally because it is degraded when taken

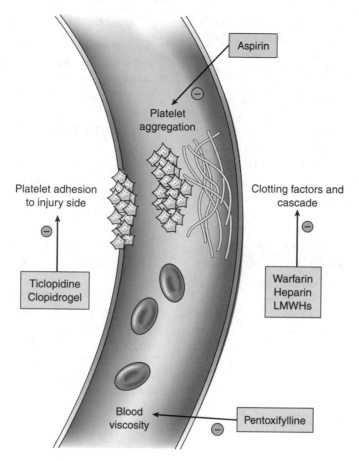

FIGURE 14–14   Mechanisms of action of anticoagulants.

orally. It has a short half-life of about one hour so it must be given frequently or as a continuous infusion. A serious adverse effect is heparin-induced thrombocytopenia whereby platelets aggregate within blood vessels resulting in clots which can lead to thrombosis.

Indications

Oral anticoagulants are indicated in the long-term management of patients with artificial heart valves and thromboembolic disorder (e.g., deep venous thrombosis, atrial fibrillation). The goal of anticoagulation therapy is to inhibit embolization and prevent the potentially fatal thrombosis. These drugs are also used in conjunction with heparin for the treatment of myocardial infarction.

Dental Treatment

The activity of warfarin is expressed using the international normalized ratio (INR). The prothrombin time (PT) test previously was used, but is not routinely used be-

cause of variability among laboratories. Dental patients taking warfarin must be routinely monitored for INR values; the patient's physician should be contacted.

There is much controversy about whether to discontinue warfarin in patients requiring dental treatment: Are they at risk of thromboembolic events if warfarin is stopped? It has been suggested that stopping warfarin can lead to a rebound hypercoagulable state, resulting in a stroke or death. Continuing warfarin therapy does increase the risk of postoperative bleeding, which usually requires intervention.

INR Values and Dental Procedures

Dental procedures   What dental procedures can be performed while taking warfarin? Ideally, the INR should be measured within 24 hours, but not more than 72 hours, before the dental procedure. For a patient not taking warfarin a normal coagulation profile is an INR of 1.0.

Nonsurgical dental procedures (e.g., periodontal debridement, endodontics, restorative) can be performed without discontinuation of warfarin if the patient's INR is within the currently recommended therapeutic range and does not exceed 3.5. Minor surgical procedures such as a single tooth extraction can be safely performed without altering the warfarin dose with an INR 3. Anticoagulation alterations are required if INR is greater than 4. The target INR differs based on the indication for taking warfarin. For example, if the patient is taking warfarin for atrial fibrillation, deep vein thrombosis or pulmonary embolus, the INR should be 2.5 (range 2.0–3.0). If the patient is taking warfarin for mechanical prosthetic heart valves or recurrence of embolism then the INR should be 3.5 (range 3.0–4.0).

Rapid Dental Hint

Assess your patients' medical history for warfarin use. Contact the patients' physician before any procedures are started. The INR level must be known.

Adverse Effects

The most common adverse effect of oral anticoagulants is bleeding, which may vary in severity from a mild nosebleed to life-threatening hemorrhage. Patients should report any signs of bleeding and ecchymoses (black-and-blue marks).

Treatment of bleeding may include a decrease in dosage and the administration of phytonadione (vitamin K_1). If bleeding is severe or the INR is markedly elevated (over 20), fresh frozen plasma or factor IX concentrate may be administered to replace clotting factors.

Drug Interactions

Warfarin is completely absorbed after oral administration. Most drug interactions occur because warfarin in about 99 percent of the drug is bound to plasma proteins, and is almost completely metabolized by CYP1A2, CYP2C9 and CYP3A4 in the liver. Erythromycin and clarithromycin (Biaxin) are inhibitors of these enzymes, which will decrease the metabolism of warfarin, thus increasing blood levels. Fluconazole (Diflucan) increases warfarin blood levels by inhibiting CYP2C9 enzymes; metronidazole inhibits enzymes that metabolize warfarin. These two drugs should be avoided.

There is an increased risk for bleeding with concomitant administration of aspirin and other nonsteroidal anti-inflammatory drugs such as ibuprofen.

Did You Know?

Tea has tannins, which reduce bleeding. Place a tea bag on the wound if there is slight bleeding after a dental procedure.

Antiplatelet drugs inhibit platelet aggregation and include:

- Aspirin (acetylsalicylic acid or ASA)
- Ticlopidine (Ticlid)
- Abciximab (ReoPro)
- Clopidogrel (Plavix)
- Dipyridamole (Perstantine)
- Aspirin-dipyridamole (Aggrenox).

Aspirin causes gastrointestinal irritation and bleeding due to inhibition of protective prostaglandins. Aspirin is used primarily to prevent arterial thrombosis in patients with ischemic heart disease and stroke, in patients with prosthetic valves, and in patients with unstable angina to prevent myocardial infarction. It is usually given in a low dose of 81 mg daily (aspirin was discussed in Chapter 5). Patients who are allergic to aspirin or who cannot tolerate its adverse effects can be prescribed ticlopidine.

Combination therapies that inhibit platelet function by more than one mechanism may be more efficacious than single-agent approaches. Aspirin/extended release dipyridamole (Aggrenox) is a combination antiplatelet agent with additive antiplatelet effects. Dipyridamole inhibits the uptake of adenosine into the platelets. It is controversial whether to prescribe both aspirin and clopidogrel for additive antiplatelet effect. In 2006, a study by the Cleveland Clinic reported that clopidogrel plus aspirin does not significantly reduce the rate of myocardial infarction, stroke, or cardiovascular death, and thus should not be recommended as a preventative therapy for such diseases.

LOW-DOSE HEPARINS

A more recently introduced group of drugs are called low-molecular-weight heparins or LMWHs, such as enoxaparin (Lovenox), ardeparin, and dalteparin (Fragmin). These drugs are used as an anticoagulant in diseases that have **thrombosis,** and for prophylaxis in situation that lead to a high risk of thrombosis. Low-molecular-weight-heparins are derivatives of heparin that are chemically altered and have once daily dosing, rather than a continuous infusion of heparin. There is also a smaller risk of bleeding and thrombocytopenia with LMWHs than heparin. Because LMWHs are administered subcutaneously and does not require coagulation monitoring, outpatient treatment of conditions such as deep vein thrombosis or pulmonary embolism is possible.

HEMATOPOEITIC DRUGS

The formation of red blood cells requires iron, vitamin B_{12}, and folic acid. Anemia develops when there is a deficiency in one of these substances. Iron is necessary for hemoglobin production. Iron deficiency anemia caused by chronic blood loss (e.g., pregnancy, menstrual problems) results in small red blood cells with insufficient hemoglobin. As a consequence, iron needs to be replaced by the administration of iron preparations. Oral therapy is continued until the normal range of hemoglobin is attained.

Orally administered iron is in the form of ferrous salts, usually ferrous sulfate, in order for the iron to be absorbed orally. Gastrointestinal upset (nausea, vomiting, and diarrhea) and extrinsic staining of teeth are common adverse side effects. There are no contraindications for dental treatment. Decreased absorption of tetracyclines and ciprofloxacin occurs if taken together.

DENTAL HYGIENE NOTES

The international normalized ratio (INR) should be recorded, and is used to monitor the patient's oral anticoagulant therapy. It is a good indicator of bleeding values. The higher the value, the greater the anticoagulant effect.

Oral anticoagulant therapy should not be discontinued; rather, the INR level should be monitored. Dental management of patients on warfarin is dependent upon the INR level. Discontinuing warfarin therapy may result in stroke or death. Dental treatment should be delayed until the INR value is within therapeutic levels of 1.0–4.0. Any dental procedure is contraindicated with INR values greater than 5.0.

Patients also may be taking aspirin prophylactically, either self-medicated or as prescribed by their physician. Aspirin inhibits platelet formation by irreversibly inhibiting cyclo-oxygenase, an enzyme found in all cell membranes of all cells, including platelets that are responsible for the formation of thromboxane A_2.

Thromboxane A_2 causes aggregation of platelets and vasoconstriction. This effect persists for the lifetime of the platelet (about 1 week). If patients are taking aspirin prophylactically, it can be stopped without consequence for dental surgery; however, if taken by order of a physician, it should not be stopped.

Although bleeding may occur if the patient is taking other drugs, such as dipyridamole, it is unlikely to interfere with dental treatment; however, a medical consult is necessary.

KEY POINTS

- Many patients are taking drugs for the heart, including aspirin.
- Take vital signs.
- Confirm that the patient took his/her medication as directed by their physician.
- Most heart drugs cause orthostatic hypotension; have patient sit upright in the dental chair for a few minutes before arising.
- Patients taking warfarin can receive dental treatment without stopping the drug; get INR levels before any treatment is started.

BOARD REVIEW QUESTIONS

1. Which of the following drugs can cause xerostomia? (p. 254)
   a. Digoxin
   b. Aspirin
   c. Furosemide
   d. Warfarin

2. Which of the following drugs *most* likely causes orthostatic hypotension? (p. 254)
   a. Diltiazem
   b. Aspirin
   c. Digoxin
   d. Niacin

3. Which of the following diseases presents with symptoms of pulmonary edema and dyspnea when lying flat, or upon exercise? (p. 253)
   a. Angina
   b. Arrhythmia
   c. Left heart failure
   d. Right heart failure

e. Hypertension

4. Which of the following drugs needs to be monitored by evaluating INR levels? (pp. 265, 266)
   a. Warfarin
   b. Atenolol
   c. Hydrochlorothaizde
   d. Nifedipine
   e. Metoprolol

5. Which of the following drugs is the first-line drug used in the treatment of heart failure in a 50-year-old male? (pp. 253, 254)
   a. Hydrochlorothiazide
   b. Furosemide
   c. Digoxin
   d. Nifedipine
   e. Captopril

6. Which of the following drugs should not be given to a patient taking naproxen (Aleve)? (pp. 242, 247)
   a. Nifedipine (Procardia)
   b. Digoxin (Lanoxin)
   c. Enalapril (Vasotec)
   d. Lidocaine (Xylocaine)

7. All of the following drugs are calcium channel blockers except one. Which one is the exception? (pp. 243, 254)
   a. Diltiazem
   b. Verapamil
   c. Amlodipine
   d. Quinapril

8. To which of the following drug classifications does atorvastatin (Lipitor) belong? (p. 262)
   a. HMG CoA reductase inhibitor (statin)
   b. Vasodilator
   c. ACE inhibitor
   d. Anticoagulant

9. A patient is taking amlodipine (Norvasc). After periodontal treatment is completed at an office visit and the patient is ready to be dismissed, which one of these procedures should be followed? (p. 254)
   a. Have the patient drink orange juice slowly.
   b. Have the patient sit upright in the dental chair a while.
   c. Administer oxygen.

d. Administer more local anesthetic.

10. A patient is self-medicating with one baby aspirin a day (81 mg) to prevent stroke. The patient has no remarkable medical history. Which of the following procedures should be followed before performing oral prophylaxis? (p. 267)
    a. It is mandatory to obtain a medical consult.
    b. Perform the dental procedure without discontinuing the aspirin.
    c. Discontinue aspirin for 2 weeks and have the patient come back.
    d. Change the patient's medication.

SELECTED REFERENCES

Budenz, A. W. 2000. Local anesthetics and medically complex patients. *Journal California Dental Association* 28:611–619.

Chobanian, A. V., H. R. Black, W. C. Cushman et al., 2003. The seventh report of the Joint National Committee on Prevention, Detection, Evaluation, and Treatment of High Blood Pressure. *JAMA* 289:2560–2571.

Horton, J. D. and B. M. Bushwick. 1999. Warfarin therapy: Evolving strategies in anticoagulation. *Am Fam Physician* 59:635–645.

Executive Summary of the third report of the National Cholesterol Education Program (NCEP) Expert Panel on Detection, Evaluation and Treatment of High Blood Cholesterol in Adults (Adult Treatment Panel III). *JAMA* 2001;285: 2486–2497.

Jeske, A. H., and G. D. Suchko. 2003. Lack of a scientific basis for routine discontinuation of oral anticoagulation therapy before dental treatment. *JADA* 134:1492–1497.

Takahashi, Y., M. Nakano, K. Sano, T. Kanri. 2005. The effects of epinephrine in local anesthetics on plasma catecholamine and hemodynamic responses. *Odontology* 93(1):72–79.

Todd, D. W. 2003. Anticoagulated patients and oral surgery. *Arch Intern Med* 163:1242.

Vlachopoulous, C., K. Aznaouridis, N. Alexopoulos, et al. 2005. Effect of dark chocolate on arterial function in healthy individuals. *American J Hypertension* 18:785–791.

Wahl, M. J. 2000. Myths of dental surgery in patients receiving anticoagulant therapy. *J Am Dent Assoc* 131:77–81.

Wahl, M. J. 1998. Dental surgery in anticoagulated patients. *Arch Intern Med* 158:1610–1616.

Weir, M. R. 1996. Angiotensin-II receptor antagonists: A new class of antihypertensive agents. *Am Acad Family Phy* 53:589–594.

QUICK DRUG GUIDE

Antihypertensive Drugs

Diuretics

(Increase elimination of water and salt, which will reduce pressure)

Thiazides
- Chlorothiazide (Diuril)
- Hydrochlorothiazide (Hydrodiuril)

Loop diuretics
- Furosemide (Lasix)
- Bumetanide (Bumex)

Potassium-sparing
- Triamterene (Dyrenium)
- Spironolactone (Aldactone)

Angiotensin Inhibitors

(Angiotensin-converting enzyme (ACE) inhibitors: Reduce blood pressure by inhibiting the conversion of angiotensin I to angiotensin II)
- Benazepril (Lotensin)
- Captopril (Capoten)
- Enalapril (Vasotec)
- Fosinopril (Monopril)
- Moexipril (Univasc)
- Quinapril (Accupril)
- Ramipril (Altace)

Angiotensin II Receptor Blockers (ARBS)

(Block angiotensin II receptor sites)
- Candesartan (Atacand)
- Eprosartan (Teveten)
- Irbesartan (Avapro)
- Losartan (Cozaar)
- Olmesartan (Benicar)
- Telmisartan (Micardis)
- Valsartan (Diovan)

Sympatholytics

β-receptor blockers

(Decrease heart rate and contractility by blocking β-receptors)
- Atenolol (Tenormin): Cardioselective
- Bisoprolol (Zebeta): Cardioselective
- Metoprolol (Lopressor): Cardioselective
- Nadolol (Corgard): nonselective
- Propranolol (Inderal): nonselective
- Timolol (Blocadren): nonselective

Centrally/peripherally α_2-agonists acting drugs
- Clonidine (Catapres)
- Methyldopa (Aldomet)
- Reserpine (generic)

α_1-adrenergic blockers
- Prazosin (Minipress)
- Terazosin (Hytrin)

Calcium Channel Blockers

(Prevent calcium from entering the cells of the coronary blood vessels and cause vasodilation)

Non-dihydropyridines
- Diltiazem (Cardizem)
- Verapamil (Calan, Isoptin)

Dihyropyridines
- Nifedipine (Procardia)
- Amlodipine (Norvasc)
- Felodipine (Plendil)

Direct Vasodilators
- Hydralazine (Apresoline)
- Minoxidil (Loniten)
- Nitroprusside (Nitropress)

Anti-Angina Drugs

Vasodilators

(Dilate Coronary Arteries)
- Nitroglycerin (Nitro-Bid, Nitrostat)
- Isosorbide dinitrate (Isordil)
- Isosorbide mononitrate (Imdur)

Calcium Channel Blockers

(Slow Heart Rate and Dilates Coronary Arteries)
- Amlodipine (Norvasc)
- Bedpridil (Vasocor)
- Diltiazem (Cardizem)

- Nicardipine (Cardene)
- Nifedipine (Procardia, Adalat)
- Verapamil (Calan, Isoptin)

β-Blockers

(Reduce Cardiac Load and thus Oxygen Demand)
- Atenolol (Tenormin)
- Metoprolol (Lopressor)
- Nadolol (Corgard)
- Propranolol (Inderal)

Heart Failure Drugs

Diuretics

(Increase Fluid Loss, thus Reducing Cardiac Load)
- Loop diuretics (furosemide)
- Thiazides (hyrochlorothiazide)

Positive Inotropic Drugs

Digitalis glycosides (Increases calcium ion concentration, which enhances heart contractility)
- Digoxin (Lanoxin)

Adrenergic Receptor Agonists

(Stimulates β-Receptors, Which Increases Cardiac Contractility)
- Dobutamine (Dobutrex)
- Dopamine

Vasodilators
- Hyralazine (Apresoline)

Angiotensin-Converting Enzyme Inhibitors

(ACE Inhibitors)
- Captopril (Capoten)
- Enalapril (Vasotec)
- Lisinopril (Prinivil, Zestril)
- Quinapril (Accupril)
- Fosinopril (Monopril)

Calcium Channel Blockers

Non-dihydropyridines
- Diltiazem (Cardizem)
- Verapamil (Calan, Isoptin)

Dihyropyridines
- Nifedipine (Procardia)
- Amlodipine (Norvasc)
- Felodipine (Plendil)

Antiarrhythmic Drugs

Class I: Sodium Channel Blockers

Class IA
- Disopyrmaide (Norpace)
- Procainamide (Pronestyl)
- Quinidine (Quinidex)

Class IB
- Lidocaine (Xylocaine)
- Mexiletine (Mexitil)

Class IC
- Flecainide (Tambocor)
- Propafenone (Rhythmol)

Class II: β-Blockers

- Acebutolol (Sectral)
- Esmolol (Brevibloc)
- Propranolol (Inderal)

Class III: Potassium Channel Blockers

- Amiodarone (Cordarone)
- Bretylium (injectable)
- Sotalol (Betapace)

Class IV: Calcium Channel Blockers

- Diltiazem (Cardizem)
- Verapamil (Calan)

Antihyperlipidemia/Hypertriglyceridemia Drugs

HMG-CoA Reductase Inhibitiors ("Statin" Drugs)

- Atorvastatin (Lipitor)
- Fluvastatin (Lescol)
- Lovastatin (Mevacor)
- Pravastatin (Pravacol)
- Rosuvastatin (Crestor)
- Simvastatin (Zocor)

Bile Acid-Binding (Sequestrants) Resins

- Cholestyramine (Questran)
- Colestipol (Colestid)

Fibric Acids

- Clofibrate (Atromid-S)
- Fenofibrate (Lofibra,Tricor)
- Gemfibrozil (Lopid)

Other Agents (Natural)

- Nicotinic acid (niacin)
- Vitamin E

Combination Drugs

- Amlodipine/atorvastatin (Caduet)
- Ezetimibe/simvastatin (Vytorin)

Anticoagulants

- Warfarin (Coumadin)
- Dicumarol

- Anisindione (Miradon)
- Heparin

Antiplatelet Drugs

- Aspirin
- Abciximab (ReoPro)
- Clopidogrel (Plavix)

- Dipyridamole ((Persantine, Pyridamole)
- Ticlopidine (Ticlid)
- Aspirin/dipyridamole (Aggrenox)

Chapter 15

Respiratory Drugs

GOALS:

- To provide an understanding of the various drugs used in the management of lung diseases and of asthma in the dental office.
- To gain knowledge of the various drugs for cough and colds.

EDUCATIONAL OBJECTIVES

After reading this chapter, the reader should be able to:

1. Classify asthma into different categories.
2. Explain the management of asthma in relation to dental treatment.
3. List and describe current medications used in asthma.
4. Discuss the management of COPD.
5. Describe the management of rhinitis.
6. Discuss the therapy for cough.
7. Discuss adverse effects of antihistamines as they relate to dentistry.

KEY TERMS

Asthma
Bronchospasm
Chronic obstructive pulmonary disease (COPD)
Corticosteroids
Rhinitis
Antihistamines
Antitussives

INTRODUCTION

Disorders of the respiratory tract include asthma, chronic obstructive pulmonary disease (COPD, which encompasses bronchitis and emphysema), and other diseases of the upper and lower respiratory tract, such as allergic rhinitis. Anti-asthmatic medications, antihistamines, decongestants, and antitussives will be reviewed in this chapter.

LUNG ANATOMY

Air entering the respiratory system travels through the nose, the pharynx, and the trachea into the bronchi, which divide into smaller passages called bronchioles (Figure 15–1). After roughly 23 generations of these airways, the tracheobronchial tree ends in sacs called alveoli. Airways are surrounded by smooth muscles. When the muscles are stimulated, they contract, narrowing the lumen (diameter; opening) of the airway.

The smooth muscle is controlled by the autonomic nervous system. When the sympathetic nervous system is activated during a stressful situation (e.g., fight-or-flight response) the bronchiolar smooth muscle relaxes and bronchodilation results. This allows more air to enter the alveoli, potentially increasing the oxygen supply to the body during stress or exercise (Figure 15–2).

PATHOGENESIS/DIAGNOSIS: ASTHMA

Asthma is a chronic lung disease characterized by inflammation of the airways and bronchoconstriction which improves either spontaneously or with treatment. Asthma affects approximately 15 million Americans. It often begins in childhood, although it can occur at any

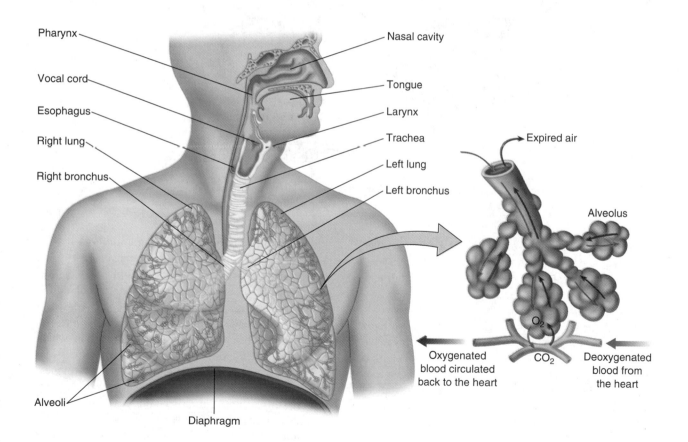

Pharynx
Nasal cavity
Vocal cord
Tongue
Esophagus
Larynx
Right lung
Trachea
Right bronchus
Left lung
Left bronchus
Expired air
Alveolus
O_2
Oxygenated blood circulated back to the heart
CO_2
Deoxygenated blood from the heart
Alveoli
Diaphragm

FIGURE 15–1 The respiratory system.

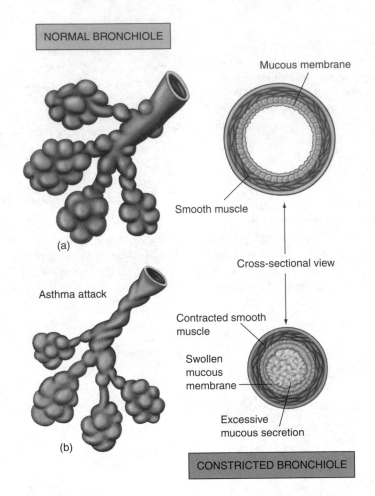

NORMAL BRONCHIOLE

Mucous membrane

Smooth muscle

(a)

Cross-sectional view

Asthma attack

Contracted smooth muscle

Swollen mucous membrane

Excessive mucous secretion

(b)

CONSTRICTED BRONCHIOLE

FIGURE 15–2   Changes in bronchioles during an asthma attack: (a) normal bronchiole; (b) in asthma attack.

age. More than 5 percent of all children younger than age 18 reported having asthma attacks. Asthma is responsible for approximately 2 million emergency department visits and 5,000 deaths per year.

Many cells and cellular elements play major roles in the pathogenesis of asthma. Cells such as T-lymphocytes (white blood cells involved in inflammatory reactions), eosinophils (white blood cells involved in allergic and inflammatory reactions), and mast cells (which make and release histamine, a substance released during allergic reaction in response to an allergen) all contribute to this response. These mediators narrow the airway by causing edema and inflammation, and cause bronchoconstriction by stimulating the airway smooth muscles to contract.

Bronchoconstriction, inflammation, and loss of lung elasticity are the three most common processes that result in airway obstruction. Airway obstruction increases airway resistance, resulting in increased work and difficulty of breathing, and wheeze and cough. Eventually the obstruction can lead to reduced blood oxygen levels. The first event that occurs is airway inflammation, which is due to the release of inflammatory mediators (e.g. histamine, prostaglandins, leukotrienes, and other cytokines) triggered by exposure to allergens such as dust, plant pollen, smoke, and animal dander; exercise; stress; changes in weather; and most frequently upper respiratory viral infection. These inflammatory mediators cause swelling of the airways, and provoke contraction of the airway smooth muscle.

Asthma in children is often associated with atopy, which is a genetic susceptibility to produce IgE (antibodies produced in the presence of an antigen or foreign body or allergen) toward allergens. This IgE antibody production is associated with the development of allergies.

When people with asthma are exposed to their triggers (the triggers vary from patient to patient) airway inflammation (mucosal edema and mucous secretions) occurs. *This inflammation may be controlled with anti-inflammatory (corticosteroids) agents, but not completely eradicated.* The airways become obstructed by the excess mucous and swelling of airway linings (Figure 15–2). A resulting contraction of the airway smooth muscle, **bronchospasm,** leads to further airway obstruction and limitation of airflow. Thus, inflammation can affect not only the size of the airway and airflow, but it causes airway hyperresponsiveness to a variety of stimuli, which results in further airway obstruction. Airway hyperresponsiveness and subsequent airway obstruction leads to cough, shortness of breath, and wheezing. Effective treatment of asthma should be geared to the reaction of airway inflammation and hyperresponsiveness.

Bronchospasm is mediated through the β_2-receptors, located on the bronchioles, and may be rapidly relieved by inhaled bronchodilators. Bronchospasm occurs within minutes, while inflammation (mucous secretions) is slower in onset, taking hours. Thus an acute exposure, such as allergy or exercise, causes acute bronchospasm, referred to as the early asthmatic response. Airway inflammation comes on more slowly, known as the late asthmatic response.

Loss of lung elasticity results from air sac enlargement (distention). Treatment to reverse this condition is more difficult, and requires long-term, high-dose drug therapy.

A clinical diagnosis of asthma may be confirmed by pulmonary function testing showing reversible air-

flow obstruction. The diagnosis is suggested by the following signs or symptoms, which may worsen at night, upon wakening in the morning, during exercise, with colds, or upon exposure to allergens:

- Wheezing
- Prolonged or troublesome cough
- Difficulty breathing
- Breathlessness (dyspnea)
- Chest tightness

Asthma is classified by severity depending on the frequency of symptoms:

- Mild intermittent (2 days a week or less; awakenings less than twice a month)
- Mild persistent (more than 2 days a week but less than one time a day; awakenings twice a month or more)
- Moderate persistent (every day)
- Severe persistent (most of the time)

Therapy is designed to decrease the frequency of asthmatic attacks or to terminate attacks in progress. Drug regimens are tailored to pattern, severity, and triggers.

Chronic obstructive pulmonary disease (COPD) encompasses diseases that cause *chronic* (long-term) obstruction of air flow. Chronic bronchitis, an inflammation characterized by excessive mucous in the bronchi, and a productive (mucous-producing) cough, and emphysema, an irreversible destruction of alveolar walls with dilation of air spaces, are the major components of COPD.

PHARMACOTHERAPY: CONTROLLING ASTHMA AND COPD

Asthma

Drug therapy is targeted toward the inflammation and relieving the bronchospasm (Figure 15–3). A problem in treating asthma is patient adherence to the drug regimens. Only about 40 percent of patients actually use their medications as prescribed. Another problem is patients that do not respond to the current therapy. In such cases there may be confounding factors making the asthma difficult to control (acid reflux disease, sinus infection, cigarette smoke, allergies) or the patients simply need higher doses of the medications. Some have genetic abnormalities which makes them less responsive to the medications.

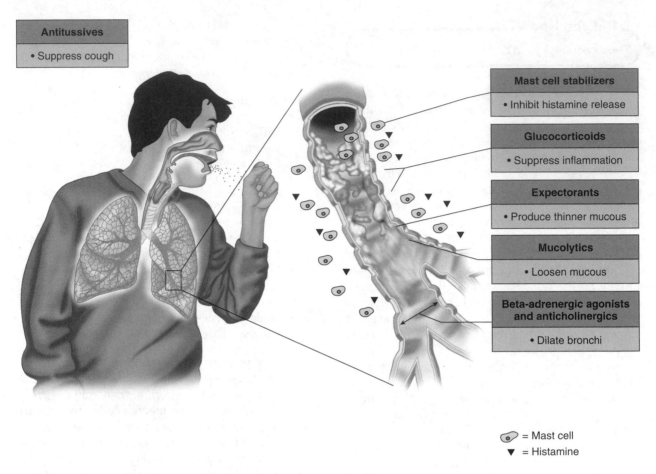

Antitussives
• Suppress cough

Mast cell stabilizers
• Inhibit histamine release

Glucocorticoids
• Suppress inflammation

Expectorants
• Produce thinner mucous

Mucolytics
• Loosen mucous

Beta-adrenergic agonists and anticholinergics
• Dilate bronchi

⬬ = Mast cell
▼ = Histamine

FIGURE 15–3   Drugs used to treat respiratory disorders.

Classification of Medications

Long-term control medications (also referred to as long-term preventive, controller, or maintenance medications) are taken daily on a long-term basis in order to achieve and maintain control of persistent asthma. Most of these have anti-inflammatory effects.

Quick-relief medications (also referred to as reliever or acute rescue medications) provide quick reversal of acute airflow obstruction and relief of bronchospasm.

Bronchodilators	Anti-Inflammatory Drugs
β_2-agonists	Corticosteroids
Methylxanthines	Mast cell stabilizers
	Leukotriene modifiers

Long-term Preventive Medications   In 2002, the National Asthma Education and Prevention Program (NAEPP) was updated by the National Institutes of Health (NIH). Asthma may be classified as mild intermittent, mild persistent, moderate persistent, and severe persistent. *Inhaled corticosteroids are the drug of choice for persistent asthma.* Safety and efficacy of these drugs has been shown down to age 1. Thus chronic inhaled corticosteroids are recommended as first-line therapy in adults and children with persistent asthma, even if it is mild (Table 15–1). Regular use of inhaled corticosteroids in adults can reduce hospitalizations and complications (e.g., death) from asthma and improve lung function and quality of life, including decreasing days of work or school missed.

Combination therapy with an inhaled corticosteroid and a long-acting β_2-agonist is the recommended treatment for adults and children over 5 years of age with

TABLE 15-1 Long-Term Control Medications

Drug Name	Route of Adminstration	Mechanism	Adverse Effects	Drug Interactions	Patient Instructions
Corticosteroids Beclomethasone dipropionate (Beclovent, Vanceril) Budesonide (Pulmicort) Flunisolide (Aerobid) Fluticasone (Flovent, Advir) Mometasone (Asmanex) Triamcinolone (Azmacort)	Inhalation (meter-dose inhalers)	Anti-inflammatory	Fewer systemic side effects because less systemic absorption. Possible reduction in growth in children, higher risk of infection	Significant drug interactions not likely to occur with inhalation steroids.	Brush teeth and rinse mouth with water after each dose to reduce the development of candidiasis.
Selective β₂-Agonists (Long-Acting) Salmeterol (Serevent) Formoterol (Foradil)	Inhalation	Bronchodilator	Tachycardia, heart palpitations, tremors	Possible Increased effect on the heart if taken with MAO inhibitors, tricyclic antidepressants, and other sympathomimetic drugs. Co-administration with theophylline may increase bronchodilation. Hyperglycemic effects when taken with corticosteroids. Cardiovascular toxicity when taken with cocaine.	Do not overuse the product.

(continued)

TABLE 15-1 (Continued)

Drug Name	Route of Administration	Mechanism	Adverse Effects	Drug Interactions	Patient Instructions
Methylxanthines	Systemic	Bronchodilator	Nausea, vomiting, headache, tachycardia, seizures (dose related: increase dose will increase side effects)	Cigarette smoke increases metabolism of theophylline, decreasing its blood levels. Erythromycin, cimetidine (Tagamet) increase theophylline blood levels. Theophylline increases toxicity of digitalis. Theophylline decreases phenytoin (Dilantin) and lithium blood levels.	Can take with food to decrease G.I. upset (pain, vomiting, nausea); avoid taking with caffeine-containing drinks.
Theophylline (Slo-Phyllin, TheoDur, Theo-24)	Oral (tablets, capsules, syrup)				
Mast Cell Stabilizers		Anti-inflammatory; used prophylactically to prevent mediator release	Throat irritation or dryness	No significant interactions	Rinse mouth with water to help prevent throat irritation or dryness.
Cromolyn sodium (Intal)	Inhalation				
Nedocromil (Tilade)	Inhalation				
Leukotriene Modifiers					
Zafirlukast (Accolate)	Tablets	Anti-inflammatory	Headache, G.I. upset	May inhibit metabolism of warfarin (anticoagulant). Erythromycin and theophylline reduces zafirlukast levels.	Take on empty stomach (1 hour before meals or 2 hours after meals).
Montelukast (Singulair)	Tablets			Decreased levels with phenobarbitol.	Take at night.
Zileuton (Zyflo)	Tablets			May inhibit metabolism of warfarin (anticoagulant).	Liver enzymes altered, soget periodic liver function tests.

moderate to severe asthma. The GOAL (Gaining Optimal Asthma ControL) study (2004) reported that when taking a combination of inhaled corticosteroids and long-acting β-agonists, most patients achieved control of their asthma.

Other drugs, such as cromolyn sodium (Intal), and leukotriene modifiers such as montelukast (Singulair) are alternative treatments with a more limited role in the treatment of asthma. Some recommend a leukotriene modifier as a controlling medication for mild persistent asthma.

The number and frequency of medications increase (step up) as the severity of asthma increases, and decrease (step down) when asthma is under control. When beginning therapy, recommendations are to start with the highest appropriate therapy and step down as the patient improves. Inhaled medications are preferred because of their high therapeutic ratio, with high concentrations of the drug being delivered directly to the airways with few systemic adverse side effects. This step-wise treatment is presented in Table 15–2 and 15–3.

Corticosteroids Corticosteroids are the most potent and effective *anti-inflammatory* agents and should to be first-line therapy for long-term management of mild, moderate and severe persistent asthma. In moderate to severe asthma the addition of a long-acting β_2-agonist may improve control (Table 15–2); although the leukotriene modifiers may serve this role, as well.

The anti-inflammatory effects of corticosteroids are due to the suppression of T-lymphocyte activation and the inhibition of mast cells and eosinophils from releasing chemical mediators of inflammation, including histamine, interleukins, leukotrienes, and prostaglandins, and other substances that cause lung tissue damage, edema, and vasodilation. Eosinophilc inflammation is a feature of the bronchial tissues; corticosteroids are most effective in reducing this type of inflammation. Clinically, corticosteroids reduce the severity of symptoms, decrease airway hyperresponsiveness, and improve lung function.

Adverse effects from inhaled corticosteroids are may include cough, oral candidiasis (thrush), and, with

TABLE 15–2   Step Wise Treatment of Asthma

Classification	Long-Term Prevention (Preferred Treatment)	(Alternative Treatment)	Quick-Relief Drugs
Step 1 Intermittent asthma	• No medications needed	• No medications needed	• Short-acting bronchodilator: inhaled β_2-agonist (e.g., Albuterol)
Step 2 Mild asthma	• Inhaled corticosteroid	• Cromolyn, leukotriene modifier, nedocromil or theophylline	• Short-acting bronchodilator: inhaled β_2-agonist as needed for symptoms
Step 3 Moderate asthma	• Inhaled corticosteroid, and long-acting inhaled β_2-agonist	• Increase dose of corticosteroid or add either a leukotriene modifier or theophylline	• Short-acting bronchodilator: inhaled β_2-agonist as needed for symptoms
Step 4 Severe persistent asthma	• Inhaled corticosteroid and long-acting β_2-agonist	• If needed, add corticosteroid tablets or syrup	• Short-acting bronchodilator: inhaled β_2-agonist as needed for symptoms

(Adapted from Expert Panel Report: Guidelines for the Diagnosis and Management of Asthma, National Asthma Education and Prevention Program, 1997; Update, 2002)

TABLE 15–3 Quick-Relief Medications for Bronchospasm

Drug Name	Route of Adminstration	Mechanism	Adverse Effects	Drug Interactions	Patient Instructions
β₂-Adrenergic (Short-Acting)					
Albuterol (Proventil, Ventolin)	Aerosol inhalation (by mouth), oral (tablet)	Bronchodilator	Although a selective β₂-receptor agonist, side effects include hypertension, tachycardia, skeletal muscle tremor, and CNS stimulation. These effects are seen more with systemic administration. Inhalation preparations have fewer systemic side effects.	Possible increased effect on the heart if taken with MAO inhibitors, tricyclic antidepressants, and other sympathomimetic drugs. Effects are antagonized with adrenergic blocking agents (e.g., metoprolol). Possible cardiovascular toxicity with cocaine. Increased bronchodilation with theophylline.	For inhalation dosage forms, rinse mouth with water after each dose to prevent dryness. May need daily home fluoride if dry mouth persists.
Pirbuterol (Maxair)	Inhalation	Bronchodilator	See above	See above	
Terbutaline (Brethine, Brethaire)	Inhalation, oral (tablet), SQ injection	Bronchodilator	See above	See above	
Metaproterenol (Alupent)	Inhalation, oral (tablet)	Bronchodilator	See above	See above	
Levalbuterol (Xopenex)	Inhalation	Bronchodilator	See above	See above	
Anticholinergics					
Ipratropium bromide HFA (Atrovent)	Aerosol inhalation (by mouth)	Bronchodilator	Few side effects because poorly absorbed into the systemic circulation (blood)	Used concomitantly with other antiasthmatic drugs	Assess salivary flow. Assess need for daily home fluoride applications; avoid oral rinses with high alcohol content such as Listerine; rinse mouth with water after each dose to prevent dryness.
Ipratropium bromide and albuterol sulfate (Combivent)	Aerosol inhalation (by mouth)	Bronchodilator	Xerostomia, bitter taste	Additive effects when used with adrenergic agonists	
Tiotropium bromide (Spiriva)	Aerosol inhalation (by mouth)	Bronchodilator	Few side effects because poorly absorbed into the	Used concomitantly with other antiasthmatic	Assess salivary flow. Assess need for daily

Name	Form	Action	Side Effects	Drug Interactions	Special Instructions
			systemic circulation (blood)	drugs. Additive effects when used with adrenergic agonists.	home fluoride applications; avoid oral rinses with high alcohol content such as Listerine®; rinse mouth with water after each dose to prevent dryness.
Corticosteroids	Systemic (oral)				
Methylprednisolone	Tablet	Anti-Inflammatory	Mask infections and higher risk of infection, peptic ulcer, increase glucose blood levels, hypertension, water retention (weight gain), psychiatric disturbances, osteoporosis	Increase insulin/oral diabetic drug requirement. Phenytoin, phenobarbital and rifampin may decrease blood levels of steroid. Steroids may decrease blood aspirin levels. Increased theophylline levels.	Take with food and at least a full glass of water to reduce G.I. (stomach) upset.
Prednisolone	Tablet	Anti-Inflammatory			
Prednisone	Tablet	Anti-Inflammatory			

very high doses, growth suppression. Lesions of candidiasis appear white on the mucosa and rub off when wiped with gauze. Patients should brush the teeth and rinse the mouth with water after every inhalation dose to prevent these infections. Some dental clinicians and physicians recommend that the patient brush the teeth after taking the inhaled steroid as a method of removing excess steroid from the mouth and pharynx, and improving dental hygiene. When a patient uses the inhaler with a valved holding chamber, the incidence of oral candidiasis drops markedly.

Long-Acting β_2-Selective Agonists (bronchodilators) Long-acting β_2-selective agonists include salmeterol (Serevent) and formoterol (Foradil) (Table 15–1). These drugs act as *bronchodilators,* causing the airway smooth muscle to relax. Both drugs have a duration of action of 12 hours or more. These drugs can used with a low or medium dosage of an inhaled corticosteroid to improve asthma control *but should not* be used alone. Long-acting β-agonists may allow a reduction of the dosage of corticosteroid used. Salmeterol is available in a fixed combination Diskus with Flovent, called Advair. In some countries formoterol and budesonide are available as a fixed combination. Adverse side effects of the long-acting β-agonists include xerostomia, tachycardia (increased heart rate), headache, tremor, and nausea. An important side effect of the long-acting β-agonists when used alone is overstimulation of the β-agonist receptors, which makes the short-acting agonists less effective. Furthermore, use of the long-acting β-agonists as a rescue

---

Guidelines for Patients Taking Inhaled Corticosteroids

BECLOMETHASONE: QVAR
FLUTICASONE: Flovent, Advair
BUDESONIDE: Pulmicort
FLUNISOLIDE: Aerobid
MOMETASONE: Asmenex
TRIAMCINOLONE: Azmacort

- Monitor for fungal infection in oral cavity
- Patients should brush their teeth and rinse the mouth with water after inhalation dose
- May require fluoride treatments at home for dry mouth
- Hoarseness may develop

Guidelines for Patients Taking Salmeterol (Serevent)

- Assess salivary flow; assess need for fluoride rinse
- Stress importance of good oral hygiene
- Monitor vital signs, especially patients with heart disease
- Keep patients in a semisupine position

---

medication has resulted in complications of altered heart rhythm. Concomitant inhaled steroids will upregulate the receptors.

Methylxanthines Methylxanthines include theophylline and aminophylline. These orally administered drugs are *bronchodilators* that relax the airway smooth muscle to control asthmatic symptoms. These drugs are no longer recommended for acute exacerbations or as a drug of choice for asthma. Decades ago, they were the mainstay of chronic therapy and when used intravenously served as the main emergent treatment of acute asthma. They have been supplanted by the drugs discussed above. Serum levels must be monitored to avoid toxicity. Caffeine is a type of methylxanthine drug. About 100 mg of caffeine is present in a cup of coffee (only about 65 mg in instant coffee), sufficient to cause mild bronchodilation in patients with asthma.

These drugs also have cardiovascular effects, stimulate secretion of gastric and digestive enzymes in the stomach, and cause insomnia. Many drug interactions occur with theophylline; for example, concomitant erythromycin or clarithromycin (Biaxin) may elevate the blood level of theophylline. A dosage adjustment of theophylline is often necessary.

Mast Cell Stabilizers Cromolyn sodium and nedocromil sodium have anti-inflammatory actions that inhibit the release of histamine and other mediators of allergic reactions leading to airway inflammation. Both medications are administered by inhalation and may be alternative treatment in mild persistent asthma.

Did You Know?

Moses Maimonides recognized the beneficial effects of strong tea in people with asthma.

Did You Know?

Cola drinks contain about 35 mg caffeine; a cup of hot chocolate contains about 4 mg.

Leukotriene Modifiers Leukotriene modifiers are orally administered agents that also may be alternative first line treatment for mild persistent asthma, and may serve as adjuncts to inhaled corticosteroids for more severe disease. These agents block the activity of arachidonic acid derivatives (e.g., leukotrienes) which are involved in the inflammatory pathway. Montelukast (Singulair) is the most prescribed because of its once a day dosing and its approval for young children. These drugs reduce the need for short-acting, inhaled β_2-agonists.

Other Agents Combination therapy of ipratropium bromide (anticholinergic) and albuterol sulfate (Duoneb) can be helpful for COPD; and, as above, fluticasone/salmeterol (Advair) is beneficial for patients with moderate or severe asthma who benefit from the addition of a bronchodilator, rather than increasing the anti-inflammatory therapy.

Quick-Relief Medications   Quick-relief medications are used for prompt relief of bronchospasm and associated symptoms including cough, chest tightness, and wheezing. These medications include *short-acting β_2-receptor selective agonists,* anticholinergics, and systemic corticosteroids (Table 15–3).

Bronchodilators SHORT-ACTING β_2-RECEPTOR SELECTIVE AGONISTS When inhaled, the β_2-agonists (Tables 15–2 and 15–3) provide the quickest onset (5–15 minutes) and relief of symptoms by *bronchodilation* (relaxation of bronchial smooth muscle). The prototype short-acting β_2-receptor selective agonist is albuterol (Ventolin, Proventil).

Beta$_2$-agonists are administered either by inhalation (with a metered dose inhaler or nebulizer) through the mouth, tablets, liquid (syrup), or by injection. These drugs should be used in all patients to treat acute symptoms. Regular daily use is not generally recommended because tachyphylaxis, due to overstimulation of the receptors, may reduce their effectiveness. When they are needed frequently, this is an indication that more controller therapy is needed. These drugs taken before exercise effectively prevent exercise-induced bronchoconstriction.

Inhaled β-adrenergic agonists produce little systemic toxicity because only small amounts of the drug

Guidelines for Patients Taking Albuterol (Proventil)

- May leave patients in a semisupine chair position
- After each inhalation, patients should rinse their mouth with water to prevent dryness
- May need daily fluoride treatments at home if dry mouth is persistent
- Use salivary substitutes if dry mouth is persistent
- Patients should have the inhalant available during dental treatment

are absorbed. When given orally, a longer duration of action is achieved, but systemic side effects such as tachycardia (increased heart rate) and tremor are more frequently experienced. Overuse of inhalation products may reduce the effectiveness of the drug and increase the side effects.

Although epinephrine is found in numerous OTC inhalation products (e.g., Primatene Mist, Bronkaid Mist), it is rarely prescribed. It causes bronchodilation by stimulation of the β_2-receptors and vasoconstriction, and decreases secretion by stimulation of the α_1-receptors. It is primarily used in emergency situations for severe bronchoconstriction, or in some cases of croup (condition of the larynx, particularly in children and infants, characterized by respiratory difficulty and brassy cough). Epinephrine is contraindicated in patients with uncontrolled hypertension, hyperthyroidism, and narrow-angle glaucoma.

The oldest oral sympathomimetic is ephedrine, which causes vasoconstriction. Over-the-counter preparations with ephedrine include Broncolate, and Primatene tablets. Although still available in many OTC products, newer selective β_2-agonists have replaced it because of possible links to stroke and heart attack because of its β_1-receptor activity.

Adrenergic agonist agents relax airway smooth muscle that results in bronchodilation. Because epinephrine and isoproterenol (Isuprel) are not β_2-receptor selective and also stimulate β_1-receptors, they cause more cardiac stimulation and are rarely used in the treatment of asthma.

ANTICHOLINERGIC AGENTS Cholinergic innervation is an important factor in the regulation of airway smooth muscle tone. Anticholinergic agents are usually used when patients cannot tolerate β_2-agonists or as an adjunct to β_2-agonists for additional relief of bronchoconstriction. These drugs reduce the symptoms of cough, wheezing, and chest tightness. Inhaled anticholinergic drugs are generally not sufficiently effective when used alone, but are beneficial when combined with β-agonists or corticosteroids. Anticholinergics are not used for allergen or exercise-induced asthma.

Ipratropium bromide (Atrovent) is the prototype anticholinergic. The mechanism of action of ipratropium is to inhibit acetylcholine receptors on smooth muscle, resulting in bronchodilation. Adverse side effects are xerostomia and taste alteration (bitter taste). The patient should rinse the mouth after each inhalation dose to prevent dryness. Anticholinergics should be used with caution in patients with narrow-angle glaucoma, prostatic hypertrophy, or bladder-neck obstruction, because they may increase pressure within the eye and cause urinary retention, respectively.

CORTICOSTEROIDS *Systemic* corticosteroids are used when asthma cannot be controlled by bronchodilators alone. Corticosteroids taken orally take more than 4 hours to have a therapeutic effect by *reducing inflammation. Systemic steroids are used for acute asthma, while for chronic, long-term maintenance therapy (prevention of attacks), inhaled steroids are used.*

Since the adverse effects of orally administered steroids include gastric irritation (ulcers), hypokalemia (low blood potassium levels), fluid retention, hyperglycemia (high blood glucose), increased appetite, acne, behavioral changes, growth suppression and, with long-term use, decreased immune function, they should be discontinued as quickly as possible.

Guidelines for Patients Taking Ipratropium (Atrovent)

- Monitor salivary flow
- Patients may need daily fluoride treatments at home if dry mouth is persistent
- Patients should use salivary substitutes if dry mouth is persistent

Guidelines for Patients Taking Systemic Corticosteroids

- Monitor patients for oral candidiasis (thrush; white areas that do not rub off)
- Monitor the patients' salivary flow
- Patients taking steroids for more than 2 weeks may require additional doses for stressful dental procedures; consult with their physician
- Patients should avoid aspirin because of gastrointestinal problems
- Frequent oral prophylaxis

Routes of Drug Administration

Medications for the management of asthma are administered either by inhaled or systemic routes. Systemic routes are oral or parenteral (intravenous, intramuscular, or subcutaneous). Medications delivered by inhalation directly to the airways have minimal adverse effects and are more effective with a shorter onset of action than when administered orally.

Inhaled drugs are delivered to the lungs by an aerosol which is a suspension of minute liquid droplets or fine solid particles suspended in a gas. Different devices are used to deliver the aerosol:

Nebulizer (small machine that vaporizes a liquid medication into a fine mist that is inhaled with a facemask or handheld device) (Figure 15–4)

Dry powder inhaler (small device that is activated by the process of inhalation to deliver a fine powder to the bronchioles)

Metered dose inhalers (use a propellant to deliver a measured dose of drugs to the lungs during each breath). Most patients who use the metered dose inhalers, the most common delivery system used, also require a valved holding chamber for optimal drug delivery.

Step-By-Step Treatment

In 1997, the publication *Expert Panel Report 2: Guidelines for the Diagnosis and Management of Asthma* was developed, revised in 2002. Table 15–4 summarizes the

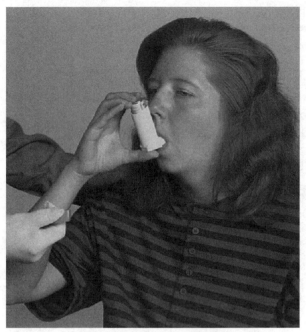

(A) Metered dose inhaler

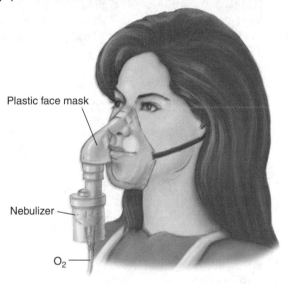

Plastic face mask

Nebulizer

O_2

(B) Nebulizer with attached face mask

FIGURE 15–4 Inhalers Used to Deliver Asthmatic Drugs: A) metered-dose inhaler. The patient times the inhalation to the puffs of drug emitted from the MDI. B) Nebulizer with a face mask. It vaporizes a liquid drug into a fine mist that is inhaled.

step-by-step treatment of asthma developed by this panel. Different medications are used depending on the severity of the disease. This table will help to determine which type of asthma the patient has and what medication is appropriate.

Severe asthma attacks are life threatening and require immediate treatment. An inhaled short-acting β_2-agonist in adequate, frequent doses is essential. Corticosteroid tablets or syrup introduced early in the course of a moderate or severe attack help to reverse the inflammation and speed recovery. Oxygen may be necessary. Theophylline or aminophylline is not recommended if it is used in addition to high doses of β_2-agonist because it provides little additional benefit and increases the likelihood of adverse side effects. Epinephrine (adrenaline) is indicated for acute treatment of anaphylaxis.

COPD (Bronchitis/Emphysema) Treatment

There is no cure for COPD. Its medication management involves a variety of step-by-step treatment regimens similar to those for asthma. The goals of treatment are to improve the chronic obstruction and to treat and prevent acute episodes. Treatment starts with smoking cessation. Pharmacotherapy begins with short-acting bronchodilators for mild disease and long-acting drugs as the disease becomes more chronic and severe (Table 15–4). The most commonly used initial drug is a β_2-agonist inhaler. Inhalation is preferred over the oral route because of increased efficacy and reduced toxicity. If chronic, mild symptoms continue then ipratropium bromide inhaler is started. Long-term oxygen therapy is occasionally required.

Rapid Dental Hint

Remind your patients who use a steroid inhaler to rinse the mouth with water after use.

DRUGS FOR COLD
Introduction

Rhinitis, inflammation of the nasal mucosa (mucous membranes in the nasal cavities) is most frequently caused by allergic reactions to pollen, mold spores, dust,

TABLE 15–4 Step-by-Step Approach for Managing COPD (Bronchitis and Emphysema)

Severity Of Disease	Clinical Symptoms	Treatment	Other
At risk	Productive cough	No bronchodilator needed	Smoking cessation
I	Productive cough	Short-acting bronchodilator as needed	Smoking cessation
II	Productive cough	Tiotropium with or without short-acting β_2-agonist	Smoking cessation, exercise
III	Productive cough, out of breath on mild exertion	Tiotropium, long-acting β_2-agonist	Smoking cessation, exercise, oxygen therapy
IV	Productive cough, out of breath on mild exertion	Tiotropium, long-acting β_2-agonist, inhaled corticosteroids	Smoking cessation, exercise, oxygen therapy

and other allergens or by viruses, such as rhinoviruses and other agents related to the common cold (Figure 15–5). Rhinitis may be seasonal in the case of allergic rhinitis or may be an acute, self-limiting condition in the case of viral rhinitis. Characteristics of both types of rhinitis are nasal congestion, rhinorrhea (runny nose), itching, sneezing, mucus production, vasodilation, and airway narrowing. Conjunctivitis (inflammation of the conjunctiva of the eye) is usually seen more in allergic rhinitis, but accompanies some viral infections.

Viral rhinitis or—as it is more often called—the common cold is a self-limiting condition and is best treated conservatively. Aches and pain are best relieved with a nonsteroidal anti-inflammatory drug (acetaminophen, ibuprofen). Nasal decongestants (e.g., psuedoephedrine, phenylephrine) may be helpful.

A distinction must be made between allergic rhinitis and the common cold. The common cold is a self-limiting condition which is caused by viruses, and is infectious and communicable. Viruses can be spread through the air by droplets from a sneeze or cough and by touching the nose, eyes, or mouth after contact. Allergic rhinitis is a risk factor for the development of asthma and nasal polyps. Cold symptoms usually last for 1 to 2 weeks.

Most of the symptoms associated with rhinitis are due to the release of histamine from mast cells and basophils (type of white blood cell). Three types of histamine receptors are found in the body: H_1, H_2, and H_3.

Did You Know?

Several clinical studies show an association between asthma and rhinitis. People with asthma have some nasal component to their disease.

• H_1-receptors are located on the smooth muscle of the bronchi, veins, capillaries, heart and gastrointestinal tract and are involved in allergic reactions that cause rhinitis. Activation of H_1-receptors causes bronchoconstriction, vasodilation, constriction of the intestinal smooth muscle, itching, and pain.

• H_2-receptors are located on the brain, stomach, heart and blood vessels. Activation of these receptors causes an increase in gastric acid production in the stomach, vasodilation (lowers blood pressure), and relaxation of smooth muscle. These receptors are not primarily involved in allergic reactions, and drugs that bind to these receptors are used for the treatment of ulcers.

• H_3-receptors are presynaptic receptors located on histamine-releasing cells which upon stimulation inhibit histamine release.

Drugs used to treat allergic rhinitis are classified into:

1. Antihistamines
2. α-adrenergic agonists
3. topical corticosteroids
4. mast cell stabilizers

Did You Know?

In 2005, the *Journal of Allergy and Clinical Immunology* found that 54 percent of people in the United States are allergic to at least one of 10 common allergens. The most common allergic reactions were to dust mites, rye grass, ragweed, and cockroaches. Men are more likely than women to have allergies.

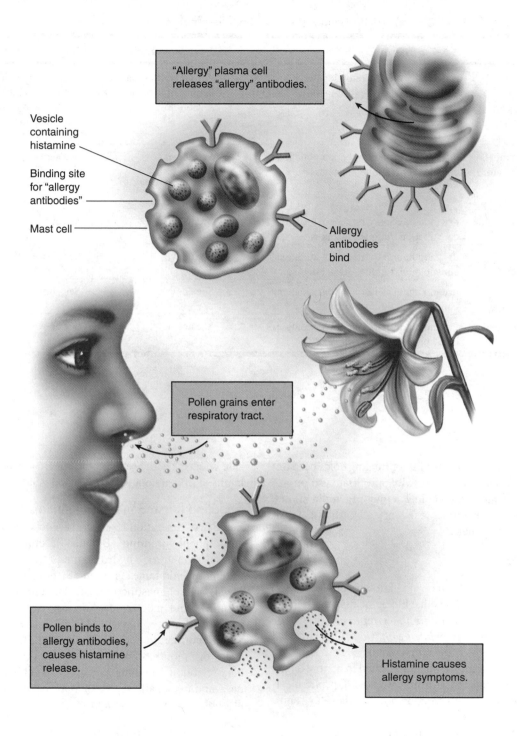

FIGURE 15–5   Development of allergic rhinitis.

TABLE 15–5   First-Generation Antihistamines (treatment of allergic rhinitis)

Drug Name	Adverse Effects	Drug Interactions	Patient Instructions
Dipheniramine (Benadryl) 25 mg tabs are OTC	dry mouth, urinary retention, sedation, constipation, fatique, dizziness	Alcohol with sedating antihistamines increases sedation (for all drugs)	Take with food if G.I. upset. If dry mouth, drink plenty of water and avoid alcohol-containing mouthrinses (for all drugs)
Chlorpheniramine (Chlor-Trimeton) 4 mg , 8 mg ext-rel, 12 mg tabs are OTC	dry mouth, urinary retention, sedation, constipation, fatique, dizziness	See above	See above
Promethazine (Phenergan)	dry mouth, urinary retention, sedation, constipation, fatique, dizziness	See above	See above
Hydroxyzine HCl (Atarax) OTC	dry mouth, urinary retention, sedation, constipation, fatique, dizziness	See above	See above
Clemastine (Tavist) OTC	dry mouth, urinary retention, sedation, constipation, fatique, dizziness	See above	See above
Cyproheptadine (Periactin)	dry mouth, urinary retention, sedation, constipation, fatique, dizziness	See above	See above

Antibiotics are not useful for treating colds because they kill bacteria, not viruses. Inappropriate use of antibiotics for the common cold is a major factor in allowing bacteria to become resistant to antibiotics that previously killed them.

Antihistamines

Histamine by itself has no known clinical use. **Antihistamines** are drugs that block the histamine (H_1)-receptors and thus *eliminate the symptoms (sneezing, itching, rhinorrhea) associated with rhinitis* but are ineffective in treating the common cold.

Antihistamines are contraindicated in narrow-angle glaucoma, prostatic hypertrophy, stenosing peptic ulcer disease, and bladder obstruction because they have anticholinergic properties.

H_1-receptor blockers are used to treat allergic reactions (allergic rhinitis) and motion sickness. Since they are not selective to the bronchioles, these drugs will bind to the receptors on other organs, producing many adverse side effects. There are two types of H_1-receptor antihistamines: first generation and second generation.

Sedating (First-Generation) Antihistamines

Some first-generation H_1-receptor blockers (Table 15–5) are diphenhydramine (Benadryl), chlorpheniramine (Chlor-Trimeton), hydroxyzine (Atarax, Vistaril), dexchlorpheniramine (Prolarmine), promethazine (Phenergan), and clemastine (Tavist). Dimenhydrinate (Dramamine) and meclizine (Antivert) are used to treat motion sickness or vertigo. Most adverse effects are due to anticholinergic activity. As a result, the drugs may cause dry mouth, blurred vision, tachycardia, and urinary retention. The most common side effect is drowsiness and/or sedation, which may be enhanced with alcohol, sedatives, or tranquilizers.

Nonsedating Antihistamines

Second-generation H_1-receptor blockers (Table 15–6) are fexofenadine (Allegra), cetirizine (Zyrtec) and loratadine (Claritin). Terfenadine (Seldane) and astemizole (His-

TABLE 15–6 Second-Generation Antihistamines

Drug Name	Adverse Effects	Drug Interactions	Patient Instructions
Cetrizine (Zyrtec)	Headache, dry mouth, dry nose and throat	No clinically significant interactions	Do not use in combination with other antihistamines
Fexofenadine (Allegra)	Headache, dry mouth, dry nose and throat	Decreased blood levels with antacids	Drug is well tolerated with few side effects
Loratadine (Claritin)	Headache, dry mouth, dry nose and throat	No clinically significant interactions	Take on empty stomach Do not use in combination with other antihistamines

manal) were taken off the market in 1999 because of the development of lethal cardiac arrhythmias. Second-generation H_1-receptor blockers do not cross the blood–brain barrier and thus cause less sedation than first-generation agents.

Intranasal Antihistamines

The antihistamines mentioned above are all given orally. Azelastine (Astelin) is an antihistmine that is applied intranasally (sprays in the nose) for the treatment of symptoms of allergic rhinitis.

α-Adrenoceptor Agonists (Nasal Decongestants)

α_1-Adrenoceptor agonists act as *nasal decongestants by constricting blood vessels in the nasal mucosa,* as well as other blood vessels throughout the body. Vasoconstriction reduces the blood supply to the nose and decreases edema.

OTC drugs include oxymetazoline (Afrin), and phenylephrine (Neo-Synephrine, Sinex). These drugs have a rapid onset of action. However, after 3–5 days of these drugs a rebound congestion occurs and may be worse than before with damage to the mucosa and severe nasal obstruction.

Since they stimulate α-adrenergic receptors causing vasodilation, they should not be used or used with caution in patients with hypertension, hyperthyroidism, diabetes mellitus, cardiovascular disease, glaucoma, urinary obstruction or if taking a beta-blocker drug or monoamine oxidase inhibitor (MAOI) for depression. Other adverse side effects include nervousness, tremor,

insomnia, dizziness and chronic mucosal inflammation (after prolonged use).

Pseudoephedrine (Sudafed) is a systemic nasal decongestion available in either tablets or in a syrup form. It is also found in anticough syrup mixtures. Since it is a sympathomimetic caution should be used in hypertensive patients.

Topical (Intranasal) Corticosteroids

Topical (intranasal) corticosteroids—which include beclomethasone (Beconase, Vancenase), mometasone (Nasonex), fluticasone (Flonase), budesonide (Rhinocort), and flunisolide (Nasalide)—reduce the inflammation. Intranasal corticosteroids are the most effective drugs for relieving symptoms of sneezing, itching, congestion, and rhinorrhea. They are administered as nasal sprays to reduce systemic absorption and adverse side effects; however, there are concerns related to diminished growth in children. Some adverse side effects include nasal irritation, burning, sneezing, sore throat, and headache. Oral antihistamines are an alternative in patients who cannot tolerate or do not want to use corticosteroids.

Guidelines for Patients Taking Antihistamines (Diphenhydramine/Benadryl)

- Anticholinergic side effects (e.g, dry mouth) are frequently seen
- Consider home fluoride applications
- Monitor patients for caries
- Stress meticulous oral hygiene

Cromolyn and Nedocromil

Cromolyn (Nasalcrom), available over the counter as a nasal spray, and nedocromil (Tiladle) have anti-inflammatory activity and are also used to treat asthma and allergic rhinitis. They are relatively safe drugs that are administered using a spinhaler or nasalmatic device.

Anticholinergic Agents

Ipratropium (Atrovent) is a bronchodilator applied as a nasal spray. It is approved for asthma and for rhinitis, but does not relieve nasal congestion.

DRUGS FOR COUGH

Cough is produced by the cough reflex. The initial stimulus for cough most likely starts in the mucosa from the nose through the branching points in the tracheobronchial tree, where irritation results in bronchoconstriction. Cough receptors in the trachea and bronchioles send nerve information to the cough center in the brain, and the cough reflex is triggered. Stimuli that start a cough include dust, pollen, and other irritants.

Antitussive drugs are used to suppress the cough. Centrally acting drugs suppress cough by depressing the cough center in the brain. This group of medications includes codeine, hydrocodone, hydromorphone, and dextromethorphan.

Codeine, a narcotic, is the gold standard to which other antitussive agents are compared. Due to the risk of respiratory depression, codeine should be used with caution in patients with pulmonary diseases such as asthma.

Dextromethorphan is a nonnarcotic agent that does not possess the same adverse effects as codeine, including low respiratory depression. Dextromethorphan should not be taken with antidepressants called monoamine oxidase inhibitors (MAOIs).

These drugs are available in various liquid cough preparations that include other agents. In the United States, cough syrups that contain codeine and hydrocodone are classified as Schedule V controlled substances and require a prescription.

Benzonatate (Tessalon), a nonnarcotic agent, is an orally administered drug that reduces the activity of peripheral cough receptors. Respiratory depression is not inhibited at recommended doses.

Expectorants

Expectorants stimulate the production of a watery, less viscous mucous. Guaifenesin is added to most oral nonprescription preparations and works by irritating the gastric mucosa, which stimulates respiratory secretions. It is a safe medication with few adverse effects.

DENTAL HYGIENE NOTES

Once it is determined that a patient has asthma, it is important to know if the patient has had recent symptoms, what therapy he/she is taking, and the date of the last severe attack. Consultation with the patient's physician may be necessary for severe asthma. If the patient is using an inhaler, it should be used just before the appointment, and it must be available throughout.

When systemic corticosteroids (e.g., prednisone) are taken, endogenous (within the body) production and secretion decrease. The patient's physician should be contacted to determine if any additional therapy is necessary. More than 20 mg a day or 2 mg/kg/d for at least 14 days may alter the patient's immunity. This should be taken into account when scheduling invasive procedures. Most routine dental procedures do not require supplemental steroids. However, patients undergoing extensive dental treatment (e.g., extraction, surgery) may need to increase the steroid dose the morning of the appointment. Consult with the patient's physician.

Aspirin and nonsteroidal anti-inflammatory drugs [e.g., naproxen (Aleve), ibuprofen (Advil, Motrin, Nuprin)] may be contraindicated in patients, especially children, with asthma and nasal polyps since these drugs can precipitate or exacerbate an aspirininduced bronchospasm that can be life threatening.

The anticholinergic side effects (e.g., xerostomia) of first-generation antihistamines have implications in dentistry. The dental clinician should educate the patient on how to reduce the symptoms of dry mouth. The patient should be informed to drink plenty of water and avoid alcohol, including alcohol-containing mouthrinses. The

---

Guidelines for Patients Taking a Nonsedating Antihistamine (Loratadine/Claritin)

- **Less incidence of dry mouth than with the sedating antihistamines**
- **Emphasize good oral hygiene**

majority of patients may be on antihistamines frequently during the year, if a seasonal allergic rhinitis is involved.

Many preparations for rhinitis and cough are over the counter. The dental clinician should interview the patient concerning *all* medications, including over-the-counter drugs.

KEY POINTS

- Asthma has both a bronchospasm component and an inflammatory component; drug therapy focuses on both of these processes. In most patients, chronic anti-inflammatory therapy is absolutely necessary.
- Bronchospasm is mediated through the β_2-receptors, located on the bronchioles, and is rapidly relieved by inhaled bronchodilators.
- Asthma-related deaths are significantly lower in patients taking inhaled corticosteroids.
- According to the NAEPP (National Asthma Education and Prevention Program) Expert Panel Report Update, 2002, chronic inhaled corticosteroids use is safe in adults and children, and is recommended as the first-line therapy in adults and children with *persistent* asthma (mild, moderate or severe).
- The addition of a long-acting β_2-agonist [e.g., salmeterol (Serevent), fluticasone propionate/salmeterol xinafoate (Advair Diskus)] to an inhaled corticosteroid is superior to all other combinations, as well as to higher doses of inhaled corticosteroids alone. However, in 2006 the FDA added a "black-box" warning to long-acting β_2-agonists (LABA); these drugs may increase the risk of asthma-related deaths. The FDA states that patients with asthma should not stop taking their LABA medications and should consult their physician with concerns regarding the new labeling changes. The new labels recommend Serevent and Advair not be the first medicine used to treat asthma, and should only be added to the treatment plan for patients whose symptoms are not controlled on other asthma drugs such as low-to-medium inhaled corticosteroids.
- For quick relief of a bronchospasm and its accompanying acute symptoms, including cough and wheezing, a short-acting β_2-selective agonist (e.g., albuterol) is the drug of choice.

- Aspirin and other nonsteroidals may be contraindicated in patients with asthma.
- Moderate/severe asthma is controlled with an inhaled corticosteroid plus a long-acting β_2-agonist.
- Brush teeth and rinse mouth after each use of a corticosteroid inhaler to help prevent Candida infection.
- Smoking cessation is a critical step in the management of COPD, and is encouraged to be done by the dental office.
- Many dental patients are taking OTC antihistamines which may cause xerostomia due to its anticholinergic effects.
- Second-generation antihistamines are not sedating and cause less xerostomia.
- Antitussives and expectorants are used to control coughs.

BOARD REVIEW QUESTIONS

1. After which of the following drugs used to treat asthma should the dental hygienist instruct the patient to rinse the mouth? (p. 277)
   a. Ipratropium
   b. Cromolyn sodium
   c. Beclomethasone
   d. Theophylline

2. Which of the following drugs *may be* contraindicated in asthmatics? (p. 290)
   a. Aspirin
   b. Acetaminophen
   c. Vitamin C
   d. Folic acid

3. Which of the following drugs is the drug of choice for the *quick relief* of bronchospasm? (pp. 280, 283)
   a. Albuterol
   b. Ipratropium
   c. Hydrocortisone
   d. Salmeterol

4. Which of the following drugs is classified as a β_2-agonist bronchodilator? (p. 280)
   a. Metaprotenol
   b. Ipratropium
   c. Hydrocortisone
   d. Montelukast

5. Which of the following drugs is used to control mild persistent asthma? (pp. 275, 277, 279)
   a. Albuterol
   b. Ipratropium
   c. Inhaled beclomethasone
   d. Salmeterol

6. Which of the following antihistamines has anticholinergic effects? (p. 288)
   a. Loratadine
   b. Fexofenadine
   c. Diphenhydramine
   d. Azelastine

7. Which of the following drugs is preferred for long-term control of asthma? (p. 277)
   a. β_1-receptor agonists
   b. β_2-receptor agonists
   c. Inhaled corticosteroids
   d. Oral corticosteroids

8. Which of the following adverse effects occurs with antihistamines? (p. 288)
   a. Dry mouth
   b. Increased salivation
   c. Dry skin
   d. Moist skin

9. Which of the following terms defines "suppressing a cough"? (p. 290)
   a. Expectorant
   b. Antitussive
   c. Antihistamine
   d. Antiasthma

10. Which of the following types of agents are nasal decongestants? (p. 289)
    a. β_1-receptor agonists
    b. β_2-receptor blockers
    c. α_1-receptor agonists
    d. α_2-receptor blockers

SELECTED REFERENCES

American Family Physician. Diagnosis and management of allergic rhinitis. Monograph No. 3. 2001.

Bateman, E. D., H. A. Boushey, J. Bousquet et al., 2004. GOAL Investigators (Group Gaining Optimal Asthma ControL) study. *Am J Respir Crit Care Med.* 170:836–844.

Guidelines for the Diagnosis and Management of Asthma, Expert Panel Report 2. 1997. NIH publication.

Guidelines for the Diagnosis and Management of Asthma, Expert Panel Report: Update on Special Topics. 2002. NIH publication.

Mintz, M. 2004. Asthma Update: Part II, Medical Management. *Am Fam Physician* 70:1061–1066.

National Guideline Clearinghouse (NGC). www.guideline.gov. Agency for Healthcare Research and Quality.

Ostrom, N. K. Asthma management: Proper uses of pharmacotherapy. *U.S. Pharmacist* 2001;26(12):53–64.

Wheeler, P. W., and S. F. Wheeler, 2005. Vasomotor rhinitis. *Am Fam Physician* 72:1057–1062.

WEB SITES

www.aafp.org
www.niaid.nih.gov/factsheets/cold.htm
www.uspharmacist.com
www.medscape.com
www.aafp.org

QUICK DRUG GUIDE

Long-Term Control of Asthma

Corticosteroids (Inhaled): for Inflammation

- Beclomethasone (QVAR)
- Budesonide (Pulmicort)
- Flunisolide (Aerobid)
- Fluticasone (Flovent, Advir)
- Mometasone (Asmanex)
- Triamcinolone (Azmacort)

Selective β$_2$-Agonists (Long-Acting): Bronchodilator

- Salmeterol (Serevent)
- Formoterol (Foradil)

Methylxanthines

- Theophylline (TheoDur)

Mast Cell Stabilizers

- Cromolyn sodium (Intal)
- Nedocromil (Tilade)

Leukotriene Modifiers

- Zafirlukast (Accolate)
- Montelukast (Singulair)
- Zileuton (Zyflo)

Quick-Relief Medications

Selective β$_2$-Adrenergic (Short-Acting): Bronchodilators (for Bronchospasm)

- Albuterol (Ventolin, Proventil): Drug of choice
- Pirbuterol (Maxair)
- Terbutaline (Brethine)
- Metaproterenol (Alupent)
- Levalbuterol tartrate (Xopenex)

Anticholinergics: Bronchodilators

- Ipratropium bromide (Atrovent)
- Ipratropium bromide and albuterol sulfate (Combivent)
- Tiotropium bromide (Spiriva)

Corticosteroids (Oral) (Anti-Inflammatory)

- Dexamethasone
- Hydrocortisone
- Methylprednisolone
- Prednisolone
- Prednisone

Drugs for Cough and Colds

First-Generation Antihistamines (H$_1$-Receptor Antagonists) (Relief of Allergy Symptoms, Motion Sickness)

- Diphenhydramine (Benadryl)
- Azatadine (Optimine)
- Chlorpheniramine (Chlor-Trimeton)
- Clemastine (Tavist)
- Cyproheptadine (Periactin)
- Dexbrompheniramine (Drixoral)

- Dexchlorpheniramine (Polaramine)
- Hydroxyzine (Atarax)
- Promethazine(Phenergan)
- Triprolidine (Actifed)

Second-Generation/Nonsedating Antihistamines

- Cetrizine (Zyrtec)
- Fexofenadine (Allegra)
- Loratadine (Claritin)

Intranasal Corticosteroids (Treating Allergic Rhinitis)

- Beclomethasone (Vancenase, Beconase)
- Budesonide (Rhinocort)
- Flunisolide (Nasalide)
- Fluticasone (Flonase)
- Mometasone (Nasonex)
- Triamcinolone (Nasacort)

Sympathomimetics (Treating Nasal Congestion Due to Allergic Rhinitis and the Common Cold)

- Epinephrine (Primatene)
- Oxymetazoline (Afrin)
- Phenylephrine (Neo-Synephrine)
- Pseudoephedrine (Sudafed)

Antitussives (Cough)

- Codeine
- Dextromethorphan (many OTC products)

Expectorants

- Guaifenesin (many OTC products)

Chapter 16

Gastrointestinal Drugs

GOAL: To introduce the fundamentals of drug therapy for common abdominal conditions.

EDUCATIONAL OBJECTIVES

After reading this chapter, the reader should be able to:

1. Describe the current theory of the etiology of peptic ulcer disease.
2. Explain the differences in treatment between peptic ulcer disease and gastroesophageal reflux disease (GERD).
3. Discuss any contraindications or precautions in dental patients with gastrointestinal disorders.
4. Discuss the pharmacologic therapy for GERD.
5. Discuss the treatments for constipation and diarrhea.

KEY TERMS

Gastrointestinal tract
Peptic ulcer disease
Helicobacter pylori
GERD

INTRODUCTION

The **gastrointestinal (G.I.) tract** comprises the stomach and the intestines. The first part of the small intestine closest to the stomach, where most absorption occurs, is called the duodenum and the large intestine is called the colon. This chapter will review the drugs that act on the gastrointestinal tract. The following conditions will be reviewed: peptic ulcer disease (PUD), gastroesophageal reflux disease (GERD), inflammatory bowel disease, constipation, diarrhea, and emesis (vomiting).

The G.I. tract is an interesting part of the body as far as drug intake is concerned. The G.I. tract is the major route for absorption into the systemic circulation of drugs taken orally. Many drugs affect the G.I. tract or its mucosal lining; for instance, salicylates (e.g., aspirin) and other nonsteroidal anti-inflammatory drugs directly affect the mucosal lining of the stomach and may cause bleeding. On the other hand, some drugs act locally and affect the G.I. tract beneficially. Antacids, for example, act locally in the stomach and duodenum to neutralize gastric acid.

GASTROINTESTINAL ACID-PEPTIC DISORDERS

Peptic-Ulcer Disease

Peptic-ulcer disease (PUD) is a general term describing a group of acid-peptic disorders of the upper G.I. tract, primarily the esophagus, stomach, and duodenum. A peptic ulcer is defined as a circumscribed loss of tissue or break that occurs in the G.I. mucosa extending through the smooth muscle that lines the G.I. tract. It occurs when there is an imbalance between gastric acid and pepsin and mucosal defense factors, including prostaglandins, which increases the production of gastric mucus and reduces the formation of gastric acid. An ulcer in the stomach is called a gastric ulcer (G.U.), a duodenal ulcer (D.U.) occurs in the duodenum; and an ulcer in the esophagus is called an esophageal ulcer (Figure 16–1). An ulcer can occur anywhere along the G.I. tract where parts of the mucosa from the tract are exposed to gastric acid and pepsin from the stomach.

Did You Know?

On average, the stomach produces two liters of hydrochloric acid daily.

The original theory of the etiology of ulcers involved excessive production and secretion of gastric juice (hydrochloric acid + pepsin) to which the deeper muscle layers of the G.I. tract are exposed. Gastric juices in the stomach are produced by either physiologic means (e.g., smell, see, and taste of food) or through the central nervous system, where the vagus nerve is stimulated. Histamine, a substance found in highest concentrations in skin, lungs, and G.I. mucosa, is found inside mast cells in the tissue and is responsible for stimulating the production of gastric juices in the stomach. It is the acidic gastric juices that cause the ulcer in the mucosa and breakdown of the protective barrier lining of the duodenum.

Thus, duodenal ulcers are due to the hypersecretion of acid, and gastric ulcers are due to a decrease in the protective lining of the stomach with a decrease in mucosal resistance and not associated with increased acid secretion.

Currently, however, excessive acid production is thought to be a secondary cause while the primary cause is due to a bacterial infection. Research has found that *Helicobacter pylori (H. pylori) is the bacterium that causes approximately 90 percent of duodenal and 80 percent of gastric ulcers.* A blood test can tell if an individual is positive for *H. pylori*. This gram-negative microorganism resides in the mucus layer overlying the gastric epithelium of infected individuals, where it damages the G.I. mucosa via releasing enzymes that degrade gastric cells and altering the inflammatory response, which may interfere with healing.

Besides *H. pylori*, PUD can usually be associated with the use of nonsteroidal anti-inflammatory drugs (NSAIDs), such as aspirin and ibuprofen, and corticosteroids which affect the mucosal defenses. Nonsteroidal anti-inflammatory drugs inhibit both forms of cyclo-oxygenase enzymes, resulting in a nonselective inhibition of COX-1, which is responsible for protecting the G.I. mucosa and COX-2, which may mediate the inflammatory response. Other risk factors are environment, cigarette smoking, alcohol consumption, caffeine, and genetics.

A duodenal ulcer is 5 to 10 times more common than a gastric ulcer. The most common symptom of PUD is epigastric pain which is more frequent at night, not in the morning when gastric secretion is the lowest, which will usually awaken the individual. Epigastric pain is usually what brings a patient to the physician. Food or antacids usually relieve the pain and the individual has a

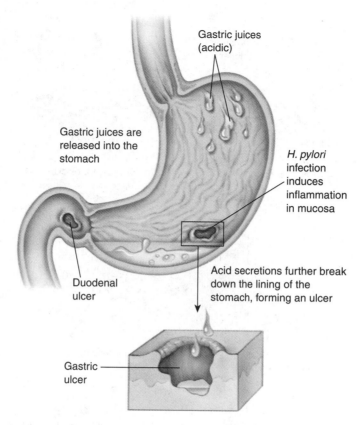

FIGURE 16-1   Mechanism of peptic ulcer formation.

feeling of being hungry. These ulcers tend to recur many times a year. Heartburn, belching, and bloating are also common symptoms. A differential diagnosis must be made between D.U. and indigestion, which has similar symptoms. A thorough patient history will determine this.

Nausea, vomiting, and weight loss is more commonly seen in gastric ulcers than duodenal ulcers. Eating usually causes pain, so that the individual does not eat and will lose weight.

Did You Know?

In 1983, Dr. J. Robin Warren and Dr. Barry Marshall reported finding a new kind of bacteria in the stomachs of people with gastritis. They hypothesized that peptic ulcers are generally caused, not by excess acidity or stress, but a bacterial infection. In 2005 they won the Nobel Prize for this work.

Pharmacotherapy

Since it has been found that PUD is primarily caused by a bacterium, therapy has changed over the years to now include antibiotics in the overall drug regimen. Lowering acid production with medications and diet is also a key outcome. Eating small, frequent meals will keep acid levels from reaching maximum levels.

There are five main types of medications used to treat PUD: antacids, antihistamines, proton pump inhibitors, mucosal defense drugs, and antibiotics (Figure 16–2) (Table 16–1). *Antacids* are used primarily for symptomatic relief of gastric pain, especially heartburn, and will not really promote healing of the ulcer. *Antihistamines (Histamine$_2$-receptor antagonists;* H$_2$RAs) will provide symptomatic relief of pain and promote healing of the ulcer. *Mucosal defense drugs* have no effect on gastric acid secretion. *Proton pump inhibitors* will provide quick pain relief and accelerated healing of the ulcer. *Antibiotics* are needed to eradicate the *H. pylori* infec-

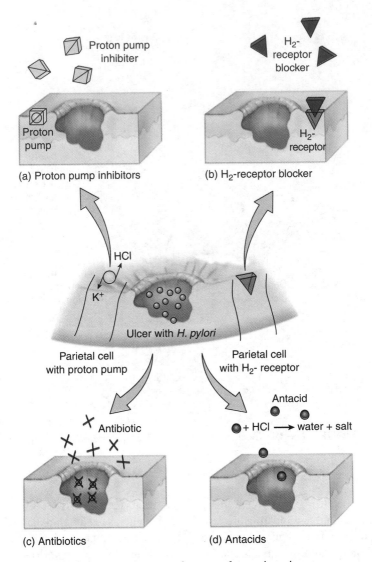

FIGURE 16–2   Mechanism of action of anti-ulcer drugs.

tion. Additionally, the patient should, if possible, stop smoking, alcohol consumption (or reduce the amount), caffeine, and use of nonsteroidal anti-inflammatory drugs.

Conventional doses of histamine$_2$-receptors, antacids, or mucosal defense drugs heal approximately 90 percent of D.U. within 8 weeks, while increasing acid suppression with higher H$_2$RA doses or proton pump inhibitors achieves healing rates within 4 weeks. Little data has been established for the efficacy of these drugs in the treatment of G.U. NSAID-induced ulcers respond to all of the drugs used for PUD, although healing is more rapid when the NSAID is discontinued.

Antacids   Antacids are primarily used in the treatment of dyspepsia (indigestion or heartburn) and to a lesser extent as adjunctive therapy for duodenal ulcers to neutralize acids. Antacids are basic salts that dissolve in acid gastric secretions and neutralize some but not all gastric hydrochloric acid, and have a greater effect of increasing the pH in the duodenum than in the stomach. Antacids neutralize or reduce the acidity of gastric juices, but they do not affect the rate or amount of gastric acid secretion by the stomach cells and do not prevent ulcer recurrence. Rather, antacids are usually used to relieve occasional duodenal ulcer symptoms on an as-need basis by the patient and systemic absorption and adverse effects.

Table 16-1 Drugs Used in the Treatment of Acid-Peptic Disorders (APD) and GERD

Drug Name	Mechanism/Indication	Adverse Effects	Drug Interactions	Patient Instructions
Antacids	Relief of epigastric (stomach) pain; indigestion; neutralizes gastric acid juices secreted in the stomach by increasing the pH of gastric secretions; primarily used in GERD (heartburn); only bismuth is recommended for duodenal ulcers	See individual drugs	• Aluminum, calcium, magnesium, and bismuth antacids form a complex with tetracyclines and fluoroquinolones (e.g., ciprofloxacin) which decrease the absorption of the tetracyclines and fluoroquinolones. • Reduced gastrointestinal absorption of: ketoconazole, Digoxin, Isoniazid (aluminum-containing antacids)	Do not take with tetracyclines or fluoroquinolones—space 2 hours between dosing
Calcium carbonate (Tums, Titralac, Maalox chewable tabs, Gaviscon)	• Preferred in the elderly (for osteoporosis risk) • Best for heartburn/indigestion (GERD); rapid onset of action and a prolonged effect	Hypercalemia (increase blood calcium)	See above	See above
Bismuth subsalicylate (Pepto-Bismol)	Best for ulcers because shown to effective against *H. pylori*	Long-term use increases risk for bismuth absorption, causing neurotoxicity (nervous system problems)	See above	See above
Magnesium hydroxide (Milk of Magnesia)	Best for GERD	Diarrhea; caution in patients with renal disease	See above	See above
Aluminum/magnesium hydroxide/simethicone (Maalox, Gelusil liquid, Mylanta liquid)	Best for GERD	Diarrhea, constipation	See above	See above
Calcium carbonate and magnesium hydroxide (Rolaids)	Best for GERD	Diarrhea	See above	See above
Sodium bicarbonate/alginic acid combination (Gaviscon extra strength tabs)	Foaming actions are good for relieving symptoms of GERD only—not indicated for PUD.		See above	Patient must take product in an uprightposition with a full glass of water.

(continued)

Drug	Uses	Side Effects	Drug Interactions	Comments
H₂-Receptor Antagonists	• Selectively blocks histamine at the histamine receptor; all H₂-receptors antagonists act equally—cost is the only deciding factor on which drug to use. • Available over-the-counter, but in a lower strength than by prescription • The OTC product is only approved for treating heartburn.	Low incidence of serious side effects with a high margin of safety	See individual drugs	Smoking decreases effectiveness of drug. Antacids can be used in conjunction.
Cimetidine (Tagamet)	For treatment of duodenal or gastric ulcer and esophagitis OTC product only approved for heartburn (100 mg tabs)	Dizziness, drowsiness, headache, nausea, diarrhea, agranulocytosis	Metabolized by and affects P450 cytochrome enzyme system; increases serum levels of: theophylline warfarin, phenytoin, carbamazepine, diazepam, lidocaine, propranolol, tricyclic antidepressants, cyclosporine	Monitor for a lot of drug–drug interactions.
Famotidine (Pepcid; Mylanta AR, Pepcid AC)	For duodenal ulcer and heartburn; OTC product only for treating heartburn (10 mg tab)	Dizziness, headache, constipation, diarrhea	Decreased absorption if taken with ketoconazole (Nizoril)	
Nizatidine (Axid)	• Treatment of duodenal or gastric ulcer and heartburn • OTC product only approved for heartburn	Dizziness, headache, constipation, diarrhea	Decreased absorption if taken with ketoconazole (Nizoril)	
Ranitidine (Zantac)	Duodenal and gastric ulcer, esophagitis, heartburn (OTC product only approved for heartburn)	Dizziness, headache, sedation, rash, nausea, constipation, diarrhea	Decreased absorption of ketoconazole Stagger doses if taking antacids with ranitidine	
Proton Pump Inhibitors	Suppress gastric acid secretion by inhibiting the gastric-ATPase enzyme pump	Generally well tolerated—can cause xerostomia	All proton pump inhibitors are metabolized by the P450 cytochrome enzyme system.	Monitor patient for caries, periodontal disease and oral candidiasis. Optimum oral hygiene. Supplemental topical fluoride and drink water is recommended. Avoid alcohol, smoking and depressants, which could aggravate the dry mouth. Smoking decreases effectiveness of the drug.
Omeprazole (Prilosec)	Healing of duodenal ulcers in 4 weeks—use in combination with antibiotics for eradication of *H. pylori*; also for maintenance of erosive esophagitis (GERD) and gastric ulcer	Nausea, headache, diarrhea	Has the most drug interactions. Inhibits metabolism of: Diazepam, warfarin, propranolol, phenytoin, cyclosporine	See above

300

Drug Name	Mechanism/Indication	Adverse Effects	Drug Interactions	Patient Instructions
Lansoprazole (Prevacid)	Duodenal ulcer treatment (in combination with other drugs to eradicate *H. pylori*) and maintenance, and NSAID-induced gastric ulcer and GERD	Nausea, headache, diarrhea	Although metabolized by the liver enzymes and known to inhibit some enzymes, there are no clinically important interactions	Take with food; see above.
Esomeprazole (Nexium)	For *H. pylori* eradication (when used with amoxicillin and clarithromycin); also for erosive esophagitis; gastroesophageal reflux disease (GERD); NSAID (nonsteroidal anti-inflammatory drug) induced ulcers	Abdominal pain, constipation, diarrhea, headache, nausea, vomiting, xerostomia	May decrease absorption of ketoconazole, itraconazole, digoxin, iron and ampicillin	See above
Rabeprazole (Aciphex)	Short-term (up to 4) weeks) treatment of the healing and symptomatic relief of duodenal ulcers; short-term (4 to 8 weeks) treatment in the healing and symptomatic relief of GERD (erosive esophagitis and heartburn)	Headache, abdominal pain, diarrhea, nausea, vomiting, dry mouth	May decrease absorption of ketoconazole, itraconazole, digoxin, iron and ampicillin; otherwise no clinical significant interactions	See above
Prostaglandin supplements Misoprostal (Cytotec)	Prevention of gastric and duodenal ulcers due to NSAIDs	Abdominal cramps, nausea, vomiting, diarrhea and uterine contractions (contraindicated in pregnant women)	No significant interactions	See above
Protective Barrier Drug Sucralfate (Carfate)	For healing of duodenal ulcers, not gastric ulcers, for GERD	Constipation, diarrhea, nausea, vomiting	Decreases absorption of: lansoprazole, ketoconazole fluoroquinolones tetracyclines	No dental-related instructions.
Prokinetic Drugs Metoclopramide (Reglan)	Dopamine antagonists; Increase lower esophageal sphincter pressure, which minimizes the number of reflux episodes	Abdominal cramping, diarrhea, fatigue, nervousness	Alcohol: increased sedation; decreases absorption of acetaminophen (Tylenol), aspirin and tetracycline	No dental-related instructions

(continued)

Table 16–1 (Continued)

FDA-Approved Antibiotic Combination Treatment Options

Helicobacter pylori **Treatment Regimen (including antibiotics, antihistamines and antacids, PPIs)**

Triple Therapy (2-Week Course)
1. Omeprazole (Prilosec) 40 mg qd OR lansoprazole (Prevacid) 30 mg bid + metronidazole (Flagyl) 500 mg bid or amoxicillin 1 g bid + clarithromycin (Biaxin) 500 mg bid*
2. Ranitidine bismuth citrate (Tritec) 400 mg bid+ clarithromycin 500 mg bid or metronidazole 500 bid + tetracycline 500 mg bid or amoxicillin 1 g bid

Quadruple Therapy (2 Week Course)
1. Bismuth subsalicylate (Pepto Bismol) 525 mg qid daily/2 tabs qid + metronidazole 250 mg qid + tetracycline 500 mg qid + H$_2$-antagonist for 28 days
2. Bismuth subsalicylate 525 mg qid/2 tabs qid + metronidazole 250 mg qid/2 tabs qid + tetracycline 500 mg qid + PPI (proton pump inhibitor) for 14 days

*Lansoprazole, amoxicillin and clarithromycin are available in a daily administration combination pack (Prevpac).
Adapted from: Antibiotic regimen: American College of Gastroenterology Guidelines. *American Journal of Gastroenterology* 1998.93:2330).

The only antacid that is used in the treatment of PUD is bismuth subsalicylate (BSS)(Pepto-Bismol), which functions to suppress *H. pylori* infection by inhibiting bacterial adherence to mucosal cells and damages bacterial cell walls. It is recommended that it be used in conjunction with antibiotics. Thus, bismuth is the antacid of choice in the treatment and maintenance of PUD.

Antihistamines (histamine-receptor antagonists)
H_2-receptor antagonists reduce histamine-stimulated gastric acid secretion by competitively inhibiting H_2-receptors on the parietal cells in the stomach. These agents have a limited effect on gastric acid secretion after food ingestion and are effective in healing ulcers in 6–12 weeks. Four H_2-receptor antagonists currently available by prescription and over the counter (the OTC drugs simply are lower doses): cimetidine (Tagamet), ranitidine (Zantac), famotidine (Pepcid), and nizatidine (Axid). These agents are indicated for the symptomatic relief and healing of ulcers and in alleviating symptoms of duodenal ulcers, gastric ulcers, and gastroesophageal reflux disease (GERD). All four agents are equally effective and are used in conjunction with antibiotics to eradicate *H. pylori* in PUD. H_2-receptor inhibitors should be taken on as-need basis to avoid the development of tolerance. Adverse effects are usually mild and include thrombocytopenia (low blood platelets), headache, diarrhea, and confusion.

Cimetidine (Tagamet) was the first H_2-receptor antagonist introduced and has since become available OTC. Cimetidine is involved with many drug–drug interactions because it inhibits CYP_1A_2 enzymes in the liver (Table 16-1). Cimetidine will decrease gastric pH for 6 hours. It is not the drug of choice for treatment of longer than 6 weeks because of the development of diarrhea, agranulocytosis [also called neutropenia, where there is a reduction in the blood neutrophil (granulocyte—white blood cell) count], which can lead to increased susceptibility to bacterial and fungal infections, and a rebound phenomenon, where new ulcers form.

Proton Pump Inhibitors Proton pump inhibitors (PPI) provide rapid symptomatic relief with accelerating healing of duodenal ulcers and GERD. Unlike H_2-receptor inhibitors, PPIs reduce peak acid output (e.g., food-stimulated acid output) without regard to administration time, although the best time to dose is 30 minutes before breakfast. PPIs achieve almost total suppression of acid secretion because they bind irreversibly to the proton pump in the membrane of the acid-producing cells in the

stomach. To restore acid secretion it is necessary either to synthesize new pumps or activate resting pumps, which takes about 3 to 5 days. The following drugs are PPIs: esomeprazole (Nexium), ilansoprazole (Prevacid), omeprazole (Prilosec), pantoprazole (Protonix), and rabeprazole (Aciphex).

These agents provide long-term and enhanced acid suppression and show high healing rates for PUD. They have been shown to achieve nearly total suppression of acid secretion. The most common adverse effects are headache, skin alterations, diarrhea, xerotomia, and nausea.

All PPIs are highly bound to plasma proteins so there will be displacement of other highly protein bound drugs including phenytoin, diazepam, and warfarin, causing elevated plasma levels. All of the PPIs are metabolized by the cytochrome P450 isoenzyme system. Drug interactions are listed in Table 16–1.

Prostaglandin Supplementation Misoprostal (Cytotec) is a synthetic prostaglandin E_2 agent that inhibits gastric acid secretion and increases gastric mucosal defense. It is indicated for the prevention of nonsteroidal anti-inflammatory drug (NSAID)–induced gastric and duodenal ulcers. This drug should not be used in pregnant women because it causes uterine contractions.

Protective Barrier Drugs Sucralfate (Carafate) is an aluminum hydroxide–sucrose complex that functions to form a protective barrier over the G.I. mucosal lining. It does not alter the pH of gastric juices or inhibit gastric acid secretion, but binds to the gastric mucosa and forms a gel that protects the ulcer from gastric acids. It is indicated for the short-term treatment of duodenal ulcers and for maintenance of healing of a D.U. Its efficacy for symptomatic relief of GERD and gastric ulcers has not been established.

Antibiotics The use of at least two antibiotics combined with an H_2-receptor antagonist or proton pump

---

Guidelines for Patients Taking Omeprazole (Prilosec)

- There are interactions with several drugs including diazepam (Valium) and phenytoin (Dilantin).
- Patients should avoid aspirin and aspirin-containing medications.
- Dry mouth is a side effect.

inhibitor and/or bismuth comprise the recommended regimen for *H. pylori* infection in PUD (Table 16–1). Using antisecretory drugs without antibiotics is not recommended because there is a high rate of ulcer recurrence and complications. Combination therapy provides better outcomes. Remember to instruct the patient to take yogurt or acidophilus gel caps when taking broad-spectrum antibiotics.

A three-drug regimen is recommended (Table 16–1) versus a two-drug regimen because it is more effective in eradicating *H. pylori*. However, there are more adverse effects, drug–drug interaction possibilities, and a lower compliance rate. Antibiotic resistance and incomplete treatment are major reasons for treatment failure. Continued therapy for 14 days has been found to be the most reliable and effective regimen.

Maintenance patients   After the acute disease is under control using antibiotics, antisecretory drugs, and/or bismuth, maintenance therapy is needed. Treatment consists of taking an H_2-receptor antagonist at a lower dosage at bedtime. Even with all of the different therapies, ulcer recurrence is up to 90 percent.

Summary

Treatment of PUD is to relieve ulcer pain, aid in ulcer healing, preventing ulcer recurrence and eliminating complications. Treatment involves changes in lifestyle, such as elimination of alcohol, spicy foods, and caffeine. Use of H_2-receptor antagonists, antacids, or sucralfate will heal the ulcer by 8 weeks. PPIs may be more effective and heal ulcers within 4 weeks. Patients positive for *H. pylori* need to take an antibiotic in addition to an antisecretory drug.

GASTROESOPHAGEAL REFLUX DISEASE (GERD)

Gastroesophageal reflux disease, commonly referred to as **GERD,** is one of the most common chronic conditions of the upper gastrointestinal tract. In GERD there is a reflux or "backing up" of gastric contents from the stomach into the esophagus, which generally occurs in many individuals without causing any complications and damage to the mucosal lining of the esophagus. The most common complaint or symptom is heartburn but the individual may also complain of epigastric pain. Most individuals with heartburn will seek therapy on their own with antacids; however, if the acidic gastric contents stay in contact for prolonged periods of time with the mu-

cosal tissue of the esophagus, a form of GERD called reflux esophagitis will develop, which is characterized by inflammation of the esophagus due to excessive acid reflux. Acid reflux into the oral cavity may cause the development of tooth erosion, particularly on the palatal surfaces of the maxillary incisors, which have the greatest contact with the acid. Esophagitis results from excessive reflux of gastric juices rather than excessive acid secretion in the stomach as seen in peptic ulcer disease. Other complications from GERD are dysphagia (difficulty in swallowing) and esophageal ulcers.

Risk factors for GERD include alcohol, smoking, spicy foods, duodenal ulcers, and some medications such as aspirin and NSAIDs, calcium channel blockers (reduce lower esophageal sphincter tone, allowing the reflux of acids), alednronate (Fosamax; for treatment of osteoporosis), and tetracycline. *Helicobacter pylori* infection does not increase the risk of GERD or reflux esophagitis, and is actually associated with a lower severity of symptoms.

Pharmacotherapy

Besides using pharmaceuticals to treat GERD, the patient must change lifestyle, which may improve the symptoms. Patients should try to lose weight, stop smoking and alcohol consumption, and avoid eating 2–3 hours before bedtime to reduce the amount of acid in the stomach available to reflux. Antacids and most H_2-receptor inhibitors are available without a prescription. Antibiotics are not used to treat GERD. Acid suppression is the cornerstone of medical therapy for GERD patients, regardless of the severity of prescence of complications. Unlike PUD, GERD responds best to profound acid suppression.

Antacids   The duration of action of antacids is short—only about 30 minutes—but if taken 1 to 3 hours after meals and at bedtime, which corresponds to the greatest gastric acid secretion that occurs during a day, the duration of action increases. Antacids are usually used in conjunction with other anti-ulcer medications. If patients with ulcers do not respond to antacids, then other drugs (e.g., antihistamines) should be used.

Adherence is low because:

1. Antacids must be taken frequently, every 2–4 hours, because of this short duration of action, to have a beneficial effect.
2. Antacids generally have a bad taste. Many products have various flavoring agents to mask the bad

taste, and refrigeration of the product may improve the taste.

3. Antacids have many adverse side effects, such as diarrhea, constipation, belching and flatulence (gas), and have many drug interactions.

The substances found in antacids that are responsible for neutralizing stomach acids are sodium bicarbonate, calcium carbonate, bismuth, aluminum salts (hydroxide, phosphate), and magnesium salts (hydroxide, chloride). Simethicone is sometimes added to antacid preparations to reduce gas bubbles that cause bloating and discomfort.

Drug–drug–food Interactions Di- or trivalent ions (Mg^{2+}, Ca^{2+}, Al^{3+}) containing antacids bind to and form an insoluble complex with tetracyclines (tetracycline HCl, minocycline HCl, and doxycycline hyclate) and fluoroquinolone (e.g., Cipro), which will decrease the absorption rate of these antibiotics. Thus, antacids should not be given concurrently with these antibiotics but 1–2 hours before or after taking the antibiotics. Other interactions are listed in Table 16–1.

Antacids with or without alginic acid and nonprescription histamine$_2$-receptor antagonists are appropriate first-line pharmacologic therapy and may provide sufficient acid neutralization/suppression for patients with mild, infrequent GERD symptoms. Because of their rapid onset of action, antacids are useful for quick relief of symptoms.

Alginic acid (which is present in Gaviscon) is not in the true sense an antacid because it does not neutralize acids in the stomach; however, it does form a thick solution of sodium alginate when in contact with gastric acids that floats on the surface of the gastric contents, minimizing the contact of acid with the esophagus. When gastroesophageal reflux occurs, it is the sodium alginate—not the acid—that is refluxed from the stomach to the esophagus, resulting in less esophageal irritation. This product works best when the patient is in an upright position, so it should not be taken at bedtime with a full glass of water. Additionally, low doses of an H$_2$-receptor antagonist can be used.

Sodium bicarbonate is available as baking soda and is combined in many OTC products (e.g., Alka-Seltzer). When taken orally it reacts with acid in the stomach to raise the pH rapidly by forming sodium chloride, carbon dioxide, and water. In patients on a sodium-restricted diet or decreased renal function, sodium bicarbonate should be taken only on a short-term basis because it is systemically absorbed into the bloodstream. Chronic use can cause alkalosis (increase in bicarbonate and pH) or the

"milk-alkali syndrome," which is difficult to diagnose because of its nondescriptive symptoms such as nausea, vomiting, and headache. This syndrome is more likely to occur in individuals who have a high intake of calcium, like pregnant women. It should be used with caution in patients with benign prostatic hypertrophy.

Magnesium hydroxide and aluminum hydroxide (Maalox) are not systemically absorbed and can be used on a long-term basis. The combination minimizes the diarrhea effect produced by the magnesium and the constipating effect produced by the aluminum.

Calcium carbonate (Tums) is a nonsystemic antacid which, when taken on a long-term basis, may cause acid rebound, with more acid being produced. It may also cause kidney stone formation and constipation.

Magnesium hydroxide (Milk of Magnesia)–containing antacids are not systemically absorbed and should be avoided in patients with a history of diarrhea (e.g., irritable bowel syndrome).

H$_2$-receptor Antagonists (H$_2$RAs)

In addition to antacids, H$_2$-receptor antagonists (Table 16–1) are the mainstays in the treatment of GERD to reduce gastric acid secretion in the stomach, reducing the chance for reflux into the esophagus. These agents are indicated for reducing symptoms of GERD and healing mild to moderate esophagitis; however, when used alone complete relief of symptoms and healing are not accomplished. Over-the-counter H$_2$-receptor antagonists generally contain about one-half of the standard prescription doses; otherwise, they are the same. In contrast to antacids, H$_2$-receptor antagonists have a similar onset of action to antacids but a much longer duration of action, up to 12 hours, and may provide nighttime relief. These agents are may be especially useful when taken before eating, when symptoms are anticipated. H$_2$-receptors antagonists are equally effective and should be taken on as-need basis to avoid the development of tolerance.

Guidelines for Patients Taking Antacids

- Patients should not take tetracyclines (doxycycline, minocycline) at the same time; they should take antacids at least 2 hours before other medications.
- Patients with hypertension should avoid sodium-based antacids.

Guidelines for Patients Taking Ranitidine (Zantac)

- Avoid prescribing aspirin and aspirin-containing medications.
- Patients with gastroesophageal reflux may present with oral symptoms, including burning mouth and tooth erosion.
- Recommend reducing acid content in the mouth with sodium bicarbonate mouthrinse.

Pepcid Complete is a nonprescription product containing famotidine, calcium carbonate, and magnesium hydroxide. The addition of the antacids has been shown to shorten the time of onset of action compared to famotidine alone.

When lifestyle changes and nonprescription products fail to relieve symptoms, acid suppression with prescription doses of H₂RAs or PPIs may be necessary (Table 16–1). Prescription H₂RAs, which were the standard of care for GERD for many years, promote healing in mild to moderate cases of esophagitis. Multiple, daily high dosing is required for symptom control, and unlike PUD, once-daily dosing at bedtime is inadequate for GERD.

Proton pump inhibitors provide the most rapid symptom relief and highest percentage of esophageal healing of all agents used in GERD management. They are the drug of choice for patients with frequent daily symptoms, moderate to severe GERD symptoms, patients not responding to H₂RAs, and those with complicated disease, including Barrett's esophagus and esophagitis. In most patients, PPIs relieve symptoms within several days of treatment.

Prokinetic Drugs

Prokinetic drugs are an alternative to standard doses of H₂RAs. The pathogenesis of GERD can be related to defects in esophagogastric motility, poor esophageal clearance, and delayed gastric emptying time. Therefore, it may be possible to promote healing with the use of a prokientic drug. A prokinetic drug is used to increase the force of the contraction of the lower esophageal sphincter, thus decreasing reflux of gastric juices and accelerating gastric emptying. Prokinetic drugs are not indicated for the treatment of PUD. Metoclopramide (Reglan) is a dopamine antagonist that blocks dopamine receptors, lowering esophageal sphincter pressure and increasing

gastric emptying. It is indicated in the symptomatic relief of GERD, but not for esophageal healing.

Summary Treatment Guidelines for PUD and GERD

Recommended therapy for *duodenal ulcers* is: two antibiotics + H₂ antagonist + antacids PRN (as needed)

Recommended therapy for *GERD* is: lifestyle modifications (e.g., change in diet, eliminating foods that aggravate GERD, losing weight, sleeping with an elevated pillow, and exercise). The first-line drug therapy is antacids and a nonprescription H₂RA such as famotidine (Pepcid), or a PPI such as omeprazole (Prilosec). Given the chronic nature of GERD and the high recurrence rates if acid suppressive therapy is discontinued, long-term maintenance therapy is appropriate and indicated for most patients.

IRRITABLE BOWEL SYNDROME

Irritable bowel syndrome (IBS) is a nonspecific disease with symptoms lasting at least 12 weeks consisting of diarrhea, constipation, and abdominal pain, which is the most common symptom. Diseases that are associated with IBS include fibromyalgia or chronic fatigue syndrome, sleep disturbance, migraines, and chronic stress.

Irritable bowel syndrome, according to the Rome Criteria, is diagnosed when there are at least 12 weeks of abdominal pain or discomfort that is relieved by defecation and/or onset is associated with change in the form of stool. Onset of IBS is usually in adolescence or early adulthood.

Since the etiology is not fully understood and the symptoms can be vague, at times, treatment of IBS is a challenge. A physical examination must be performed to rule out other conditions. Constipation is a side effect of certain medications including antacids, nonsteroidal anti-inflammatory agents, calcium channel blockers (verapamil), iron, and antipsychotics and antidepressants. Diarrhea is a side effect of certain medications, including antacids, antibiotics (e.g., tetracyclines, clindamycin, ampicillin, amoxicillin), and antilipemic agents (gemfibrozil). Psychological issues must be addressed. Dietary modifications should be made to avoid fatty foods, gas-producing foods such as beans, alcohol, and caffeine.

Pharmacotherapy

Pharmacologic treatment utilizes any of the following drugs:

1. Antidiarrheal agents: loperamide (Imodium), cholestyramine (use in patients with high cholesterol levels)

2. Antispasmodic agents: An anticholinergic drug is used to treat the pain and bloating (abdominal distention) caused by IBS. These drugs work by suppressing intestinal contractions after meals or during stressful periods. The following are anticholinergics/antispasmodics: dicyclomine (Bentyl), hyoscyamine (Levsin), donnatal tablets or elixir (phenobarbital, hyoscyamine, atropine, and scopolamine), chlordiazepoxide/clidinium bromide (Librax)

3. Anticonstipation agents: osmotic laxative (lactulose, polyethylene glycol), or other laxatives and increase dietary fiber intake either with foods or supplements which will act as bulk-forming agents.

NAUSEA AND VOMITING

Emesis (vomiting) is defined as the expulsion of gastric contents through the mouth, whereas nausea is the feeling in the throat that vomiting may happen. Numerous causes of nausea and vomiting include gastrointestinal, cardiovascular (HF: heart failure: MI: myocardial infarction or heart attack; psychogenic causes (self-induced as seen in bulimia); drug-induced (opiates, antibiotics, radiation therapy); pregnancy; changes in position; and many other causes.

Chronic vomiting may cause the enamel on the palatal surfaces of the maxillary incisors to erode, creating a "shiny, smooth" surface (Figure 16–3). A sodium bicarbonate mouthrinse may be recommended to reduce acid content.

Most cases of nausea and vomiting are self-limiting. Treatment is aimed at preventing or eliminating the nausea and vomiting to prevent dehydration. There are many OTC and prescription antiemetic drugs. Some preparations are listed in Table 16–2.

CONSTIPATION

Constipation is defined as a reduced number of bowel movements and frequently occurs with straining without effect. The patient may complain of abdominal distention or pain. Several risk factors associated with constipation include: narcotics (opiates), anticholinergics, calcium channel blockers (especially verapamil), aluminum-containing antacids, and iron products.

Pharmacotherapy

The causative drug can be discontinued, changed to another drug without constipating side effects or if possi-

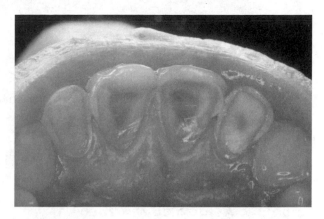

FIGURE 16–3   Erosion of palatal surfaces of maxillary teeth due to chronic vomiting.

ble, the dose may be reduced. Chronic constipation can be managed with increasing dietary fiber intake to 20–30 grams/day with an increase in fluid intake. Prune juice contains a substance which helps with constipation.

There are different types of laxatives available:

1. Bulk-forming agents that soften the stool: methylcellulose, polycarbophil, psyllium
2. Emollients that soften the stool: docusate (sodium, calcium, potassium), lactulose, sorbitol, and mineral oil
3. Drugs that cause soft or semisoft stool: disacodyl, senna, magnesium sulfate
4. Drugs that cause watery evacuation: magnesium (citrate, hydroxide, sulfate)

DIARRHEA

Diarrhea is a term used to describe watery or loose stools, or excessive stool frequency or amount. Loose or watery stools may be a sign of pathology. Causes may be contaminated food or water, infection (bacterial, viral, protozoa), disease (malabsorption syndrome, inflammatory

Table 16–2   Common Antiemetics

- Meclizine (Antivert)
- Promethazine (Phenergan)
- Metoclopramide (Reglan)
- Trimethobenzamide (Tigan)
- Prochlorperazine (Compazine)
- Ondansetron (Zofran)

bowel disease such as ulcerative colitis or Crohn's disease), immunocompromised individuals (HIV/AIDS), drugs, irritable bowel syndrome, colon carcinoma, or traveler's diarrhea.

Acute diarrhea lasting less than 3 weeks is most often due to bacterial or viral infection, food poisoning, or drugs. The most common bacteria involved in food poisoning are *Salmonella* and *Escherichia coli* (*E. coli*). Chronic diarrhea lasting more than 4 weeks can lead to dehydration and loss of important minerals and electrolytes.

Antibiotic-Associated Diarrhea

Diarrhea due to antibiotic use, especially broad-spectrum antibiotics (e.g., tetracyclines, amoxicillin) (Table 16–3) is usually caused either by a direct irritant of the drug on the gastrointestinal mucosa (such as tetracycline) or the disruption of normal bowel flora (bacteria that normally live in the gut) leading to the overgrowth of a bacterium called *Clostridium difficle* which releases toxins that cause inflammation and damage to the intestinal mucosa, resulting in diarrhea.

If diarrhea that results from taking antibiotics is very severe and is watery with exudative mucosal plaque, then it is called pseudomembranous colitis. Pseudomembranous colitis usually is the major cause of hospitalized (noscomial) diarrhea.

The offending drug should be discontinued, if possible, even if diarrhea is a common adverse side effect. Antidiarrhea medication should not be given because it is necessary for the bacterial toxins to be eliminated from the body and giving antidiarrhea medications will not allow this. Yogurt, which has *Lactobacillus acidophilus* culture or acidophilus, is given to replace bowel flora.

Besides antibiotics, other drugs that can cause diarrhea include diuretics, histamine$_2$-receptor inhibitors, digoxin, and nonsteroidal anti-inflammatory drugs.

Treatment of Acute Diarrhea (Other than Antibiotic-Associated Diarrhea)

Once infection, carcinoma, or antibiotic-induced diarrhea is ruled out, acute diarrhea can be treated with many different types of medications (Table 16–4), keeping in mind to prevent dehydration:

1. Loperamide (Imodium), which is available without a prescription, slows down G.I. motility with few side effects. If diarrhea does not stop within 2 days, then further medical evaluation is needed.
2. Diphenoxylate hydrochloride and atropine sulfate (Lomotil) are available without a prescription. Diphenoxylate is a synthetic opiate, and atropine is an anticholinergic drug which slows down G.I. motility. This drug can cause dry mouth, blurred vision, urinary retention, tachycardia, and drowsiness. Alcohol and other CNS depressants should be avoided when taking this drug.
3. Tincture of opium (Paregoric) is a liquid narcotic that is used when other antimotility drugs have failed. This drug is also used in AIDS-associated diarrhea.
4. Bismuth subsalicylate (Peto-Bismol, Kaopectate) is available without a prescription. It has an antisecretory effect on the colon. Antidiarrheal properties make it good in preventing traveler's diarrhea.
5. Yogurt or acidophilus tablets can be taken before the antibiotic is given to re-establish the normal bacterial flora of the intestinal tract. However, with tetracycline HCl, yogurt (a dairy product) should be taken 1 hour before the antibiotic because insoluble complexes are formed which would decrease the absorption of tetracycline. Yogurt can be taken concurrently with doxycycline and minocycline.
6. Octreotide acetate (Sandostatin) is used for refractory diarrhea when all other medications have

Table 16–3 Common Antibiotics Causing Antibiotic-Associated Diarrhea

- Clindamycin
- Amoxicillin
- Ampicillin
- Cephalosporins
- Tetracyclines

Table 16–4 Therapy for Nonspecific Diarrhea

- Ioperamide (Imodium)
- Diphenoxylate hydrochloride and atropine sulfate (Lomotil)
- Tincture of opium (Paregoric - Rx)
- Bismuth subsalicylate (Peto-Bismol; Kaopectate)
- Yogurt or acidophilus tablets
- Octreotide acetate (Sandostatin)

failed to relieve the diarrhea. It is administered subcutaneously or intravenously, and is very expensive.

INFLAMMATORY BOWEL DISEASE: ULCERATIVE COLITIS

Ulcerative colitis is a chronic disease resulting in inflammation of the mucosa of the colon and rectum with an un-known etiology. Common symptoms of ulcerative colitis include bloody diarrhea and abdominal pain. Differential diagnoses are irritable bowel syndrome, colon polyps, and colon cancer.

Pharmacologic treatment of ulcerative colitis is to reduce the inflammation of the tissues of the colon by using anti-inflammatory drugs which inhibit leukotriene and prostaglandin synthesis (Table 16–5). The type of

Table 16–5 Drugs Used in the Treatment of Ulcerative Colitis

Drug Name	Adverse Effects	Drug–Drug Interactions	Dental Notes
5-Aminosalicylates (5-ASA)			
Sulfasalzine (Azulfidine)	**Dose-dependent:** Nausea, vomiting, headache, hair alopecia (loss of hair; baldness), anorexia **Non–dose-dependent:** Rash, anemia, pancreatitis, hepatotoxicity (liver disease), blood disorders (agranulocytosis), male infertility	Increased photosensitivity when taken with tetracycline	Avoid antibiotics that could aggravate colitis
Mesalamine (Asacol-tabs, Rowasa—enema, Pentasa—caps)	Newer non–sulfa-containing aminosalicylate reduces incidence of adverse effects; expensive	No significant drug-drug interactions	Monitor for oral ulcerations, xerostomia and candidiasis. Avoid antibiotics that could aggravate colitis
Olsalzine (Dipentum)	Diarrhea, skin rash	No significant drug-drug interactions	Avoid antibiotics that could aggravate colitis
Glucocorticoids			
Prednisone	Glucose intolerance (hyperglycemia), spread of herpes infection, cataracts, peptic ulcers, osteoporosis, adrenal suppression, psychosis, masks infections	Increase glucose blood levels, thus increase dosage of antidiabetic drugs; decrease salicylate serum levels The following drugs increase metabolism of glucocorticoids: phenytoin, phenobarbital, rifampin.	Consult with patient's physician to determine the need to change dosage. Routine dental procedures including periodontal scaling and root planing does not need to have increased dosage.
Immunosuppressives			
Cyclosporine (Neoral, Sandimmune)	Use in refractory cases of ulcerative colitis and Crohn's disease, hypertension, gingival overgrowth, nausea, vomiting, xerostomia parathesias (numbness, tingling), nephrotoxicity (kidney), hepatotoxicity (liver), hypertrichosis (excessive hair growth in areas that usually don't have hair), seizures	Increased effect of anti-cholinergic drugs	Gingival overgrowth occurs; maintain periodontal health

drug used depends on the severity of the condition and where in the G.I. tract the drug is released (e.g., colon, distal ileum, or jejunum). For a mild form of the disease, topical therapy using suppositories, enema, or foam results in a more rapid response, fewer adverse side effects, and less frequent dosing than oral therapy. For mild-to-moderate active disease, or for maintenance of remission, oral drugs are used which include aminosalicylates (e.g., sulfasalazine and mesalamine) and corticosteroids (prednisone). Mesalamine (Asacol) does not contain the sulfa component of sulfasalzine and thus has fewer adverse side effects. Immunosuppressive drugs (e.g.,cyclosporine) have fewer adverse side effects than glucocorticosteroids and are used in refractory (resistant to other drugs) cases.

An antibiotic such as metronidazole has been used as an alternative treatment of ulcerative colitis. Supplemental therapy includes the use of antidiarrheal agents and, for those patients in remission, a change in dietary habits to include low-roughage foods.

RDH Rapid Dental Hint

Patients with ulcerative colitis cannot take clindaymcin (Cleocin), an antibiotic frequently prescribed for dental infections.

DENTAL HYGIENE NOTES

There are no contraindications or precautions to follow for dental treatment of patients with peptic ulcer disease or gastroesophageal reflux disease. Some gastrointestinal drugs such as cimetidine have many drug interactions about which the dental hygienist should be aware, whether related to dental drugs or not. Since H_2-receptor antagonists are available over the counter without a prescription, many patients will be taking them for heartburn or indigestion.

Patients with GERD may experience symptoms when lying down in the dental chair. The patient may prefer to be lying half-way up and not in a totally supine position.

Since antacids are also available over the counter, many patients may be taking them. When reviewing the medical history with the patient, ask if they are taking antacids. Antacids (aluminum, calcium, and magnesium) interact with certain antibiotics such as tetracyclines and fluroquinolones. These antibiotics should be taken either 1 hour before or 2 hours after taking the antacid.

Xerostomia may be a side effect of anticholinergics, antiemetics, and proton pump inhibitors (PPIs), so the patient must be counseled on prevention, including maintenance of optimum oral hygiene.

H_2-receptor inhibitors can inhibit the metabolism of some drugs metabolized by the P450 cytochrome enzyme system, which will increase plasma levels of diazepam, theophylline, warfarin, phenytoin, carbamazepine, lidocaine, propranolol, phenytoin, and tricyclic antidepressants.

KEY POINTS

- *Helicobacter pylori* (*H. pylori*) is a bacterium that causes approximately 90 percent of gastric and duodenal ulcers.
- Xerostomia may be a side effect of anticholinergics, antiemetics, and proton pump inhibitors (PPIs), so the patient must be counseled on prevention, including having optimum oral hygiene.
- Many drug–drug interactions occur with medications for ulcers.
- Diarrhea associated with antibiotic use is caused by *Clostridium difficile*.

BOARD REVIEW QUESTIONS

1. Which of the following gastrointestinal drugs should not be given concurrently with doxycycline? (p. 299)
   a. Omeprazole
   b. Cimetidine
   c. Antacids
   d. Lansoprazole

2. Which of the following risk factors are primarily involved in causing peptic ulcer disease? (p. 296)
   a. Smoking and alcohol consumption
   b. Caffeine and smoking
   c. *Helicobacter pylori* and NSAIDs
   d. *Streptococcus mutans* and alcohol consumption

3. Which of the following drugs is best for starting initial treatment of mild, intermittent heartburn? (p. 305)
   a. Sodium bicarbonate/alginic combination
   b. Cimetidine
   c. Omeprazole
   d. Lansoprazole

4. Which of the following drugs can cause xerostomia? (p. 303)
   a. Omeprazole
   b. Cimetidine
   c. Ranitidine
   d. Maalox

5. Which of the following drugs has the potential to cause severe diarrhea? (p. 308)
   a. Clindamycin
   b. Ciaspride
   c. Diazepam
   d. Metronidazole
   e. Vancomycin

SELECTED REFERENCES

Engstrom, P. F. and E. B. Goosenberg. 1999. *Diagnosis and Management of Bowel Diseases.* Philadephia: Professional Communications Inc. pp.15–58, 63–90.

Henderson, R. P. 2004. In: *Handbook of Nonprescription Drugs.* Edited by J. V. Allen et al. 14th ed. Washington, DC: American Pharmaceutical Association, pp. 243–272.

Mears, J. M., B. Kaplan. 1996. Proton pump inhibitors: New drugs and indications. *Am Family Phy* 53:285–292.

Meurer, L. N., D. J. Bower. 2002. Management of *Helicobacter pylori* Infection. *Am Fam Physician* 65:1327–1336, 1339.

Pham, C. Q. D., L. M. Sadowski-Hayes and R. E. Regal. 2006. Prevalent prescribing of proton pump inhibitors: Prudent or pernicious? *Pharmacy and Therapeutics* 31(*3*):159–167.

Smith, C. 1999. Gastroesophageal reflux disease. *U.S. Pharmacist* 24:77–88.

Weart, C. W. 2002. Opportunities for pharmacist in managing GERD and peptic-ulcer disease. *U.S. Pharmacist* supplement.

Wells, B. G., J. T., Dipiro, T. L. Schwinghammer, and C. W. Hamilton. 2000. *Pharmacotherapy Handbook.* 2nd edition. New York: McGraw Hill, pp. 251–261; 314–312.

WEB SITES

www.cdc.gov/ulcer/
www.medscape.com
www.uspharmacist.com

Q U I C K   D R U G   G U I D E

Antacids

Bismuth subsalicylate
- Pepto-Bismol

Magnesium hydroxide
- Milk of Magnesia

Aluminum hydroxide/magnesium hydroxide/simethicone
- Maalox liquid
- Gelusil liquid
- Mylanta liquid

Sodium bicarbonate/alginic acid combination
- Gaviscon

Calcium carbonate/magnesium hydroxide
- Rolaids

Calcium Carbonate
- Tums
- Titralac
- Gaviscon

Antihistamines

H_2-Receptor Antagonists
- Cimetidine (Tagamet)
- Famotidine (Pepcid)
- Nizatidine (Axid)
- Ranitidine (Zantac)

Proton Pump Inhibitors
- Omeprazole (Prilosec)
- Lansoprazole (Prevacid)
- Esomeprazole (Nexium)
- Pantoprazole (Protonix)
- Rabeprazole (Aciphex)

Prostaglandin supplements
- Misoprostal (Cytotec)

Protective Barrier Drug
- Sucralfate (Carfate)

Prokinetic Drugs
- Metoclopramide (Reglan)

Antibiotic Combination Treatments

H. pylori Treatment Regimen (including antibiotics, antihistamines, and antacids)

- Lansoprazole + clarithormycin + amoxicillin (PrevPac) *or*
- Omeprazole + clarithromycin + amoxicillin *or*
- Lansoprazole or omeprazole + clarithromycin + metronidazole *or*

- Lansoprazole or omeprazole + Bismuth + metronidazole + tetracycline *or*
- Famotidine or ranitidine or nizatidine + bismuth + metronidazole + tetracycline (Helidac)

Adapted from: Antibiotic regimen: American College of Gastroenterology Guidelines. *American Journal of Gastroenterology* 1998, 93:2330.

Chapter 17

Neurologic Drugs

GOAL: To gain knowledge of the various drugs used to control seizures, Parkinson's disease, and migraine headaches.

EDUCATIONAL OBJECTIVES

After reading this chapter, the reader should be able to:

1. List the different types of epilepsy.
2. Describe the management of a patient undergoing an epileptic seizure in the dental chair.
3. List and discuss drug–drug interactions with antiepileptic drugs.
4. List and discuss drugs used in the treatment of Parkinson's disease.
5. Discuss the drug management of headaches.

KEY TERMS

Seizures
Antiepileptic drugs
Parkinson's disease
Extrapyramidal
Migraine

EPILEPSY

Pathophysiology

Epilepsy is a relatively common central nervous system disorder affecting about one in 200 individuals. This disorder is characterized by the repeated occurrence of **seizures,** defined as the abnormal, excessive synchronous discharges of certain populations of cerebral neurons and changes in the electrical activity in the brain. Convulsions or violent, involuntary contractions of the voluntary muscles may or may not occur with a seizure. If a seizure occurs, it is often intermittent and brief. Drooling is a common problem due to difficulties in swallowing.

Seizures may result from hypoxia (lack of oxygen), birth injury to the brain, fever, alcohol intoxication/withdrawal, brain tumors, head trauma or stroke. In some patients, epilepsy may be genetic.

Classification of Seizures

There are three classifications of seizures (Table 17–1):

- Partial (focal) seizures
- Generalized seizures
- Unclassified epileptic seizures

A partial seizure originates in one cerebral hemisphere in the brain; the patient does not lose consciousness during the seizure. A generalized seizure originates in both cerebral hemispheres, with a loss of consciousness. Seizures are accompanied by characteristic changes in the electroencephalogram (EEG). Most seizures last for about 10 seconds to 5 minutes. Seizures may be preceded by an aura, a warning similar to a light, noise, or feeling to the individual that a seizure is going to occur.

The two main types of generalized seizure are tonic-clonic seizures and absence seizures. Absence seizures (formerly known as petit mal seizures) most often occur in children and last less than 20 seconds.

Tonic-clonic seizures (formerly known as grand mal) are the most common type of seizure in all age groups. During these seizures tongue biting may occur. A tonic-clonic seizure usually lasts 1 to 2 minutes, after which the patient becomes confused, drowsy, and sleepy. Seizures may be preceded by an aura; intense muscle contractions indicate the tonic phase. A cry may occur after the onset of the seizure due to air being forced out of the lungs. The clonic phase is characterized by alternating contraction and relaxation of muscles.

Status epilepticus is a medical emergency that occurs when a seizure is repeated continuously. It could

Table 17–1 Classification of Seizures (Commission of Classification and Terminology of the International League Against Epilepsy)

Partial Seizures (Seizures are Localized to One Part of the Brain)
- Simple partial seizure (no loss of consciousness)
- Complex partial seizure (impairment of consciousness)
- Secondarily generalized seizure

Generalized Seizures (Seizures are Bilaterally Symmetrical or Generalized Involving Both Cerebral Hemispheres; there is Loss of Consciousness)
- Absence seizures (formerly called petit mal; in young children and adolescents ages 2 to 12; many seizures a day with a momentary loss of consciousness with eye blinking and muscle jerks)
- Tonic-clonic seizures (formerly called grand mal; an aura or symptoms may appear before the seizure occurs; jerking of the extremities with loss of consciousness)
- Myoclonic seizures (sudden, short jerks or muscle contractions of the extremities that can occur at any age; associated with hereditary disorders)
- Clonic seizures (contraction and relaxation of muscles of the entire body)
- Tonic seizures (increased muscle tone; loss of bladder and bowel control)
- Atonic seizures (sudden loss of muscle tone similar to slumping to the ground)
- Febrile seizures (in children, and last for just a few minutes; the child has a fever)

Unclassified Seizures
- Includes all seizures that cannot be classified because of inadequate or incomplete data and some that defy classification in any of the above categories. This includes some neonatal seizures, e.g., rhythmic eye movements, chewing and swimming movements
- Status epilepticus (emergency situation characterized by continuous, prolonged seizures longer than 20 minutes)

occur with any type of seizure, but usually generalized tonic-clonic seizures are seen.

Antiepileptic Drug (AED) Therapy

Many hypotheses have been proposed to explain the mechanism by which **antiepileptic drugs** attenuate or prevent seizures. Such theories include:

1. Acting on ion channels: changes in transmembrane (across the cell membrane) movement of sodium and calcium
2. Changes in the activity of (sodium and potassium) ATPase, protein phosphorylation
3. Changes in the reuptake of neurotransmitters such as GABA (gama-aminobutyeric acid), NE (norepinephrine), ACh (acetylcholine), and glutamate (excitatory chemical in the brain). It has been shown that neurotransmitters affect seizure threshold. Gamma-aminobutyric acid (GABA) inhibits nerve impulse transmissions. In epilepsy there is a blocking of GABA's actions, causing a seizure.

The objective of treatment is to suppress seizures by maintaining an effective concentration of the drug in the blood and brain cells at all times. Since individuals are chronically taking these drugs, adherence is a problem. Thus, administration of the drug should be kept as infrequent as possible. Most antiepileptics are taken once or twice a day.

The selected agent should be a first-line antiepileptic drug (AED) specific to the seizure type diagnosed. The usual approach to antiepileptic drug therapy is to maximize seizure control while minimizing adverse drug effects, keeping costs lower and adherence higher. *Monotherapy* is desirable rather than polytherapy which has not been found to be more effective than the use of one drug. Problems with adverse events increase in direct proportion to the number of drugs used. Sometimes adjunctive therapy is needed which is an add-on to existing AED therapy.

Drugs

Treatment or control of seizures depends on the type of seizure. There are specific first-line drugs for each type.

> ### Did You Know?
>
> Modern treatment of seizures started in 1850 with the introduction of bromides, on the basis of the theory that epilepsy was caused by an excessive sex drive.

First-Generation/Traditional Drugs

Phenobarbital In 1910, phenobarbital, a type of barbiturate which was then used to induce sleep, was found to have antiseizure activity and was the first antiepileptic drug. Although it is among the oldest and safest antiepileptic drugs, its use has declined in favor of newer drugs. It is a second-line drug in adults with partial and generalized seizures except absence seizures. The mechanism of action is to enhance the effects of GABA, prolonging the chloride channel opening, and blocking the sodium channel. The half-life of phenobarbital is long, between 72 and 125 hours, so it takes a long time (about 3 weeks) to get to steady state levels. Phenobarbital is rapidly and completely absorbed following oral doses.

Its high incidence of adverse effects, including sedation, high abuse potential, dizziness, and respiratory depression have precluded its use as a primary antiepileptic drug. In children, phenobarbital may cause hyperactivity and aggression. It is about 70% metabolized in the liver by CYP2C9 and CYP2C19. Phenobarbital is a potent CYP enzyme inducer.

By inducing liver microsomal P450 enzymes, phenobarbital is involved in many drug–drug interactions; see Table 17–2.

Phenytoin Phenytoin (Dilantin) was first introduced in 1938 for the treatment of seizures and is still widely used. It was the first nonsedating antiepileptic drug. Phenytoin decreases passive sodium influx across brain cell membranes by blocking sodium channels, decreasing excessive abnormal discharge of neurons.

Phenytoin is the first-line therapy for partial (both simple and complex) seizures, generalized tonic-clonic seizures, and status epilepticus, but is ineffective in absence seizures. Phenytoin combined with diazepam (Valium), a benzodiazepine, are the drugs of choice in the maintenance of patients with status epilepticus.

Table 17-2 Drugs Used in the Treatment of Seizures

Drug Name	Use	Adverse Effects	Dental Drug Interactions	Patient Instructions
Phenytoin (Dilantin)	Used in tonic-clonic seizure and complex partial seizures	Gingival enlargement, megaloblastic anemia, CNS depression, hyperglycemia	No significant dental drug interactions Metabolized by the liver microsomal enzymes. Increased phenytoin blood levels if taken with: isoniazid, cimetidine. Decreased phenytoin blood levels if taken with: carbamazepine Antacids decrease absorption of phenytoin. Warfarin increases phenytoin levels.	• Monitor for gingival enlargement or overgrowth. Keep meticulous oral hygiene. • Medical consult may be necessary to assess level of seizure control. Be aware of the adverse effects
Carbamazepine (Tegretol, Carbitrol)	For tonic-clonic and partial seizures and for trigeminal neuralgia Also used in dental patients with chronic orofacial pain	Respiratory depression or coma in acute toxication, liver function altered, aplastic anemia, agranulocytosis, drowsiness, vomiting	Metabolized by the P450 enzyme system Dental drug interaction: Increases metabolism of doxycycline, decreasing blood levels. Erythromycin and clarithromycin may inhibit metabolism of carbamazepine. Other interactions: Metabolism of carbamazepine is inhibited by (increased carbamazepine blood levels): Isoniazid, Propoxyphene, Verapamil, Cimetidine, Carbamazepine decreases blood levels of the following drugs (by increasing metabolism): Oral contraceptives theophylline warfarin	• Carbamazepine should not be given with erythromycin or doxycycline. • Medical consult may be needed to assess control. • Be aware of the adverse effects. • Maintain optimum oral hygiene.
Oxcarbazepine (Trileptal)	Monotherapy partial/mixed seizures Adjunctive treatment of children and adults with refractory partial seizures	Rash, nausea, vomiting, abdominal pain	No dental drug interactions	• Medical consult may be needed to assess control.
Levetiracetam (Keppra)	Partial seizures generalized tonic-clonic Adjunctive refractory	Headache, weakness, drowsiness	No significant dental drug interactions	• Medical consult may be needed to assess control.

Drug Name	Use	Adverse Effects	Dental Drug Interactions	Patient Instructions
Phenobarbital (Luminal)	Alternative drug for partial seizure and tonic-clonic seizures; the drug of choice in febrile seizures in children	Sedation, dizziness, rash, nausea, vomiting, headache	• No significant dental drug interactions metabolized by P450 enzymes. • Alcohol increases phenobarbital metabolism, decreasing blood levels. • Increases metabolism or systemic corticosteriods	• Medical consult may be needed to assess control. • Be aware of the adverse effects • Maintain optimum oral hygiene.
Primidone (Mysoline)	Complex partial and generalized tonic–clonic seizures	Same as for phenobarbital	No significant drug interactions	• Medical consult may be needed to assess control. • Be aware of the adverse effects. • Maintain optimum oral hygiene.
Valproic acid (Depakene) Divalproex sodium (Depakote)	For complex partial seizures	Nausea, vomiting, sedation, unsteadiness, tremor, behavior changes	Dental drug interaction: Salicylates (aspirin) increase valproic acid levels. Other drug interactions: Cimetidine increases valproic acid levels.	• Medical consult may be needed to assess control. • Be aware of the adverse effects. • Maintain optimum oral hygiene. • Possible gingival enlargement.
Ethosuximide (Zarontin)	Generalized Absence (petit mal)	Dizziness, nausea, vomiting, lethargy, hiccups, headaches	No significant drug interactions	• Medical consult may be needed to assess control; no specific patient instructions pertaining to dentistry. • Be aware of the adverse effects. • Maintain optimum oral hygiene.
Benzodiazepines (e.g., diazepam, lorazepam, clonazepam)	Lorazepam is drug of choice in status epilepticus; clonazepam for treating myoclonic seizures in children.	CNS depression (sedation), respiratory depression, drug dependence, Contraindicated in acute angle-closure glaucoma	Significant dental drug interactions: Increased CNS depression with alcohol, narcotics, barbiturates. Cimetidine increases benzodiazepine level.	• Medical consult may be needed to assess control. Be aware of the adverse effects. • Maintain optimum oral hygiene.
Gabapentin (Neurontin) Pregablin (Lyrica)	• Partial seizures adjunctive in adults and children with refractory partial seizures . • Used in dental patients with chronic orofacial pain	Dizziness, fatigue, drowsiness, tremor	Decreased levels if taken with antacids	• Medical consult may be needed to assess control. Be aware of the adverse effects. • Maintain optimum oral hygiene.

(continued)

317

Table 17-2 Continued

Drug Name	Use	Adverse Effects	Dental Drug Interactions	Patient Instructions
Lamotrigine (Lamictal)	Partial seizures in combination with other drugs adjunctive in adults and children with refractory partial seizures	Include diplopia (double vision), drowsiness, rash and headache, cleft lip or cleft palate	Decreased lamotrigine levels when taken with the other antiepileptics	• Be aware of the adverse effects. • Maintain optimum oral hygiene.
Zonisamide (Zonegran)	Partial seizures adjunctive in refractory	Xerostomia, vomiting, weight gain, dizziness, constipation, tremor, cough	No dental drug interactions	• Xerostomia • Maintain oral hygiene • Use caution when patient is getting up from dental chair.
Tiagabine (Gabitril)	Adjunctive in refractory partial seizures	Dizziness, accidental injury, tremor, nervousness	No dental drug interactions	• Be aware of adverse effects.
Topiramate (Topamax)	• Partial/tonic-clonic seizures • Adjunctive therapy in adults and children with refractory partial seizures	Paraesthesia in the extremities, disturbance of memory, dizziness	May decrease topiramate plasma levels if taken with carbamazepine; alcohol increases CNS side effects. No other dental interactions	• Photosensitivity: caution with dental light. • Caution when patient arises from dental chair.

318

Guidelines for Patients Taking Phenytoin (Dilantin)

- Monitor for gingival enlargement.

- Monitor and emphasize oral hygiene; difficult for patients to adequately maintain oral hygiene because of tissue overgrowth.

- Place patients on frequent recall appointments to monitor gingival condition.

Adverse effects Phenytoin has a narrow therapeutic index so that even small fluctuations in plasma levels can cause toxicity. Overdose usually occurs after IV loading. Missed doses will result in a marked change in plasma concentration. Since different drug formulations from various manufacturers can affect absorption, it is best to use the same drug manufacturer and not to change brands because severe changes in the serum levels can occur. Frequent blood level monitoring is best for optimal dosing.

Many adverse effects can occur, which are concentration dependent, including gingival enlargement (Figure 17–1), nausea, vomiting, anorexia, blurred vision, slurred speech, incoordination anemia, fatigue, acne and cardiac arrhythmias and arrest. An erythematous morbilliform skin rash occurs frequently. There is some evidence that phenytoin is teratogenic; it has a pregnancy category of D.

The patient should be informed that if gingival enlargement occurs it will remain as long as the patient is

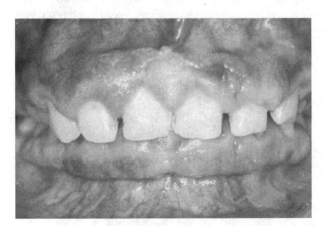

FIGURE 17–1 Gingival enlargement in a patient taking phenytoin.

taking phenytoin. Surgical removal of the excessive gingival tissue may be necessary but the enlargement most likely will recur. Meticulous oral home care is important for these patients.

Phenytoin can cause fetal hydantoin syndrome, where there is a deficiency in prenatal growth, mental retardation, cleft palate, and heart deformities.

Drug–drug interactions Phenytoin is metabolized in the liver by the P450 cytochrome enzyme (CYP2C9) system so many drugs interact with phenytoin (Table 17–2). Antacids decrease its absorption.

Carbamazepine Carbamazepine is the drug of choice for controlling partial and generalized tonic-clonic seizures. It was originally developed for the treatment of trigeminal neuralgia, a painful inflammation of the trigeminal nerve (fifth cranial nerve) and it is also effective for bipolar disorder.

The mechanism of action is similar to phenytoin—blocking sodium channels and prolonging the inactivation state of these channels, allowing the drug to inhibit the development of an action potential or firing of the neurons involved in the seizure.

RDH Rapid Dental Hint

Remember to assess patients taking phenytoin for gingival enlargement. It is difficult for patients to maintain effective oral hygiene. Gingivectomy/gingivoplasty may be indicated.

Adverse effects Severe blood disorders may develop such as aplastic anemia, the failure of the bone marrow to produce red blood cells, white blood cells, and platelets. This can result in bleeding gingiva and agranulocytosis (decreased number of circulating neutrophils or white blood cells). A medical consult from the patient's physician is needed for dental treatment; lab tests are necessary when taking carbamazepine.

Carbamazepine is much less sedating than phenobarbital, but commonly causes dizziness, diplopia (double vision), unsteadiness, and headache, which make this drug difficult initially to take.

Drug–drug interactions Carbamazepine is metabolized by the P450 liver cytochromes (CYP3A4) and can reduce effectiveness of oral contraceptives (Table 17–2). When taken with erythromycin and clarithromycin, carbamzepine levels become elevated. Carbamazepine induces the metabolism of doxycycline (a tetracycline type

Guidelines for Patients Taking Carbamazepine

• Patients should avoid erythromycin, clarithromycin (Biaxin), and doxycycline.

• Monitor for xerostomia.

• Monitor for blood disorders: infections, spontaneous bleeding (not provoked with an instrument), and poor healing.

• Monitor blood lab values.

• Look for oral ulcerations and glossitis.

• Tell patients to maintain good oral hygiene.

of antibiotic), resulting in lower blood levels of the antibiotics.

Oxcarbazepine   Oxcarbazepine (Trileptal) is a recently developed analog of carbazepine, but has fewer adverse effects. Like carbamazepine, oxcarbazepine blocks the neuronal sodium channel during sustained rapid repetitive firing. It is used as monotherapy for partial-mixed epilepsy and as monotherapy in patients with refractory partial seizures. It does not increase the metabolism of warfarin, cimetidine, or erythromycin.

Valproic acid   The preferred agent to use is divalproex (Depakote) rather than valproic acid (Depakene) for controlling all types of generalized seizures (including absence, myoclonic, and partial seizures), because it is available as delayed-release tablets which cause fewer G.I. side effects by releasing valproic acid slowly over 24 hours until it reaches the small intestine. It blocks sodium channels and increases GABA synthesis, inhibits GABA degradation in the brain, and is metabolized in the gut to valproic acid.

Adverse effects   There are many side effects, including xerostomia, inhibition of platelet aggregation (which may be reflected in altered bleeding time and frank hemorrhage), G.I. complaints, nausea, vomiting, weight gain, hair loss, drowsiness, behavior changes, and tremor. There are three black box warnings associated with valproate: (1) Severe, fatal hepatotoxic reactions may occur especially in infants under 2 years; (2) it can produce teratogenic effects such as neural tube defects, and has a pregnancy category of D; and (3) cases of life-threatening pancreatitis have been reported in both children and adults.

Drug–drug interactions   Valproic acid is extensively metabolized by the liver cytochrome P450 enzyme (CYP2C9) system and inhibits the metabolism of many drugs, including phenytoin, carbamazepine, and phenobarbital. Aspirin should be avoided since it increases plasma levels of valproic acid by displacement from protein-binding sites.

Ethosuximide   Ethosuximide (Zarotin) is the drug of choice in controlling absence (petit mal) seizures. Its mechanism of action is inhibiting calcium influx into the brain cell by blocking the T-type calcium channels.

Common side effects include nausea, vomiting, anorexia, dizziness, confusion, and leukopenia (low white blood cell count).

Ethosuximide is metabolized in the liver the cytochrome P450 enzyme system. Carbamazepine decreases plasma levels of ethosuximide.

Benzodiazepines   Lorazepam, administered intravenously (IV), is the drug of choice in status epilepticus and in alcoholic-related seizures. Clonazepam (Klonopin) can be used for controlling myoclonic seizures in children.

Common side effects include drowsiness, and respiratory and cardiac depression.

Second-Generation Drugs

Newer antiepileptic drugs are called second-generation drugs and tend to have more specific sites of action and fewer adverse effects (Table 17–2).

Levetiracetam   Levetiracetam (Keppra) was developed in the 1980s for the treatment of anxiety. It is well tolerated, with minimal adverse effects. It is useful in patients with hepatic or renal insufficiency and in patients on concomitant medications, because it has no drug interactions. It is indicated for partial seizures and recently in April 2007 approved as adjunctive (add-on to

Guidelines for Patients Taking Valproic Acid (Depakote)/Valproate (Depakene)

• Emphasize good oral hygiene.

• Evaluate for blood clotting ability during periodontal debridement, since inhibition of platelet aggregation may occur.

• Monitor for xerostomia.

existing AED therapy) therapy for primary generalized tonic-clonic seizures in patients 6 years of age and older.

Tiagabine Tiagabine (Gabitril) is a derivative of the GABA uptake inhibitor nipecotic acid. The exact mechanism of action is unknown, but it is believed to enhance the activity of GABA. It use is limited to adjunctive therapy in refractory partial epilepsy. If used for absence or partial seizures, it can worsen seizure control or cause status epilepticus.

Lamotrigine Lamotrigine (Lamictal) blocks sodium channels, inhibiting the release of glutamate and aspartate. It is approved as adjunctive or monotherapy therapy in partial-mixed epilepsy and in children and adults with partial epilepsy refractory to other agents. It has been used as monotherapy and appears to be effective against many generalized seizures types and in children. It is also used in the treatment of bipolar disorder.

Common adverse side effects include diplopia (double vision), drowsiness, headache, and a serious rash (a black box warning), including Stevens-Johnson syndrome. It has also been reported to be teratogenic, causing cleft palate, maxillary-mandibular hypoplasia, and median facial cleft.

Lamotrigine is metabolized in the liver, but by glucuronidation (Phase II metabolism) rather than through the P450 enzymes.

Gabapentin Gabapentin (Neurontin) is indicated as monotherapy or adjunctive therapy for partial seizures in children 3–12 years and adults and in children with refractory partial seizures. Gabapentin blocks sodium channels and increases GABA release in brain cells. Another FDA-approved indication is for the management of postherpetic neuralgia (PHN). Increasing use for chronic orofacial pain management has shown good initial effects. It is not metabolized in the liver, and approximately 80 percent is excreted unchanged in the urine.

Common side effects include dizziness, fatigue, drowsiness, and tremor. When taken concurrently with antacids, serum levels of gabapentin are reduced. Otherwise, there are no significant drug–drug interactions.

Pregabalin Pregabalin (Lyrica) is indicated for the adjunctive treatment in patients with partial seizures. It is also approved for the treatment of postherpetic neuropathy and diabetic peripheral neuropathy and for orofacial pain (off-label use). Common side effects include peripheral edema and dizziness

Felbamate Felbamate (Felbatol) is effective in the treatment of partial seizures, primary tonic-clonic seizures, and atonic seizures in patients with Lennox-

Gastaut syndrome. When it was first put on the market, it was associated with aplastic anemia and hepatotoxicity, which restricted its use. The drug is still available and is used as monotherapy or adjunctive therapy in refractory patients.

Topiramate Topiramate (Topamax) is a very potent AED. It is effective in treating partial and primary generalized tonic-clonic seizures and as adjunctive treatment of children and adults with refractory partial seizures. It is derived from D-fructose and initially was developed as an antidiabetic drug. It is also approved for the prophylaxis of migraine headaches.

Rapid Dental Hint

Remember that one of the most important complications of antiepileptic drugs is to increase congential malformations.

Zonisamide Zonisamide (Zonegran) is chemically unrelated to any of the other AEDs. It is structurally related to sulfonamide antibiotics. It was FDA approved in March 2000. It is used for adjunctive therapy for patients with partial seizures. Since it has a long half-life it is a good alternative for patients with compliance problems.

Other Indications for Antiepileptic Drugs

Besides being used in the management of seizures, AEDs are also used in the treatment of;

1. anxiety disorders
2. bipolar disorder
3. migraines
4. neuropathic pain (e.g. diabetic peripheral neuropathy, postherpetic neuralgia)

Table 17–3 summarizes the drugs of choice and alternative drugs for the treatment/control of epileptic seizures.

Dental Hygiene Notes

Reviewing the patient's medical history and interviewing the patient allows the dental hygienist to determine the type of seizure the patient has, cause of seizures, the age

Table 17–3 Drugs Used in the Treatment of Epileptic Seizures

Type of Seizure	Drug of Choice	Alternative Drug
Partial seizures	Carbamazepine Valproic acid Phenytoin	Phenobarbital Primidone Gabapentin Lamotrigine
Generalized tonic-clonic (grand mal) seizures	Carbamazepine Valproic acid Phenytoin	Phenobarbital Frimidone Gabapentin Lamotrigine
Absence (petit mal) seizures	Ethosuximide	Clonazepam Valproic acid
Febrile seizures in children	Phenobarbital	
Myoclonic seizures	Valproic acid	Clonazepam
Status epilepticus	lorazepam (IV)	

of onset, medications used, and degree of control. It is important to determine the patient's adherence in taking the drug. If the patient is not routinely taking his/her medication, a consult with the physician may be needed. The patient should be asked when his/her last epileptic episode was and if there was a loss of consciousness.

PARKINSON'S DISEASE

Parkinson's disease, a chronic, progressive, degenerative central nervous system disorder first described by Dr. James Parkinson, affects about 1 million people in the United States. Parkinson's disease occurs in men more often than women, with an average age of onset at 65 years. It is characterized by a reduction in the neurotransmitter *dopamine* in a specific area of the brain called the basal ganglia, a collection of cell bodies in the central nervous system.

Clinical Presentation

Symptoms of Parkinsonism develop due to depletion of dopamine. The classic four symptoms of Parkinsonism are a resting tremor, muscle rigidity, bradykinesia, and postural instability.

Resting Tremor
In 75 percent of patients, a resting tremor is the first notable symptom. The tremor begins as a fine "pin rolling" of one hand at rest where the patient rubs the thumb and forefinger together in a circular motion. With purposeful movement, the tremor may disappear. This is different from an essential tremor, which is seen during muscle movement.

Muscular Rigidity
Stiffness may resemble symptoms of arthritis. Some patients have difficulty in bending over or moving extremities. A stiff "poker face" may develop later on in the disease.

Bradykinesia
Bradykinesia, which is the most noticeable of all symptoms, is displayed as difficulty initiating movement (slowness of movements) and controlling fine muscle movements. Patient may have difficulty in chewing, swallowing, and speaking. Walking often becomes difficult and the patient has a slow moving shuffle or "short step" gait.

Postural Instability
Poor posture and imbalance may result in falls.

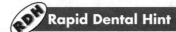

Rapid Dental Hint

Parkinson's tremor may begin in the jaw; monitor elderly dental patients.

The diagnosis of Parkinson's disease is made clinically because there are no diagnostic laboratory tests.

Pathophysiology

Functionally in the brain, the initiation of muscle movement is through the pyramidal system, and the control of muscle movement is through the **extrapyramidal** system. Manifestations of Parkinson's disease are seen as an increase in extrapyramidal side effects due to a *decreased synthesis and release in dopamine (DA),* which is responsible for "turning off the extrapyramidal system." Low production of dopamine is due to the degeneration and destruction of dopamine-producing neurons found within an area of the brain known as the *substantia nigra.* Loss of dopaminergic cells in the substantia nigra is the hallmark of Parkinson's disease. So, when dopamine is not being produced it cannot reach other areas of the brain that require it. The most important area in the brain for dopamine contact is the *corpus striatum,* which is responsible for controlling unconscious muscle movement. Additionally, there is an *elevated level of acetylcholine (ACh)* which causes an excitatory action that is associated with muscle movement. Thus, Parkinson's disease is associated with an imbalance between the dopaminergic and cholinergic systems in the brain. Balance, posture, and involuntary muscle movement depends on an equilibrium between dopamine (inhibitory) and acetylcholine (stimulatory) in the *corpus striatum.* If dopamine is absent, ACh can stimulate this area of the brain.

Drug-Induced Parkinsonism

Drug-induced parkinsonism may have identical clinical signs to Parkinson's disease. Drugs most commonly implicated in inducing parkinsonian symptoms are antagonistic to dopaminergic response. These drugs include some antipsychotics, and metoclopramide (Reglan; for gastroesophageal reflux disease, GERD).

Drug-induced parkinsonism is reversible, but it may take up to a few months after discontinuing the drug before symptoms disappear completely.

Pharmacologic Treatment

Unfortunately, there is no cure for Parkinson's disease; however, drugs focus on reducing symptoms in some patients by restoring the balance between dopamine and ACh. This is accomplished by *increasing the activity of DA or decreasing the activity of ACh.* Dopamine activity is increased either by giving dopamine (dopamine agonists) or increasing the endogenous (within the body) levels of dopamine. Anticholinergic drugs will block the effect of ACh within the *corpus striatum* (Table 17–4).

Dopaminergic Drugs
Dopaminergic drugs are used to increase dopamine levels in the *corpus striatum.* The drug of choice is levodopa and is most effective in relieving muscle rigidity and bradykinesia. Since dopamine cannot get through the blood–brain barrier and get into the brain, it must be given in the form of levodopa which, once past the blood–brain barrier, converts into dopamine. Thus, levodopa or L-dopa is changed into dopamine in the brain, replacing the missing dopamine (Figure 17–2). It undergoes extensive first-pass metabolism so that an extensive amount of the drug is metabolized in the liver before it reaches general circulation.

There are many adverse effects of L-dopa. Nausea and vomiting are due to action of DA in the stomach and on the chemotrigger zone in the CNS (controls vomiting). Food will decrease these side effects. Cardiac arrhythmias, which occur due to beta-adrenergic stimulation, can be controlled by administering a beta-blocker such as propranolol. Other adverse effects include orthostatic (postural) hypotension, psychiatric disturbances (e.g., hallucinations, nightmares, depression) and involuntary oral-facial movements and "swings." Dark color may appear in the saliva, urine, or sweat.

To decrease the amount of L-dopa used and thus reduce the incidence of adverse effects and to maximize levodopa in the brain another drug, carbidopa, is added. Carbidopa, which is given in a combined formulation with L-dopa, increases the CNS penetration of L-dopa so that an effective dose is attained more rapidly while reducing side effects. Carbidopa does not cross the blood–brain barrier and does not affect the metabolism of L-dopa. The combination of L-dopa and carbidopa is the foundation and the drug of choice for moderate to severe disease.

L-dopa therapy is most effective during the first year of the disease, with a marked decrease in effectiveness by 3 years; by 5 years the signs and symptoms are back to the predrug level. This phenomenon, where the patient experiences fluctuations in their response to L-dopa with an increase in involuntary muscle movement of the orofacial and limb muscles, is referred to as the "on–off effect."

Drug–drug Interactions L-dopa undergoes extensive first-pass metabolism so that a lot of the drug is degraded or metabolized in the small intestine before reaching the site of action. Drugs that may alter gastrointestinal motility may also alter the degree of metabolism of L-dopa.

Patients should not be taking an MAOI (monoamine oxidase inhibitor) for depression during or within 14 days of use. There is an increased risk of postural hypotension when taken with antihypertensive agents.

Dopamine Agonists
Dopamine agonists when used in combination with L-dopa are helpful in treating the "on–off effect," including the involuntary muscle movements caused by using L-dopa.

Table 17-4 Drugs Used in Parkinson's Disease

Drug Name	Features	Adverse Effects	Dental Drug Interactions	Patient Instructions
Dopamine Precursor Carbidopa/levodopa (generics; Parcopa—orally disintegrating tabs) L-dopa/carbidopa/entacapone (Stalevo)	Mainstay of current therapy for moderate to severe disease; carbidopa added to L-dopa, thus decreasing side effects; carbidopa lowers dosage of L-dopa, thus decreasing side effects; most effective drug; effective for only 2–5 years, then signs and symptoms reappear	Anorexia, nausea, orthostatic hypotension, hallucination, nightmares, dry mouth	No significant dental drug interactions	• Anti-Parkinson's drugs have a high incidence of causing dry mouth and other anticholinergic side effects. • Monitor dental patient for caries, periodontal disease, and oral candidiasis. • Optimum oral hygiene. • Supplemental topical fluoride and drink water is recommended. • Avoid alcohol, smoking, and depressants, which could aggravate the dry mouth. • For orthostatic hypotension, have patient remain upright in dental chair a few minutes before rising • Since these drugs also cause dizziness and confusion, monitor the patient for these signs.
MAO-B Inhibitor Selegiline (Eldepryl)	• Use as adjunctive treatment with levodopa/carbidopa • Useful when on–off effects are seen from levodopa use	Insomnia, nausea, orthostatic hypotension, abdominal pain	Do not use in conjunction with meperidine (Demerol). Selegiline + selective serotonin reuptake inhibitor SSRI (e.g., nefazodone, venlafaxine) Do not use with other MAO inhibitors (antidepressants).	See above
Rasagiline (Azilect)	See above	Depression, anorexia, vomiting, weight loss	Ciprofloxacin (Cipro) increases rasagiline plasma levels Do not use with meperidine. Do not use with other MAO inhibitors. Do not take with SSRI (antidepressant).	See above

Drug Name	Features	Adverse Effects	Dental Drug Interactions	Patient Instructions
COMT Inhibitor			Do not use with other MAO inhibitors. Do not take with SSRI (antidepressant).	
Entacapone (Comtan) Tolcapone (Tasmar)	Used in conjunction with L-dopa/carbidopa in patients with on—off symptoms	Liver failure, diarrhea, orthostatic hypotension	No dental drug interactions Do not use with MAOIs (monoamine oxidase inhibitors).	See above
Dopamine Agonists				Anti-Parkinson's drugs have a high incidence of causing dry mouth and other anticholinergic side effects. Monitor patient for caries, periodontal disease and oral candidiasis. Optimum oral hygiene. Supplemental topical fluoride and drink water is recommended. Avoid alcohol, smoking, and depressants, which could aggravate the dry mouth.
Bromocriptine (Parlodel)	Directly activate dopamine receptors in the brain; best to use later on in the disease when response to levodopa diminishes or on—off effects are seen	Nausea, nasal congestion, orthostatic hypotension, constipation, headache, sleeping problems, hallucinations	Dental drug interactions: Erythromycin may increase bromocriptine serum levels.	For the orthostatic hypotension, have patient remain upright in dental chair a few minutes before rising
Pergolide (Permax)	Used as adjunctive treatment to L-dopa/ carbidopa	Hypotension, hallucinations, sleep problems, nausea, vomiting	No significant dental drug interactions	See above
Pramipexole (Mirapex)	For mild to severe disease	Sleep disorders, hallucinations, dry mouth, nausea and constipation	No significant dental drug interactions	See above

(continued)

325

Table 17-4 Continued

Drug Name	Features	Adverse Effects	Dental Drug Interactions	Patient Instructions
Ropinirole (Requip)	So special features	Slow heart beat (brady-cardia), syncope, hallucinations	Dental drug interactions: Increased levels when taken with erythromycin.	See above
Anticholinergic Agents	Decreases levels of ace-tylcholine in the brain by blocking muscarinic re-ceptors; for mild disease	Dry mouth, urinary reten-tion, constipation, blurred vision		• Monitor for caries, periodontal dis-ease and oral candidiasis. • Drink plenty of water, use topical fluoride supplement, and practice good oral hygiene. • Avoid alcohol, depressants, and smoking, which could aggravate the dry mouth.
Amantadine (Symmetrel)	Antimuscarinic; may in-crease dopamine activity	Edema (fluid) of lower limbs, confusion, nausea, vomiting, orthostatic hypotension	No significant dental drug interactions Increase in CNS side effects when used with anticholinergic drugs such as antihistamines	• For the orthostatic hypotension, have patient remain upright in dental chair a few minutes before rising
Benztropine (Cogentin)	Muscarinic antagonists; used for tremor rather than rigidity and brady-kinesia	Dry mouth, blurred vision, drowsiness, urinary reten-tion, postural hypotension, dry mouth, constipation	No significant dental drug interactions Alcohol will increase sedation and drowsiness; increase CNS side effects when used with other anticholinergics	See above
Trihexylphenidyl (Artane)	Muscarinic antagonists; best for the tremor and not for muscle rigidity and bradykinesia	Urinary retention, postural hypotension, dry mouth, constipation	See above	See above

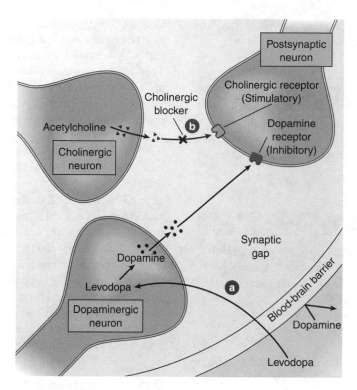

FIGURE 17-2   Mechanism of Action of Antiparkinsonism Drugs. (a) levodopa therapy increases dopamine production; (b) cholinergic blocker decreases acetylcholine reaching receptor.

The dopamine agonist agents act directly to stimulate dopamine receptors. There are four dopamine agonists used to treat Parkinson disease: bromocriptine (Parlodel), Pergolide (Permax), pramipexole (Mirapex), and ropinirole (Requip). These drugs are commonly used with levodopa to delay the onset of levodopa-motor complications. The most frequent side effects are orthostatic hypotension, daytime sleepiness, mental confusion, hallucinations, and nightmares, which are greater than seen with L-dopa.

The newest FDA approved drug, ropinirole (Requip) significantly reduces "wearing-off" time. Requip should be added into the patient's regular medication if it is not reducing symptoms consistently throughout the day.

Anticholinergic Agents

Anticholinergic drugs are used either in the early or mild stages of the disease or later on in combination with levodopa/carbidopa, and are primarily effective for tremors. These drugs block cholinergic receptors to balance acetylcholine and dopamine levels. Commonly used anticholinergics include benztropine mesylate (Cogentin), trihexyphenidyl (Artane), and amantadine (Symmetral), which is used with levodopa. Anticholinergic agents are not commonly used to treat Parkinson's disease due to adverse effects and inability to improve bradykinesia. Amantadine is also used prophylactically for prevention of influenza A viral infection.

Common adverse effects   As with all types of anticholinergic drugs, common adverse effects include

Did You Know?

Amantidine was originally used as an antiviral drug to prevent the Asian flu. When it was given to a Harvard Medical School patient who also had Parkinson's disease, the condition improved. Today, amatadine is still given to high-risk patients to prevent influenza A virus respiratory infections.

xerostomia, urinary retention, constipation, blurred vision, dry skin, and drowsiness.

Rapid Dental Hint

Remember to assess your patients with Parkinson's disease for xerostomia.

Rapid Dental Hint

The main symptoms of Parkinson's disease are usually stiffness, tremor (shaking), and slowness of movement. Your patients may have difficulty getting in and out of the dental chair.

Drug–drug Interactions Anticholinergic drugs taken with other anticholinergic drugs (or drugs with anticholinergic side effects such as sedating antihistamines, including diphenhydramine) will have additive anticholinergic side effects.

Alcohol will have an additive oral drying effect. CNS depressants increase the sedative side effect.

Monoamine Oxidase B (MAO-B) Inhibitor and COMT (catechol-O-methyltransferase) Inhibitor

Selegiline (Eldepryl) and rasagiline (Azilect) are MAO-B inhibitors that block the enzyme MAO-B, which metabolizes dopamine and increases levels in the brain. Rasagiline is used alone or in combination with L-dopa. The main advantage of rasagiline is that it does not have the toxic metabolic breakdown products of selegiline.

The newest class of anti-Parkinson drugs is COMT (catechol-O-methyltransferase) inhibitors. These drugs are used as an adjunct to carbidopa/levodopa to help with motor complications due to levodopa.

ALZHEIMER'S DISEASE

Like Parkinson's disease, Alzheimer's is a neurodegenerative disease characterized by the destruction of cholinergic and other neurons in the central nervous system. As the disease progresses less acetylcholine is produced. The etiology is unknown and there is no cure. In the United States, Alzheimer's accounts for about 60 percent of all cases of dementia in people over 65 years of age, and is associated with about 100,000 deaths per year. This disease has overwhelming effects on the individual's emotional, memory, and physical function.

There are currently four prescription drugs approved by the FDA to treat people with Alzheimer's disease. Treating the symptoms can provide patients with comfort, dignity, and independence for a longer period of time. These medications do not stop the progress of the disease.

Galantamine (Razadyne), rivastigmine (Exelon), and donepezil (Aricept) are cholinesterase inhibitors that function to prevent the breakdown of acetylcholine, important for memory and thinking.

Memantine (Namenda) is an N-methyl D-aspartate (NMDA) antagonist indicated for moderate to severe Alzheimer's disease. This drug works by regulating glutamate, which is produced in excessive amounts and may cause brain cell death. Cholinersterase inhibitors can be prescribed in combination with Namenda.

Dental Hygiene Notes

Most antiparkinson drugs cause anticholinergic side effects and orthostatic (postural) hypotension. The patient must be counseled by the dental clinician about xerostomia.

The vital signs of the patient should be monitored. After supine positioning to avoid orthostatic hypotension, have the patient remain in an upright position in the dental chair for a few minutes before arising.

Aggregated mouth and tongue movements and drooling may be a sign of a serious adverse side effect of the medication or the disease process. A physician's consult may be needed.

There are no specific precautions needed with regard to the use of vasoconstrictors in local anesthetics.

HEADACHE

The International Classification of Headache Disorders identifies 165 headache types, divided into primary and secondary headaches depending on the underlying risk factors. Primary headache disorders, which account for 97–98 percent of all headaches, are characterized by the lack of an identifiable and treatable underlying cause. Examples of primary headache disorders include migraine, tension-type, and cluster headaches. Secondary headache disorders are associated with an identifiable cause such as headache or facial pain attributed to disorders of the neck, eyes, ears, nose, sinuses, teeth, mouth or other facial or cranial structures; head or neck trauma; drug substance or its withdrawal; infection; cranial neuralgias; brain tumors; meningitis; temporal arteritis; intracranial lesions; and primary angle closure glaucoma.

Migraine

In the United States, approximately 24 million people (18 percent of women, 6 percent of men) suffer from **migraine** headache. Migraine is a recurring, episodic, and often severe headache disorder, with attacks lasting 4 to 72 hours. Migraine is further divided into several subtypes including, among others, migraine without aura and migraine with aura.

To establish a diagnosis of migraine without aura, five attacks lasting 4–72 hours must have occurred. It is usually associated with photophobia (sensitivity to or intolerance of light) and phonophobia (fear of sounds, including your own voice), nausea and vomiting, and cutaneous allodynia, a nonpainful stimulus on the skin which is perceived as painful, and is experienced by some patients during an attack.

Migraine with aura, experienced by about 20 percent of patients, is characterized by episodes of headache with features similar to those of migraine without aura in addition to aura symptoms that precede or occur with the onset of pain. Most aura symptoms develop gradually over 5 to 20 minutes and last less than 60 minutes. Aura represents a transient episode of focal neurologic dysfunction caused by an imbalance between excitatory and inhibitory neuronal activity at different levels in the central nervous system. A visual aura may be bright flashing lights and a sensory aura may take the form of a paresthesia that involves the arm, face, hands and body. About 25 percent of people experience a postdrome, which involves changes in mood and behavior after the migraine attack. Precipitating factors include caffeine (and caffeine withdrawal), menstruation, stress, smoking, lack of sleep, certain foods, and strenuous exercise. Attacks are commonly unilateral.

A migraine attack develops over 4 phases:

- prodrome (hours to days before the attack),
- aura,
- headache, and
- postdrome (recovery)

Pain during the headache phase is due to vasodilation of cerebral blood vessels which is caused by the neurons in the trigeminal nerve releasing substance P.

Additionally, low levels of vascular $5\text{-}HT_{2B}$ (serotonin), could hypothetically result in dilation of cerebral blood vessels and concomitant activation of sensory trigeminovascular nerves, initiating the manifestation of head pain. At this stage in the migraine process, activation of specific subtypes of $5\text{-}HT_1$ receptors which will increase levels of serotonin has proven clinically effective in relieving migraine pain.

Substance P is a chemical messenger that signals the brain to feel pain when it is released.

Medication-Overuse Headaches

Medication-overuse headache (MOH) is a syndrome/cycle that starts when a patient takes too much headache medication, which contributes to the headache rather than easing it. Anyone with a history of migraine headache is at risk for developing a MOH. Unfortunately, drug companies and advertisements contribute to the development of medication-overuse headaches. Many over-the-counter pain relievers that contain caffeine are the culprits (e.g., Excedrin Migraine and Excedrin Tension Headache). Caffeine present in coffee and sodas and pain relievers may all contribute to medication-overuse headaches. To stop rebound headaches, the amount of pain medication should be reduced or stopped. Signs and symptoms of rebound headache include nausea, anxiety, insomnia, and restlessness.

Drug Therapy

Drug therapy is aimed at aborting a migraine at the time it occurs, symptomatic pain relief, and preventing a migraine from occurring. The use of any symptomatic therapy, either prescription or OTC, should not be more than twice a week. Beyond that, the patient should be taking preventative medications. Therapy should start by eliminating all products containing caffeine, which causes vasoconstriction. The following are classifications of drugs used in the treatment of acute migraine attacks and for prophylaxis (chronic therapy) (Table 17–5):

- Triptans stimulate $5\text{-}HT_1$ receptors (e.g., sumatriptan)
- Analgesics (e,g., Excedrin, Fioricet) and nonsteroidal anti-inflammatory drugs (e.g., NSAIDs such as naproxen sodium)

Table 17–5 Drugs Used in the Treatment of Headaches

Drug Name	Dosage Form and Indication
Triptans	Acute treatment of migraine; not for prevention
• Almotriptan (Axert)	Tablet
• Eletriptan (Relpax)	Tablet
• Frovatriptan (Frova)	Tablet
• Naratriptan (Amerge)	Tablet
• Rizatriptan (MAXALT, MAXALT-MLT)	Tablet, orally disintegrating tablet
• Sumatriptan (Imitrex)	Tablet, nasal spray, injection (for immediate relief)
• Zolmitriptan (Zomig)	Tablets, orally disintegrating tablets, nasal spray
Non-narcotic Analgesics	Acute symptoms, abort attack
• Acetaminophen (Tylenol)	Tablet, capsule, caplet
• Aspirin, acetaminophen and caffeine (Excedrin Migraine)	Tablet
• Ibuprofen (Advil, Motrin, Nuprin)	Tablet
• Naproxen (Aleve)	Tablet
Narcotic Analgesics	Acute symptoms, abort migraine
• Codeine, acetaminophen, caffeine, butalbital (Fioricet)	Tablet
Ergot	Acute symptoms, abort attack
• Ergotamine (Ergomar) Ergotamine, caffeine (Carfergot)	Sublingual tablet, tablet, suppositories
Anticonvulsants	Prophylaxis
• Topiramate (Topamax)	Tablet, sprinkle capsule
• Valproic acid (Depakote)	Tablet, sprinkle capsule, capsule
Calcium Channel Blockers	Prophylaxis
• Diltiazem (Cardizem)	Tablet
• Nifedipeine (Procardia)	Tablet
• Verapamil (Calan, Isoptin)	Tablet
Beta-Blockers	Prophylaxis
• Atenolol (Tenormin)	Tablet
• Metoprolol (Lopressor)	Tablet
• Propranolol (Inderal)	Tablet
• Timolol (Blocadren)	Tablet
Tricyclic Antidepressants	Prophylaxis
• Amitriptyline (Elavil)	Tablet
• Imipramine (Tofranil)	
• Nortipytyline (Pamelor)	
• Protriptyline (Vivactil)	
Botulinum Toxin	Prophylaxis
• Botulinum toxin Type A (Botox)	injection

- Beta-blockers (e.g, propranolol)
- Anticonvulsants (e.g, valproate)
- Ergot (e.g., ergotamine),
- Drugs that inhibit 5-HT reuptake into the nerve (e.g., tricyclic antidepressants such as amitriptyline or calcium channel blockers)
- Drugs that inhibit sodium and calcium channels (e.g., antiepileptics)
- Botulinum toxin type A (Botox)

Treatment of Acute Migraines (Abortive)

Triptans Triptans, the newest drugs for migraine management, are effective and well tolerated drugs for the *treatment of acute migraine* to abort the attack, but are not used prophylactically. Triptans bind with high affinity to the 5-HT$_1$ (serotonin) receptors and are referred to as selective serotonin agonists. Activation of these receptors results in cranial vessel constriction, inhibition of neuropeptide release, and reduction transmission in trigeminal pain pathways. They have a rapid onset of action. Formulations available include: oral, suppositories, injections, and nasal sprays. Orally administered triptans provide pain relief within 30 minutes. Injected sumatriptan has an onset of action of less than 15 minutes.

Triptans are metabolized primarily by monoamine oxidase enzymes, similar to monoamine oxidase inhibitors (MAO; drugs for depression). Thus, taking triptans and MAO-A inhibitors together generally leads to an increase of triptan blood levels. It is necessary to wait 2 weeks after the MAO inhibitor is discontinued.

Triptans are contraindicated in patients with ischemic heart disease (e.g., angina pectoris, history of myocardial infarction, or silent ischemia) or in patients who have symptoms of ischemic heart disease and coronary artery vasospasm. Triptans may increase blood pressure and should not be given to patients with uncontrolled hypertension. Caution should be used when using local anesthetics containing epinephrine. The patient's blood pressure should be monitored.

The combined use of triptans and antidepressants, including selective serotonin reuptake inhibitors (SSRIs) such as Prozac or Zoloft or selective serotonin/norepinephrine reuptake inhibitors (SNRIs) such as Cymbalta or Effexor, *may* result in a serotonin syndrome resulting from excessive blood levels of serotonin. Symptoms include: restlessness, hallucinations, fast heartbeat, diarrhea, nausea, vomiting, and rapid changes in blood pressure. Serotonin syndrome *may* be more likely to occur when starting or increasing the dose of a triptan, SSRI, or SNRI. This combination is *not contraindicated, but care should be taken when the two drugs are taken concurrently.*

Common adverse reactions include head and jaw discomfort, flushing, dizziness, sleepiness, and tiredness.

Ergot Derivatives Drugs such as ergotamine (Ergomar) and dihydroergotamine nasal spray (Migranal) are -adrenergic blockers and vasoconstrictors of cranial smooth muscle.

Elevated blood levels occur when taken with erythromycin and clarithromycin. Many adverse effects, including nausea, localized edema and itching, and numbness and tingling in fingers and toes, preclude its long-term use and for prevention. Ergotamine derivatives are contraindicated in pregnancy (FDA pregnancy category X)

Treatment of Acute Migraine Symptoms

Analgesics For mild migraine attacks, analgesics alone or in combination with caffeine have been used. Overuse of analgesics and caffeine can aggravate the migraine (medication-overuse headaches). Most of the pain relievers that patients use are over the counter. Excedrin Migraine (which is the same as regular Excedrin) contains acetaminophen, aspirin, and caffeine. Caffeine, a vasoconstrictor, is added to pain relievers to make them more effective in relieving headaches. Two tablets contain the same amount of caffeine as a cup of coffee. Long-term use of analgesics is discouraged, as this may lead to medication-overuse headaches on withdrawal. Adverse side effects include gastrointestinal upset and bleeding, and nausea. Nonsteroidal anti-inflammatory drugs including ibuprofen and naproxen; these reduce the release of serotonin and can be used in combination with triptans.

Narcotic analgesics containing codeine are used for more severe pain. These prescription products include Fiorinal (a combination of codeine, aspirin, butalbital, and caffeine) and Fioricet (acetaminophen, butalbital and caffeine). These drugs are also available without codeine.

There are many adverse side effects including dependency constipation, sedation, and drowsiness that preclude long-term use.

Migraine Prophylaxis

Choosing a drug for prevention is based upon the adverse effect profile of the drug and on the medical status of the patient.

Anticonvulsants   Topiramate (Topamax) is approved for migraine prevention in adults and not for the acute treatment. It is a sulfamate-substituted monosaccharide with a broad spectrum of anticonvulsant activity. Its precise mechanism of action is unknown. Common adverse effects include lowered bicarbonate levels in the blood, resulting in an increase in the acidity of the blood (metabolic acidosis) and hyperventilation (rapid, deep breathing) or fatigue. Maintenance of adequate fluid intake is important to minimize the risk of renal stone formation. Other side effects are tingling in arms and legs, loss of appetite, nausea, diarrhea, taste change, and weight loss. There are no contraindications with epinephrine.

Valproic acid (Valproate) is approved for migraine prophylaxis and can take up to 2–3 weeks to be effective. Common adverse effects, including weight gain, sedation and xerostomia, may preclude its use in certain patients.

Also, levetiracetam (Keppra) and zonisamide (Zonegran) work off label.

Beta-Blockers   The use of beta-blockers for the treatment of migraines started in the 1960s when people being treated for heart problems found that their migraines lessened. The mechanism of action may be due to limiting the tendency for cranial blood vessels to overdilate. It may take up to 4 to 6 weeks to see a reduction in migraine frequency. Timolol and propranolol are FDA approved.

Nonselective beta blockers are contraindicated in patients with asthma. The amount of epinephrine should be limited to 0.04 mg (two cartridges of 1:100,000) when taking a nonselective beta-blocker.

Calcium Channel Blockers   Similar to beta-blockers, calcium channel blockers were originally used to treat cardiovascular conditions. These drugs may also work by stabilizing blood vessel membranes by preventing them from overdilating. It can take up to 2 months to see effects.

Tricyclic antidepressants   Antimigraine action is separate from antidepressant effect. For migraine prevention, a lower dose is prescribed than would be used for the treatment of depression and it can take up to 3–4 weeks before the drug is effective. The dose of epinephrine should be limited to 0.04 mg.

Botulinum toxin type A   Injection of botulinum toxin type A (Botox), derived from the bacteria *clostridium difficle*, besides being used cosmetically and for dystonia (sustained contraction of muscles) has been used in the prevention of migraines for up to 6 months. Although the exact mechanism is unclear, it has been hypothesized that it works by inhibiting the release of transmitters from pain-sensitive nerve endings.

Alternative Treatments

Some alternative medications used in the prophylaxis of migraine include feverfew, petasites, magnesium, riboflavin, coenzyme Q10 and melatonin. There are no randomized, controlled studies using melatonin. There is concern with the lack of standardization regarding the contents and purity of herbal supplements.

A number of alternative treatments have been recommended in the treatment and prevention of migraine including: hypnosis, biofeedback, meditation, acupuncture, massage, transcutaneous electrical nerve stimulation, and magnesium supplements.

Dental Hygiene Notes

Migraine is the most common headache disorder, affecting approximately 28 million people in the United States, and is present in one in four households. During a migraine, stimulation of the trigeminal nerve (the fifth cranial nerve, carrying sensory information from the face) may cause referral of pain to any of the nerve's three branches, resulting in facial pain.

Many dental patients will be taking one type of headache medication. There are no precautions for using local anesthetics with epinephrine in patients taking migraine drugs, except for nonselective beta-blockers and triptans.

KEY POINTS

- Take a complete medical history.
- Determine when the patient's last epileptic seizure was and what brought it on.
- Monotherapy is the preferred treatment option for epilepsy.

- What medication does the patient take, and is it taken regularly?
- Be prepared if the patient has a seizure in the dental chair.
- Get a medical consultation and lab blood tests.
- Patient management in the dental chair is an important part of treatment.
- Monitor the patient for xerostomia.
- There are no special precautions for using vasoconstrictors in local anesthetics.

BOARD REVIEW QUESTIONS

1. Which of the following antiepileptic drugs decreases doxycycline serum levels? (p. 316)
   a. Phenytoin
   b. Carbamazepine
   c. Valproic acid
   d. Primidone
   e. Phenobarbital

2. Which of the following antiseizure drugs increases the incidence of gingival enlargement? (p. 316)
   a. Phenobarbital
   b. Lamotrigine
   c. Carbamazepine
   d. Phenytoin
   e. Ethosuximide

3. Which of the following drugs is used to treat trigeminal neuralgia? (p. 316)
   a. Phenytoin
   b. Carbamazepine
   c. Phenobarbital
   d. Valproic acid
   e. Primidone

4. Which of the following drugs are used to treat migraines? (p. 330)
   a. Triptans
   b. Anticonvulsants
   c. Beta-blockers
   d. All of the above

5. Which of the following are two common adverse side effects of drugs used to treat Parkinson's disease? (p. 328)
   a. Hypertension and diarrhea
   b. Xerostomia and orthostatic hypotension
   c. Orthostatic hypotension and nasal congestion
   d. Hypertension and constipation

SELECTED REFERENCES

American Academy of Neurology and the American Epilepsy Society. AAN Guideline Summary for Clinicians. Efficacy and Tolerability of the New Antiepileptic Drugs, I: treatment of New Onset Epilepsy. April 2004.

American Academy of Neurology and the American Epilepsy Society. AAN Guideline Summary for Clinicians. Efficacy and Tolerability of the New Antiepileptic Drugs, II: Treatment of Refractory Epilepsy. April 2004.

American Academy of Neurology and the American Epilepsy Society. AAN Guideline Summary for Clinicians. Treatments for Refractory Epilepsy. April 2004.

DeVane, C. L. 2001. Substance P: A new era, a new role. *Pharmacotherapy* 21(9):1061–1069.

Dodick, D. W., A. Mauskop, A. H. Elkind, et al. 2005. Botulinum toxin type A for the prophylaxis of chronic daily headache: Subgroup analysis of patients not receiving other prophylactic medications: A randomized double-blind, placebo-controlled study. *Headache,* 45:315–324.

Evans, R. W., F. R. Taylor, 2006. "Natural" or alternative medications for migraine prevention. *Headache,* 46:1012–1018.

Faulkner, M. A. 2006. The role of the pharmacist in the management of Parkinson's disease: Its symptoms and comorbidities. *U.S. Pharmacist,* Continuing Education Series.

French, J. A., A. M. Kanner, J. Bautista, B. Abou-Khalil, T. Browne, C. L. Harden, et al. 2004. Efficacy and tolerability of the new antiepileptic drugs. I. Treatment of new onset epilepsy: Report of the Therapeutics and Technology Assessment Subcommittee and Quality Standards Subcommittee of the American Academy of Neurology and the American Epilepsy Society. Neurology 62;1252–1260.

Hamel, E. 1999. The biology of serotonin receptors: focus on migraine pathophysiology and treatment. *Can J Neurol Sci* 26:S2-6.

Hargreaves, R. J., S. L. Shepheard. 1999. Pathophysiology of migraine-new insights. *Can J Neurol Sce* 26(Suppl 3): S12–S19.

Headache Classification Subcommittee of the International Headache Society. The International Classification of Headache Disorders. 2nd ed. 2003. *Cephalalgia* 2004; supplement 1:1–150.

LaRoche S. M. 2004. The new antiepileptic drugs. *JAMA* 291:605–614.

Lipton, R. B., W. R. Stewart, D. D. Celentano, et al. 1992. Undiagnosed migraine headaches—a comparison of symptom-based and reported physician diagnosis. *Arch Intern Med* 152:1273–1278.

Merck. 2005. Monographs in Medicine: A Study of Migraine. Whitehouse Station, NJ: Merck & Co., Inc.

Ochoa, J. G. 2006. Antiepileptic drugs: An overview. www.emedicine.com.

Padmanabhan, R., Y. M. Abdulrazzaq, S. M. Bastaki, M. Shafi-ullah, and S. I. Chandranath. 2003. Experimental studies on reproductive toxicologic effects of lamotrigine in mice. *Birth Defects Res B Dev Reprod Toxicol* 68(5):428–438.

Parks, B. R. Jr, V. G. Dostrow, S. L. Noble. 1994, Drug therapy for epilepsy. *American Fam Physician.* 50:639–648.

Parmet S., C. Lynm, R. M. Glass. Epilepsy. *JAMA* 2004; 291:654.

Schapira, AhV., C. W. Olanow. 2004. Neuroprotection in Parkinson's Disease. *JAMA* 291:358–364.

Schuumans, A., C. van Weels. 2005. Pharmacologic treatment of migraine: comparison of guidelines. *Can Fam Physician* 51(6):838–843.

Serge J., C. Pierre-Louis. 2000. New drugs: Which should be included in the formulary? All new drugs should be included. *Arch Neurol* 57:272–273.

Silberstein, S. D., J. Olesen, M-G. Bousser, H-C. Diener, et al., 2005. The International Classification of Headache Disorders, 2nd Edition (ICHD-II)-revision of criteria for 8.2 *Medication-overuse* headache. *Cephalalgia* 25:460–465.

Tea, C. P., B. R. Williams, R.Atkinson, M. A. Gill. 2003. Management and treatment of Parkinson's disease. *U.S. Pharmacist* 28:93–100.

Wenzel, R. G., C. A. Sarvis, M. L. Krause, 2003. Over-the-counter-drugs for acute migraine attacks: Literature review and recommendations. *Pharmacotherapy* 23(4):294–505

WEB SITES

www.Parkinson's.org

www.nia.nih.gov/Alzheimers/Publications/medicationsfs.htm

QUICK DRUG GUIDE

Drugs for Epilepsy

- Carbamazepine (Tegretol, Carbiarol): first line therapy—oxcarbazepine; partial/mixed and refractory partial (Trileptal); partial/tonic-clonic/mixed seizures
- Ethosuximide (Zarontin): petit mal only
- Gabapentin (Neurontin): partial seizures
- Lamotrigine (Lamictal): partial seizures and refractory partial
- Levetiracetam (Keppra): partial seizures and primary generalized tonic-clonic seizures in patients 6 years of age and older
- Phenytoin (Dilantin): first line therapy; tonic-clonic and complex partial seizures
- Phenobarbital (Luminal): tonic-clonic seizures, partial seizures

- Pregabalin (Lyrica): partial seizures
- Primidone (Mysoline): grand mal
- Tiagabine (Gabitril): partial mixed & refractory partial seizures
- Topiramate (Topamax): partial/tonic-clonic seizures & refractory partial
- Valproic acid (Depakene): first line therapy; complex and simple partial seizures
- Zonisamide (Zonegran): partial seizures
- Benzodiazepines: Diazepam (Valium); lorazepam (Ativan) not commonly used—only used for status epilepticus

Drugs for Parkinson's Disease

Dopamine Replacement

- Carbidopa/levodopa (Parcopa)
- Carbidopa/levodopa/entacapone (Stalevo)

Monoamine Oxidase Inhibitor

- Rasagiline (Azilect)
- Selegiline (Eldepryl)

Dopamine Agonists

- Bromocriptine (Parlodel)
- Pergolide (Permax)
- Pramipexole (Mirapex)
- Ropinirole (Requip)

COMT (Catechol-O-Methyltransferase) Inhibitor

- Entacapone (Comtan)
- Tolcapone (Tasmar)

Anticholinergic Agents

- Amantadine (Symmetrel)
- Benztropine (Cogentin)
- Trihexylphenidyl (Artane)

Drugs for Alzheimer's Disease

- Donepezil (Aricept)
- Galantamine (Razadyne)

- Memantine (Namenda)
- Rivastigmine (Exelon)

Drugs for Migraine

Triptans (Serotonin Receptor Agonists)

- Almotriptan (Axert)
- Eletriptan (Relpax)
- Frovatriptan (Frova)

- Naratriptan (Amerge)
- Rizatriptan (MAXALT, MAXALT-MLT)
- Sumatriptan (Imitrex)
- Zolmitriptan (Zomig)

Antiepileptics

- Levetiracetam (Keppra)
- Topiramate (Topamax)

- Valproic acid (Depakene)
- Zonisamide (Zonegran)

Ergot Derivatives

- Ergotamine (Ergomar)
- Ergotamine, caffeine (Carfergot)

- Dihydroergotamine (Migranal Nasal Spray)

Calcium Channel Blockers

- Diltiazem (Cardizem)
- Nifedipeine (Procardia)

- Verapamil (Calan, Isoptin)

Beta-Blockers

- Propranolol (Inderal)

- Timolol (Blocadren)

Tricyclic Antidepressants

- Amitriptyline (Elavil)
- Imipramine (Tofranil)

- Nortipytyline (Pamelor)
- Protriptyline (Vivactil)

Analgesics

- Acetaminophen (Tylenol)
- Aspirin, acetaminophen and caffeine (Excedrin, Migraine)

- Ibuprofen (Advil, Motrin, Nuprin)
- Naproxen (Aleve)

Narcotic Analgesics

- Codeine, acetaminophen, caffeine, butalbital (Fioricet)

Botulinum Toxin

- Botulinum toxin Type A (Botox)

Chapter **18**

Psychotropic Drugs

GOAL: To provide an understanding of psychotropic medications used to treat psychiatric and dental disorders and how to manage these patients in the dental office.

EDUCATIONAL OBJECTIVES

After reading this chapter, the reader should be able to:

1. Discuss the biochemical etiology of the various psychiatric disorders.
2. Describe the major classes of psychotherapeutic medications.
3. Discuss the adverse effects of psychotropic medications.
4. Discuss the impact of these adverse side effects during dental treatment.

KEY TERMS

Antipsychotics
Antidepressants
Anxiolytic agents
Sedative/hypnotics
Psychopharmacology
Extrapyramidal side effects
Major depression

INTRODUCTION

Psychopharmacology is one of the most rapidly growing areas of clinical pharmacology. There are three major symptoms of psychiatric/emotional disorders: anxiety, depression (mood disorders), and psychosis. *Psychotropic* medications are classified according to therapeutic applications including:

- **Antipsychotics** for the treatment of psychoses such as schizophrenia
- **Antidepressants** (**mood-elevating agents**) for the treatment of depression, and mood-stabilizing agents for the treatment of manic or bipolar disorders (formerly known as manic-depressive disorder)
- **Anxiolytic agents** for the treatment of anxiety disorders
- **Sedative/hypnotics** (e.g., barbiturates) for the induction of sleep

Many dental patients may be taking one or more of these medications either for a psychiatric disorder, alleviating anxiety before a dental procedure, nocturnal bruxism, or chronic orofacial pain. The majority of these drugs cause xerostomia, which may lead to the development of caries and periodontal disease. Thus it is important for the dental hygienist to be familiar with psychotropic medications, to monitor patients taking these medications, and to instruct patients on proper oral home care.

A publication from the American Psychiatric Association entitled the *Diagnostic and Statistical Manual of Mental Disorders,* 4th ed., 1994 (DSM-IV), allows the physician to diagnose a wide range of psychiatric disorders. Essentially, the DSM-IV is organized by symptoms which are related to specific diagnoses.

Psychopharmacology deals with drugs used to treat psychosomatic disorders which have a biochemical origin in the brain. In psychiatric disorders of the central nervous system, many CNS neurotransmitters are involved in causing signs and symptoms of the disease.

BASIC PHARMACOLOGY

For a drug to be effective there must be equilibrium among absorption, distribution, metabolism, and excretion. Especially for psychiatric drugs to reach the brain, the drug must also effectively cross the blood–brain barrier. Since most psychotropic drugs are weak bases, they are readily absorbed from the intestine and best absorbed on an empty stomach. Psychotropic drugs have numerous adverse oral side effects which may interfere with adequate management of the dental patient.

Rapid Dental Hint

Patients taking any type of psychiatric drug should be monitored for xerostomia, which may lead to caries and periodontal diseases.

ANTIPSYCHOTIC DRUGS
Clinical Symptoms of Schizophrenia

Psychosis is a mental disorder characterized by gross impairment of thought and behavior, in which a person cannot differentiate between real and unreal thoughts. *Positive symptoms* add on to normal behavior and consist of hallucinations, delusions, paranoia, and suspiciousness. *Negative symptoms* consist of emotional and social withdrawal and lack of interest. *Schizophrenia,* the most common type of psychosis, affects only approximately 1 percent of the American population. It usually occurs in males and begins in adolescence or early adult life.

Etiology
The etiology of schizophrenia is essentially unknown; however, there are several hypotheses, including a strong genetic predisposition and a chemical imbalance in the brain. It is a chronic disease for which there is no cure. Treatment can decrease symptoms and optimize functioning between psychotic episodes.

Dopamine Receptors

Dopmaine receptors play a role in the etiology of schizophrenia and in the mechanism of action and side effects of antipsychotics. In schizophrenia too much dopamine is produced in the brain which overexcites the D_2 dopamine receptors and causes the positive symptoms, while a deficiency in dopamine causes the negative symptoms.

Medications

All antipsychotic drugs act by binding to the D_2 receptor, preventing dopamine from attaching. This results in decreased dopamine activity in the neuronal synapse. Antipsychotics are often referred to as *dopamine antagonists.* When about 65 percent of the D_2 receptor is blocked by the drug, psychotic behavior is reduced. The older theory of the pharmacodynamics of antipsychotics stated that the stronger an antipsychotic was in binding and blocking the D_2 receptor, the more potent it was as an antipsychotic. However, the current theory is that the *strength (affinity) to the receptor is not correlated with efficacy.* For example, clozapine is the weakest binding antipsychotic, but it has the most efficacy on positive symptoms.

Adverse Effects

Besides binding to dopamine receptors, which is responsible for their antipsychotic action, antipsychotics also bind nonspecifically to muscarinic receptors (anticholinergic), α_1-adrenergic receptors, and histamine (H_1) receptors (antihistaminic), resulting in a variety of side effects.

Binding to Muscarinic Receptors
Binding to muscarinic receptors causes a*nticholinergic effects,* including xerostomia, constipation, blurred vision, tachycardia, sexual dysfunction, and urine retention. The mouth can be extremely dry, causing the dental mirror to stick to the oral mucosa. The decrease in salivary flow may lead to dental and root caries, periodontal disease, and oral candidiasis. Drugs to increase salivary flow, salivary substitutes, and moisturizers may be required.

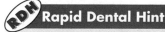 **Rapid Dental Hint**

Monitor patients who are taking psychiatric drugs for xerostomia, periodontal disease, and root caries.

Binding to Dopamine Receptors
Binding to the D_2 receptors correlates not only to antipsychotic effects but also to movement disorders called **extrapyramidal side effects (EPS).** It has been esti-

mated that between 50 and 75 percent of patients on antipsychotics eventually develop some form of EPS. This can be permanent, even when the drug is discontinued.

The extrapyramidal side effects which can occur within days from starting the medication include:

- Dystonia (abnormal muscle contraction)
- acute akathisia (the most common EPS; sense that the patient must keep moving; swaying from foot to foot)
- parkinsonism (tremors, impaired gait); benztropine (Cogentin) may help relieve the early onset side effects
- Tardive dyskinesia, an EPS which is not always reversible and is characterized by involuntary, persistent movements of the tongue (rolling), and lips (lip smacking), lateral jaw movements, chewing movements, blinking, rocking back and forth, and facial muscle movement. Oral dyskinesias may result in bruxism, broken teeth, tongue trauma, and ulcerations. Since the patient cannot remain "still" and is always moving, dental management of these patients is difficult. Approximately 20 percent of patients and 50 percent of the elderly on long-term neuroleptics experience tardive dyskinesia. There is no recognized treatment.
- Blocking D_2 receptors also may cause prolactin elevation, which can suppress ovarian and testicular function, causing infertility, reduced libido, breast tenderness, and gynecomastia (enlarged breasts) in men.

Rapid Dental Hint

Dental patients with extrapyramidal side effects may be difficult to manage.

Binding to Histamine Receptors
Binding to H_1 receptors results in antihistamine side effects including sedation, drowsiness and weight gain (and serotonin receptor blockade).

Binding to α_1-Adrenergic Receptors
Another concern of neuroleptics is cardiac safety. Binding to the α_1-adrenergic receptors causes postural hypotension, dizziness, syncope, palpitations and reflex tachycardia.

Most neuroleptics cause a prolongation of the QT interval, which can lead to a potentially fatal ventricular tachycardia. The highest incidence occurs with thioridazine, followed by ziprasidone, quetiapine, risperidone, olanzapine and holoperidol. It also occurs in atypical antipsychotics, but to a lesser extent. Because of this, it is important to question the patient about all medications, prescription as well as OTC, to avoid cardiac problems. Precautions should be taken when using local anesthetics containing epinephrine, which could increase the cardiac side effects.

Antipsychotics (also called *neuroleptics*) are classified as *typical antipsychotics* and *atypical antipsychotics*.

Typical Antipsychotics

The older, typical, or conventional antipsychotics treat the positive symptoms, but not the negative symptoms. These drugs have been the treatment of choice for psychoses for 50 years. Typical antipsychotics (Table 18–1) act by binding to both D_1 and D_2 (dopamine) receptor sites, but *more at D_2 receptors,* which is responsible for their many side effects, which create an adherence problem and many treatment failures. These older dopamine antagonists are being replaced by newer, atypical antipsychotic drugs. The typical antipsychotics are subclassified into:

- High-potency, such as haloperidol (Haldol), or low-potency drugs such as chlorpromazine (Thorazine), and promethazine (Phenergan), used for relief of allergic conditions rather than as an antipsychotic.

Table 18–1 Common Typical "Older" Antipsychotics: Adverse Effects

Typical Antipsychotics
Low Potency
- Chlorpromazine (Thorazine)
- Thioridazine (Mellaril)

High Potency
- Trifluoperazine (Stelazine)
- Fluphenazine (Prolixin)
- Thiothixene (Navene)
- Haloperidol (Haldol)
- Loxapine (Loxitane)
- Molindone (Moban)

Potency is based on the affinity to the D_2 receptors and is related to the amount of drug needed to cause a therapeutic response or effect. Thus, high-potency drugs have a greater affinity to D_2 receptors and low-potency drugs have a lower affinity to the D_2 receptors. *Note:* This was the older theory with the typical antipsychotics, but theory has changed with the newer, atypical antipsychotics as discussed below
- whether they are phenothiazines or nonphenothiazines or
- incidence of adverse effects

Atypical or Novel Antipsychotics

With the limitations of the traditional antipsychotic agents (e.g., adverse effects, treatment failure, adherence problems and limitation in treating negative symptoms), the introduction of newer, atypical antipsycotics has broadened the therapeutic spectrum to include negative symptoms and fewer serious adverse effects, although there are still many adverse effects. Atypicals bind weakly to D_2 receptors (Figure 18–1) and then quickly detach to allow normal dopamine transmission in a matter of hours. Weaker D_2 receptor effects minimize EPS; however, there is a stronger binding to D_4 receptors. These drugs are called atypical because they were discovered, by Dr. H. Meltzer, also to block *serotonin* 5-HT_2 (5-hydroxytrytamine) receptors. Thus, there is a reorientation of the traditional approach to schizophrenia as a dopamine-related disease. There must be interactions among dopamine, serotonin, histamine, and adrenergic systems. *Each atypical has unique properties* in addition to whether each has a tight or loose binding to the D_2 receptor. For example, clozapine has more sedative effects than risperidone. Some agents have no appreciable affinity for cholinergic muscarinic receptors, thus no anticholinergic side effects. Table 18–2 lists the atypical antipsychotics currently available in the United States.

With a better drug profile, the atypical antipsychotics have become the first line of treatment of schizophrenia. Although these newer antipsychotics greatly reduce the risk of developing adverse effects, especially anticholinergic and EPS, there are still numerous side effects related to the atypical antipsychotics including weight gain, diabetes mellitus, increased serum lipid levels, daytime sedation, and cardiac problems.

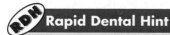
Rapid Dental Hint

Patients taking atypical antipsychotics are at increased risk for diabetes. Monitor periodontal disease status.

Atypical antipyschotics include:

- Risperidone (Risperidal), considered to be first-line therapy
- Olanzapine (Zyprexa)

- Ziprasidone (Geodon)
- Quetiapine (Seroquel)
- Clozapine (Clozaril)

Clozapine (Clozaril) was the first atypical antipsychotic available in the United States. Clozapine causes seizures and blood disorders such as agranulocytosis (white blood cell count decreases to under 1,000 mm^3), which is a FDA black box warning. Clozapine is usually used for refractory cases where other treatments have failed. It is necessary to take a blood test weekly to check on white blood cells levels.

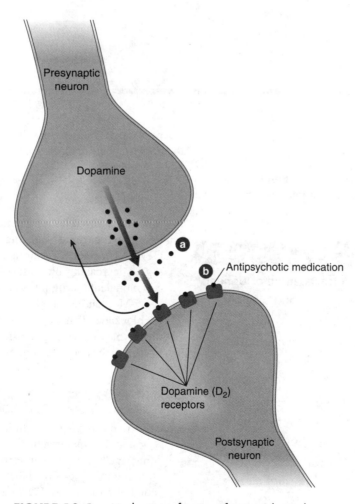

FIGURE 18-1 Mechanism of action of antipsychotic drugs. (a) (overproduction of dopamine; (b) antipsychotic medication occupies D_2 receptors, preventing dopamine from stimulating the postsynaptic neuron.

Table 18-2 Adverse Effects of Atypical Antipsychotics

Drug Name	Sedation	Extrapyramidal Side Effects (EPS)	Anticholinergic	Orthostatic Hypotension	Dental Patient Instructions
Atypical Antipsychotics					
Clozapine (Clozaril; Clozapine USP; FazaClo)	High	Very Low	High	High	Fewer adverse side effects. Orthostatic hypotension may still occur in some patients. Reported to have much less xerostomia
Risperidone (Risperdal)	Moderate	Moderate	Low	Low	
Olanzapine (Zyprexa)	High	Low	Moderate	Low	
Quetiapine (Seroquel)	High	None	Low	Low	
Aripiprazole (Abilify)	Low	Low	Low	Low	
Ziprasidone (Geodon)	Low	Low	Low	Low	

Adjuncts to Antipsychotics

Because psychosis involves the expression of multiple symptoms and many patients respond only partially to antipsychotics, combination pharmacotherapy may be necessary. Thus, antipsychotics can be used with other drugs such as valproate, an anticonvulsant drug.

Drug Interactions of Dental Significance

Since all antipsychotics are metabolized in the liver, the P450 cytochrome enzymes (CYP2D6, CYP1A2, CYP3A4) will affect their metabolism either by increasing or decreasing blood levels. Table 18–3 lists some common dental drug interactions.

Most antipsychotics can cause α-adrenergic receptor blockade. Thus, epinephrine-containing local anesthetics may cause hypotension and reflex tachycardia. Epinephrine should be administered cautiously. The den-

---

Guidelines for Patients Taking Antipsychotics

- Anticholinergic side effects; monitor patients for xerostomia, root caries, and oral candidiasis.

- Monitor patients for orthostatic hypotension: Patients should remain in an upright position in the dental chair before standing.

- Greater incidence of hyperglycemia (diabetes mellitus) in patients with schizophrenia; monitor patient for periodontal disease.

- Tardive dyskinesia: Dental management may be difficult due to abnormal muscle movement.

- Limit the use of epinephrine; avoid use of epinephrine-impregnated retraction cord.

Rapid Dental Hint

The Food and Drug Administration (FDA) has requested that manufacturers of atypical antipsychotic drugs include a warning on the label of these drugs describing the risk of off-label use (using the drug for a condition that is not FDA indicated) to older patients with dementia. These patients who have dementia and take an atypical antipsychotic show a greater mortality (death) rate.

Table 18–3 Significant Drug-Drug Interactions: Antipsychotics

Drug Name	Drug–Drug Interactions
Atypical Antipsychotics	Epinephrine: antipsychotics block α-adrenergic receptors allowing increased beta activity (e.g., vasodilation and increased heart rate). Monitor blood pressure when epinephrine is given to hypotensive patients taking neuroleptics, because hypotension and tachycardia may occur.
Aripiprazole (Abilify)	Carbamazepine (Tegretol) will decrease aripiprazole levels. Ketoconazole (Nizoril) will increase levels.
Clozapine (Clozaril) Clozapine USP (FazaClo)	Inducers of metabolism causing lowered plasma levels of clozapine: Smoking Carbamazepine (Tegretol) Phenytoin (Dilantin) Inhibitors of metabolism causing elevated clozapine plasma levels: Erythromycin Ketoconazole (Nizoril) Fluroquinolones (Cipro)
Risperidone (Risperdal)	No significant dental drug interactions Inducers: Carbamazepine Inhibitors: Fluoxetine (Prozac) Paroxetine (Paxil) Nefazodone (Serzone)
Olanzapine (Zyprexa)	Erythromycin, ciprofloxacin (Cipro) may inhibit the metabolism of olanzapine, thus increasing blood levels. Inducers: Smoking Carbamazepine Phenytoin Inhibitors: Fluvoxamine (Luvox)
Quetiapine (Seroquel)	Inducers: Smoking Carbamazepine Inhibitors: Ketoconzole Erythromycin Thioridazine
Ziprasidone (Geodon)	Inducers: Carbamazepine Inhibitors: Ketoconazole

tal hygienist should monitor vital signs in patients taking antipsychotics. The maximum number of cartridges that should be used is two of 1:100,000 epinephrine. Levonordefrin should be avoided because of high toxicity.

DRUGS FOR MOOD DISORDERS

Mood disorders are characterized by marked mood swings and include major depressive episode (depression), dysthymia, and bipolar disorder. Mood disorders can be treated by nonpharmacologic methods (e.g., psychotherapy, hypnosis, electroconvulsive therapy), pharmacotherapy, or a combination of both.

Depression

Antidepressants: Etiology/Diagnosis of Major Depression

Major depression is a common illness, affecting approximately 5–10 percent of the population. Depression is a mood state with diagnostic criteria found in DMS-IV. In order to diagnose depression, a certain number of symptoms (at least five) must be present every day for at least 2 weeks. These symptoms include depressed mood, markedly diminished interest or pleasure in activities, weight gain, sleep changes, feelings of worthlessness or guilt, poor concentration, thoughts of death, and fatigue or loss of energy. Dysthymia is a milder type of depression, causing less impairment.

Mechanism of Action   There are many theories about how antidepressants work. It is known that a biochemical imbalance occurs in depression. It is believed that depression causes *decreased levels of norepinephrine and/or serotonin* in the brain which occurs either because of an increased breakdown of these neurotransmitters by enzymes, a decrease in their synthesis in the presynaptic neuron, or reuptake of the neurotransmitter back into the presynaptic axon terminal that released it. In any case, there are reduced levels of norepinephrine and serotonin (regulates mood) in the neuronal synapse junction.

Thus the purpose of some *antidepressant medication is to increase the concentration of norepinephrine and/or serotonin by inhibiting or blocking the reuptake* into synaptic terminals on the neuron. The subsequent increase in the amounts of these neurotransmitters available at the synapse may compensate for their deficit seen in depressed individuals. Other antidepressants act by inhibiting monoamine oxidase (MAO), an enzyme responsible for the breakdown of catecholamine neurotransmitters such as epinephrine and norepinephrine.

There is usually a delay of onset of action of antidepressants, taking at least 2–3 weeks until therapeutic effects are seen. Full recovery from depression may take several months.

Classification of Antidepressants   There are different classifications of antidepressant drugs, each with a specific mechanism of action (Table 18–4):

- Monoamine oxidase inhibitors (MAOIs)
- Tricyclic antidepressants (TCAs)
- Selective serotonin reuptake inhibitors (SSRIs)

Monoamine oxidase inhibitors   Monoamine oxidase is an enzyme that metabolizes catecholamine neurotransmitters. There are two isoenzymes of MAO: A and B. MAO-A inactivates norepinephrine and serotonin that leak out of the presynaptic storage vesicles, MAO-B is responsible for the metabolism and inactivation of dopamine. These enzymes are found in the G.I. tract, liver, and central nervous system.

Monoamine oxidase inhibitors (MAOIs) are antidepressant drugs that inhibit the actions of MAO, resulting in increased activity of NE within the brain and other places in the body (Table 18–4). Generally the MAOIs, including tranylcypromine (Parnate) and phenelzine (Nardil), nonselectively and irreversibly inhibit and destroy monoamine oxidase. Selegiline transdermal system (Emsam) is the first antidepressant patch approved for major depressive disorder.

At one time, these drugs were widely used, but have not been popular in many years because of adverse side effects. They are reserved for more severely depressed patients or atypical depression (e.g., depression with phobia). Monoamine oxidase is required to metabolize tyramine, found in certain foods. MAOIs inhibit this metabolism, allowing the accumulation of tyramine, a sympathomimetic, which may cause a hypertensive episode (increased heart rate, elevated blood pressure, and headache). Since these drugs inhibit both MAO-A and MAO-B, the body is left without a mechanism for metabolizing ingested tyramine. While the patient is taking an MAOI, they must not eat any foods containing tyramine, including aged cheeses, bananas, raisins, avocados, aged meat, soy sauce, yeast, beer, wines, yogurt, sour cream, bologna, salami, hot dogs, green figs, sauerkraut, and pickled herring.

The "newest" MAOIs are classified as COMT inhibitors.

Table 18-4 Classification of Antidepressants: Treatment of Major Depressive Disorder

Drug Name	Adverse Effects	Dental Drug–Drug Interactions	Patient Instructions
Tricylic Antidepressants (TCAs) Amitriptyline (Elavil) Comipramine (Anafranil) Desipramine (Norpramin) Doxepin (Adapin, Sinequan) Imipramine (Tofranil) Nortriptyline (Pamelor) Protriptyline (Vivactil) Trimipramine (Surmontil)	Sedation, weight gain, xerostomia, urinary retention, orthostatic hypotension, constipation, memory dysfunction, sexual impairment, increased changes for arrhythmias and cardiac conduction disturbances	• May increases action of sympathomimetics (e.g., epinephrine in lidocaine, phenylephrine, pseudoephedrine)—not necessary to avoid using EPI, but treat as a cardiac patient and give 0.04 mg of EPI which is present in two cartridges of lidocaine 2% with 1 : 100,000 epinephrine; avoid levo-nordefrin • Other interactions: Do not use with MAOIs. • Additive effect with anticholinergic drugs (e.g., antihistamines, anti-parkinsonian drugs, antipsychotic drugs) • Increased sedative effects if taken with alcohol and other drugs that cause sedation • Cimetidine (Tagamet) inhibits elimination of TCAs	• Monitor vital signs at each visit (before and after treatment) because of cardiac side effects. • Avoid orthostatic hypotension by having the patient sit upright for a few minutes before getting out of the dental chair. • Assess salivary flow. • Recommend salivary substitutes and/or fluoride supplements to decrease incidence of caries.
Monoamine oxidase inhibitors (MAOIs) Isocarboxazid (Marplan) phenelzine (Nardil) Tranylcypromine (Parnate)	Agitation, tremors, insormnia, postural hypotension, headache, dry mouth, weight gain, sexual dysfunction	• Carbamazepine is contraindicated. • Other interactions: Hypertensive crisis possible with OTC preparations containing symphomimetics (e.g., phenylephrine, pseudoephedrine) • Hypertensive crisis with foods containing tyramine (e.g., aged cheeses) • When taken with a TCA, a hypertensive crisis can occur • Additive sedation and CNS depression if taken with alcohol, opoids (narcotic analgesics such as codeine), barbiturates • If taken with SSRIs, can cause elevated serotonin levels (serotonin syndrome), which can result in cardiovascular collapse	• Tyramine-free diet • Monitor vital signs • Instruct on dealing with dry mouth • Orthostatic hypotension

Table 18–4 (Continued)

Drug Name	Adverse Effects	Dental Drug–Drug Interactions	Patient Instructions
Selective Serontonin Reuptake Inhibitors (SSRIs)		No special precautions using epinephrine No vasoconstrictor (epinephrine) interactions Other interactions: Do not use concurrently with MAOIs or TCAs (during or within 14 days of therapy). All SSRIs inhibit various CYP450 (CYP2D6) drug metabolizing enzymes but some are less involved. SSRIs, especially fluoxetine, increase blood levels and effects of β-blockers, benzodiazepines, antiseizure drugs, codeine, antipsychotics, carbamazepine, TCAs, dextromethorphan. Alcohol—increased CNS effects	Less zerostomia than with TCAs Xerostomia counseling: drink water, salivary substitutes, avoid alcohol-containing mouthrinses, fluoride supplement Increased risk of gastrointestingal bleeding especially if also taking an NSAID (e.g., ibuprofen), aspirin, warfarin
Citalopram (Celexa)	Dry mouth, nervousness, sweating, nausea, insomnia, sexual dysfunction	Less effect on P450 enzymes	See above
Escitalopram (Lexapro)	Nervousness, sweating, nausea, insomnia, sexual dysfunction	Less effect on P450 enzymes	See above
Fluoxetine (Prozac)	Gastrointestinal upset (nausea, diarrhea), dry mouth, restlessness, nervousness, sexual dysfunction, weight loss, insomnia, headache	The most drug interactions because it inhibits cytochrome P450 enzymes Increases toxicity of diazepam	See above
Fluvoxamine (Luvox)	Highest incidence of nausea, headache, tremor, insomnia; less incidence of dry mouth	High effect on inhibiting P450 enzymes	See above
Paroxetine (Paxil)	Nausea, dizziness, insomnia, sexual dysfunction, more anticholinergic effects (constipation, dry mouth) and more sedation than fluoxetine	High effect on inhibiting P450 enzymes	See above
Sertraline (Zoloft)	Relatively few side effects than the other SSRIs; highest incidence of tremors and nervousness; xerostomia	Less effect on P450 enzymes; avoid grapefruit juice	See above
Duloxetine (Cymbalta)	Nausea, xerostomia, constipation hepatotoxicity	Effect on inhibiting P450 enzymes Most atypical antidepressants have little effect on the P450 enzymes.	See above

Drug Name	Adverse Effects	Dental Drug–Drug Interactions	Patient Instructions
Atypical Antidepressants			
Amoxapine (Asendin)	Few G.I. effects; low sedation; sexual dysfunction, low orthostatic hypotension; dry mouth, constipation, blurred vision	Additive sedative effects with narcotics, alcohol, barbiturates, and other CNS depressants • See above • No precautions with epinephrine	• See above • Slight orthostatic hypotension

Bupropion (Wellbutrin)	Similar to SSRIs: nausea, agitation, insomnia; not anticholinergic, seating or cardiotoxic; seizures are common
	Used in smoking cessation therapy (Zyban)
		• See above
		• No precautions with epinephrine
		• Bupropion inhibits the CYP2D6 isoenzyme in the liver. Thus drugs metabolized by this enzyme will have elevated levels:
		  TCAs
		  SSRIs
		  Antipsychotics (haloperidol, risperidone) Beta-blockers
			• See above

Maprotiline (Ludiomil)	Less anticholinergic and sedation than TCAs—no advantage over TCAs	• No significant dental drug interactions	• See above
Mirtazapine (Remeron)	Sedation, weight gain, increased appetite, potential orthostatic hypotension	• Limit use of epinephrine-containing local anesthetics to two cartridges of 2% lidocaine with 1 : 100,000 epi (because of alpha$_1$ receptors blockade)	• See above • Caution with patient going from supine to upright position (because block alpha$_1$ receptors)
Nefazodone (Serzone)	No sexual dysfunction, high sedation, no anticholinergic effects; liver toxicity	• Limit use of epinephrine-containing local anesthetics to two cartridges of 2% lidocaine with 1 : 100,000 epi (because of alpha$_1$ receptors blockade)	• See above
Trazodone (Desyrel)	Xerostomia, nausea, constipation, dry mouth, postural hypotension	• No precautions with epinephrine	• Monitor vital signs at each visit (before and after treatment) because of cardiac side effects • Moderate orthostatic hypotension
Venlafaxine (Effexor)	Nausea, headache, insomnia, sweating, sexual dysfunction, increase in systolic blood pressure with increased dose	• No precautions with epinephrine	• Monitor for increases in blood pressure; monitor for signs of xerostomia • No orthostatic hypotension
Herbal remedies			
St. John's wort	Nausea, diarrhea, allergic reaction, dizziness, dry mouth, photosensitivity (sensitive to sunlight—itching, red lesion)	• No precautions with epinephrine	• Caution use of non-FDA approved drugs; counseling for dry mouth

DRUG INTERACTIONS OF DENTAL SIGNIFICANCE
There is no reported evidence of a drug–drug interaction between the older MAOIs and epinephrine-containing anesthetic.

Tricyclic antidepressants The **tricyclic antidepressants** (TCAs) were first introduced in 1957 and are used in the treatment of depression. The TCAs work by inhibiting the reuptake (inactivation) of norepinephrine and/or serotonin from the synapse, resulting in elevated levels of these neurotransmitters, which would improve the depression (Figures 18–2). There is little effect on dopamine reuptake. Thus, TCAs are termed norepinephrine/serotonin reuptake inhibitors. Besides depression, TCAs are indicated for the dental management of nocturnal bruxism and chronic orofacial pain.

ADVERSE SIDE EFFECTS The biggest problem when deciding which antidepressant to use is its side effect profile (Table 18–5). Adverse side effects of TCAs are due to the *nonselective* affinity and blockade of other receptors, including muscarinic (cholinergic), histaminic, and α-adrenergic receptors.

- Binding to and blockading of muscarinic receptors results in anticholinergic effects such as sedation, xerostomia, constipation, tachycardia, urinary retention, sexual dysfunction, and blurred vision. These anticholinergic effects are the most troublesome side effects.
- Affinity to and blockade of histaminic H_1 receptors result in sedation and weight gain.

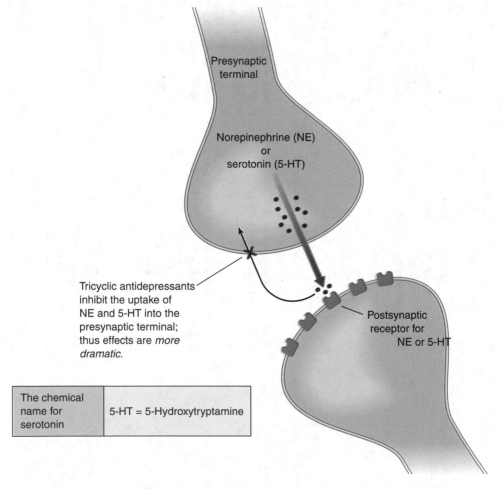

Presynaptic terminal

Norepinephrine (NE) or serotonin (5-HT)

Tricyclic antidepressants inhibit the uptake of NE and 5-HT into the presynaptic terminal; thus effects are *more dramatic.*

Postsynaptic receptor for NE or 5-HT

The chemical name for serotonin	5-HT = 5-Hydroxytryptamine

FIGURE 18–2 Tricyclic antidepressants produce their effects by inhibiting the reuptake of neurotransmitters into the nerve terminal. The neurotransmitters particularly affected are norepinephrine and serotonin.

Table 18–5 Major Side Effects of TCAs

Muscarinic Blockade	Histaminic Blockade	α-adrenergic blockade
Xerotomia	Drowsiness, sedation	Postural hypotension, dizziness
Blurred vision	Weight gain	Reflex tachycardia
Urinary retention	Hypotension	Sexual dysfunction
Constipation		
Increased heart rate		
Memory dysfunction		

- Affinity to and blockade of α-adrenergic receptors causes postural (orthostatic) hypotension and reflex tachycardia.

These side effects can best be managed either by changing the medication or reducing the dosage. Xerostomia may be severe enough that it causes difficulty in swallowing or speech and can lead to the development of dental/root caries and periodontal disease.

Because TCAs increase heart rate, they should not be used in patients with heart conduction disorders or those recovering from a heart attack. TCAs may precipitate arrhythmias in patients with pre-existing conditions.

TCAs must be discontinued slowly to avoid withdrawal symptoms. Since the advent of newer antidepressants, TCAs have been used less frequently, primarily because of their low margin of safety in overdose and numerous adverse drug effects.

DRUG INTERACTIONS OF DENTAL SIGNIFICANCE TCAs are extensively bound to plasma proteins so other highly protein bound drugs such as aspirin and phenytoin (Dilantin) can increase TCA levels by binding to the protein, "knocking off" the TCA from the protein and elevating blood levels. TCAs also increase the effects of other CNS depressants agents, including alcohol (Table 18–4).

It is not necessary to avoid using epinephrine-containing local anesthetics, but to limit the amount to 0.04 mg, which is present in about two cartridges of lidocaine 2% with 1 : 100,000 epinephrine. Epinephrine, from the local anesthetic solution, is inactivated by either the enzyme catechol-O-methyl transferase (COMT) or by reuptake into the nerve terminal. TCAs block the reuptake of both NE and EPI, allowing accumulating levels (Figure 18–3).

Levonordefrin-containing local anesthetic (carbocaine) is *contraindicated* in patients taking a tricyclic antidepressant because accidental intravascular (into the arteries) can result in acute hypertension and cardiac arrhythmias.

TCAs are metabolized in the liver by the cytochrome P450 enzymes, primarily by CYP2D6. The degree of inhibition of metabolism of drugs via the P450 cytochrome enzymes in the liver varies between individuals. If a TCA needs to be co-administered with a drug that inhibits these enzymes (e.g., cimetidine) or inducers of these enzymes (e.g., dexamethasone), then space the dosing of each drug.

Selective serotonin reuptake inhibitors (SSRIs) The neurotransmitter serotonin (5-hydroxytryptamine; 5-HT) was discovered in 1954 to be present in the brain and that the synthesis or function was reduced in depressed individuals. In order to improve the profile of antidepressants, research started in the late 1960s, aimed at developing more potent and more *selective* drugs for the *inhibition of serotonin reuptake*. This was desirable, since many of the adverse effects of tricyclic antidepressants are thought to be due to their nonselective binding to and blocking of receptors for acetylcholine and histamine.

Selective serotonin reuptake inhibitors (**SSRIs**) are a type of antidepressant drug first introduced in 1988 (Table 18–4). The prototype SSRI is fluoxentine (Prozac). SSRIs work to normalize serotonergic imbalances, which may contribute to both depression and anxiety. Development of SSRIs was intended to focus more on the increasing serotonin levels in the brain while producing fewer adverse effects. These drugs selectively inhibit serotonin reuptake into the neuron vesicles by blocking the reuptake serotonin receptor site on the presynaptic neuron, without affinity for the uptake inhibition of norepinephrine and other neurotransmitter amines (Figure 18–4). Besides depression, some SSRIs are used to treat anxiety disorders, eating disorders (anorexia nervosa or bulimia), fibromyalgia, premenstrual syndrome, obsessive-compulsive disorder, and panic disorder.

The SSRIs are not as lethal in an overdose and do not have the anticholinergic side effects (sedation) of TCAs. The SSRIs are equally effective as the TCAs in the treatment of mild to moderate depression. However, the TCAs are still most effective for severe depression and in patients with insomnia (because these drugs cause sedation) and agitation.

ADVERSE EFFECTS SSRIs do not have the same affinity to other receptors, so they do not exert the same

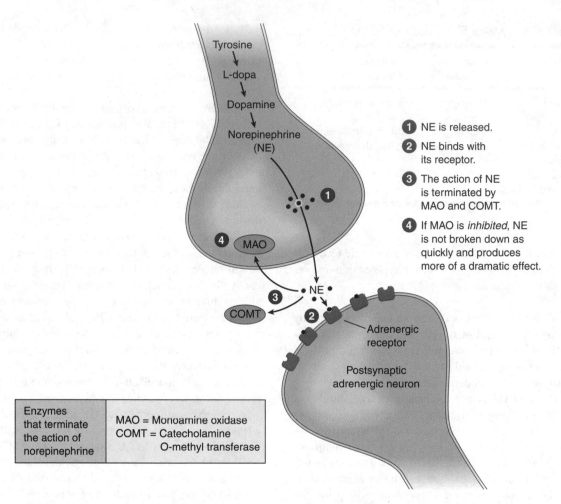

FIGURE 18–3   Terminiation of norepinephrine activity through enzyme activity in the synapse.

anticholinergic, antihistaminic, antiadrenergic effects. Thus, the SSRIs have a different adverse side effect profile that includes gastrointestinal discomfort (nausea, diarrhea), nervousness, headache, reduced appetite, sexual dysfunction, and weight loss. Additionally, SSRIs can induce bruxism. There is an increased risk of gastroin-

---

Did You Know?

Antidepressants were originally developed as antihistamines. They were discovered in the 1950s. The first modern antidepressant, iproniazid, was originally developed to treat tuberculosis, but it was found that it was mood elevating and stimulated activity in patients. The first tricyclic antidepressant was imipramine.

---

testinal bleeding, especially if the patient has preexisting risk factors or is taking other drugs (e.g., nonsteroidal anti-inflammatory drugs such as ibuprofen, aspirin, warfarin) that increase risk. SSRI use increases risk of bleeding by 3.6 times, compared with the risk in the general population for those who don't use SSRIs, but there is a twelve-fold risk increase when nonsteroidal anti-inflammatories and SSSRIs are combined.

In general, these drugs do not cause drowsiness or sedation because they do not bind to the histamine receptors. Fluoxetine (Prozac) can alter blood glucose levels in diabetics. When any antidepressant drug is discontinued, the dose must be decreased gradually to prevent any harmful withdrawal symptoms or rebound responses such as dizziness, nausea, or headache.

DRUG–DRUG–FOOD INTERACTIONS   In January 2006, the FDA-approved safety labeling revisions for venlafax-

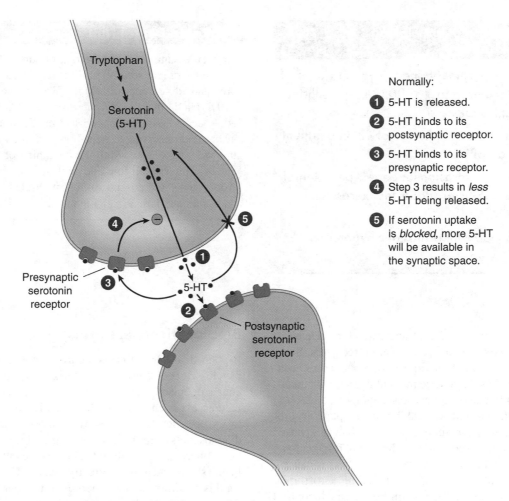

Normally:

1. 5-HT is released.

2. 5-HT binds to its postsynaptic receptor.

3. 5-HT binds to its presynaptic receptor.

4. Step 3 results in *less* 5-HT being released.

5. If serotonin uptake is *blocked*, more 5-HT will be available in the synaptic space.

FIGURE 18–4   SSRIs block the reuptake of serotonin into nerve terminals, resulting in increased serotonin levels.

ine (Effexor and Effexor XR) to warn of the risk for sustained hypertension associated with their use in some patients.

The SSRIs have many drug interactions, but there are no significant dental drug interactions. The SSRIs are metabolized by the cytochrome P450 system in the liver and thus are affected either by induction or inhibition by other drugs metabolized the same way. Some SSRIs such as sertraline may have less cytochrome P450 inhibition action than others.

Grapefruit juice is a potent CYP3A4 inhibitor of the metabolism of fluvoxamine and sertraline.

A "serotonin syndrome" can occur due to elevated serotonin blood levels which are potentially very dangerous and fatal. This usually is caused by a combina-

tion of two or more drugs, one of which is an SSRI and the other an MAOI. Symptoms include severe hypertension, rapid eye movement, rapid muscle contraction, feeling drunk, dizziness, confusion, diarrhea, and eventually cardiovascular collapse and death.

Since serotonin reuptake blockade has no effect on the disposition of EPI because EPI uses the NE reuptake pump, there are no precautions or concerns for using EPI in patients taking SSRIs.

Atypical antidepressants There are other types of antidepressants that have action similar to the TCAs but are classified as atypical. These drugs include nefazodone (Serzone), venlafaxine (Effexor), bupropion (Welbutrin), maprotiline (Ludiomil) and trazodone (Desyrel) (Table 18–4).

Guidelines for Patients Taking Antidepressants

- Limit use of epinephrine to two cartridges of 2% lidocaine with 1 : 100,000 epinephrine if patient is taking a TCA.

- No concerns with the use of EPI in a patient taking a SSRI.

- Monitor for xerostomia: caries, periodontal disease (SSRIs produces less xerostomia than TCAs).

- Use caution with orthostatic hypotension (usually with TCAs).

 Rapid Dental Hint

Antidepressants increase the risk of suicidal thinking and behavior (suicidality) in short-term studies in children and adolescents with Major Depressive Disorder (MDD) and other psychiatric disorders. Children and adolescents taking antidepressant medication must be aware and observed closely for suicidality. In 2004, this warning was added to the beginning of the package insert in bolded font and enclosed in a black box. Additionally, there is a warning for clinical worsening and suicide risk in adult patients with MDD.

Nefazodone (Serzone) and trazodone (Desyrel) block both serotonin and α-adrenergic receptors. Since trazodone lacks anticholinergic action but causes sedation, it is used as a hypnotic in combination with an antidepressant that does not cause sedation (e.g., SSRI).

Venlafaxine (Effexor) inhibits the reuptake of serotonin, NE, and to a lesser extent, dopamine, and is used for severely depressed patients who do not respond to an SSRI. The most common adverse side effect is nausea, but there are other side effects including xerostomia, dizziness, sweating, tremor, anorexia and increased supine diastolic blood pressure. Venlafaxine does not have a high incidence of drug interactions; however, it should not be given with an MAOI. It is metabolized by the cytochrome P450 (2D6) enzymes and thus should not be given with cimetidine, which would inhibit the metabolism of venlafaxine, leading to increased blood levels.

Herbal Remedies Herbal remedies for the treatment of depression are not approved by the U.S. Food and Drug Administration. There are concerns over the "purity" of the ingredients in the formulations as well as their efficacy. An example of an herbal supplement that is not FDA approved for the management of depression is St. John's wort, which comes from the flowering plant *Hypericum perforatum*. There are may adverse side effects, including xerostomia, G.I. disturbances, restlessness, headache, dizziness, and confusion.

Bipolar Disorders (BPD)

Bipolar disorder (BPD) is a chronic common, serious psychiatric condition characterized by an irregular course of episodes of mania and depression. An individual can experience manic, hypomanic, depressive and mixed episodes. Bipolar disorder is most commonly misdiagnosed as unipolar (major) depression because patients often present while at the depressive rather than the manic stage, and thus incorrectly treated. The older term for this condition is manic-depression. Patients with undiagnosed bipolar disorder are at increased risk for suicide. To be diagnosed with BPD the individual must have the following episodes for a specific duration of time:

- *Manic episodes* (or mania) are characterized by an abnormally elevated or irritable mood, aggressiveness, happy, euphoric, impulsive behavior, decreased sleep, increased activity, and grandiosity (exaggerated sense of self-importance). Must have symptoms for at least 1 week.

- *Hypomanic episodes* are not full-blown mania but a milder form that does not interfere with an individual's daily functioning. At least 4 days with three or more symptoms.

- *Depressive episodes* are characterized by feeling sad, decreased interest (low mood), low self-esteem, sleep disturbance, and appetite disturbance.

At least 2 weeks with five or more symptoms most of the day/nearly every day.

Mixed episodes are characterized by both mania and depression (both high and low mood) over a 1-week period.

DSM-IV classifies bipolar disorders as:

- *Bipolar I disorder:* Considered the classic form of manic depression, in which manic, depressive, hypomanic, or mixed states can occur. There must be a full manic episode for a diagnosis of bipolar I.
- *Bipolar II disorder:* Patients never experienced a full manic episode, but have experienced at least one hypomanic episode and at least one episode of major depression.
- *Cyclothymic disorder:* chronic (more than 2 years), fluctuating mood disturbances involving many periods of mild hypomanic and depressive symptoms that do not meet the criteria for either mania or major depression.

In most cases, patients with major depression/ mood disorder have shown a tendency toward certain comorbid conditions in which there is another illness associated with the depression/mania, such as substance abuse or anxiety.

Phases of Treatment:

Standard pharmacologic treatment of symptoms of bipolar disorder involves: (Table 18–6)

- Acute therapy: treatment of the acute episode of the manic and depressed stage
- Maintenance therapy: prevention of the relapse of these episodes

Many types of drugs are used to treat BPD, including mood stabilizers antidepressants and antipsychotics. *Mood stabilizers* to treat the mania exert their effects by "stabilizing from above," and *antidepressants* to treat the depression exert their effects by "stabilizing mood from below." In 2002, the American Psychiatric Association (APA) updated its guidelines for the treatment of patients with bipolar disorder. The main changes reflected the shifts in the evidence for use of treatment other than lithium.

Treatment of the manic/mixed (acute) episode Although most of the data of the effectiveness of mood stabilizers in bipolar illness come from studies using monotherapy (one drug), in clinical practice most bipolar patients are treated with more than one drug. Combination therapy also has the potential to improve the therapeutic: side effect ratio and for long-term stabilization.

The American Psychiatric Association (APA) recommends as stage 1 primary agents:

- For *mild* acute manic (agitated) episode (monotherapy): lithium, divalproex (valproate/valproic acid), or an atypical antipsychotic such as risperidone (Risperdal), ziprasidone (Geodon), aripiprazole (Abilify), olanzapine (Zyprexa), or quetiapine (Seroquel).
- For mixed episode: divalproex, aripiprazole, risperidone, or ziprasidone
- For *severe* manic or mixed episodes (Two-drug combination): lithium + atypical antipsychotic *or* valproate plus an atypical antipsychotic

Lithium (Lithobid) Discovered in 1949, lithium is the gold standard mood stabilizer. The specific mechanism of action in mania is relatively unknown. By decreasing or preventing manic episodes, subsequent depression episodes may be avoided. Lithium may also help to reduce rapid cycling (four or more episodes of mania, hypomania, or depression in the preceding 12 months) experienced by some patients. Patients taking lithium alone had significantly fewer suicide attempts.

Since lithium has an FDA black-box warning for a *narrow therapeutic index,* blood tests must be taken to find the optimal therapeutic dosage and to avoid toxicity even at doses close to therapeutic levels. Chronic lithium

---

Did You Know?

Napoleon and Beethoven are just a few of the famous people diagnosed with bipolar disorder.

Did You Know?

When the soda 7-UP was originally introduced in the 1930s, it contained lithium.

Table 18-6 Common Bipolar Disorder Medications

Drug Name	Mechanism	Adverse Effects	Dental Drug–Drug Interactions	Patient Instructions
Lithium carbonate (Eskalith)	Manic episodes; mechanism of action is unclear Maintenance therapy	Many; cardiac arrhythmias, fine hand tremor, increase in thirst, increased urination (polyuria), drowsiness, dizziness, tongue movements, dry skin, hypothyroidism, diarrhea, and neutropilia (increase white blood cell count).	Increased lithium serum levels with: Nonsteroidal anti-inflammatory drugs Metronidazole (Flagyl)	• Medical consult with the patient's physician may be necessary. • Have patient sit in upright position in dental chair before getting up. • Dry mouth: Advise patient to drink water, avoid alcohol containing mouth rinses, use artificial saliva (if needed) and brush frequently. • Lithium can cause orthostatic hypotension; patient should sit in upright position in dental chair before standing.
Carbamazepine (Equetro)	Anticonvulant drugs to treat manic and mixed episodes	Fatigue, headache, sedation, rash, leukopenia, liver toxicity, GI upset	• Metabolism of carbamazepine is decreased by activation of P450 liver enzymes when taken with: Erythromycin Clarithromycin (Biaxen) • Increased liver toxicity with acetaminophen • Carbamazepine stimulates the metabolism of: Anticoagulants (e.g., warfarin) Oral contraceptives Doxycycline Corticosteroids Cyclosporine Other interactions: • Increased leukopenia (low WBCs) if taken with:Clozapine (Clorazil) • Increased sedation with alcohol, other CNS depressants	• Monitor for a decrease in WBC counts. • Monitor cardiovascular signs at each visit.

Drug Name	Mechanism	Adverse Effects	Dental Drug–Drug Interactions	Patient Instructions
Gabapentin (Neurontin)	Anticonvulsant drug; refractory for acute mania	Sedation, dizziness, fatigue, weight gain, xerostomia	• No significant dental interactions • Other interactions: Minimal drug interactions with other psychotropics; antacids other psychotropics; antacids decrease levels; cimetidine (Tagamet) increases levels; oral contraceptives decreases levels	• Monitor for xerostomia
Lamotrignine (Lamictal)	Anticonvulsant drug; bipolar I depression; Maintenance therapy	Dizziness, headache, sedation, tremor, nausea, vomiting, rash	• No significant dental interactions • Other interactions: Oral contraceptives decreases levels.	• First trimester exposure may cause cleft lip or palate. • Serious rashes requiring hospitalization
Valproic acid (Depakene), Divalproex sodium (Depakote)	Anticonvulsant drugs to treat manic states and mixed episodes. Increases levels of the inhibitory neuro-transmitter GABA in the brain.	Sedation, nausea, vomiting, dizziness, hair loss, confusion, agitation, stomach pain, prolonged bleeding (inhibits platelet aggregation), weight gain, liver toxicity, pancreatitis	• Increased valproic acid levels: Magnesium- and aluminum-containing antacids Aspirin and naproxen • Inhibits microsomal liver enzymes, thus increasing blood levels of: phenobarbital Phenytoin Carbamazepine	• Monitor the patient's clotting.

toxicity generally occurs after long-term therapy with high dosages.

There are several preparations of lithium. Lithium carbonate is the most frequently used, and lithium citrate is a liquid preparation for patients who can not tolerate swallowing pills. Generally, a reduction in manic symptoms occurs within 1 to 3 weeks.

ADVERSE EFFECTS   Since lithium is widely distributed throughout the body, there are numerous adverse effects, involving the central nervous system, gastrointestinal tract, cardiovascular system, kidneys (renal), blood system (hematologic), urinary tract, and skin. Some of these side effects include cardiac arrhythmias, fine hand tremor, polydipsia (increase in thirst), polyuria (increase urination), dizziness, drowsiness, tongue movements, xerostomia, metallic taste, dry skin, hypothyroidism, diarrhea, and an increase in white blood cell count (neutrophilia).

Lithium should not be given to patients with renal or cardiovascular disease.

DRUG–DRUG INTERACTIONS OF DENTAL SIGNIFICANCE   There are multiple drug–drug interactions with lithium. Since lithium is 100 percent orally absorbed from the gastrointestinal tract and excreted unchanged in the urine there are many drugs that alter its clearance. Metronidazole taken with lithium may increase lithium toxicity. Since lithium is not metabolized in the liver, the cytochrome P450 enzymes are not involved in these drug interactions.

Nonsteroidal anti-inflammatory drugs (e.g., ibuprofen) increase lithium blood levels by decreasing its clearance in the urine.

SPECIAL DENTAL CONSIDERATIONS   Since lithium can decrease salivary flow, it is important to assess the patient for caries, periodontal diseases, and oral candidiasis. A lichenoid drug reaction can occur with lithium. Since lithium can cause orthostatic hypotension, the dental hygienist should monitor vital signs and have the patient remain in the dental chair in an upright position for a few minutes before standing up.

Divalproex sodium (Depakote)   In 1995, divalproex sodium (Depakote) was the first anticonvulsant approved as a mood stabilizer, and is most effective in treating mixed episodes. Often it is combined with lithium in lower doses to reduce side effects and improve therapeutic response.

Divalproex sodium is a compound comprised of sodium *valproate* and valproic acid, and dissociates to the valproate ion in the gastrointestinal tract. Divalproex

acts by increasing levels of γ (gamma)-aminobutyric acid (GABA), a neurotransmitter in the brain, either by inhibiting its metabolism or by enhancing postsynaptic GABA activity.

The most commonly reported gastrointestinal adverse effects reported at the beginning of therapy are nausea, vomiting, and indigestion. *Inhibition of platelet aggregation may cause altered bleeding times.* It is recommended that valproate blood concentration and platelet counts be monitored once weekly during acute treatment with maintenance monitoring as clinically indicated. Valproate can produce teratogenic effects such as neural tube defects. Divalproex is available as enteric coated tablets and extended-release tablets which allow for absorption in the small intestine and not the stomach, where GI adverse effects occur. Additional adverse effects include weight gain and hair loss.

It is well absorbed orally from the gastrointestinal tract and is about 90 percent bound to plasma proteins so that it displaces and is displaced by other drugs highly protein bound such as warfarin, aspirin, and phenytoin.

The FDA has a black box warning for hepatic failure which may result in death. The drug is extensively metabolized in the liver by the cytochrome P450 system. It inhibits the metabolism of phenytoin, carbamazepine, and phenobarbital, increasing the serum levels of these drugs.

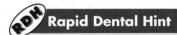

Rapid Dental Hint

Patients taking lithium, valproate, and carbamazepine should have blood values monitored and reported.

DRUG INTERACTIONS OF DENTAL SIGNIFICANCE   There is increased chance of bleeding if taken with aspirin or a nonsteroidal anti-inflammatory drug.

Atypical Antipsychotics   The APA recommends the use of an atypical antipsychotic as monotherapy for less ill patients or in combination with lithium for more severely ill patients.

Olanzapine   Olanzapine (Zyprexa), the first atypical antipsychotic drug approved as a mood-stabilizing drug, has been FDA approved since 2000. It is used either as monotherapy for manic episodes or as an add-on agent for mania partially responsive to conventional mood-stabilizing drugs. Olanzapine and aripiprazole are the only drugs FDA approved for relapse prevention of manic episodes. There are no established blood levels associated with antimanic response, so there is no need for blood level monitoring. It is metabolized by CYP1A2 and CYP2D6 isoenzymes in the liver. There are no dental drug interactions involving these isoenzymes.

Quetiapine Quetiapine (Seroquel) is an antipsychotic agent that is FDA approved for acute manic episodes. Since it may cause orthostatic hypotension, use caution with dental patients when uprighting from the dental chair.

Antiepileptic Mood Stabilizers *Carbamazepine* Carbamazepine (Equetro) is an anticonvulsant drug used to treat acute bipolar I mania and mixed episodes, and is better for long-term use. Fatigue is a common and annoying adverse effect, which makes adherence a problem. Because of its similarity in chemical structure to tricyclic antidepressants, MAOIs should not be given concurrently. Carbamazepine is metabolized by the CYP3A4 isoenzymes in the liver. Many dental drugs such as erythromycin, clarithromycin, and ciprofloxacin inhibit the metabolism of carbamazepine, causing increased blood levels. Carbamazepine stimulates liver enzymes, resulting in lowered blood levels of certain drugs (Table 18–6).

Other antiepileptics drugs for treatment of bipolar disorder If the patient does not respond to these drugs, several newer anticonvulsants such as lamotrigine (Lamictal) and gabapentin (Neurontin) may be effective. Lamotrigine is indicated in the depressed phase of bipolar disorder or as adjunctive add-on in acute mania. It has been associated with development of a severe systemic rash. On September 29, 2006, the FDA announced that first-trimester exposure to lamotrigine may increase the risk for cleft lip or palate in newborns.

Treatment of the depressive episodes of bipolar disorder As mentioned early, bipolar depression can be difficult to recognize and distinguish from generalized depression. Currently, lithium is the only proven agent for treatment of bipolar depression, but lamotrignine is also shown good results. Other drugs include a combination of olanzapine and fluoxetine (Prozac). Antidepressant monotherapy is not recommended due to the chance of starting a manic episode or inducing a pattern of rapid cycling, the evidence of long-term effectiveness of antidepressant therapy is also weak.

If the acute depressive episode does not respond to these medications, the next step would be to add on bupropion (Wellbutrin) or paroxetine (Paxil). Alternative secondary steps include adding an SSRI or venlafaxine (Effexor). For patients who are severely depressed, electroconvulsive therapy should be considered.

Maintenance phase for bipolar I disorder Once the acute crisis is over, patients may remain at particularly high risk of relapse for up to 6 months. This phase of treatment, also referred to as continuation treatment, is aimed at preventing recurrences of mood

APA Guidelines for Treating Manic and Depressive Episodes in Bipolar Disorder

Episodes	*Drugs*
Manic/Mixed	
Severe	*Two-drug combination:* Lithium or valproate + atypical antipsychotic (such as olanzapine or risperidone) (Alternative to lithium or valproate: carbamazepine)
Moderate (less severe)	*Monotherapy:* Lithium, valproate, or an atypical antipsychotic (olanzapine)
Depressive	
First-line pharmacological treatment	Lithium *or* lamotrigine
Alternative, especially for severely ill	Lithium + antidepressant
Depressive episode that does not respond to first-line treatment	ADD: lamotrigine, buproion *or* paroxetine Alternative steps: Add an SSRI.
Maintenance	Lithium, valproate (Alternatives: lamotrigine, olanzapine, carbamazepine)

episodes (depression, mania, hypomania, mixed episodes) and maximizing the patient's quality of life.

Drugs approved for maintenance therapy in bipolar illness (American Psychiatric Association, 2005) include lamotrigine (Lamictal), lithium, or valproate. Lamotrigine is especially effective in preventing relapse into depression; lithium is more effective in preventing relapse of mania. The addition of an antidepressant to lithium maintenance therapy has failed to prevent bipolar depression.

ANXIOLYTICS (ANTI-ANXIETY AGENTS)

Introduction

Anxiety disorders are the most common type of psychiatric disorder, but less than 30 percent of people will seek treatment. Anxiety is an emotion experienced by almost everyone. It is important to distinguish normal fears from abnormal anxiety. Usually, if an individual is in a situation that may be conceived as threatening or dangerous, a state of anxiety is produced; however, if anxiety occurs without sufficient reason and interferes with an individual's health, then it is referred to as pathologic anxiety. Only pathologic anxiety needs to be treated.

Anxiety has an effect on the body (somatic) as well as psychological changes. Symptoms of anxiety include chest pain, tachycardia, trembling, tremors, restlessness, abdominal pain, diarrhea, fatigue, palpitations, insomnia, irritability, headache, dizziness, shortness of breath, profuse sweating, apprehension, headache, and nausea. Chronic stress and anxiety may contribute to increase acid production and development of ulcers. The individual appears to be nervous, frightened, and has a feeling of impending doom. The individual actually enhances his/her somatic symptoms into a serious medical condition.

The DSM-IV-TR™ divides clinical anxiety into the following components:

- Generalized anxiety disorder (GAD)
- panic disorder
- phobias
- posttraumatic stress disorder (PTSD)
- obsessive compulsive disorder
- other anxiety disorders (e.g., alcohol-induced anxiety disorder, substance-induced anxiety disorder, or separation anxiety)

To be diagnosed as generalized anxiety disorder (GAD), the anxiety must be present continuously for at least 6 months. Obsessive-compulsive disorder is characterized by the presence of persistent thoughts and impulses that need to be carried out purposively. Panic disorder is characterized by unexpected, recurrent periods of intense fear that last several minutes. Post-traumatic stress disorder occurs after exposure to a psychologically distressing event where physical harm is anticipated.

There are many theories as to the etiology of anxiety. Normal arousal occurs with antagonism of the inhibitory neurotransmitter called GABA (gamma-aminobutyric acid), resulting in elevated GABA levels in the brain. If this arousal is consistent and GABA is continuously fired, a clinically apparent anxiety state develops. Serotonin is also involved in the pathogenesis of anxiety.

Pharmacology

Benzodiazepines

Benzodiazepines are the drug of choice in the pharmacologic treatment of generalized anxiety disorder because they are the most rapidly acting and effective anxiolytic agents. But they do have side effects, including sedation and physical dependency. Some states (including New York) require that benzodiazepines be a Schedule II controlled drug just like narcotics because of its abuse potential.

Benzodiazepines are used for short-term treatment for the acutely anxious patient experiencing functional disability, and should not be used for the treatment of mild anxiety or depression. Duration of therapy is usually 2–6 months. For long-term treatment, an antidepressant such as an SSRI (selective serotonin reuptake inhibitor) or SNRI (selective mixed reuptake inhibitor) should be considered.

Mechanism of Action Benzodiazepines bind to receptors on GABA and stimulate or activate them by increasing membrane permeability to chloride ions. This results in an increased effect of GABA, which is an inhibitory neurotransmitter. Decreased GABA levels in the brain are supposed to reduce/eliminate anxiety symptoms.

Indications Benzodiazepines have a wide range of indications due to their different dose levels, onset, and duration of actions. Benzodiazepines are classified as anxiolytics (relief of anxiety), sedatives (tranquilizing), hypnotics (sleep-inducing drugs), muscle relaxants, and anticonvulsants. The anti-anxiety effect is caused by sedation, while the hypnotic effect produces insomnia. The short-acting, rapid onset benzodiazepines (e.g., lorazepam, alprazolam) at low doses relieve dental anxiety with little sedation, which is unique with these drugs. But at higher doses, lorazepam is a sedative/hypnotic taken at bedtime. A benzodiazepine that has an onset of 15–45 minutes and is intermediate/long acting is best to induce sleep in insomniacs. These drugs are classified as hypnotics. Benzodiazepines are also used in the treatment of alcohol withdrawal. Thus deciding which drug to use depends on the condition being treated and the pharmacokinetics of the drug.

Drugs with a long elimination half-life such as diazepam (Valium) should not be given to elderly patients because they have a reduced metabolism and may not be able to metabolize the drug efficiently, resulting in elevated blood levels and toxicity. However, an advantage of benzodiazepines is the wide margin of safety between therapeutic and toxic doses, so that there is less likely chance of overdosing.

Adverse Effects   All of the benzodiazepines are similar in effects, with the most common side effect being CNS depression, including sedation, drowsiness, and respiratory depression. Sedation is dose related: The higher the dose, the more sedation occurs. Xerostomia is a dental-related side effect that should be monitored in patients.

Tolerance does occur within 3 to 14 days; more and more of the drug is needed to get a therapeutic response. Because of this, overdosing is also less likely to occur. Dependence is most likely to occur in patients with a past history of alcoholism or substance abuse if taken for prolonged periods of time (even normal doses, dependence may occur as soon as within 4–6 weeks of starting the drug. Excessive ingestion (overdose) is not likely to result in respiratory depression.

Withdrawal symptoms occur if benzodiazepines are taken for long periods. When discontinuing the drug, the dose should be decreased slowly over time. Benzodiazepines with short half-lives such as alprazolam have the greatest tendency for dependency and withdrawal symptoms. Thus the lowest possible dose for the shortest period of time is the best regimen, which may be difficult since many patients with anxiety or panic disorder may be in treatment for months to years. Intravenous flumazenil (Romazicon) antagonizes the effects of benzodiazepines on the CNS, including sedation and psychomotor impairment.

The benzodiazepines should not be given to women in the first trimester of pregnancy, or in patients with alcohol intoxication, acute angle glaucoma, and a history of substance abuse.

Drug–Drug Interactions of Dental Significance (Table 18–7):   Alcohol and other CNS depressants should be avoided to prevent additional drowsiness and sedation. Benzodiazepines are metabolized by the liver P450 enzymes (CYP3A4). They are either transformed by oxidative pathways in the liver or metabolized by conjugation into water-soluble products in the liver, whereby the metabolite products formed are inactive. Epinephrine is not contraindicated with benzodiazepines.

Other Drugs: GAD

Drugs other than benzodiazepines have been used to treat anxiety. All drugs with serotonin reuptake inhibiting properties are effective in treating GAD. Buspirone (Buspar) is a nonbenzodiazepine that is an agonist at serotonin type 1A receptors and is effective in the treatment of some anxiety disorders. It is very well tolerated by patients. Buspirone should not be given to patients also taking MAOIs.

Propranolol, a β-blocker, has also been used to relieve anxiety. Propranolol does not act centrally in the brain to relieve symptoms of anxiety, but reduces the autonomic symptoms of anxiety (e.g., the tachycardia that results from anxiety).

SEDATIVE-HYPNOTIC DRUGS

Barbiturates

Barbiturates at one time were used in the treatment of anxiety, but are no longer because of their ability to cause overdosing, tolerance (more of the drug is needed to produce the same therapeutic effect), and dependence (increased need to want a psychoactive drug), and have been replaced by the benzodiazepines. Barbiturates are used mainly as hypnotics (tranquilizing, sleep inducing) in the short term (2 weeks) treatment of insomnia (sleep disturbance), as anticonvulsants in the treatment of seizures, and preoperatively to relieve anxiety and provide sedation. The benzodiazepines are also used as sedatives/hypnotics and anticonvulsants and have fewer adverse side effects than barbiturates. When taken for insomnia (difficulty in sleeping), barbiturates can cause hangover and daytime sedation and if used longer than 2 weeks, the

Table 18-7 Commonly Used Anxiolytics: Drugs for Treatment of Generalized Anxiety Disorders

Drug Name	Mechanism	Adverse Effects	Dental Drug–Drug Interactions	Patient Instructions
Benzodiazepines	Stimulates the inhibitory neurotransmitter GABA	Tolerance develops rapidly, drowsiness, sedation, disorientation, blurred vision, dry mouth, nausea, difficulty in swallowing, decrease in respiratory rate, possible seizures Contraindicated in open angle glaucoma, alcohol and substance abuse, first trimester pregnancy	Increased sedation and drowsiness with alcohol and other CNS depressants; Erythromycin, clarithromycin and cirprofloxacin inhibit metabolism of benzodiazepines Other drug interactions: Fluoxetine and fluvoxamine increase blood levels of alprazolam and diazepam Oral contraceptives inhibit the metabolism of diazepam and chlordiazepoxide	Dry mouth: Advise patient to drink water, avoid alcohol-containing mouthrinses, use artificial saliva (if needed) and brush frequently.
Short-acting				
Alprazolam (Xanax; Niravam—orally dissolving)	Panic disorder; dental anxiety	See above	See above	See above
Lorazepam (Ativan)	Dental anxiety	See above	See above	See above
Intermediate-acting				
Chlordiazepoxide HCl (Librium, Libritabs)	Antianxiety; alcohol withdrawal; preoperative sedation; sedative/hypnotic	See above	See above	See above
Clonazepam (Klonopin)	Panic disorder	See above	See above	
Diazepam (Valium)	Dental anxiety, alcohol withdrawal; anticonvulsant (IV), skeletal muscle relaxant; very rapid onset	See above	See above	See above
Halazepam (Paxipam)	Antianxiety; treat phobias	See above	See above	See above
Long-acting				
Clorazepate (Tranxene)	Very rapid onset	See above	See above	See above

Drug Name	Mechanism	Adverse Effects	Dental Drug–Drug Interactions	Patient Instructions
Other anti-anxiety drugs				
Buspirone (Buspar)	Selective serotonin receptor agonists; only has anxiolytic properties	Dizziness, drowsiness, nausea, headache, fatigue	Decreased metabolism with erythromycin and clarithromycin	Dry mouth: Advise patient to drink water, avoid alcohol-containing mouthrinses, use artificial saliva (if needed) and brush frequently.
Hydroxyzine (Atarax)	Antihistamine; pruritus; preoperative and postoperative sedation	Sedation; anticholinergic (xerostomia, urine retention)	Potentiates CNS depression with narcotics (codeine), barbiturates (phenobarbital); may increase alcohol effects	See above
Antidepressants:	Inhibit reuptake of serotonin	Nausea, sexual dysfunction	No significant dental interactions (e.g., xerostomia)	Fewer anticholinergic side effects
SSRIs: Fluoxetine (Prozac), sertraline (Zoloft)				

drugs lose their effectiveness in producing sleep. Today, it is preferred to use the benzodiazepines as sedative-hypnotics and anxiolytics because benzodiazepines have a higher therapeutic index, making them a safer drug.

When taken orally, barbiturates pass the blood–brain barrier into the brain and produce changes in CNS moods, ranging from excitation, to mild sedation, to hypnosis (altered state of awareness), and anesthesia in high doses. Barbiturates produce respiratory and brain depression. Death can occur in an overdose.

Pharmacology

Barbiturates are derived from barbituric acid and are combined with a salt, which makes it more rapidly absorbed. The mechanism of action of these drugs is to depress central nervous system activity in the brain, producing drowsiness, sedation, deep coma, and even death. A level of excitation usually occurs before drowsiness begins. These drugs work similarly to the benzodiazepines by enhancing the binding of GABA to GABA receptors, increasing GABA activity, and allowing chloride ion channels to open.

In usual dosages, barbiturates also suppress respiratory activity, such as seen in sleep.

Barbiturates are classified according to their lipid solubility and duration of action (Table 18–8). Ultrashort-acting barbiturates are highly lipid soluble and have a very short duration of action. They are used as IV anesthetics, and are not given orally.

Short- and intermediate-acting barbiturates [pentobarbital (Nembutal)] are less lipid soluble and their effects last longer than the ultrashort-acting barbiturates. These drugs are used for sleep induction (sleeping pills).

Long-acting barbiturates are the least lipid soluble, with much longer duration of action. These drugs are used as sedatives for a tranquilizing effect or anti-anxiety.

Barbiturates are slowly metabolized in the liver by the liver P450 microsomal enzymes.

Adverse Effects

Adverse side effects include drowsiness, headache, nausea, and vomiting, impaired consciousness, excitement, and CNS depression. In toxic doses, death occurs by respiratory depression. With continued use, development of tolerance and dependency are likely, which makes the ultrashort-acting barbiturates, such as pentobarbital, a frequently intentionally abused drug. Dependency presents a clinical picture similar to alcoholism. Ingestion of excessive quantities of barbiturates usually results in a respiratory depression and coma.

These drugs are addicting. Abrupt discontinuation of barbiturates can cause withdrawal symptoms consisting of tremors, nausea, vomiting, seizures, and cardiac arrest.

Barbiturates used for insomnia are only given for short-term usage because chronic use can cause rebound insomnia.

Drug–Drug Interactions of Dental Significance

Barbiturates induce P450 enzymes in the liver, which increases the metabolism of many drugs, including phenytoin, digoxin, coumadin (warfarin), and their own metabolism.

After barbiturates are absorbed into the blood they are highly protein bound to albumin in the blood. Thus, many drug–drug interactions can occur whereby other highly protein-bound drugs compete for binding sites on the protein molecule displacing the other drug. This results in higher drug concentrations in the blood and subsequent toxic effects.

Other Sedative-Hypnotic Medications

Chloral Hydrate Chloral hydrate (Noctec) is a prodrug; it must be metabolized in the liver to its active form. It is used primarily for sedation in children and is frequently used in the dental office as pre-anesthetic sedation before a dental procedure. It has an unpleasant taste and has a low therapeutic index, indicating it has a high incidence of toxicity.

Zolpidem Zolpidem (Ambien) is used as a hypnotic in patients with problems with early morning awakening. It is used only for short-term treatment of insomnia.

Zaleplon Zaleplon (Sonata) is used on a short-term basis in patients who have difficulty with falling asleep or morning grogginess. Possible drug interactions occur with rifampin, phenytoin, carbamazepine, and phenobarbital.

ATTENTION DEFICIT-HYPERACTIVITY DISORDER (ADHD)

Many children seen in the dental office may be diagnosed with attention deficit-hyperactivity disorder. Attention deficit/hyperactivity disorder affects 3–5 percent of all children, and approximately 2 million American children. Children with ADHD have difficulty concentrat-

Table 18-8 Sedative-Hypnotics: Induction of Sleep

Drug Name	Uses	Adverse Effects	Significant Drug Interactions	Notes
Benzodiazepines *Short-acting Hypnotics*	To induce sleep (conscious/ preoperative sedation) Used for sedation in dental offices	Tolerance develops rapidly, drowsiness, sedation, disorientation, blurred vision, dry mouth, nausea, difficulty in swallowing, decrease in respiratory rate, possible seizures Contraindicated in open angle glaucoma, alcohol and substance abuse, first trimester pregnancy	Increased sedation and drowsiness with alcohol and other CNS depressants Nefazodone inhibits alprazolam and triazolam metabolism. Fluoxetine and fluvoxamine increase blood levels of alprazolam and diazepam. Oral contraceptives inhibit the metabolism of diazepam and chlordiazepoxide. Disulfiram and cimetidine inhibit metabolism of alprazolam, diazepam, and chlordiazepoxide.	
Midazolam (Versed)	Intravenous	See above	Erythromycin inhibits metabolism.	IV sedation: monitor vital signs
Triazolam (Halcion)	Very rapid onset	See above	Erythromycin inhibits metabolism.	Monitor vital signs
Intermediate-acting Hypnotics	To induce sleep	See above	See above	Dry mouth: advise patient to drink water, avoid alcohol-containing mouthrinses, use artificial saliva (if needed) and brush frequently.
Estazolam (Prosom)	Rapid onset			
Temazepam (Restoril)	Rapid onset			
Long-acting Hypnotics Flurazepam (Dalmane)	To induce sleep Very rapid onset			
Quazepam (Doral)	Rapid onset			
Non-Benzodiazepines Saleplon (Sonata)	Rapid onset, very short duration; short-term treatment of insomnia—must dose during the night	Drowsiness, headache, eye pain, abdominal pain	Increased effect with alcohol, antihistamines and other CNS depressants; increased effect with cimetidine (Tagamet)	Avoid alcohol and other CNS depressants.
Zolpidem (Ambien)	Selectively binds to serotonin-1 receptor; short-term treatment of insomnia (2–3 weeks); Rapid onset	Drowsiness, dizziness, head-ache, nausea, confusion, dependence	Increased effect with alcohol and other CNS depressants (e.g., TCAs); Rifampin (for treatment of TB) may decease effects	

(continued)

Table 18-8 (Continued)

Drug Name	Uses	Adverse Effects	Significant Drug Interactions	Notes
Others Chloral hydrate (Noctec)	Rapid onset; short-term sedative/hypnotic to allay anxiety or induce sedation preoperatively; reduce anxiety; associated with drug withdrawal	Gastrointestinal irritation; avoid with gastric or duodenal ulcers; suicidal tendencies; skin eruptions; diarrhea, dizziness	Reduces effectiveness of anti-coagulants (coumarin); additive CNS depressants	Available as a syrup; especially used in dental offices for sedation of children; must calculate dosage according to weight of child. As a hypnotic use 50 mg/kg.

Barbiturates	All barbiturates increase GABA activity and are sedative-hypnotics.	All barbiturates can cause drowsiness, early morning (residual) "hangover," daytime sedation, headache, nausea, vomiting, diarrhea, excitement	• Many because barbiturates increase the metabolism of themselves and other drugs.
			• Increased metabolism of:
			  Cyclosporine
			  Doxycycline
			  Estrogens
			  Ketoconazole
			  Phenothiazine
			  Quinidine
			  Oral contraceptives
			  Increased CNS depression with:
			  Alcohol
			  Antidepressants
				• Drowsiness occurs, but since the patient is not taking it chronically, no special instructions are required.
				• Avoid alcohol and other CNS depressants.

Long-Acting Phenobarbital (Luminal)	Sedative-hypnotic; epilepsy (anticonvulsant)	See above	See above	See above
Intermediate/Short Acting Amobarbital (Amytal)	Insomnia (sleep disorder) Sedation (insomnia), anxiety, preanesthetic medication (for hypnotic effects)	See above	See above	See above
Butabarbital (Butisol)	Sedative	See above	See above	See above
Pentobarbital (Nembutal)	Sedative/hypnotic (insomnia) (short-term use only)	See above	See above	See above
Secobarbital (Seconal)	Sedative/hypnotic (insomnia) (short-term use only)			

ing on certain tasks, do not have a wide attention span, and are easily distracted. Adults are now being diagnosed with ADHD. Signs and symptoms include forgetting appointments, difficulty staying seated, and constantly losing things.

The goal of treatment is to improve behavior and academic performance in children. If diagnosed properly, these children are taking a CNS stimulant (Schedule II drugs) such as an amphetamine (Adderall XR). These drugs have sympathomimetic effects, and the amount of epinephrine-containing local anesthetics should be kept to a minimum. Vital signs should be monitored. Methylphenidate (Concerta, Ritalin) and atomoxetine (Strattera) are other drugs used in the management of ADHD.

USE OF PSYCHOTROPIC DRUGS IN THE DENTAL OFFICE

Dental clinicians can prescribe psychotropic drugs for sedation of the apprehensive dental patient, treatment for bruxism, and orofacial pain (Table 18–9).

Anxious Dental Patient

Benzodiazepines are considered the drug of choice for relieving anxiety associated with dental procedures. Benzodiazepines are anti-anxiety drugs. The most commonly used oral benzodiazepines are diazepam (Valium), triazolam (Halcion), chlorazepate (Tranxene), and lorazepam (Ativan). Generally, these drugs are given in a single dose either the night before or one hour before the dental procedure. An adverse side effect of benzodiazepines is sedation. Triazolam, which has a more rapid onset of action and shorter half-life, shows less postoperative sedation. The patient should have a designated driver taking them to and from the dental office.

Intravenous benzodiazepines such as diazepam (Valium) and midazolam (Versed) are used in the dental office for conscious sedation. Complications may arise during intravenous administration of these drugs, and must be recognized early and appropriate treatment rendered. Venipuncture complications include hematoma, fluid extravasation, and intra-arterial drug injection. Drug-related side effects such as nausea and vomiting

Table 18–9 Psychotropic Drugs Used in the Dental Office

Condition	Drug	Dose	Effects
Apprehensive patient	*Benzodiazepines:*		Postoperative sedation; abuse/dependence issues
	Diazepam (Valium)	5–10 mg one hour before dental treatment	Do not give to patients who are also taking phenytoin (Dilantin) and cimetidine (Tagamet).
	Lorazepam (Ativan)	1–2mg one hour before dental procedure	Avoid with alcohol and other CNS depressants.
	Triazolam (Halcion)	0.25–0.5 mg one hour before dental treatment	Diazepam and triazolam decreased metabolism with erythromycin.
Bruxism	*Benzodiazepines:*		
	Diazepam (Valium)	5–10 mg at bedtime (limited therapy to 2 weeks)	Abuse/dependence issues
			Do not give to patients who are also taking phenytoin (Dilantin) and cimetidine (Tagamet).
			Avoid with alcohol and other CNS depressants.
	Antidepressants:		
	Amitriptyline (Elavil) Doxepin (Sinequan)	Starting dose: 10 mg at bedtime, then gradually increase	Anticholinergic side effects, including xerostomia
Chronic Orofacial Pain	*Antidepressants* Amitriptyline (Elavil)	Initial dosing 10–25 mg at bedtime with weekly increments to a target dose of 25–150 mg	

can occur. Practitioners must have emergency drugs and equipment available in the dental office at all times.

Bruxism

Many patients who have nocturnal bruxism also have anxiety problems. The management of bruxism is using appliances and in some cases medications. A benzodi-azepine such as diazepam (Valium) 5–10 mg, chlo-razepate (Tranxene) taken at bedtime can be effective in these patients. Benzodiazepines should not be used for more than 2 weeks because of the potential for abuse and dependency. Tricyclic antidepressants such as amitripty-line (Elavil) can also be used when appliance therapy has failed. The starting dose is 10 mg at bedtime and gradu-ally increases every few days.

Table 18–10 Summary

Disease	Therapy	Transmitter Receptor Actions
Schizophrenia	Antipsychotics	Dopamine (DA), 5-HT$_{2A}$ receptor antagonism
Depression	Antidepressants	Serotonin and/or norepinephrine reuptake blockade
Anxiety	Anxiolytics	GABA receptor blockade; serotonin reuptake inhibition

Chronic Orofacial Pain

As discussed in Chapter 5, besides analgesics, many psy-chotropic drugs are used in the treatment of orofacial pain, including tricyclic antidepressants such as amitriptyline (Elavil), which have been reported to relieve chronic facial pain. The exact mechanism is unclear. Anticholinergic side effects including xerostomia are frequently seen in these patients. The selective serotonin reuptake inhibitors (SSRIs) have fewer side effects but appear to be less effec-tive than the TCAs for the treatment of facial pain.

DENTAL HYGIENE NOTES

Drugs used in psychiatry have many adverse effects that are implicated in dental treatment. There is a high inci-dence of dry mouth, which can be so severe that a mouth mirror can stick to the oral mucosa. Instruct the patient to drink plenty of water and use a saliva substitute avail-able at the pharmacy. Examples of saliva substitutes are Optimoist Liquid and Salivart Synthetic Saliva Solution. Reduction in salivary flow can also cause candidiasis. The patient should be instructed to avoid alcohol, smok-ing, and antihistamines, which also reduce salivation.

Since patients with dry mouth are prone to caries, regular in-office fluoride treatment and/or self-applied fluorides may be indicated. A 0.05% sodium fluoride over-the-counter rinse (e.g., PreviDent) or 0.4% stannous fluoride over-the-counter gel (e.g., GelKam) may be use-ful for home use.

To prevent dental/root caries, foods that are high in sugar and acid should be avoided; sugar promotes bacte-rial growth and acid causes demineralization. Instruct the patient to use a soft or extra-soft toothbrush.

The extrapyramidal side effects seen with antipsy-chotics may pose a patient management problem. The patient may be in constant motion, moving the lips, tongue, and head. Unfortunately, nothing can be done to eliminate this, the dental clinician has to be aware of it so that injuries are avoided.

Many antipsychotics block α-adrenergic receptors, resulting in hypotension (postural), angina, and diarrhea. Patients should remaining sitting upright in the dental chair for a few minutes before rising.

There is no compelling evidence that antipsychotic drugs cause diabetes, but there is a greater prevalence of hyperglycemia in patients with serious mental illness. Patients with schizophrenia have an eight-fold to ten-fold higher risk of diabetes than the general population. It has been documented that diabetes is an established risk fac-tor of periodontal diseases. Thus patients taking antipsy-chotic medications for schizophrenia should be monitored for the periodontal diseases.

There is much controversy regarding the use of local anesthetics containing vasoconstrictors. The ques-tion arises as to whether the use of EPI in cardiac pa-tients and in patients taking antidepressants (other than SSRIs and drugs that do not affect the levels of NE/EPI) will increase blood pressure and heart rate. The use of epinephrine in local anesthetics as a vasoconstrictor is *not* contraindicated in patients taking antidepressants, antipsychotics, anxiolytics, or barbiturates. Since some antidepressants (e.g., TCAs) inhibit the reuptake of norepinephrine, it was presumed that there would be an additive effect with epinephrine (from the local anesthetic) in the synaptic area, which could possibly result in a hypertensive crisis (extremely elevated blood pressure). Since MAOIs inhibit the enzyme that breaks down NE and serotonin, use of these drugs with EPI is not of much concern. Some newer antidepressants (e.g., SSRIs) do not affect the levels of NE. Epinephrine contained in local anesthetics functions as a vasoconstrictor to delay systemic absorption, which then increases the duration of anesthesia. Using vasoconstrictors in these types of patients may actually prevent the release of endogenous epinephrine. Thus patients taking tricyclic antidepressants that elevate NE levels should be treated like cardiac patients in terms of EPI administration. One to two cartridges of 2% lidocaine with 1 : 1000,000 epinephrine (0.04 mg epinephrine) should be used in a patient taking a TCA. Retraction cords containing epinephrine are contraindicated.

Levonordefrin, the vasoconstrictor in carbocaine, should be avoided in patients taking tricyclic antidepressants due to enhanced sympathomimetic effects. Also, retraction cord containing epinephrine should be avoided in these patients.

KEY POINTS

- Most psychotropic drugs cause xerostomia, which may lead to carious lesions. Monitor patients; advise patients to drink plenty of water, use sugarless gum, and use salivary substitute such as Optimoist, Salivart, or Moi-Stir Swabsticks.
- Xerostomia is due to a decreased salivary flow (anticholinergic effects).
- Epinephrine may be given in limited amount to patients taking TCAs. Retraction cord containing EPI is contraindicated.
- No contraindications for EPI in patients taking SSRIs.
- Tardive dyskinesia (repetitive involuntary movements of the tongue, lips and jaw) are adverse effects of antipsychotic drugs. These movements make management of dental patients difficult.

- TCAs and SSRIs have cardiac side effects (e.g., tachycardia, increased blood pressure and arrhythmias).
- Most psychotropic drugs cause orthostatic hypotension. The patient should sit in an upright position in the dental chair for a few minutes before getting out of the chair.
- Patients taking divalproex (Depakote) should have a medical consult regarding platelet counts.
- Benzodiazepines are used for sedation of the anxious dental patient and in the management of nocturnal bruxism.
- TCAs are used in the management of nocturnal bruxism when appliance therapy has failed.
- Lithium, used in the treatment of the acute manic phase of mixed bipolar disorder, may cause a metallic taste in the mouth due either to the taste of the lithium tablet or due to the secretion of lithium in the saliva. There are increased lithium blood levels if taken with nonsteroidal anti-inflammatory drugs [ibuprofen (Advil, Motrin), naproxen (Aleve)].
- Carbamazepine (Tegretol), used in the treatment of seizures and non–FDA-approved in the treatment of manic-depressive disorder, may cause sores in the mouth, which may be an early sign of a blood disorder. Do not prescribe erythromycin or clarithromycin,

BOARD REVIEW QUESTIONS

1. Which of the following drugs requires regular blood tests to determine the white blood cell levels? (p. 341)
   a. Thorazine
   b. Resperidone
   c. Clozapine
   d. Ziprasidone

2. Which of the following adverse side effects makes treating a patient difficult? (p. 339)
   a. Dystonia
   b. Akathisia
   c. Drug-induced parkinsonism
   d. Tardive dyskinesia

3. Which of the following drugs does tolerance and dependency develop quickly? (p. 359)
   a. Diazepam

b. Haloperidol
c. Fluoxetine
d. Paroxetine

4. Local anesthetics containing epinephrine are contraindicated in the dental patient taking fluoxetine requiring local anesthesia because epinephrine will cause orthostatic hypotension. (p. 352)
   a. The first statement is true and the reason is correct.
   b. The first statement is true and the reason is incorrect.
   c. The first statement is not true but the reason is correct.
   d. The statement and the reason are not correct.

5. Which of the following is a common adverse effect of psychiatric drugs and requires patient counseling in the dental office? (p. 338)
   a. Tardive dyskinesia
   b. orthostatic hypotension
   c. weight gain
   d. xerostomia
   e. sedation

SELECTED REFERENCES

ADA Guide to Dental Therapeutics, 3rd ed. 2003. Chicago: American Dental Association.

American Academy of Family Physicians. 2000. Diagnosis and management of depression. *American Family Physician* Monograph No. 2. Kansas, MO: American Academy of Family Physicians.

American Psychiatric Association. 1994. Task Force on DSM-IV. Diagnostic and statistical manual of mental disorders: DSM-IV. Washington, DC: American Psychiatric Association.

American Psychiatric Association. 2005. *Annual Meeting Highlights.* Bipolar disorder management: A new edition. May 21–26, Atlanta, GA.

American Society of Health-System Pharmacists. *AHFS Drug Information 2001.* Edited by G.K. McEvoy. Bethesda, MD: American Society of Health-System Pharmacists,

Citrome, L. and J. F. Goldberg. 2005. Bipolar disorder is a potentially fatal disease. *Postgrad Med* 117:9–11.

Gentile, S. 2007. Atypical antipsychotics for the treatment of bipolar disorder. *CNS Drugs* 21(5):367–387.

Goldberg, J. F. and L. Citrome. 2005. Latest therapies for bipolar disorder: looking beyond lithium. *Postgrad Med* 117:25–26,29–32, 35–36.

Gonzales-Pinto, A., M. Gutierrez, J. Ezcurra, et al. 1998. Tobacco smoking and bipolar disorder. *J Clin Psychiatry* 59:225–228.

Hawton, K. 2005. Suicide risk and attempted suicide in bipolar disorder: A systematic review of risk factors. *J Clin Psychiatry* 66:693–704.

Henin, A., E. Mick, J. Biederman et al. 2007. Can bipolar disorder-specific neuropsychological impairments in children be identified? *J Consult Clin Psychol* Apr; 75(2):210–220.

Hirschfeld, R. M., L. A. Vornik. Bipolar disorder—Costs and comobidity. *Am J Manag Care* 2005;11(suppl).

Kastrup, E. 2005. *Drug Facts and Comparison.* St. Louis: J.B. Lippincott.

Muzyka, B. C., M. Glick. 1997. The hypertensive dental patient. *JADA* 1997;128:1109–1120.

Sanger, T. M., Tohen, M., Vieta, E., et al. 2003. Olanzapine in the acute treatment of biopolar I disorder with a history of rapid cycling. *J Affect Disord* 73:155–161.

Suppes, T., E. B. Dennehy, R. M. A. Hirschefld, et al. 2005. The Texas Implementation of Medication Algorithms: Update to the algorithms for treatment of bipolar I disorder. *J Clin Psychiatry* 2005:66:870–886.

WEB SITES

www.medscape.com
www.psychiatrictimes.com
www.psych.org
www.psychiatryonline.org

Q U I C K   D R U G   G U I D E

Antipsychotics

Typical Antipsychotics

Phenothiazines

- Chlorpromazine (Thorazine)
- Mesoridazine (Serentil)
- Thioridazine (Mellaril)
- Fluphenazine Prolixin)
- Perphenazine (Trilafon)
- Trifluoperazine (Stelazine)

Non-Phenothiazines

- Thiothixene (Navane)
- Haloperidol (Haldol)
- Loxapine (Loxitane)
- Molindone (Moban)

Atypical Antipsychotics

- Clozapine (Clozaril)
- Risperidone (Risperdal)
- Olanzapine (Zyprexa)
- Quetiapine (Seroquel)
- Ziprasidone (Geodon)

Drugs for Mood Disorders: Antidepressants

Tricylic Antidepressants (TCAs)

- Amitriptyline (Elavil)
- Imipramine (Tofranil)
- Trimipramine (Surmontil)
- Doxepin (Adapin, Sinequan)
- Desipramine (Norpramin)
- Nortriptyline (Pamelor)
- Protriptyline (Vivactil)
- Comipramine (Anafranil)
- Amoxapine (Asendin)

Monoamine oxidase inhibitors (MAOIs)

- Phenelzine (Nardil)
- Isocarboxazid (Marplan)
- Tranylcypromine (Parnate)

Selective Serontonin Re-uptake Inhibitors (SSRIs)

- Fluoxetine (Prozac)
- Paroxetine (Paxil)
- Sertraline (Zoloft)
- Citalopram (Celexa)
- Fluvoxamine (Luvox)

Atypical Antidepressants

- Mirtazapine (Remeron)
- Reboxetine (Edronax)
- Bupropion (Wellbutrin)
- Trazodone (Desyrel)
- Nefazodone (Serzone)
- Venlafaxine (Effexor)

Drugs for Mood Disorders: Mood Stabilizers (Bipolar Disorder)

Mood Stabilizing: Acute Mania

- Lithium carbonate (Eskalith)
- Valproic acid (Depakene), divalproex sodium (Depakote)
- Olanzapine (Zyrexa)
- Carbamazepine (Equetro)

Depressive Disorder

- Lithium carbonate
- Lamotrigine (Lamictal)
- Nonresponsive: addition of
- Bupropion (Wellbutrin),
- Paroxetine (Paxil)

Anxiolytics/Hypnotics

Benzodiazepines

Short-acting Anxiolytics

- Alprazolam (Xanax)
- Lorazepam (Ativan)
- Oxazepam (Serax)

Long-acting Anxiolytics

- Prazepam (Centrax)

Short-acting Hypnotics

- Midazolam (Versed)
- Triazolam (Halcion)
- Zolpidem (Ambien)

Intermediate-acting Hypnotics

- Estazolam (Prosom)
- Temazepam (Restoril)
- Chlordiazepoxide HCl (Librium, Libritabs)
- Clorazepate (Tranxene)
- Diazepam (Valium)
- Halazepam (Paxipam)

Long-acting Hypnotics

- Flurazepam (Dalmane)
- Quazepam (Doral)

Other anti-anxiety drugs

- Buspirone (Buspar)
- Sertraline (Zoloft)
- Venlafaxine extended-release (Effexor XR)
- Paroxetine (Paxil)

Barbiturates

Long-Acting

- Phenobarbital (Luminal)

Intermediate/Short-Acting

- Amobarbital (Amytal)
- Butabarbital (Butisol)
- Pentobarbital (Nembutal)
- Secobarbital (Seconal)

Ultra-short Acting

- Thiopental (Pentothal)

Drugs for Attention Deficit/Hyperactivity Disorder (ADHD)

Amphetamine

- Dextroamphetamine sulfate
- Dextroamphetamine saccharate
- Amphetamine aspartate monohydrate
- Amphetamine sulfate (Adderall XR) CII
- Methylphenidate (Concerta, Ritalin) CII
- Atomoxetine (Strattera)

Chapter 19

Endocrine and Hormonal Drugs

GOALS

- To provide knowledge of the various medications used in the treatment of diabetes mellitus.
- To provide an understanding of thyroid conditions and how to manage these patients in the dental office.
- To gain knowledge about the dental management of patients taking corticosteroids.
- To provide the dental professional with a basic understanding of the various hormonal drugs, including oral contraceptives, and their relationship to dental treatment.

EDUCATIONAL OBJECTIVES

After reading this chapter, the reader should be able to:

1. Illustrate the pathogenesis of diabetes mellitus.
2. Compare the indications and effects of the available medications used to treat diabetes mellitus.
3. Explain the dental management of diabetic patients.
4. Describe the various drug-drug interactions of diabetic medications.
5. State the dental management of patients with thyroid disorders.
6. State the management of dental patients taking corticosteroids.
7. Describe the dental indications of topical corticosteroids.
8. Describe important dental concerns of corticosteroids.
9. Summarize the components of oral contraceptives and dental concerns.

KEY TERMS

Diabetes mellitus
Hyperglycemia
Insulin
Insulin resistance
Thyroid gland
Corticosteroids
Glucocorticoids
Gonadocorticoids
Adrenal crisis
Sex hormones
Anti-inflammatory

DIABETES MELLITUS

Introduction

Diabetes mellitus makes up a group of hormonal diseases characterized by alterations in carbohydrate, protein and lipid metabolism resulting in elevated levels of blood glucose. This **hyperglycemia** is due to a lack of insulin secretion by the pancreas, a reduction in insulin action, or a combination of both. Plasma glucose concentrations are usually maintained between 40 and 160 mg/dL. Glucose is a sugar that is taken up into the cells by insulin and is used as energy by the cells. **Insulin** is a hormone made and secreted by the beta cells of the islets of Langerhans in the pancreas. When insulin does not function properly or is not produced in efficient amounts to take up the glucose into the cells, glucose remains in the blood and causes a condition called hyperglycemia or diabetes mellitus, which is characterized by glucose intolerance. The liver, however, continues to make glucose (gluconeogenesis) and additional glucose is secreted into the blood stream (Figure 19–1). The elevated glucose levels affects almost all organs in the body, including the cardiovascular system, eyes, nerves, kidney, and the periodentum.

Over the years the classification of diabetes mellitus has changed. Diabetes mellitus is no longer referred to as juvenile- or adult-onset diabetes, nor is it referred to as insulin-dependent and non–insulin-dependent. In 1997, new terms used to classify diabetes mellitus were developed. Diabetes mellitus is now classified as type 1 and type 2.

Type 1

Type 1 diabetes mellitus (formerly juvenile-onset or insulin-dependent diabetes) is due to an *absolute* insulin deficiency as a result of destruction of pancreatic islet beta-cells. Without adequate insulin to allow glucose from the blood to enter cells, the cells starve while glucose accumulates in the blood. The cells do not have glucose as a source of energy, so they begin to break down fat. Free fatty acids accumulate in the blood which are converted into ketones, which may result in ketoacidosis, a potentially life-threatening condition. Diabetic ketoacidosis occurs when there is hyperglycemia (more than 250 mg/dL) and urinary ketone bodies, which results in a metabolic acidosis characterized by drowsiness, nausea, sweating, tachycardia and coma. Type 1 diabetes is primarily an autoimmune process whereby insulin autoantibodies in the body are involved in pancreatic cell

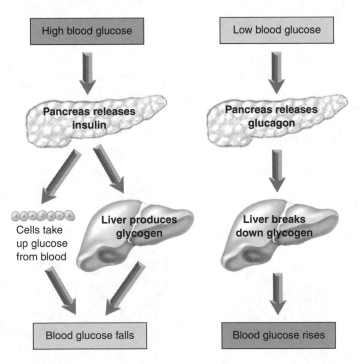

FIGURE 19–1   Insulin, glucagon, and blood glucose.

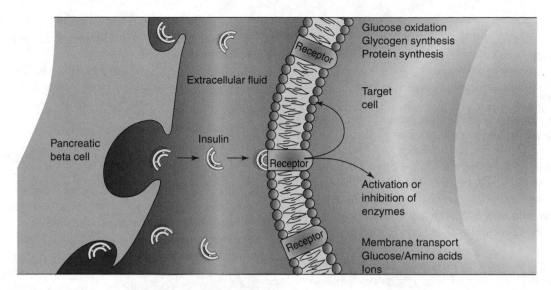

FIGURE 19–2   Plasma insulin binds to receptors on target cells to enter the cells, which starts actions that lead to insulin's biologic effects.

destruction. The onset of type 1 diabetic symptoms is usually quick.

Type 2

Type 2 diabetes mellitus (formerly adult-onset diabetes mellitus or non–insulin-dependent diabetes mellitus) is the more prevalent form of diabetes, and its incidence is increasing due to increased aging population and obesity. Type 2 diabetes mellitus is characterized by insulin resistance with adequate or near adequate and, perhaps even excessive, amounts of insulin. Unlike type 1 diabetes, autoimmune destruction of the beta-cells does not occur in type 2 diabetes mellitus but rather genetics (heredity—family history) play a major role in its development. The typical type 2 diabetic is usually obese and symptoms of the disease are seen gradually. Diabetic ketoacidosis is not usually seen in type 2 diabetics because adequate endogenous insulin is produced to keep ketone formation low.

Insulin Resistance: Type 2 Diabetic

Understanding the concept of insulin resistance is necessary for managing the type 2 diabetic. **Insulin resistance** is defined as decreased insulin effectiveness with a reduced sensitivity of the cells to respond to insulin. After insulin is secreted by the beta cells, it binds to insulin receptors on adipose, liver, and muscle cells, as well as other cell types. Insulin must bind with these receptors and become active in bringing glucose into the cell and stimulating glucose metabolism (Figure 19–2). In type 2 diabetes, insulin receptors in the target tissues have become insensitive or resistant to insulin so that insulin may bind to the receptor, but there is a defect in both insulin action and secretion, making the insulin ineffective in glucose uptake into the tissues. When insulin resistance develops, the beta cells are forced to compensate by secreting more insulin (*hyperinsulinemia*). Over time, the beta cells of the pancreas lose their ability to produce insulin in sufficient quantities to overcome insulin resistance. This condition is referred to as *impaired glucose tolerance* or prediabetes. This results in high blood glucose levels, especially after meals, which is called postprandial hyperglycemia. The degree of insulin defects is influenced by many factors, including obesity, smoking, and decreased physical activity. Continued insulin resistance and insulin deficiency ultimately will result in type 2 diabetes.

Diagnosis

Common signs and symptoms of type 1 diabetes include:

1. Polyphagia (increased appetite)
2. Polyuria (increased urination)
3. Polydipsia (increased thirst)

4. Weight loss
5. Weakness
6. Xerostomia
7. Burning tongue/mouth
8. Periodontal disease (also seen in type 2 diabetes)

Symptoms may not be apparent in type 2 diabetics because the disease is slow in development. Most individuals are obese, and most are diagnosed with diabetes because of an abnormal random blood glucose test.

There are other types of diabetes, including gestational diabetes, when pregnant women have hyperglycemia. Diabetes can result from taking drugs such as corticosteroids, or from other diseases such as Cushing's syndrome.

Criteria for diagnosing diabetes mellitus have changed over the years from those previously recommended by the National Diabetes Data Group (NDDG) and the World Health Organization (WHO). The following are different ways to diagnosis diabetes mellitus:

1. *Random (not fasting) plasma glucose.* If ≥200 mgdL, then a fasting plasma glucose (FPG) test should be done.
2. A subsequent (FPG) test should be performed to confirm the results of the random plasma glucose test. Diabetes is characterized by the presence of a fasting hyperglycemia: plasma glucose of 126 mg/dL after fasting (no caloric intake for at least 8 hours) overnight.
3. In patients with an abnormally high FPG value, an *oral glucose tolerance test* (OGTT) may be performed; however, since it is an expensive test and many false positives can occur, patients have to follow strict preparation rules. Patient preparation for an OGTT involves a carbohydrate diet and 10–12 hour fasting before the test. Plasma glucose levels are taken at different times after taking a carbohydrate (glucose) solution. A 2-hour postprandial (2 hours after consuming the carbohydrate solution) glucose of 200 mg/dL is diagnostic of diabetes. Many drugs that can produce a false positive (getting positive results when they should be

negative) include thiazide diuretics, corticosteroids, propranolol, oral contraceptives, and phenytoin.

Impaired glucose tolerance (IGT) is diagnosed by an OGTT, with the 2-hour postprandial (after a meal) value of 140 mg/dL, but > 200 mg/dL.

Complications

Individuals with diabetes are at an increased risk for microvascular (the terminal ends of blood vessels: arterioles, capillaries and venules) complications of the eye (retinopathy), gingiva, kidneys, nerves (neuropathy), and extremities (e.g., foot ulcers). Macrovascular (arteries) complications include coronary artery disease. Diabetics are at increased risk for congestive heart disease (CHD) and peripheral vascular disease and stroke. Coronary artery disease is the major cause of death in both type 1 and type 2 diabetics. All of these conditions are associated with insulin resistance (increased production of insulin by the beta cells). Other diseases associated with insulin resistance and diabetes are hyperlipidemia and hypertension. *Diabetes is a risk factor for developing periodontal diseases, and individuals with periodontal disease are at risk for developing diabetes mellitus.* (Figures 19–3 and 19–4)

 Rapid Dental Hint

Remember to screen and monitor your diabetic patients for periodontal disease.

Control and Management

The ultimate goal for diabetic control and reduction in complications is glycemic control. Glycosated hemoglobin, or HbA1c, is a test that monitors how the patient is controlling the diabetes. This test measures the percentage of hemoglobin in the red blood cells that is bound to glucose. When hemoglobin becomes glycosated it will stay bound to that red blood cell for the life of that cell. HbA1c levels reflect glycemic control over the preceding 2–3 months and thus are useful in determining the efficacy of treatment. The goal is to have a HbA1c of 7 percent or lower and a preprandial (before meals) blood glucose of 80–120 mg/dL. This test should be done about every 3 months.

Did You Know?

Diabetes also occurs in animals, including cats.

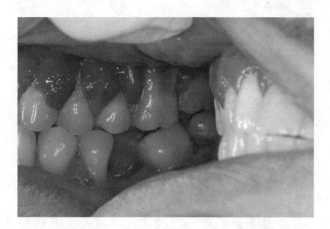

FIGURE 19–3 *Patient diagnosed with type 2 diabetes mellitus. Periodontal examination revealed deep periodontal pockets & bleeding. Radiographic bone loss was evident.* (Courtesy, Dr. David Lefkowitz)

Patients usually self-monitor blood glucose and urinary glucose. Accu-Check® is one type of monitoring devices available.

Diet modification is critical for type 1 diabetics and can be used as monotherapy in type 2 diabetics. Weight loss in type 2 diabetics will improve insulin secretion, which may reduce the risk of microvascular and macrovascular complications. Exercise may improve insulin sensitivity and reduce plasma glucose. The importance of smoking cessation should be reinforced. These patients may need exogenous insulin to help maintain type 2 status.

RDH **Rapid Dental Hint**

Make sure your patients eat and take diabetic meds prior to dental treatment.

Pharmacology

Oral Hypoglycemics

Antidiabetic drugs are classified into oral and injectable agents (Tables 19–1 and 19–2). The decision to use a specific drug is based on whether there is an absolute insulin deficiency of insulin (as seen in type 1 diabetes) or a defect in insulin action and secretion (as seen in type 2

diabetes). Thus, for type 1 diabetes, insulin is essential because there is no insulin being produced by the beta-cells. In type 2 diabetes, rather than an absolute insulin deficiency, insulin is being produced even in excess (hyperinsulinemia), but there is a problem with its action and secretion. If monitoring and lifestyle modifications (e.g., weight loss/exercise, smoking cessation) are not successful in glucose control of type 2 diabetes, oral antidiabetic agents must be used. Proper diet and exercise can sometimes increase the sensitivity of insulin receptors to the point that drug therapy is not needed.

Oral Antidiabetic Agents

All oral antihyperglycemic agents reduce blood glucose levels by different methods and/or degrees, but all need insulin in order to be effective. Intact beta cells are needed for these drugs to work. Therapy is usually initiated with a single agent. If therapeutic goals are not achieved, two agents are given. Oral antidiabetic agents are divided into six classifications:

1. *Sulfonylureas* have been around for over 40 years and were the first oral agents used in the treatment of type 2 diabetes mellitus, particularly in patients in whom diet fails to control the hyperglycemia. Sulfonylureas, or insulin secretion stimulators, work by stimulating the release of insulin from the pancreatic beta cells and to increase the binding of insulin to the receptors on target tissues (cells), increasing insulin sensitivity and increasing glucose transport in the tissues. These agents are used by al-

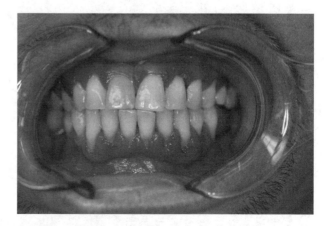

FIGURE 19–4 *Severe periodontitis in a patient with uncontrolled diabetes.* (Courtesy, Dr. David Lefkowitz)

Table 19–1   Agents Used in the Treatment of Diabetes Mellitus

Drug Name	Mechanism of Action	Common Adverse Events	Significant Dental Drug Interactions	Dental Notes
Sulfonylureas **First-Generation Agents** Chlopropamide (Diabinese) Tolazamide (Tolinase) Tolbutamide (Orinase) **Second-Generation Agents** Glipizide (Glucotrol) Glyburide (DiaBeta, Micronase) Glyburide, micronized (Glynase) Glimepiride (Amaryl)	Stimulates release of insulin from pancreatic beta cells. Use in type 2 diabetics with endogenous (body) insulin still being produced and secreted.	Hypoglycemia, jaundice, gastrointestinal upset, weight gain, skin reactions	Significant dental drug interactions: If taken with aspirin or other nonsteroidal anti-inflammatory drugs (e.g., ibuprofen), increased incidence of hypoglycemia Epinephrine-containing local anesthetics: May need increased dose of antidiabetic agent Other interactions: The following drugs increase the effects of sulfonylureas causing hypoglycemic (low blood glucose) effects: MAOIs Tricyclic antidepressants Ethanol (alcohol) Allopurinol Anticoagulants H₂-antagonists The following drugs reduce the hypoglycemic effects of sulfonylureas: Phenobarbital β-adrenergic blockers rifampin loop and thiazide diuretics	Monitor blood glucose levels of patient. Drug is best taken 30 minutes before breakfast to get maximum absorption into the bloodstream. Ask the patient what their blood glucose (sugar) level was today, and if they took their medication as directed. A random plasma glucose level of ≥200 mg/dL and a FPG (fasting plasma glucose)of ≥126 mg/dL should be consulted with the patient's physician before dental treatment is started. Early morning appointments should be scheduled to avoid stress-induced hypoglycemia. Monitor for periodontal infections and delayed
Biguanides Metformin (Glucophage)	Shuts off the liver's excess glucose production; insulin secretion is not affected	Hypoglycemia is not a risk because insulin secretion is not affected; minor gastrointestinal side effects (anorexia, diarrhea, nausea, abdominal pain), metallic taste	Epinephrine-containing local anesthetics: May need increase dose antidiabetic agent Other drug interactions: Increased metformin effects (hypoglycemic) with: Contraceptives Phenytoin Niacin Calcium channel blockers (e.g., diltiazem) Thiazide diuretics	

Combination Drugs Glyburide/metformin (Glucovance) Metformin/glipizide (Metaglip) Metformin/rosiglitazone (Avandamet)	See above	See above	Decreased metformin effects (hyperglycemia) with: Digoxin Morphine Procainabmide Quinidine Cimetidine (Tagamet)	See above
Thiazolidinediones Pioglitazone (Actos) Rosiglitazone (Avandia)	The newest agents. Act specifically to target insulin sensitivity. Mechanism unclear. Does not stimulate endogenous insulin secretion. Decreases insulin resistance and improves beta cell response. Additionally, may lower serum lipids, triglycerides, and LDL cholesterol.	Severe liver damage, fluid retention (edema), weight gain	Epinephrine-containing local anesthetics: May cause hyperglycemic effects	See above
Alpha-glucosidase Inhibitors Acarbose (Precose) Miglitol (Glyset)	Slows postprandial (after meals) carbohydrate absorption in the blood. Used in type 2 diabetics that cannot be managed on diet alone. Can be used in combination with metformin or insulin.	Gastrointestinal (diarrhea, abdominal pain)	Epinephrine-containing local anesthetics: May cause hyperglycemic effects; may need increased dose antidiabetic agent	See above
Meglitinides Repaglinide (Prandin) Nateglinide (Starlix)	Increases insulin secretion from beta cells, which reduces glucose levels. Usually used in combination with metformin.	Headache, hyperglycemia/hypoglycemia	Metabolized by CYP3A4: Erythromycin and clarithromycin may increase serum levels Precautions with EPI	See above

Table 19–2 Insulin Preparations

Drug Name	*Dental Drug Interactions*
Rapid-Acting Insulins *Recombinant Human Insulin Preparations* Insulin regular (human insulin) (Humulin R; Novolin R, Regular Iletin II)	Drugs that decrease insulin effect (hyperglycemia) or augment the glucose-lowering effect of insulin • epinephrine • corticosteroids • aspirin/NSAIDs • MAO inhibitors • tetracyclines • Alcohol
Insulin Analog Preparations Insulin human inhalation powder (rDNA origin) (Exubera) Insulin glulisine (rDNA original) (Apidra) Insulin aspart (rDNA origin) (NovoLog FlexPen; NovoLog Mix 70/30; Novolog FlexPen) Insulin lispro (rDNA origin) (Humalog; Humalog Pen)	see above
Intermediate- and Long-Acting Insulins *Recombinant Human Insulin Preparations* NPH Insulin (human insulin) (Humulin N; Novolin N, NPH Iletin I, NPH Iletin II) Human regular and human NPH mixture (Humulin 70/30, Humulin 50/50, Novolin 70/30) Insulin zinc human (Humulin L) Insulin isophane human (NPH) (Humulin N, Novolin N) Insulin zinc human (Humulin L, Novolin L)	see above
Analog Preparations Insulin glargine (Lantus) Insulin determir (Levemir) PZI—insulin lispro protamine 75%/insulin lispro 25% (Humalog Mix)	see above

most 30–40 percent of all individuals with type 2 diabetes mellitus. Sulfonylureas can cause hypoglycemia because of their ability to increase insulin secretion. First-generation agents are no longer the first-line drugs being replaced by second-generation sulfonylureas and other newly introduced (within the last 12 years) drugs. Second-generation sulfonylureas (including glime-

pride, glipizide and glyburide) also work by stimulating the release of insulin from the beta cells but are more potent (smaller doses are used) with fewer adverse effects, including less weight gain, less hypoglycemia, and fewer drug–drug interactions. Patients recently diagnosed (less than 5 years) and older than 40 years of age and obese who cannot control their glucose levels with exercise or diet respond well with sulfonlyureas. Dosage adjustment is necessary in patients with liver disease. In patients who do not respond to sulfonylureas alone, another antidiabetic drug is added or used.

2. *Biguanides* work by decreasing glucose production and release by the liver, and stimulating glucose uptake into tissues. Metformin is an example of a biguanide. Unlike the sulfonylureas, biguanides alone do not cause weight gain or hypoglycemia. In obese individuals, they increase insulin sensitivity, resulting in weight loss. Since metformin does not affect insulin production or secretion (release), it does not cause hypoglycemia or hyperinsulinemia. It is generally used in combination with insulin or a sulfonylurea. Adverse side effects include anorexia, diarrhea, nausea, and abdominal discomfort. Gastrointestinal side effects can be reduced if the medication is taken with food. Metformin reduces triglyceride and LDL cholesterol. Metformin is contraindicated and should not be used in patients with renal (kidney) disease, respiratory disease, or cardiac insufficiency.

3. *Alpha-glucosidase inhibitors* reduce postprandial (after eating) hyperglycemia by reversibly inhibiting the alpha glucosidase enzymes in the small intestine, delaying carbohydrate absorption and delaying and reducing a rise in blood glucose after meals. Gastrointestinal discomfort is the most common side effect and is contraindicated in patients with inflammatory bowel disease or any obstructive bowel conditions. Acarbose (Precose) and miglitol (Glyset) are in this category. These medications do not cause weight gain or hypoglycemia when used alone. But, when used with a sulfonylurea, side effects may occur.

4. *Thiazolidinediones* (TZDs) are a relatively new class of drugs used to reduce insulin resistance by enhancing the effects of circulating insulin by improving insulin sensitivity in muscle and fat cells. These agents are used only as a second-line therapy and some in combination with other antidiabetic agents such as a sulfonylurea or metformin. Three thiazolidinedoines currently approved in the United States are rosiglitazone (Avandia) and pioglitazone (Actos). Adverse side affects include fluid retention (which may exacerbate heart failure), weight gain, and severe liver damage. Since they do not stimulate insulin secretion, hypoglycemia does not occur.

More drug interaction studies need to be conducted with these drugs and other drugs metabolized by the cytochrome P450 isoenzyme system. These drugs have been reported to decrease triglyceride blood levels.

5. *Meglitinides* are the newest class of oral hypoglycemics. They increase insulin secretion from beta cells of the pancreas, but from a different site than the sulfonylureas. These drugs are taken before meals to stimulate insulin release and control the rise in postprandial glucose plasma levels. Two drugs in this category are repaglinide (Prandin) and nateglinide (Starlix). Weight gain is a common adverse side effect. Hypoglycemia and effects on blood lipids are not seen.

6. *Combination Drugs* combine metformin with glipizide (Metaglip), glyburide (Glucovance) and rosiglitazone (Avandamet). Various oral hypoglycemic drugs have different mechanisms of action. As diabetes progresses, more metabolic disorders arise. Combination therapy is needed to treat the more complex and varied complications. For example, a patient may be taking a sulfonylurea to enhance insulin secretion and a TZD to reduce insulin resistance and hyperglycemia.

Guidelines for Patients Taking Oral Hypoglycemic Agents—Glipizide (Glucotrol)

- Monitor the periodontal condition of diabetic patients.
- Stress meticulous home care.
- Patients should have frequent recall appointments.
- Patients should avoid aspirin and nonsteroidal anti-inflammatory drugs (e.g., ibuprofen).
- Question patients about self-monitoring of their diabetic condition.
- Encourage patients to follow a prescribed diet and regularly take the medication to avoid hypoglycemic episodes.

Insulin Pharmacology: History

Insulin is required in type 1 diabetics because there is an absolute or total deficiency of insulin and it needs to be replaced from an exogenous source to prevent ketoacidosis. Although not used as a first-line treatment in type 2 diabetes, insulin (with oral agents) can be used to supplement deficient levels of insulin in the blood, especially in patients who have had diabetes for a long time and are unable to achieve adequate glycemic control (more than 350 mg/dL) with oral agents alone. Diet, exercise, and oral agents are usually tried first in type 2 diabetics. About 30 percent of diabetics in the United States are taking insulin.

As mentioned previously, insulin is a hormone (protein) produced by and secreted from the beta cells in the pancreas. When endogenous insulin is not being produced or in ineffective amounts, exogenous insulin must be introduced into the blood to maintain adequate blood levels. Insulin regulates plasma glucose levels by decreasing liver glucose production and increasing glucose uptake into the cells. Insulin is biologically inactive until it is bound by specific receptors located in target cells.

Insulin Secretion and Absorption

Endogenous insulin is normally released from the pancreas when blood glucose levels are elevated. *Prandial insulin* is released into the blood sporadically in two phases in response to elevated blood glucose after a meal. In phase 1, insulin is released within seconds of eating and lasts for about 10 minutes. Phase 2 insulin release occurs within 15 minutes of phase 1 and last for about 2 hours, and is responsible for lowering the postprandial rise in blood glucose. *Basal insulin* is released continuously during the day at low levels in response to continuous liver glucose output.

Did You Know?

In 1921, Dr. Frederick Grant Banting and Charles Best discovered insulin by tying string around the pancreatic ducts of several dogs. When they examined the pancreases of these dogs several weeks later, all of the pancreas cells were gone and only pancreatic islets were left. These islets contained a protein they called insulin.

Goal of Insulin therapy

The goal of insulin therapy is to mimic prandial and/or basal insulin production so that blood glucose can be controlled continuously during the day and night, and limit the potential for hypoglycemic effects.

Formulations

A different amino acid sequence than human insulin allows for a more predictable action in the body and more closely mimics physiologic insulin secretion. All insulin analogs are available as clear solutions and are indicated for use in insulin pump therapy.

Insulin Regimen

Insulin preparations (Table 19–2) are classified as rapid, intermediate or long acting. The regimen for controlling hyperglycemia is a basal-bolus regimen, which includes an intermediate- or long-acting insulin injected once or twice daily to mimic basal insulin secretion, and a rapid- or short-acting insulin injected at mealtime to mimic prandial insulin secretion. The use of an insulin pump can accomplish this.

Some patients may not like to have multiple injections during the day, so an alternative choice includes premixed insulin formulations that contain both a rapid- or short-acting insulin and an intermediate-acting insulin that can be administered in one injection twice daily (see Table 19–2). Older insulin products do not need a prescription; however the newer analog insulin does require a prescription.

FORMULATIONS
Recombinant Human Insulin Preparations

Short- or Rapid-Acting Insulin
In the past, insulin preparations came from animal sources, primarily pork because beef caused allergic reactions in humans. In 1986, *recombinant human insulin* first emerged. Today, recombinant human insulin is produced from either genetically altered bacteria (*Escherichia coli*) or yeast and has the same amino acid chain sequence as human insulin. Recombinant human insulin has fewer impurities, limiting significant allergic reactions, and is more rapid in onset and shorter in duration than pork insulin. Regular human insulin (R) and neutral protamine Hagedorn (NPH) are types of human insulin formulations.

Regular human insulin (R) is FDA approved for the treatment of type 1 and type 2 diabetes and mimics post-prandial pancreas insulin release to reduce meal-related glucose levels (Table 19–2). It has a quick onset and short duration, which allows for postprandial glucose control. It should be injected about 30 minutes before meals. Regular insulin can be mixed with another type of insulin. Regular insulin can be administered in a subcutaneous injection. It is the only insulin preparation that may be administered as an intramuscular or intravenous injection. It is available in a vial or a prefilled pen.

Intermediate-Acting Insulin

Isophane insulin suspension (NPH; neutral protamine Hagedorn) was developed to reduce the number of injections required to achieve glycemic control. It is formulated as a crystalline suspension (cloudy). It is FDA approved for the treatment of type 1 and type 2 diabetes. It has a longer duration of action than rapid-acting insulin and is injected once or twice daily to mimic endogenous basal insulin release throughout the day.

NPH is available in a vial and a prefilled pen. It can be mixed with other insulin preparations including regular, insulin lispro, insulin aspart, and insulin glulisine, or a premixed formulation (available with regular).

Insulin Analog Preparations

Because of the pharmacologic limitations of the human insulin formulations, various insulin analogs have been developed. In 1996, the first *insulin analog,* insulin lispro was introduced. Insulin analogs are synthetically derived preparations based on the human insulin structure but slightly modified, resulting in altered pharmacokinetics that mirror the pharmacokinetics of endogenous insulin. Insulin aspart (NovoLog), insulin glulisine, and insulin lispro (Humalog) are insulin analog preparations. Today, only recombinant human insulin and insulin analog preparations are available. Beef and pork insulin were discontinued in 2003 and 2005, respectively.

Rapid-Acting Insulin Analog Preparations

Insulin lispro (Humalog), insulin aspart (NovoLog), and insulin glulisine (Apidra) are rapid-acting insulin analogs. These formulations are being used more frequently because they are absorbed more quickly (10 to 15 minutes) and have a shorter duration of action (less than 5 hours) than human insulin (onset: 30 to 60 minutes). They are usually used with insulin infusion pumps.

Intermediate-Acting Analog Preparations

There are no intermediate-acting analog preparations.

Long-Acting Analog Preparations

Insulin glargine was the first long-acting insulin analog, introduced in the United States in 2003, and requires only one injection during the day which avoids nocturnal (nighttime) hypoglycemia (low glucose), whereas most other insulins require multiple injections daily. It should not be mixed in the syringe with any other insulin.

Adverse effects include injection site reactions and limitations for mixture with other insulin preparations.

Insulin detemir (Levemir) was FDA approved in 2005. It has a duration of action of up to 24 hours and is injected either once or twice daily.

Mixing Insulin Preparations and Premixed Insulin Preparations

Multiple daily dose insulin (MDI) therapy using a basal-bolus regimen offers tight glycemic control by mimicking endogenous insulin activity. However, it requires frequent blood glucose monitoring and multiple injections during the day. Different insulin preparations can be mixed together in the same syringe to deal with the different onset and duration of action of the insulin. When insulin is mixed, regular insulin, which is clear, must be drawn first into the syringe followed by another type of insulin which is cloudy.

Many people have difficulty mixing the different insulin preparations or are unable to do multiple injections. Premixed insulin preparations are available that minimize the number of injections while offering both postprandial and basal insulin control. However, if patients require tight glycemic control and have not modified their lifestyle, these premixed preparations should not be used because dose adjustment cannot be done with premixed preparations. Premixed formulations contain both a rapid-acting and an intermediate-acting insulin that can be administered in one injection twice daily. It is administered as a subcutaneous injection in the abdomen, arm, buttocks, or thigh.

Insulin Delivery Devices

Insulin is available in vials as well as in a prefilled pen device. Rapid-acting insulin can also be used in an insulin pump, which delivers intensive insulin therapy with better absorption, decreased risk of nighttime and activity-related hypoglycemia, and allows a more flexible lifestyle. The pump is placed on the abdomen and is programmed to give small doses of insulin subcutaneously into the abdomen at predetermined intervals, with larger doses (boluses) at mealtime.

Newest Insulin Formulation

In 2006, inhaled (nasal spray) insulin (Exubera) was approved by the FDA. The inhaled powder is a form of recombinant human insulin that is used in the treatment of type 1 and type 2 diabetes. Peak levels were achieved in about 30 to 90 minutes. In type 1 diabetes, inhaled insulin may be added to a longer acting insulin as a replacement for short-acting insulin taken with meals. In type 2 diabetes, inhaled insulin may be used alone, along with oral hypoglycemics or with longer acting insulin.

Adverse Effects

The most common side effect of insulin is hypoglycemia, due either to too much insulin being injected or improper timing of the injections with meals. Patients and dental offices should have a source of simple sugar in case of hypoglycemic reactions. Hypoglycemia progresses rapidly, whereas hyperglycemia is slow in progression. Glucagon (GlucaGen Hypokit) given IV, IM, or SC is administered

for some diabetic patients when they are in hypoglycemic shock.

Other adverse effects include hyperglycemia, weight gain, pain at injection site, lipohypertrophy [proliferation of subcutaneous fat (adipose) tissue] at the injection site and allergic reaction. Insulin therapy is especially prone to hypoglycemia (more susceptible to hypoglycemia than patients taking oral agents) and is managed by adjusting the insulin dosage to the proper levels. Patients taking insulin should be advised of the possibility of hypoglycemic attacks at any time, and be prepared to treat them by taking sugar or glucose tablets. Patients using inhaled insulin may develop a cough and xerostomia.

Drug interactions with insulin are related to medications that can cause hypoglycemia or hyperglycemia. Significant dental drug interactions are listed in Table 19–2. Epinephrine can cause hyperglycemia by stimulating glucose formation. Thus precautions should be taken when injecting a local anesthetic containing epinephrine.

 Rapid Dental Hint

To prevent insulin shock (hypoglycemia), make sure patients have taken medication as usual and an adequate intake of food.

 Rapid Dental Hint

Instruct your patients if they feel symptoms of an insulin reaction occurring. Have orange juice or other form of sugar available in the clinic/office.

Guidelines for Patients Taking Insulin

- Patients must be adequately controlled.
- Common side effect is hypoglycemia.
- Determine if patients are self-monitoring blood glucose.
- Make early dental appointments.
- Make sure patients took insulin as directed.
- Assess and monitor for periodontal disease, caries, and candidiasis.
- Aspirin and NSAIDs (e.g., ibuprofen) increase hypoglycemic effects.
- Epinephrine decreases the effect of insulin due to epinephrine-induced hyperglycemia; caution in amount of epinephrine-containing local anesthetic.

DENTAL HYGIENE NOTES

Patients in the dental office should be screened and monitored for periodontal disease, since diabetes mellitus is a documented risk factor for periodontal diseases. On the other hand, patients with periodontal disease should be cognizant of the development of diabetes mellitus. Thus patient education is an integral part of treatment of the periodontal patient with diabetes.

Other oral manifestations of diabetes mellitus include xerostomia, burning tongue/mouth, and *Candida* (fungal) infections. These factors must be monitored in the diabetic patient because xerostomia can lead to increased incidence of caries.

As diabetes progresses, many organs become affected and the patient most likely will be taking many other different types of drugs such as antihypertensives and drugs to lower cholesterol (antihyperlipidemic drugs). A review of all medications a diabetic is taking is important to determine adverse side effects and drug interactions.

Patients should be asked at the beginning of every appointment if they took insulin/oral agents as directed that day, since many diabetic patients (especially those taking insulin) are susceptible to hypoglycemic reactions (profuse sweating, nervousness, fainting, palpitations, hunger, nervousness, or unconsciousness). The dental clinician should ask patients if they are prone to hypoglycemic reactions. If patients become hypoglycemic, sugar, orange juice, or glucose tablets can be given if patients are conscious. If patients become unconscious, then additional medical assistance should be called. Most diabetic patients monitor their blood glucose levels at home with a finger-stick test. Ask patients the results of the test for that day.

Epinephrine decreases the effect of insulin due to epinephrine-induced hyperglycemia. Thus, epinephrine counters the effect of insulin, which may interfere with diabetic control. Precautions should be taken to minimize the amount of epinephrine used in local anesthetics.

THYROID DRUGS

Introduction

Thyroid Gland Hormones

The **thyroid gland** (Figure 19–5), located on the front side of the neck, produces and releases a hormone (protein) called *thyroxine* (T_4, levothyroxine). At the target tissues, thyroxine is converted to the active form, *triiodothyronine* (T_3), which enters the cells and binds to receptors. About 87 percent of T_3 is derived from T_4 and the remaining 13 percent is synthesized by the thyroid gland. Iodine is required for the synthesis of T_4 and is provided by dietary intake of iodized salt. For therapeutic purposes (medications for replacement of thyroid hormone), T_4 is used because more constant blood levels can be achieved due to its longer duration of action with a half-life of 7 days than T_3 with a half-life of 1 day.

Thyroid gland hormones regulate the *basal metabolic rate,* which is the baseline speed at which cells perform their functions and are essential for carbohydrate,

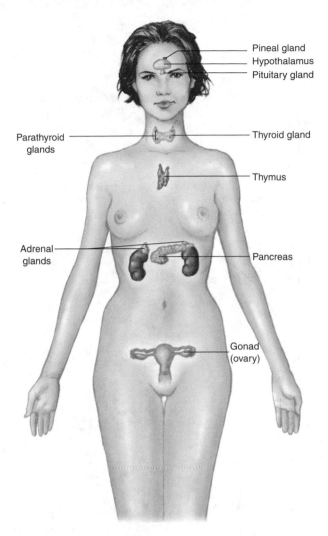

FIGURE 19–5   Location of the thyroid gland.

protein, and lipid metabolism in the body. As cellular metabolism increases, thyroid hormone increases body temperature. The gland also regulates blood pressure and growth and development.

Thyroid stimulating hormone (TSH), which comes from the hypothalamus, stimulates growth of the thyroid gland and synthesis and secretion of the thyroid hormones (Figure 19–6). The thyroid forms a *negative feedback loop:* Secretion of TSH declines as the blood level of thyroid hormones rises, (T_4) and vice versa (e.g., peaks at night and lower levels during the day.)

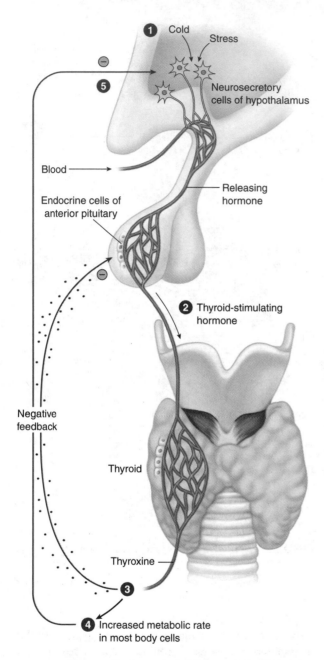

FIGURE 19–6 Mechanism of the thyroid gland showing a stimulus (1) which causes the release of TSH (2) and then the release of thyroid hormone (3). There is an increase in basal metabolic rate (speed by which cells perform their functions (4). This effect creates a negative feedback loop (5) where TSH production is suppressed when T4 levels are high, and vice versa.

Once released into the bloodstream, thyroid hormones can exist in the bound (to a protein) or unbound form. Thyroid hormones are highly protein bound (99.9 percent for T_4 and 99.5 percent for T_3) so that only a little of the free unbound form is actually binding to receptors and producing an effect in the body. The conversion to T_3 is critical because T_3 has greater biological activity than T_4.

To determine if an individual has a thyroid disorder, hyperthyroidism, or hypothyroidism, a blood test is taken that measures unbound T_4 and TSH levels.

Pharmacology: Antithyroid Drugs

Hyperthyroidism (thyrotoxicosis) or excessive production of thyroid hormones must be treated by reducing the levels of the thyroid hormones. The most common type of hyperthyroidism is called Graves' disease, an autoimmune disease in which the body develops antibodies against its own thyroid gland. Other causes of overactivity includes multinodular goiter or Plummer's disease (enlargement of thyroid gland), and tumors. Pharmacologic treatment options include the following antithyroid drugs (Table 19–3):

1. *Thioamide drugs:* Propylthiouracil (PTU) and methimazole (Tapazole) work by inhibiting thyroid hormone production by interfering with in the incorporation of iodine. These drugs are used as short-term treatment of Graves' disease. There is a high incidence of agranulocytosis (blood disorder of the neutrophils; a reduction of the white blood cells).

2. *Radioactive iodine (RAI):* Another first-line treatment for Graves' disease. The patient drinks an oral liquid containing sodium iodide that concentrates and destroys the overactive thyroid gland. After RAI, the patient usually becomes hypothyroid and must take thyroid supplements for the rest of his/her life.

3. *Iodine:* Iodine-containing compounds including Lugol's solution (5% iodine (I_2) 10 percent potassium iodide (KI)). These agents are primarily used for the treatment of thyrotoxic crisis or, as it is sometimes called, thyroid storm, a life-threatening condition featuring acute manifestations of thyrotoxicosis including hypertension, tachycardia, confusion, vomiting, and coma. Surgical removal of the gland is also a recommended treatment for thyroid storm.

Table 19–3 Disorders and Treatment of the Thyroid Gland

Disorder	Signs and Symptoms	Drug Treatment	Drug-drug Interaction
Hyperthyroidism	Sweating, weight loss, nervousness, oversensitivity to heat, fatigue, moist skin, tachycardia (in Graves' disease there is exophthalmos, or bulging of the eye) Plummer's disease (toxic multinodular goiter): symptoms of hyperthyroidism but without exophthalmos	Goal: to reduce thyroid levels. Thiourea drugs: Propylthiouracil (PTU) Methimazole (Tapazole) Radioacative iodine (RAI) Beta-blockers: Propranolol Nadolol Iodine compounds: Lugol's solution Potassium iodide (SSKI)	• Altered pharmacokinetics to the following drugs may cause a change in dosing: Aminophylline Dicumarol Digoxin Metoprolol Propranolol Theophylline Warfarin
Hypothyroidism	Cold intolerance, weakness, tiredness, fatigue, hoarseness, constipation, aches, pains	Thyroid USP L-thyroxine (Levoxyl, Synthroid, Levothroid) L-triiodothyronine (Cytomel) Liotrix (Thyrolar)	• Decreases absorption of levothyroxine from the G.I. tract: Chloestryramine Sucralfate aluminum hydroxide ferrous sulfate • Drugs that increase T_4 excretion, reducing blood levels: Rifampin, Carbamazepine, phenytoin

Lugol's solution is available over-the-counter in the United States as of January 2007, although the DEA is considering a public ban on all iodine solutions of greater than 2.2% because iodine is required for the production of methamphetamine. Lugol's is available over-the-counter in Canada.

4. Beta-blockers (propranolol, nadolol) are not approved in the United States by the FDA for the treatment of thyrotoxicosis.

5. Other drugs include calcium channel blockers (diltiazem or verapamil), which block the effects of thyroid hormone, but do not have an effect on the underlying disease. Corticosteroids can be used for treating thyroid storm but there are many adverse effects which preclude its use as the first line of treatment.

Pharmacology: Hypothyroidism

Hypothyroidism is a common disorder that results from a deficiency in secretion of T_4 and T_3 from the thyroid gland. It frequently occurs after a patient is treated with radioactive iodine, whereby the thyroid gland become inactive (hypothyroid) and requires replacement therapy.

It can be caused by thyroid gland failure, autoimmune thyroiditis (Hashimoto's disease), cretinism (congenital hypothyroidism), tumors, excessive iodide intake (e.g., from kelp), or be drug induced (e.g., lithium, iodides, sulfonylureas). Diagnosis is based on elevated levels of TSH. Initially, T_4 levels may be normal, but later on in the disease there are decreased levels. Symptoms of hypothyroidism in adults, also known as myxedema, include slowed body metabolism, slurred speech, bradycardia, weight gain, low body temperature, and intolerance to cold environments. Treatment goals for hypothyroidism are to return thyroid hormone levels to normal with the used of medications. Periodic (monthly) blood tests should be performed while the patient is taking thyroid replacement medications to monitor for TSH and T_4 levels.

1. Thyroid, USP (Armour) is manufactured from desiccated (dry) pig, beef, or sheep thyroid gland, and contains iodine. This product has unpredictable hormonal stability.

2. Levothyroxine (Synthroid, Levothroid) is synthetic T_4 hormone that is identical to the T_4 secreted from

the thyroid gland and is one of the most commonly prescribed drugs in the United States. This is the drug of choice for thyroid hormone replacement. This product has predictable absorption, is stable, potent, has a long duration of action, is less expensive than the other products and can be administered once daily. Although T_3 has greater biological activity than T_4, administration of L-thyroxine results in a concentration of T_4 that is converted to T_3.

3. L-triiodothyronine (Cytomel) is synthetic T_3 hormone. Daily multiple dosing is required. Hard to monitor blood levels.

4. Liotrix (Thyrolar) is synthetic T_4 : T_3. This product is not really necessary because T_4 is converted to T_3 in the peripheral tissues and it is expensive.

 Rapid Dental Hints

Dental treatment modifications may be necessary for patients with thyroid disorders; assess your patient.

Adverse Effects

Adverse effects include irritability, nervousness, insomnia, headache, palpitations, and weight loss. Excessive doses can lead to heart disorders, including congestive heart failure and myocardial infarction.

Liothyronine has a high incidence of cardiac side effects. Thyroid USP may cause allergic reactions, since it is derived from animal sources.

Dental Hygiene Notes

There are no special precautions to following when treating dental patients who are well controlled with thyroid medication. Most patients presenting to the dental office will be controlled and under the care of a physician; however, patients may be seen with undiagnosed hypothyroidism or hyperthyroidism, where routine dental treatment may result in adverse outcomes. If there is no documentation on the patient's medical history about thyroid disorders but several signs and symptoms point to thyroid disease, it is prudent to get a medical consult from the patient's physician. Epinephrine is contraindicated in hyperthyroid patients; however, patients with thyroid storm will most likely not be seen in the dental office, since it is a life-threatening disorder and patients

are very ill. Monthly blood tests should be done to maintain normal thyroid hormone levels.

ADRENAL (STEROID) HORMONES

Introduction

Adrenal Glands

The adrenal glands are located next to the kidneys (Figure 19–5). One part of the adrenal gland, the adrenal medulla, produces and secretes epinephrine and norepinephrine, which stimulate the sympathetic division of the central nervous system. Epinephrine is responsible for converting stored glycogen (carbohydrates) into glucose in the liver. This process is called glycogenolysis.

The other part of the adrenal gland is the adrenal cortex. The adrenal cortex produces and releases steroid hormones into the circulation. When released into the circulation, these natural hormones have many effects on the body and are essential for life. These hormones allow the body to endure stresses put upon it such as injury, disease, and mental strain.

The release of **corticosteroids** by the adrenal cortex is controlled by the hypothalamus and anterior pituitary gland via ACTH (adrenocorticotropic hormone), which stimulates corticosteroid release. All human steroids are synthesized from cholesterol found in the body. Three natural corticosteroids that the body produces and secretes are classified by their actions:

1. **Mineralocorticoids.** The primary mineralocorticoid is aldosterone. Mineralocorticoids have the responsibility of maintaining the levels of sodium and potassium in the body. They conserve or maintain the body's concentration of water at a near constant level. They exert most of their effect on the kidneys, causing selective excretion of excess potassium in the urine and at the same time retain sodium. The medical use of mineralocorticosteroids is limited.

2. **Glucocorticoids.** Hydrocortisone (cortisol) is the primary glucocorticoid. **Glucocorticoids** or glucocorticosteroids regulate energy metabolism by causing proteins (e.g., muscles) and lipids (e.g., body fats) to be broken down and converted into glucose (glycogenolysis). They cause carbohydrates stored in the form of glycogen to be converted back to glucose and deposited into the blood, where they are available for the tissues in the body. About 15–30 mg of cortisol is secreted in

the body daily. Glucocorticoids also suppress inflammatory processes (anti-inflammatory) within the body (e.g., bee sting, arthritis), have anti-allergic properties, and are important to the body's immunological defense reactions.

3. **Gonadocorticoids,** or sex hormones. Male and female sex hormones produced by the adrenal cortex supplement those produced by the testes and ovaries. The female hormones are called estrogen and progesterone, and the male androgens include testosterone; the androgens are referred to as anabolic steroids.

Systemic Adrenocortical Steroids

Naturally occurring cortisol is not used, but is substituted for by others that can be produced more economically for the treatment of specific systemic medical conditions.

Mineralocorticoids: Indications

Clinically, synthetic mineralocorticoids affect the kidneys by increasing sodium retention and potassium loss. Thus, mineralocorticoids are used primarily in patients with a medical condition called hypoadrenalism to replace and maintain loss of fluids and electrolytes. Fludrocortisone (Florinef) is the drug that is used for mineralocorticoid replacement.

Glucocorticoids: Indications

Clinically, synthetic glucocorticosteroids are used primarily as anti-inflammatory agents in the treatment of the following medical conditions:

- Asthma
- Rheumatoid arthritis
- Bursitis
- *Pneumocystis jiroveci* pneumonia in HIV infected patients
- Viral croup (upper airway obstruction with cough in children)
- Systemic lupus erythematosus (SLE)
- Ulcerative colitis
- Antirejection for organ transplant
- Inflammatory conditions of the eye and skin
- Bullous disorders (e.g., pemphigus vulgaris and erythema multiforme)
- Stress-induced shock syndrome

- Severe allergic reactions
- Joint diseases (given as intra-articular injections every 1–6 weeks)

Its immunosuppressive actions allow it to be used in the management of organ transplant patients to prevent organ rejection. Corticosteroids are also used in the treatment of Addison's disease (adrenal insufficiency) and in the treatment of dental-related ulcerative inflammatory lesions such as lichen planus, burning tongue, and aphthous stomatitis (canker sores). Corticosteroids are known to be beneficial in treating herpes zoster infection, but their effectiveness in the treatment of recurrent herpes labialis infection is unknown; however, corticosteroids in combination with an antiviral agent may be safe and beneficial for herpes labialis. Corticosteroids by themselves are not so effective in reducing inflammation in viral lesions, and will mask symptoms of infection.

Steroid hormones act by controlling the rate of protein synthesis inside cells. When taken systemically, glucocorticosteroids are absorbed into the circulation and enter sensitive cells, where they bind to protein receptors and regulate the levels of specific proteins and enzymes, which result in its anti-inflammatory effects. Corticosteroids also exert an anti-inflammatory effect by inhibiting the release of histamine from mast cells.

Glucocorticoids: Systemic Products

Table 19–4 lists the more commonly used systemic glucocorticosteroids, which are classified according to their duration of action:

1. Shorting-acting
2. Intermediate-acting
3. Long-acting

Corticosteroids are also classified according to their anti-inflammatory potency. Hydrocortisone has the least anti-inflammatory activity, while betamethasone and dexamethasone are the most potent anti-inflammatory steroids.

Adverse Effects

Short-term, low-dose steroid therapy rarely results in any adverse effects. However, as the dosage and duration of therapy increases so does the risk of unwanted side effects. Long-term therapy is more related with severe adverse events including suppressing normal adrenal gland function, osteoporosis, hyperglycemia, hypertension, candidiasis (including intraoral), peptic ulcers,

Table 19–4   Systemic Glucocorticosteroids

Drug Name	Mechanism of Action	Significant Drug Interactions	Dental Notes
Short-acting (8–12 hours) Cortisone (generic, Cortone) Hydrocortisone, Cortisol (Cortef, various names)	After absorption into the bloodstream the drug enters the cell, where it binds to receptors, allowing change in certain proteins and enzymes, resulting in anti-inflammatory effects.	Decreased corticosteroid levels (P450 cytochromes) when taken with: Barbiturates Carbamazepine Phenytoin Rifampin NSAIDs: Increased GI side effects Antacids: Decreased steroid absorption.	Consult with the patient's physicians if they are taking corticosteroids. Long-term therapy may need to have supplemental steroids to avoid stressful situations.
Intermediate-acting (12–36 hours) Methylprednisolone (generic, Medrol) Prednisolone (generic, Orapred, Prelone) Prednisone (generic, Meticorten, Deltasone) Triamcinolone (Aristocort, Kenacort, generics)	Predisone is usually the first drug of choice because of low cost and fewer adverse side effects (sodium and water retention).	See above	See above
Long-acting (36–54 hours) Betamethasone (Celestone) Dexamethasone (Decadron, generic)	Dexamethasone has the greatest anti-inflammatory activity.	See above	See above Syrup can be used in the management of some oral diseasses (e.g., aphthous ulcers, lichen planus) Oral solution can be used in the management of some oral diseases (e.g., aphthous ulcers, lichen planus)

psychiatric disorders, poor/delayed wound healing, and immune suppression. With prolonged use there is a reduction in protein production and fat deposition in areas that were previously occupied by muscle, producing the characteristic "moon face" and "buffalo hump." These features simulate the disease called Cushing's syndrome. Corticosteroids also cause water and sodium retention (except for prednisone), calcium excretion, and potassium imbalance (Table 19–5).

In long-term therapy, alternate-day dosing should be used. Doubling the dosage and administering the drug every other day in the morning mimics the endogenous

 Rapid Dental Hint

Look for intraoral candidiasis in patients taking systemic corticosteroids.

(body's own) corticosteroid circadian rhythm. The goal of steroid therapy should be to maintain the lowest dosage possible while obtaining the desired clinical response.

Corticosteroids should be used with caution or not be given to patients with herpes simplex, glaucoma, diabetes mellitus, peptic ulcer disease, osteoporosis, con-

Table 19–5   Common Adverse Effects of Corticosteroids

Short-Term Therapy (1 Week or Less)	Long-Term (Chronic) Therapy
Peptic ulcer (gastro-intestinal bleeding)	Cushing's syndrome (moon face; buffalo hump)
Psychosis (psychiatric disorders)	Peptic ulcers
Hypertension	Psychosis
Hyperglycemia (diabetes mellitus)	Potassium imbalance (cardiac problems)
Sodium and water retention	Diabetes mellitus Sodium and water retention

gestive heart failure, hypertension, infections (fungal, bacterial, viral), and psychiatric disorders.

Withdrawal of Corticosteroids

When corticosteroids are to be withdrawn, there is a "tapering" period so that patients do not experience withdrawal syndrome. This allows the body to recover the normal secretion of endogenous corticosteroids. In most patients the dosage is tapered over 2 months or more. Symptoms of adrenal insufficiency that are seen if the steroid is withdrawn rapidly include: headache, fatigue, joint pain, nausea, vomiting, weight loss, fever, and peeling of the skin.

 Rapid Dental Hint

For certain less stressful procedures (e.g., periodontal debridement, restorative), no dosage adjustment is necessary. When necessary, consult with your patients' physicians.

Drug Interactions

Corticosteroids (e.g., hydrocortisone, methylprednisolone) are metabolized by the CYP3A4 isoenzymes in the liver. Metabolism of corticosteroids is enhanced, decreasing plasma levels, when taken with carbamazepine (Tegretol), phenobarbital, phenytoin (Dilantin), and rifampin. Glucocorticoids may increase the dosage requirement for insulin.

Topical Corticosteroids

Synthetically produced steroid agents are also used topically (e.g., cream, ointment) for skin and oral lesions (e.g., aphthous stomatitis, vesiculo-bullous diseases on the oral mucosa, burning mouth/tongue) as well as ear, nose, and throat conditions. Table 19–6 lists the common topical steroid preparations according to the degree of potency. For example, hydrocortisone is the least potent and best to use in infants and children because of minimal systemic absorption. Local and systemic adverse effects from topical corticosteroids are minimal. Absorption through the skin varies with the different formulations. Some formulations are fluoridated (a fluorine atom is added to the molecule), which prolongs the duration of action and increases the anti-inflammatory action, but unfortunately increases the incidence of adverse effects, including mineralocorticoid activity (e.g., sodium and water retention). Over-the-counter topical corticosteroids are available as hydrocortisone 0.5% and 1%.

For dental application on oral mucosa, a special formulation is available, a type of oral paste made from carboxymethycellucose, gelatin, and pectin dispersed in a plasticized hydrocarbon gel that is composed of 5% polyethylene in mineral oil. This oral paste or adhesive is available as Orabase (Colgate Oral Hoyt, Canton, MA). Different compounds are added to this adhesive paste including benzocaine (topical anesthetic) and hydrocortisone acetate 5 mg (0.5%) which is available under the name Orabase HCA Oral Paste (Colgate Oral Hoyt). The HCA paste, available only by prescription, is indicated for any ulcerations or irritations of the oral mucosa (e.g., oral lichen planus, lupus erythematosus, and recurrent aphthous ulcers—canker sores).

Corticosteroids alone are not effective against viral infections, and they are immunosuppressive, which would further aggravate the lesions or increase the incidence of herpes simplex infections. In addition to using Orabase HCA, formulations of high-potency gels or very high-potency ointments (see Table 19–6) such as fluocinonide gel 0.05% (Lidex, Lidex-E), or clobetasol propionate 0.05%, can be used for shorter periods of time. The affected area in the mouth should be dried and then the paste should be "dabbed" on, not rubbed, with a clean finger or cotton swab.

Systemic absorption occurs when topical corticosteroids are applied to oral mucosa. Absorption increases with increased potency of the steroid and with prolonged usage.

Table 19–6 Selected Topical Corticosteroids for Dermatologic and Oral Lesions

Drug Name (Generic)

Low-potency, Group IV
- Hydrocortisone (generic; Cortef, Synacort)
- Hydrocortisone (various brand names—Cortaid, Cortizone—OTC; 0.5% and 1%)
- Hydrocortisone acetate (in Orabase)
- Alclometasone (Aclovate)
- Flurandrenolide (Cordran 0.0125%) F
- Dexamethasone (Decadron) F
- Triamcinolone acetonide (Aristocort, Kenalog 0.025%) F
- Triamcinolone acetonide F dental paste

Medium-potency, Group III
- Betamethasone benzoate (Uticort) F
- Desoximetasone (Topicort 0.05%) F
- Flurandrenolide (Cordran) F
- Flucoinolone acetonide (Synlar) F
- Halcinonide (Halog 0.025%) F
- Hydrocortisone valerate (Westcort 0.2%) F
- Mometasone furoate (Elocon) F
- Triamcinolone acetonide (generic, Aristocort, Kenalog 0.1%) F

High-potency, Group II
- Amcinonide (Cyclocort) F
- Betamethasone dipropionate F (diprosone)
- Desoximetsone (Topicort 0.25%) F
- Fluocinolone (Synalar HP 0.2%) F
- Fluocinonide (Lidex) F
- Triamcinolone acetonide (generics, Aristocort, Kenalog 0.5%) F

Very high-potency, Group I
- Betamethasone dipropionate (Diprolene 0.05%) F
- Clobetasol propionate (generic, Temovate) F
- Diflorasone diacetate (Psorcon) F
- Halobetasol propionate (Ultravate) F

All are available by prescription only except for those listed as OTC.
Hydrocortisone acetate in Orabase is used orally.
*High-potency gel or very high-potency ointment can also be used orally.
F denotes fluorinated (increased potency).

Topical corticosteroids are available in different formulations and strengths. Since creams are oil in water emulsions, they must be rubbed in well until the cream is not seen. Ointments provide more occlusive covering than creams and are best suited for dry skin. Lotions are made of suspensions of powder or liquid in a water (aqueous) vehicle and are best for inflamed and tender areas because they are "cooling" and lubricate the area.

DENTAL HYGIENE NOTES

When exogenous glucocorticosteroids are taken systemically, the internal or endogenous production of these hormones by the adrenal cortex may be "turned off," resulting in adrenal gland suppression. There is concern regarding dental patients who may be at risk of experiencing **adrenal crisis** (acute adrenocortical insufficiency) during or after stressful invasive procedures; however, literature suggests that this is a rare event in dentistry.

Patients' physicians should be contacted for any dental surgical procedures.

The usual recommended dose of predisone is 5–60 mg/d in single or divided doses. Short-term treatment usually does not present with any adverse effects, including adrenal suppression. More than 20 mg a day or 2 mg/kg/d for at least 14 days may alter the patients' immunity. This should be taken into account when scheduling invasive procedures (e.g., extractions, periodontal surgery, implant surgery, incision and drainage of infections). The clinician should confirm that patients took the recommended dose of steroid within 2 hours of the procedure. It may be advantageous to increase the dose so as not to exacerbate the medical condition. The normal dose may need to be increased and tapered back to the normal dosage after the procedure; however, some studies no longer support routine recommendations for corticosteroid supplementation (Miller, C.S., J.W. Little, D.A. Falace. 2001. Supplemental corticosteroids for dental patients with adrenal insufficiency. *JADA* 132(*11*):1570–1579.). For minor, less stressful procedures such as periodontal probing, scaling and root planing, restorative, and orthodontics, no corticosteroid adjustments are required.

SEX HORMONES AND CONTRACEPTIVES

Sex hormones or steroids are specific proteins produced and secreted by male and female organs called gonads (ovaries and testes), the adrenal cortex and the placenta, during pregnancy that affect the growth or function of the reproductive organs and the development of secondary sex characteristics. The female sex hormones are estrogens and progestins, which include progesterone;

the major male sex hormone are androgens, which include testosterone.

The gonadotropins, secreted by the anterior pituitary gland, are responsible for controlling the activity of the reproductive organs and controlling the synthesis of the hormones produced by the male and female. The primary gonadotropins are FSH (follicle stimulating hormone), LH (luteinizing hormone), ICSH (interstitial cell stimulating hormone), PL (prolactin), and GH (growth hormone).

Estrogens control contractility of the myometrium and contribute to the development of the primary female sexual characteristics (ovaries and uterus) and secondary characteristics (cervix, vagina, mammary gland). Estrogens also control the menstrual cycle. Sex hormones are used to treat various medical conditions. These hormones can be used alone or in combination with other sex hormones.

Estrogens

Indications and Mechanism of Action

Estrogens are available naturally or synthetically with estrogenic activity (Table 19–7). Three natural estrogens the female body produces are estradiol (the main estrogen secreted by the ovary), estrone, and estriol. Estrogen is used as:

1. Hormone replacement therapy (estrogen alone or in combination with progestins) to reduce the symptoms of menopause in postmenopausal women
2. Oral contraceptives in combination with progestins
3. Treatment of uterine bleeding due to a hormone imbalance
4. Amenorrhea (lack of menstruation)
5. Vulvar and vaginal atrophy (postmenaupausal symptoms)
6. Prevention and treatment of osteoporosis
7. Treatment of skin lesions (e.g., acne)

Estrogens also increase HDL and triglyceride levels, and decrease LDL cholesterol levels. Estrogen products are available in different formulations including oral tablet, vaginal tablet, vaginal ring, vaginal cream, and transdermal (skin) system.

Estrogen acts by diffusing through the cell membranes and binding to estrogen (protein) receptors to activate it. This activated receptor binds to specific DNA sequences, eliciting a hormone response.

Older formulations of estrogens underwent first-pass metabolism through the liver where they were extensively converted to inactive metabolites. Today, newer formulations using small particles (micronized estradiol) allow estradiol to be absorbed rapidly and undergo little first-pass metabolism. Additionally, the development of nonoral administration (patch, vaginal, implant, and intramuscular injection) of estradiol bypasses the oral route and avoids the first-pass effect so that a smaller dosage can be used. The development of conjugated estrogens allowed the drug to be metabolized in the gastrointestinal tract rather than undergoing extensive first-pass metabolism in the liver. Estradiol is metabolized in the liver to sulfate and glucuronide conjugates by intestinal bacteria. This allows for more rapid reabsorption into the circulation and back into the liver. This process of enterohepatic circulation prolongs the action of the drug and reduces elimination. It has been suggested that some bactericidal antibiotics (e.g., amoxicillin, metronidazole, tetracycline, and ampicillin) that kill bacteria in the intestines may reduce the enterohepatic circulation of estrogen, resulting in a decrease in serum levels and reducing effectiveness of the contraceptive. It is advisable to inform patients of such interaction and discuss with the patients' physicians additional or alternative methods of contraception.

Adverse Effects

Estrogens are contraindicated and should never be given to patients with breast cancer (uterine, cervical, and vaginal cancer), pregnant patients, patients with liver disease, or patients with a vascular thromboembolic (blood clot) condition. There can be an increased risk for blood clots if patients smoke and take oral contraceptives. Many oral contraceptives are being taken off the market due to high mortality.

Estrogens may increase the risk, especially if used long term, of cerebral vascular accident (stroke)—especially in smokers, certain carcinomas (endometrial), endometrial hyperplasia, and gallbladder disease. Increased incidence of breast cancer in patients taking estrogens on a long-term basis is controversial. Additionally, estrogens cause nausea and vomiting, headache, dizziness, and breast tenderness.

Did You Know?

The birth control pill was first patented in 1960.

Table 19-7 Sex Hormone Products

Drug Name	Indications	Adverse Effects	Significant Drug Interactions	Dental Notes
Estrogens Estradiol, micronized (Estrace); oral, vaginal cream	Estrogen replacement therapy (ERT) Estrogen replacement	Edema, endometrial hyperplasia, nausea, vomiting, breast tenderness/enlargement, bloating, headache, hypertriglyceridemia, liver problems, gallbladder disease Transdermal estrogen has fewer adverse effects (less headache, nausea, and rise in triglycerides).	Reduced effects of: Tricyclic antidepressants Warfarin Increased metabolism of estrogen if taken with: Phenytoin (Dilantin) Barbiturates Carbamazepine (Tegretol) Rifampin Decrease metabolism resulting in increase serum levels of: Corticosteroids Diazepam (Valium)	Glucose tolerance may be decreased (monitor serum/urine glucose). Take with food to reduce G.I. irritation. Use caution when patient gets up from supine position (dizziness or fainting can occur)
Estradiol transdermal system (Estraderm, Climara, Vivelle, Esclim, generics); skin patch	therapy (ERT). Patch may provide more constant levels of estrogen.	See above	See above	See above
Conjugated estrogens (generics; Premarin); oral, IM, vaginal cream	ERT	See above	See above	See above
Ethinyl estradiol (Estinyl); oral	ERT; oral contraceptive	See above	See above	See above
Estradiol Cypionate (Depo-Estradiol, generics)	ERT; oral contraceptives	See above	See above	See above
Quinestrol (Estrovis)	ERT	See above	See above	See above
Progestins		Breakthrough bleeding, edema, change in weight, acne, depression, headache, breast tenderness, masculinization	Effectiveness of progestins may be decreased when taken with: Phenytoin Barbiturates Rifampin GriseofluIvin (antifungal)	No significant notes

Drug Name	Indications	Adverse Effects	Significant Drug Interactions	Dental Notes
Hydroxyprogesterone caproate (Duralutin, Pro-Depo, generics); injectable	Abnormal uterine bleeding, amenorrhea (no menstru-ation), and endometriosis	See above	See above	See above
Medroxyprogesterone acetate (Provera, generics); oral	Abnormal uterine bleeding, amenorrhea (no menstru-ation), and endometriosis	See above	See above	See above
Medroxyprogesterone acetate (Depo-Provera); injectable	Contraception	See above	See above	See above
Megestrol (Megace); oral	Advanced breast cancer and endometrial cancer	See above	See above	See above
Norethindrone (Norlutin); oral	Abnormal uterine bleeding, amenorrhea (no menstru-ation), and endometriosis	See above	See above	See above
Norethindrone acetate (Aygestin, Norlutate); oral	Abnormal uterine bleeding, amenorrhea (no menstru-ation), and endometriosis	See above	See above	See above
Progesterone micro-nized (Prometrium); oral	Hormone replacement to prevent endometriosis	See above	See above	See above
Hormone Replace-ment Therapy: Estrogen + Proges-terone Products Activella (estradiol/ norethindrone); oral CombiPatch (estradiol/norethin-drone); patch Estratest (esterified estrogens/methyl-testosterone); oral Estratest H.S. (esterified estrogens/ methyltestosterone); oral FemHRT 1/5 (ethinyl estradiol/ norethindrone); oral	Replacement of estrogen with progesterone in women with menopause	Edema, endometrial hyperplasia, nausea, vomiting, breast tenderness/ enlargement, bloating, headache, hypertriglyceridemia, gallbladder disease Transdermal estrogen has fewer adverse side effects (less headache, nausea, and rise in triglycerides)	**Estrogens:** **Reduced effects of:** Tricyclic antidepressants **Warfarin** Increased metabolism of estrogen if taken with: • Phenytoin (Dilantin) • Barbiturates • Carbamazepine (Tegretol) • Rifampin • Decrease metabolism resulting in increase serum levels of: • Corticosteroids • Diazepam (Valium) **Progesterones:** Effectiveness of progestins may be decreased when taken with: • Phenytoin	• Estrogens may exacerbate gingi-val inflammation. • Monitor gingival condition and oral hygiene care at dental appointments.

(continued)

Table 19-7 (Continued)

Drug Name	Indications	Adverse Effects	Significant Drug Interactions	Dental Notes
Ortho-Prefest (estradiol/norgestimate); oral Premphase (conjugated estrogens/medroxyprogesterone); oral Prempro (conjugated estrogens/medroxyprogesterone); oral			• Barbiturates • Rifampin • Griseoflulvin (antifungal)	
Oral Contraceptives	To prevent pregnancy (ovulation)	To minimize the risk of thromboembolism, the least amount of estrogen should be used. Thrombophlebitis, embolisms, hypertension, gallbladder disease, liver tumors, nausea, vomiting, abdominal cramps, breakthrough bleeding, breast tenderness, rash, depression, migraine headache, edema, weight change Contraindications: Thromboembolic disorders, pregnancy, liver cancer, myocardial infarction (heart attack), coronary artery disease Warnings: Cigarette smoking increases the risk of cardiovascular side effects, glucose tolerance may decrease, triglycerides may increase	Decreased effectiveness of oral contraceptive when taken with: • Antibiotics (penicillin V, tetracycline, sulfonamides, methronidazole, ampicillin) • Barbiturates • Phenytoin • Corticosteroids • Carbamazepine • Isoniazid • Antidepressants • Oral anticoagulants • Hypoglycemic agents	• Although newer contraceptive formulations contain less steroid than the older ones, it still is important to monitor gingival changes in patients taking oral contraceptives. • Monitor blood pressure, since oral contraceptives may cause hypertension within months of starting them. • Remember that the effectiveness of oral contraceptives (estrogen component) may be reduced when taken with certain antibiotics prescribed in dentistry, including penicillin V and tetracyclines.
Estrogen + progestin *Monophasic* Loestrin (ethinyl estradiol/norethindrone acetate) Lo/Ovral (ethinyl estradiol/norgestrel) Demulen (ethinyl estradiol/ethynodiol diacetate)	See above	See above	See above	See above

Drug Name	Indications	Adverse Effects	Significant Drug Interactions	Dental Notes
Modicon, Brevicon (ethinyl estradiol; norethindrone)				
Ovcon (ethinyl estradiol; norethindrone)	See above	See above	See above	See above
Norinyl, Ortho-novum (ethinyl estradiol; norethindrone)				
Norlestrin (Ethinyl estradiol; norethindrone acetate)				
Ovral (ethinyl estradiol; norgestrel)				
Ortho Evra (norelgestromin/ethinyl estradiol)				
Norinyl (Mestranol; norethindrone)				
Enovid (Mestranol; norethynodrel)				
Biphasic				
Ortho-novum (Ethinyl estradiol; norethindrone)	See above	See above	See above	See above
Triphasic				
Tri-Levlen; Triphasil (ethinyl estradiol; levonorgestrel)				
Ortho-novum (ethinyl estradiol; norethindrone)	See above	See above	See above	See above
Tri-Norinyl (ethinyl estradiol; norethindrone)				

(continued)

Table 19-7 (Continued)

Drug Name	Indications	Adverse Effects	Significant Drug Interactions	Dental Notes
Androgens				
Fluoxymesterone (Halostestin, generics); oral	Inoperable breast cancer in women	Menstrual irregularities, hirsutism (excessive hair growth in areas on the body that usually don't have hair)	Decrease blood glucose and insulin/oral hypoglycemic levels May increase oral anti-coagulant effects	Oral forms take with food to reduce G.I. irritation No dental implications
Methyltestosterone (Android, generic); oral	Inoperable breast cancer in women	See above; hypertension	See above	See above
Testosterone (Androderm, generic); IM	Treatment for male hypogonadism	See above	See above	See above
Anabolic Steroids		See above	May increase oral anticoagulant effects Decrease blood glucose and insulin/oral hypoglycemic levels	See above
Nandrolone decanoate (Deca-Durabolin); injectable	Postmenopausal osteoporosis	See above	See above	See above

Nonsteroidal Estrogens

Nonsteroidal estrogens, such as diethylstilbesterol (DES), were first introduced to prevent miscarriages, but it was found that the fetus was affected and that the children had a high incidence of development of vaginal cancer. Today, they are used only in the treatment of inoperable breast cancer.

Anti-Estrogens

Anti-estrogens are drugs that inhibit the actions of estradiol by binding to the estrogen receptor, preventing estradiol from binding. Tamoxifen (Nolvadex), anastrozole (Arimidex), exemestane (Aromasin), and toremifene (Fareston) are anti-estrogen drugs used in the treatment of breast cancer. Clomiphene (Clomid) is used to treat infertility by stimulating ovulation, causing the release of multiple mature ova.

Progestins

Progestins modify some of the effects of estrogens and may reduce the incidence of endometrial hyperplasia. There are two main groups of progestins: progesterone (naturally occurring; includes dydrogesterone, hydroxyprogesterone, and medroxyprogesterone) and testosterone (norethindrone and norethynodrel). Progestins are used as antifertility agents (contraceptives) by decreasing ovulation, treatment of menstrual disorders, treatment of endometriosis (ovarian suppression), and in hormone replacement therapy (HRT) with estrogens (Table 19-7).

Adverse Effects

Because of the similar structure in progesterone and testosterone, progesterone may cause masculinity in females. Other adverse side effects of progestins include weight gain, hypertension, edema, cervical and breast changes, depression, acne, and thrombophlebitis.

Progestin Inhibitors

Progestin inhibitors inhibit the action of progestin at the progesterone receptors. Mifepristone (RU 486), called the "morning after" pill is used to abort the embryo.

Estrogen/Hormonal Replacement Therapy

Estrogens are used for estrogen replacement therapy in menopausal and postmenopausal women for the prevention of osteoporosis. Additionally, estrogens may lower the incidence of menopausal symptoms, such as hot flashes, mood changes, and vaginitis, and reduce the incidence of cardiovascular disease. Estradiol, estropipate, and conjugated estrogens are primarily used in ERT. When estrogen only is used it is called estrogen replacement therapy (ERT), when estrogen is used in combination with progestins it is referred to as hormonal replacement therapy (HRT). In women without a hysterectomy (with a uterus), progesterone should be added to the estrogen, which may reduce the incidence of endometrial hyperplasia.

There is controversy concerning the preventive values of using ERT or HRT in menopausal/postmenopausal women. While there may be a reduction in the risk of bone fractures, with long-term therapy there may be an increased risk of breast cancer, stroke, and thromboembolism. HRT is contraindicated in women who are pregnant, or have liver disease, breast cancer, thromboembolic disorders, and vaginal bleeding. Smoking may decrease the effectiveness of estrogen on bone and may increase the risk of thromboembolic disease.

Table 19-7 lists some estrogen-only ERT products, which include transdermal estradiol, conjugated estrogens, and micronized estradiol and estrogen plus progesterone HRT products.

Phytoestrogens, which are plant-derived products with so-called natural estrogen activity, are available in the health stores and should be used with caution, since the purity of the product as well as its side effects are unknown.

Oral Contraceptives

Estrogens + Progestins; Progestin Only

Estrogens are used in oral contraceptives in combination with progestins to suppress the FSH (follicle stimulating hormone) and thus inhibit ovulation (Table 19-1). Essentially, contraceptives work by mimicking pregnancy. Oral contraceptives are also used to treat endometriosis. Although most contraceptives are given orally, a few products are administered through a transdermal patch or a long-lasting depot, a long-lasting formulation which requires only weekly or monthly dosing.

Estrogen + Progestin

Combination oral contraceptives contain estrogen, generally in the form of ethinylestradiol, and a progestin (Table 19–7). They are taken for 20–21 days and then discontinued for the following 6–7 days when menstruation occurs. The newer generation of oral contraceptives contains newer progestins that have no estrogenic effect and less androgenic (acne, depression, hirsutism, weight gain) effect. Combination oral contraceptives are available as monophasic, biphasic, and triphasic, corresponding to the progestin content. All of the oral contraceptives are taken orally (pill formulation) except a new formulation, Ortho Evra, which is delivered by a patch.

Adverse effects of combination contraceptives include vaginal yeast infections, depression, headache, nausea, weight gain, leg, chest or abdominal (stomach) pain, shortness of breath, and breast tenderness.

Oral contraceptives are contraindicated in pregnancy, liver disease, breast cancer, history of myocardial infarction, thromboembolism, and thrombophlebitis (especially in smokers). Oral contraceptives should be used with caution in women with gallbladder disease, and in women over age 35 who are smoking.

The newer progestins, such as norgestimate and desogestrel, cause fewer side effects than the older progestins.

Progestin Only

The so-called "minipill" (norethindrone) is a type of progestin-only contraceptive. Progestin oral contraceptives are given continuously, with no days off. Progestin-only contraceptives are indicated in women who smoke, where estrogen is contraindicated, and in older women. It is indicated in patients at high risk to side effects from estrogen.

Drug Interactions: Sex Hormones

Tobacco smokers taking estrogen alone or in combination with progestins have an increased risk of stroke. Estrogens reduce the effects of oral anticoagulants (e.g., warfarin), resulting in bleeding; adjustment of warfarin may be needed. Barbiturates (e.g., phenobarbital) may increase the metabolism of estrogens. Estrogens may inhibit the metabolism of benzodiazepines (Valium, Xanax), resulting in increased serum levels of benzodiazepines. Broad-spectrum antibiotics (e.g., tetracyclines, ampicillin, amoxicillin, rifampin) have been stated in medical literature to interact with oral contraceptives (mainly the estrogen part), resulting in a decreased effectiveness of the oral contraceptive. Phenytoin may decrease the estrogen effect by increasing its metabolism.

Male Sex Hormones/Androgens and Anabolic Steroids

Male sex hormones have androgenic and anabolic effects. Androgens (testosterone) are used in the treatment of hypogonadism—which increases development of male puberty and growth when it is delayed—and inoperable breast cancer in women. Most testosterone products undergo extensive first-pass metabolism in the liver, reducing the oral bioavailability. Thus most products are given parentally (IM), or transdermal (Table 19–7).

Anabolic steroids are testosterone-like compounds with hormonal activity used to hasten weight gain after severe trauma or surgery, and alleviate postmenopausal osteoporosis. They are taken (inappropriately) by athletes to increase muscle mass and strength.

Did You Know?

Some athletes abuse anabolic steroids as performance-enhancing drugs to build muscle. These are deadly drugs, and many athletes die.

DENTAL HYGIENE NOTES

During a medical history interview, it is important to note if patients are taking contraceptives. Ethinyl estradiol, which is the primary drug used in contraceptives, may become ineffective in preventing pregnancy if patients are also taking bactericidal/broad-spectrum antibiotics such as tetracyclines, amoxicillin, or metronidazole (Flagyl). Consultation with the patient's physician may be necessary to change the method of contraception.

It has been stated in older dental literature that estrogens may cause increased gingivitis and gingival bleeding. Most of these studies were done in the 1960s and 1970s. The formulation of oral contraceptives has changed over the years resulting in less estrogen, which causes less gingival tissue change.

KEY POINTS

- Adrenal crisis is rare in dentistry.
- Increases in systemic corticosteroid doses are not usually necessary in dental patients undergoing routine dental care (e.g., oral prophylaxis, scaling/ root planing, operative).

- An increase in dose is necessary for patients undergoing stressful dental procedures such as extractions, periodontal surgery, and implant surgery.
- Systemic and topical corticosteroids are used in the treatment of many dental/oral conditions.
- A preparation containing hydrocortisone acetate in a paste (Orabase®) is used in patients with oral mucosa ulceration or irritation.
- Human insulin preparations: Regular insulin (rapid-acting) and NPH (intermediate-acting). All other insulin formulations are insulin analog preparations.
- Diabetics are more prone to the development of periodontal disease, and patients with periodontal disease have an increased incidence of development of diabetes.
- Other oral manifestations of diabetes mellitus include xerostomia, burning tongue/mouth, and *Candida* (fungal) infections.
- Epinephrine increases blood glucose. Patients who are not well controlled, with fluctuating blood glucose levels, or taking high doses of insulin should have the amount of epinephrine limited.
- Interview patients about the type of diabetic medication being taken. Make sure the medication is taken as directed and patients have eaten before dental treatment.
- There are no special precautions to follow regarding the use of epinephrine in patients taking thyroid medication as long as the condition is controlled and not hyperthyroid.
- Oral manifestations of undiagnosed thyroid disease can be recognized during a dental exam.
- There is a possible drug–drug interaction between broad-spectrum antibiotics (e.g., tetracyclines) and oral contraceptives. Alternative contraceptive methods may have to be used.
- Oral contraceptives usually do not cause gingival inflammation because current formulations contain less estrogen.

BOARD REVIEW QUESTIONS

1. Which of the following medications is most susceptible in causing hypoglycemia? (pp. 380–382)
   a. Microsnase
   b. Metformin
   c. Insulin
   d. Pioglitazone
   e. Repaglinide

2. Which of the following medications should *not* be given to a diabetic taking insulin? (p. 378)
   a. Ibuprofen
   b. Aspirin
   c. Penicillin
   d. Acetaminophen
   e. Vitamin C

3. To which of the following classifications does metformin belong? (p. 376)
   a. Alpha-glucosidase inhibitors
   b. Biguanides
   c. Meglitindies
   d. Thiazolidinediones
   e. Insulin

4. Which of the following adverse effects is seen with insulin and should be carefully monitored while seeing a dental patient? (p. 382)
   a. Hypoglycemia
   b. Anorexia
   c. Constipation
   d. Hyperlipidemia
   e. Liver enzyme problems

5. In which of the following organs is insulin produced and secreted? (p. 372)
   a. Heart
   b. Kidney
   c. Liver
   d. Pancreas
   e. Lung

6. Which of the following substances should be given in limited amounts to uncontrolled diabetics? (p. 382)
   a. Water
   b. Epinephrine
   c. Lidocaine
   d. Benzocaine

7. Which of the following oral conditions occurs more frequently in a diabetic? (p. 374)
   a. Tooth decay
   b. Lip numbness
   c. Periodontal disease
   d. Increased salivation

8. If a conscious patient becomes hypoglycemic in the dental chair, which of the following substances should be administered? (p. 383)
   a. Sugar
   b. Water
   c. Coffee
   d. Tea

9. Which of the following systemic conditions could a diabetic also have? (p. 374)
   a. Hyperlipidemia
   b. Sinusitis
   c. Headaches
   d. Depression

10. Most of the insulin used today is: (p. 381)
    a. Animal
    b. Plant
    c. Recombinant human
    d. Combination plant and animal

11. Which of the following drugs may interact with Ortho-novum? (pp. 394–396, 398)
    a. Aspirin
    b. Tetracycline
    c. Chlorhexidine
    d. Ibuprofen
    e. Vitamin C

12. Which of the following statements is true concerning replacement of hormones in postmenopausal women? (p. 397)
    a. When estrogen is used alone, it is referred to as hormonal replacement therapy (HRT).
    b. Progesterone is usually combined with estrogen in women with a uterus.
    c. When estrogen is combined with progesterone, it is referred to as estrogen replacement therapy.
    d. An adverse side effect of estrogen therapy is depression.
    e. Patients taking estrogen may complain of xerostomia.

13. There is a high incidence of gingival overgrowth in patients taking oral contraceptives *because* most products on the market today contain lower concentrations of estrogen. (pp. 397–398)
    a. Statement is true and the reason is correct.
    b. Statement is true and the reason is incorrect and not related.

c. Statement is false but the reason is correct.
d. Both the statement and reason are incorrect.

14. Which of the following hormones consists of the minpill? (p. 398)
    a. Estrogen
    b. Progestin
    c. Estrogen/progestin
    d. Androgen

15. Which of the following is an anti-estrogen drug? (p. 397)
    a. Tamoxifen
    b. Progestin
    c. Estrogen
    d. Metronidazole

16. Which of the following is the most common medication used to treat patients with hypothyroidism? (pp. 385, 386)
    a. Levothyroxine
    b. Thyroid USP
    c. Liotrix
    d. Iodide
    e. Propranolol

17. Which of the following blood markers are used to monitor for thyroid function? (pp. 383, 388)
    a. T_3 and T_4
    b. T_4 and TSH
    c. T_4 and pituitary stimulating hormone
    d. Iodine and T_3

18. All of the following are signs and symptoms of hyperthyroidism *except* one; which is the exception? (p. 385)
    a. Dry skin
    b. Nervousness
    c. Sweating
    d. Heat intolerance
    e. Palpitations

19. Which of the following medications is derived from animals? (p. 385)
    a. Thyroid USP
    b. Levothyroxine
    c. Liotrix
    d. Liothyronine

20. The primary classification of hydrocortisone is (p. 387)
    a. Anti-inflammatory
    b. Antihypertenisve

c. Antimicrobial
d. Antifungal
e. Antiviral

21. Which of the following steroid hormones is naturally occurring? (p. 387)
    a. Prednisone
    b. Prednisolone
    c. Cortisol
    d. Betamethasone
    e. Triamcinolone

22. All of the following are adverse effects of corticosteroids *except* one. Which one is the exception? (pp. 387, 388)
    a. Hypertension
    b. Psychosis
    c. Peptic ulcers
    d. Water retention
    e. Heat tolerance

23. All of the following conditions are acceptable for use of a topical corticosteroid *except* one; which one is the exception? (p. 389)
    a. Herpes labialis
    b. Aphthous stomatitis
    c. Ulcerative lichen planus
    d. Burning mouth

24. A patient is taking prednisone 10 mg/day and will have periodontal scaling and root planing (1 quadrant per visit). The dose of systemic corticosteroids should be increased to avoid prolong healing following the scaling. (p. 390)
    a. Both statements are true.
    b. The first statement is true and the second is not.
    c. The first statement is false and the second is true.
    d. Both statements are false.

SELECTED REFERENCES

Evans, A., and A. J. Krentz. 1999. Benefits and risks of transfer from oral agents to insulin in type 2 diabetes mellitus. *Drug Saf* 21:7–22.

Fletcher, S.W., and G. A. Colditz. 2002. Failure of estrogen plus progestin therapy for prevention. *JAMA* 288(*3*): 366–367.

Grossi, S. G., and R. J. Genco. 1998. Periodontal disease and diabetes mellitus: A two-way relationship. *Ann Periodontol* 3(*1*):51–61.

Haines, S. T., L. M. Cushenberry, D. LeRoith, and C. F. Steil. 2001. New approaches to insulin therapy for diabetics. In:

Special Report: A Continuing Education Program for Pharmacists. American Pharmaceutical Association.

Haupt, B. A. Management of thyroid disorders. *U.S. Pharmacist* suppl. July 2000.

Koda-Kimble, M. A., L. Y. Young, W. A. Kradjan, and B. J. Guglielmo. 2002. Thyroid disorders. In: *Handbook of Applied Therapeutics,* 7th ed. Baltimore: Lippincott Williams & Wilkins. Chapter 46.

Mattson, J. S., and D. R. Cerutis. 2001. Diabetes Mellitus: A review of the literature and dental implications. *Compendium Dent Educ* 22(*9*):757–773.

Miller, C. S., J. W. Little, and D. A. Falace. 2001. Supplemental corticosteroids for dental patients with adrenal insufficiency. *JADA* 132(*11*):1570–1579.

Muzyka, B. C. 2000. Revisiting the use of glucocorticosteroids in dentistry. *Practical Perio Aesthetic Dent* 2:814.

Pinto, A., and R. Glick. 2002. Management of patients with thyroid diseases. *JADA* 133:849–858.

Moritz, A. J., and B. L. Mealey. 2006. Periodontal disease, insulin resistance, and diabetes mellitus. *Grand Rounds in Oral-Systemic Medicine 1(2):* 13–20.

Takiya, L. and T. Dougherty. Pharmacist's guide to insulin preparations: A comprehensive review. *Pharmacy Times.* Continuing education program 290-000-05-016-H01.

Thorstensson, H., J. Kuylensteirna, and A. Hugoson. 1996. Medical status and complications in relation to periodontal disease experience in inuslin-dependent diabetics. *J Clin Periodontol* 23:194–202.

Webb, M. R. 2000. Treatment options for type 2 diabetes. *American Family Physician.* monograph no. 1.

Wells, B. G., J. T. DiPiro, T. L. Schwinghammer, and C.W. Hamilton. 2000. Thyroid disorders. *Pharmacotherapy Handbook,* 2nd ed. p. 213–225: Appleton & Lange.

White, J. R. Jr., and R. K. Campbell. 2003. Type 2 diabetes and insulin resistance: Counseling patients in the pharmacy. *U.S. Pharmacist* 28:65–87.

Wilson, G. R., and W. R. Curry Jr. 2005. Subclinical thyroid disease. *Am Fam Physician* 72:1517–1524.

World Health Organization. 1985. *Diabetes Mellitus: Report of a WHO Study Group.* Geneva: World Health Org., tech. rep. ser., no. 727.

Zoorob, R. J., and D. Cender. 1998. A different look at corticosteroids. *Am Fam Physician* 59:443–452.

WEB SITES

www.diabetesmonitor.com
www.diabetes.org
www.medscape.com
www.thyroid.org
www.medscape.com

QUICK DRUG GUIDE

Antidiabetic Drugs

Sulfonylureas
First-Generation Agents

- Chlopropamide (Diabinese)
- Tolazamide (Tolinase)
- Tolbutamide (Orinase)

Second-Generation Agents

- Glipizide (Glucotrol)
- Glyburide (DiaBeta, Micronase)
- Glyburide, micronized (Glynase)
- Glimepiride (Amaryl)
- Glipizide ext-rel (Glucotrol XL)

Biguanides and Combinations

- Metformin (Glucophage, Fortamet)
- Metformin/rosiglitazone (Avandamet)
- Metformin/glyburide (Glucovance)
- Metformin/glipizide (Metaglip)
- Rosiglitazone/glimepiride (Avandaryl)

Thiazolidnedoines

- Rosiglitazone (Avandia)
- Pioglitazone (Actos)

Glucosidase Inhibitors

- Acarbose (Precose)
- Miglitol (Glyset)

Insulins
Rapid-Acting

- Insulin human inhalation powder (rDNA origin) (Exubera)
- Insulin glulisine (rDNA original) (Apidra)
- Insulin aspart (rDNA origin) (NovoLog FlexPen; NoVoglog Mix 70/30; NovoLog FlexPen)
- Insulin lispro (rDNA origin) (Humalog; Humalog Pen)
- Insulin regular (human insulin) (Humulin R; Novolin R, Regular Iletin II)

Intermediate- and Long-Acting

- Isophane insulin suspension (human insulin) (NPH, Humulin N; Novolin N, Iletin I, NPH Iletin II)
- Insulin zinc human (human insulin) (Humulin L, Novolin L)
- Human regular and human NPH mixture (Humulin 70/30, Humulin 50/50, Novolin 70/30)
- Insulin Glargine (Lantus) (analog)
- Insulin Determir (Levemir) (analog)
- PZI: Insulin lispro protamine 75%/insulin lispro 25%

Thyroid Drugs

Hyperthyroidism
Thiourea Drugs

- Propylthiouracil (PTU)
- Methimazole (Tapazole)

Radioacative Iodine (RAI)

Iodine Compounds

- Lugol's solution/potassium iodide (SSKI)

Hypothyroidism

- Thyroid USP
- L-thyroxine (Levoxyl, Synthroid, Levothroid)
- L-triiodothyronine (Cytomel)
- Liotrix (Thyrolar)

Systemic Corticosteroids

Short-acting (8–12 hours)

- Cortisone (generic, Cortone) (tabs)
- Hydrocortisone, Cortisol (Cortef, various brand names) (tabs)

Intermediate-acting (12–36 hours)

- Methylprednisolone (generic, Medrol) (tabs)
- Prednisolone (tabs, syrup) (generic, Orapred, Prelone)
- Prednisone (generic, Meticorten, Deltasone)
- Triamcinolone (Aristocort, Kenacort, generics)

Long-acting (36–54 hours)

- Betamethasone (Celestone) (tabs, syrup)
- Dexamethasone (Decadron, generic)

Topical Corticosteroids (Drug Name/Generic)

Low-potency Group IV

- Hydrocortisone (generic; Cortef, Synacort) Rx
- Hydrocortisone (various brand names—
- Cortaid, Cortizone—OTC; 0.5% and 1%)
- Hydrocortisone acetate (in Orabase®)
- Alclometasone (Aclovate)
- Flurandrenolide (Cordran 0.0125%) F
- Dexamethasone (Decadron) F
- Triamcinolone acetonide (Aristocort Kenalog 0.025%) F
- Triamcinolone acetonide F dental paste

Medium-potency Group III

- Betamethasone benzoate (Uticort) F
- Desoximetasone (Topicort 0.05%) F
- Flurandrenolide (Cordran) F
- Flucoinolone acetonide (Synlar) F
- Halcinonide (Halog 0.025%) F
- Hydrocortisone valerate (Westcort 0.2%) F
- Mometasone furoate (Elocon) F
- Triamcinolone acetonide (generic, Aristocort, Kenalog 0.1%) F

High-potency Group II

- Amcinonide (Cyclocort) F
- Betamethasone dipropionate F (diprosone)
- Desoximetsone (Topicort 0.25%) F
- Fluocinolone (Synalar HP 0.2%) F
- Fluocinonide (Lidex) F
- Triamcinolone acetonide (generic, Aristocort, Kenalog 0.5%) F

Very High-Potency Group I

- Betamethasone dipropionate (Diprolene 0.05%) F
- Clobetasol propionate (generic, Temovate) F
- Diflorasone diacetate (Psorcon) F
- Halobetasol propionate (Ultravate) F

F denotes if the formulation is fluoridated which prolongs the duration of action.

Estrogens

- Estradiol, micronized (Estrace); oral, vaginal cream
- Estradiol transdermal system (Estraderm, Climara, Vivelle, Esclim, generics); skin patch
- Conjugated estrogens (generics; Premarin); oral, IM, vaginal cream
- Ethinyl estradiol (Estinyl); oral
- Estradiol Cypionate (Depo-Estradiol, generics)
- Quinestrol (Estrovis)

Progestins

- Hydroxyprogesterone caproate (Duralutin, Pro-Depo, generics); Injectable
- Medroxyprogesterone acetate (Provera, generics); oral
- Medroxyprogesterone acetate (Depo-Provera); injectable
- Megestrol (Megace); oral
- Norethindrone (Norlutin); oral
- Norethindrone acetate (Aygestin, Norlutate); oral
- Progesterone micronized (Prometrium); oral

Hormone Replacement Therapy

Estrogen + Progesterone Products

- Activella (estradiol/norethindrone); oral
- CombiPatch (estradiol/norethindrone); patch
- Estratest (esterified estrogens/ methyltestosterone); oral
- Estratest H.S. (esterified estrogens/ methyltestosterone); oral
- FemHRT 1/5 (ethinyl estradiol/ norethindrone); oral
- Ortho-Prefest (estradiol/norgestimate); oral
- Premphase (conjugated estrogens/ medroxyprogesterone); oral
- Prempro (conjugated estrogens/ medroxyprogesterone); oral

Oral Contraceptives

Estrogen + progestin

Monophasic

- Loestrin (ethinyl estradiol/norethindrone acetate)
- Lo/Ovral (ethinyl estradiol/norgestrel)
- Demulen (ethinyl estradiol/ethynodiol diacetate)
- Modicon, Brevicon (ethinyl estradiol; norethindrone)
- Ovcon (ethinyl estradiol; norethindrone)
- Norinyl, Ortho-novum (ethinyl estradiol; norethindrone)
- Norlestrin (ethinyl estradiol; norethindrone acetate)
- Ovral (ethinyl estradiol; norgestrel)
- Ortho Evra (Norelgestromin/ethinyl estradiol)
- Norinyl (Mestranol; norethindrone)
- Enovid (Mestranol; norethynodrel)

Biphasic

- Ortho-Novum 10/11 (ethinyl estradiol; norethindrone)

Triphasic

- Tri-Levlen; Triphasil (ethinyl estradiol; levonorgestrel)
- Ortho-novum 7/7/7 (ethinyl estradiol; norethindrone)
- Tri-Norinyl (ethinyl estradiol; norethindrone)

Androgens

- Fluoxymesterone (Halostestin, generics); oral
- Methyltestosterone (Android, generic); oral
- Testosterone (Androderm, generic); IM

Anabolic Steroids

- Nandrolone decanoate (Deca-Durabolin); injectable

Chapter 20

Infectious Disease Drugs

GOAL: To provide an understanding of the pharmacology of drugs used to treat HIV, tuberculosis, and hepatitis C.

EDUCATIONAL OBJECTIVES

After reading this chapter, the reader should be able to:

1. Describe the pharmacology of currently approved drugs used in the treatment of HIV infection.
2. Describe selected drugs with adverse effects related to dentistry and how to manage them.
3. Explain dental implications of patients taking anti-HIV drugs.
4. List the characteristics of the bacterium that causes tuberculosis.
5. List the various antimycobacterial drugs.
6. Discuss the dental adverse side effects of antimycobacterial drugs.
7. Explain the role of interferons and herbal supplements in the treatment of hepatitis C.

KEY TERMS

Human immunodeficiency virus (HIV)
Acquired immune deficiency syndrome (AIDS)
Antiretroviral therapy
HAART
Tuberculosis
Interferons

ANTIRETROVIRAL AGENTS: HIV/AIDS

Since the first cases were reported in the United States in 1981, the AIDS epidemic has been the subject of much clinical research. The end stage of infection with **human immunodeficiency virus** is **acquired immune deficiency syndrome (AIDS).** HIV (Figure 20–1) attacks the body's immune system, resulting in life-threatening infections and cancers. Once one has developed AIDS, the immune system is weakened enough to allow for unusual or prolonged infections.

AIDS is caused by a transmissible RNA retrovirus known as HIV type 1. A related but antigenically distinct retrovirus, HIV type 2, causes some cases of AIDS in western Africa but is rare in the United States. The primary immune cells involved are the T-lymphocytes (CD4). HIV "hunts" for CD4 cells and fuses to the cell membrane allowing viral RNA from the HIV to be released into the CD4 cell. Once inside the cell, the HIV converts viral RNA into proviral DNA by an enzyme called *reverse transcriptase,* which then incorporates into the host cell (CD4) DNA. The proviral DNA enters the nucleus of the host cell and inserts into the cell's DNA. The cell then makes copies of HIV (Figure 20–2).

A decreased CD4 T-cell count occurs as the disease progresses, and serves as a good predictor of risk of opportunistic infections. These opportunistic infections include tuberculosis, fungal infections (oral candidiasis, esophageal candidiasis), *Pneumocystis jiroveci* (formerly *Pneumocystis carinii*) pneumonia (PCP), recurrent bacterial pneumonia, diarrhea, meningitis, and cancers such as Kaposi's sarcoma and non-Hodgkin lymphoma. Additionally, the wasting syndrome occurs, where there is tremendous amount of weight loss.

Diagnosis

The Centers for Disease Control (CDC) defines AIDS as a CD4 count of under 200/μL or CD4+ T under 14 percent of total lymphocytes in the presence of HIV infection. As the amount of virus in the plasma (viral load) increases, the CD4+ count decreases. A combination of CD4 + T counts and plasma HIV RNA (viral) loads is the best overall disease marker. A medical consult is necessary for this type of patient.

Antiretroviral Pharmacology

The objective of **antiretroviral therapy** is to reduce the viral (RNA retrovirus) load, thereby improving survival. HIV viral load is the most sensitive marker for disease control and should be monitored, as well as CD4+ counts. Past guidelines for the initiation of treatment in asymptomatic patients depended upon the CD4+ count. However, new information indicates that quantitation of HIV RNA in plasma (viral load) is a better indicator for the start of drug therapy. Drug therapy should be started if the patient is symptomatic or if the asymptomatic patient has a CD4+ count of under 500 per mm^3 or a viral load of more than 30,000 copies per mL. Lack of adherence to drug treatment is a major cause of failure of treatment and the emergence of resistant strains of the virus, which makes it more difficult to treat.

Antiretroviral Drugs

Four classes of drugs are currently available for the treatment of HIV infection (Table 20–1):

- Nucleoside/nucleotide reverse transcriptase inhibitors (NRTI/NtRTIs)
- Nonnucleoside reverse transcriptase inhibitors (NNRTIs)
- Protease inhibitors (PIs)
- Fusion (entry) inhibitors

Three or four drug combinations for initial therapy are termed highly active antiretroviral therapy (**HAART**)

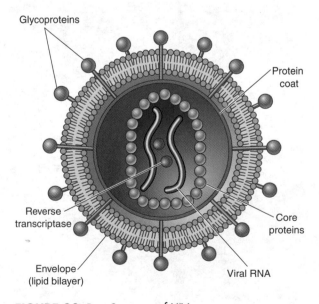

Glycoproteins

Protein coat

Reverse transcriptase

Core proteins

Envelope (lipid bilayer)

Viral RNA

FIGURE 20–1 Structure of HIV.

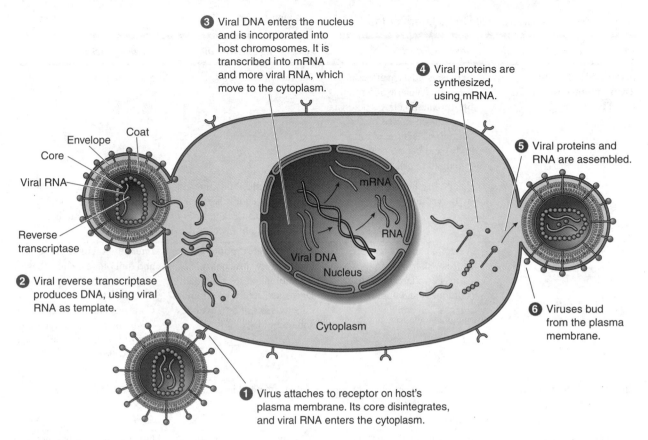

3 Viral DNA enters the nucleus and is incorporated into host chromosomes. It is transcribed into mRNA and more viral RNA, which move to the cytoplasm.

4 Viral proteins are synthesized, using mRNA.

5 Viral proteins and RNA are assembled.

Envelope

Coat

Core

Viral RNA

mRNA

RNA

Reverse transcriptase

Viral DNA

Nucleus

2 Viral reverse transcriptase produces DNA, using viral RNA as template.

Cytoplasm

6 Viruses bud from the plasma membrane.

1 Virus attaches to receptor on host's plasma membrane. Its core disintegrates, and viral RNA enters the cytoplasm.

FIGURE 20–2 Replication of HIV.

and are the preferred initial regimen. The purpose of HAART is to improve both survival and quality of life with a regimen using three or four drugs to suppress viral replication and management or prevention of opportunistic infections. The goal of therapy is to use a HAART that reduces plasma levels of HIV RNA to below detectable limits (fewer than 50 copies/mL). There are currently 20 FDA-approved drugs in the United States used to treat HIV. Drug toxicity and HIV resistance toward these drugs makes adherence a critical issue. Approximately 78 percent of patients are becoming resistant to at least one HIV drug. Current treatment guidelines recommend the use of two or more of these drugs to suppress viral replication and management, or prevention of opportunistic infections. Usually, two nucleoside reverse transcriptase inhibitors (NRTI) or nucleoside analogs and a highly active protease inhibitor drug are used. Alternative regimens include two RTIs and a nonnucleoside reverse transcriptase inhibitor (NNRTI), or two RTIs and a protease inhibitor.

To understand the actions of these drugs, refer to Table 20–1; all of these drugs are related to the events of the HIV on the CD4+ cell. For example, the nonnucleoside reverse transcriptase inhibitors (NNRTIs) bind to a different site on the reverse transcriptase than the NRTIs, preventing the virus from transcribing viral RNA into viral DNA.

The nucleoside reverse transcriptase inhibitors (NRTIs), the first drugs approved by the FDA in the 1980s, embed themselves into virus DNA and inhibit the conversion of RNA to DNA by binding to the reverse transcriptase enzyme. Since the NRTIs do not undergo extensive liver cytochrome P450 metabolism, other drugs that are metabolized that way are not affected by the NRTIs.

Did You Know?

The first antiretroviral drug, zidovudine, is no longer given by itself except as prophylaxis in exposed newborns; it loses its effectiveness against HIV over time.

Table 20–1 Antiretroviral Drugs Used for the Treatment of HIV/AIDS

Drug Name	*Adverse Effects*	*Drug-Drug Interactions*	*Dental Notes*
Nucleoside Reverse Transcriptase Inhibitors (NRTIs)	Extensive adverse effect profile. All can cause potentially life-threatening lactic acidosis (a condition caused by the buildup of lactic acid in the body) and hepatomegaly (enlarged liver).	See individual drugs	See individual drugs
Abacavir (Ziagen)	Potentially fatal hypersensitivity reaction	Decreased metabolism resulting in elevated levels when given with disulfiram, isoniazid, and ethanol (alcohol)	No significant dental notes Monitor viral load and CD4 counts through medical consultations.
Didansoine (ddl, Videx)	Anemia, pancreatitis, G.I. distress (diarrhea, abdominal pain), peripheral neuropathy (numbness and tingling of toes, finger), *xerostomia*	Decreased absorption of ketoconazole and itraconazole Alcohol increases pancreatitis Decreased serum levels and effectiveness of tetracyclines and quinolones	Interaction with tetracyclines and quinolones—take these drugs 2 hours before or 4 hours after ddL. Can cause xerostomia—maintain good oral hygiene, fluoride supplementation, and drink water.
Emtricitabine (Emtriva)	Nausea, diarrhea, rash, hyperpigmentation of palms and soles of feet	No documented interactions	No significant dental notes
Lamivudine (3TC, Epivir)	Better tolerated than the other drugs; fatigue, headache, G.I. distress, neuropathy, insomnia	No documented interactions	No significant dental notes Monitor viral load and CD4 counts through medical consultations.
Stavudine (d4T, Zerit) Zidovudine (Retrovir)	Bone marrow suppression, resulting in severe anemia (low blood iron), granulocytopenia (low neutrophils/white blood cells), thrombocytopenia (low platelets), myopathy (muscle weakness), and hepatitis Minor side effects: headache, anorexia, nausea, vomiting dizziness, insomnia	Rifampin increases ZDV metabolism. Increased incidence of blood disorders with prolonged administration of acetaminophen	Monitor viral load and CD4 counts through medical consultations.
Tenofovir disoproxil fumerate (Viread)	Lactic acidosis and hepatomegaly (enlarged liver)	Increased toxicity if taken with probenecid (antigout)	No significant dental notes
Zalcitabine (ddC) —HIVID	Peripheral neuropathy; no G.I. or blood problems, *oral ulcerations (stomatitis, aphthous ulcers)*	Decreased absorption of ddC when given with antacids Additive toxicity when given with metronidazole and isoniazid. Decreased clearance when given with cimetidine	Monitor for oral ulcerations—apply Orabase with benzocaine (OTC) or lidocaine 2% viscous (Rx) for pain relief. Don't give metronidazole and ddC together.

Drug Name	Adverse Effects	Drug-drug Interactions	Dental Notes
NonNucleoside Reverse Transcriptase Inhibitors (NNRTI)		NNRTIs are metabolized by cytochrome P450 liver enzymes.	Monitor viral load and CD4 counts through medical consultations.
Efavirenz (Sustiva)	Dizziness, headache, rash, insomnia, hallucinations, nightmares, altered concentration	Increases levels of clarithromycin.	See above
Nevirapine (Viramune)	Rash is very common, fatal liver damage		See above
Delavirdine (Rescriptor)	Less incidence of rash compared to other NNRTIs, headaches, increase in liver enzymes	Phenobarbital decreases delavirdine levels; Increases levels of clarithromycin.	See above; do not give clarithromycin (Zithromax) and delavirdine together. An alternate antibiotic should be used.
Protease Inhibitors (PIs):		Metabolized by CYP450, predominately CYP3A4 (many drug interactions) Do not give with lidocaine, ketoconazole (antifungal), antihistamines	Monitor viral load and CD4 counts through medical consultations.
Amprevavir (Agenerase)	*Oral paresthesia* (numbness), rash	See above St. John's wort, rifampin, triazolam	See above; monitor for oral paresthesia.
Atazanavir (Reyataz)	*Dental pain, taste changes*	See above	
Fosamprenavir (Lexiva)	*Perioral paresthesia* (numbness around the mouth), *taste disorders,* skin rash, nausea, vomiting, diarrhea	See above	Many drug interactions
Indinavir (Crixivan)	*Metallic taste in mouth,* blurred vision, thrombocytopenia, alopecia	See above	See above Monitor for metallic taste in mouth.
Lopinavir + Ritonavir (Kaletra)	Potentially fatal hypersensitivity reaction	See above	See above
Nelfinavir (Viracept)	Paresthesias	See above	See above
Ritonavir (Norvir)	Pancreatitis, hepatitis, *taste impairment,* paresthesias	See above	See above
Saquinavir (Fortovase; formerly Invirase)	Increase in liver enzymes	Decreased serum levels with dexamethasone	See above
Fusion (Entry) Inhibitors Enfuvirtide (Fuzeon)	Injection only; hypersensitivity, skin reactions	None documented	No specific instructions

The protease inhibitors (*PIs*) prevent breakdown of proteins produced by the virus into infectious mature viruses, and are the most potent of the antiretroviral drugs. These drugs are extensively metabolized by the cytochrome P450 enzymes so there are many potential drug interactions. For example, rifampin should not be given concurrently with any PI except for ritonavir.

The *fusion (entry) inhibitors* interfere with the entry of HIV-1 into hosts (lymphocytes) by inhibiting fusion of the virus and cell membranes. For HIV-1 to enter and infect the CD4+ cell, the viral glycoprotein must bind the cell membrane. Then the glycoprotein changes its shape, which helps in the fusion of the viral membrane with the cell. Enfuvirtide (Fuzeon) works by binding to the viral glycoprotein and preventing a change in the shape of the glycoprotein required for membrane fusion and viral entry into the target cell.

Pharmacologic Treatment of Systemic Opportunistic Infections

There may be an association between CD4 count and the increased incidence of specific opportunistic infections in HIV+ patients.

HIV/AIDS patients may also be taking medications to prevent or treat opportunistic infections. If the patient has or had *Pneumocystis jiroveci* pneumonia, he/she will most likely be taking trimethoprim/sulfamethoxazole. The drug of choice for various forms of systemic candidiasis includes fluconazole (Diflucan).

 Rapid Dental Hint

Many HIV-infected patients present with oral lesions. Monitor those patients.

Pharmacologic Treatment of Oral Opportunistic Lesions/Conditions

Table 20–2 lists common opportunistic oral lesions/conditions associated with HIV, with the appropriate treatment. Many oral infections develop in the immunocompromised patients, including:

- Fungal infections: oral candidiasis, angular cheilitis
- Viral infections: herpes simplex, human papilloma virus, hairy leukoplakia

- Bacterial infections: periodontal infections. It is important to emphasize that not all patients with HIV disease necessarily have gingival or periodontal infections. These infections are associated with immunodeficiency.
- Intraoral pain: Intraoral pain from the lesions can be so severe that eating becomes difficult, resulting in weight loss.
- Aphthous ulcers
- Xerostomia: common, may predispose to fungal infections
- Oral neoplasms: Kaposi's sarcoma (KS) is a neoplasm that causes both intraoral and skin lesions
- Infections of unknown etiology

Rapid Dental Hint

There are no contraindications for using local anesthetics in HIV-infected patients.

Dental Hygiene Notes

Certain laboratory tests and values associated with HIV infection may be useful in the dental management of the patient. CD4+ lymphocyte counts range from 500 to 1,600 cells/mm^3 in the HIV-negative patient whereas initial signs and symptoms of immune suppression occur at CD4+ counts of under 500 cells/mm^3. When the CD4 counts fall to this level, many major and life-threatening opportunistic infections and malignancies develop. Patients with CD4+ lymphocyte counts above 200 cells/mm^3 usually have their immunologic status assessed every 6 months by their physician, whereas patients with counts of under 200 cells/mm^3 usually are assessed every 3 months.

Thrombocytopenia (under 150,000 platelets/mm^3) is often seen with HIV infection. Platelet counts are used to assess the patient for bleeding tendencies. Oral signs usually present as small, blood-filled petechiae or larger ecchymoses. Excessive bleeding during surgery may occur in these patients. Anemia is common in HIV-infected patients, either due to the medications or the infection; it is important to obtain laboratory blood values from the patient's physician.

Local anesthesia has not been associated with increased risk of intraoral infections. However, deep block injections can result in medical complications in patients

Table 20-2 Common Oral Lesions/Conditions Associated with HIV Infections and Treatment Guidelines.

Condition	*Treatment (Common Drugs)*
Fungal Infections Candidiasis (oral, pharyngeal)	Antifungal agents: choose one of the following regimens. Clotrimazole (Mycelex) troches, 10 mg: Dissolve 1 troche in mouth 5 times a day. Nystatin pastilles, 200,000 units: dissolve one pastille in mouth 5 times a day. Nystatin (Mycostatin) vaginal troches, 100,000 units: dissolve in mouth 1 troche 6–8 times per day. Nystatin oral suspension: Take 4–6 ml 4 times a day. Retain in mouth as long as possible before swallowing. Ketoconazole (Nizoral) tab 200mg: Take 2 tabs orally on the first day, followed by 1 tab per day for 14 days. Fluconazole (Diflucan) tab 100mg: Take two tabs orally on the first day, followed by one tab per day for 14 days.
Angular chelitis	Clotrimazole topical (Lotrimin, Gyne-Lotrimin) cream 1%. Apply to lesion 4 times a day. Ketoconazole cream 2%: Apply to area 4 times a day; Nystatin ointment 100,000 units; apply to area 4 times a day.
Viral Infections Herpes simplex lesions	Acyclovir topical ointment 5%; Acyclovir cap 800mg, 1 cap 5 times a day.
Hairy leukoplakia (Epstein-Barr virus infection)	Treatment is elective: acyclovir cap 800 mg—1 cap 4 times a day.
Bacterial Infections Linear gingival erythema (LGE)	Periodontal debridement Chlorhexidine gluconate 0.12% (Peridex, Periogard) (rinse with 20 ml of rinse for 30 seconds twice a day)
Necrotizing ulcerative gingivitis (NUG)	Periodontal debridement Chlorhexidine gluconate 0.12% oral rinse plus Systemic antibiotic: Metrondiazole 250 mg qid or Amoxicillin 500 mg tid or Clindamycin 300 mg tid
Necrotizing ulcerative periodontitis (NUP)	Chlorhexidine gluconate 0.12% oral rinse Systemic therapy: Metrondiazole 250 mg qid or Amoxicillin 500 mg tid or Clindamycin 300 mg tid
Other Oral Conditions Minor aphthous ulcers (canker sores)	Fluocinonide gel (Lidex) 0.05% mixed with equal parts of Orabase (it is a methylcellulose inert ingredient that is a vehicle to carry the gel; Colgate Oral Pharm): Apply to ulcer 4 times a day. Orabase; Lidocaine viscous 2%: Swish with solution until the pain goes away and spit out (expectorate) (shake well before use).
Oral pain: acute due to oral lesions	Lidocaine viscous 2% (mild to moderate pain) or NSAIDs For severe pain: narcotic analgesics
Chronic neurologic pain	Psychotropic drugs (e.g., tricyclic antidepressants)
Xerostomia	Chew or suck on sugarless candy; avoid alcohol, which further dries the mucosa Saliva substitutes (carboxymethylcellulose or hydroxyethylcellulose): Biotene Dry Mouth Relieving Gel, Optimoist, Salivart, Salix, Xero-Lube, Moi-Stir® Oral Swabsticks, MouthKote) Systemic: Cevemeline (Evoxac) 30 mg 3 times a day Pilocarpine (Salagen) 5 mg 3–4 times a day

(Adapted from Dental Management of the HIV-Infected Patient. 1995. Supplement to *JADA*. American Dental Association and American Academy of Oral Medicine.)

with a recent history of increased bleeding tendencies. In these cases, use infiltrations.

There are generally no special restorative treatment precautions for the immunocompetent HIV-infected patient.

HIV-infected patients may be taking many different types of medications for the HIV infection itself as well as for opportunistic infections. Thus, many drug–drug interactions can occur. Many antiretroviral drugs have oral adverse side effects; for instance, indinavir causes a metallic taste, ritonavir causes taste impairment, and amprevnavir causes oral paresthesias. Additionally, many opportunistic infections are found in the mouth.

Antibiotic prophylaxis may be necessary, although not definitive, when the CD4+ count falls below 200 cells/mm^3. HIV infection itself is not a contraindication to procedures likely to cause bleeding. However, due to the systemic nature of the disease, the need for antibiotic prophylaxis should be assessed.

Meticulous oral hygiene should be reinforced with the HIV+ patient at every office visit. At least twice a year the patient should have a recall; if oral lesions are present, more frequent visits are necessary. Patients should be placed on a topical fluoride supplement such as PreviDent 1.1% neutral sodium fluoride to prevent dental caries. Chlorhexidine gluconate as an oral rinse is effective as an antiplaque and anticaries by reducing *lactobacillus* counts.

TUBERCULOSIS

In 1993, the World Health Organization declared **tuberculosis** (TB) a world-wide emergency. Tuberculosis affects all mammals, with the most common form in humans being pulmonary tuberculosis. About 9 million people are estimated to be infected or will develop active TB disease this year.

Tuberculosis is a bacterial infection caused by *Mycobacterium tuberculosis,* a tubercle bacillus (MTB). Its name indicates its formation of firm nodules (tubercles) throughout the body. The micro-organism is inhaled into the lungs through aerosol droplets from coughing, sneezing, or similar close contact with an infected individual. MTB is slow growing, with an optimum growing temperature of 37 degrees centigrade, which is body temperature. An individual may be "exposed" to MTB, but not clinically show signs of the disease because of the body's defense mechanism. However, inactive tubercle bacilli in the body may be activated, resulting in active TB under favorable conditions such as malnutrition, disease (diabetes mellitus, HIV/AIDS), corticosteroid or other immunosuppressive therapy, or chronic alcoholism.

About 4–6 weeks after the first contact with the infection, symptoms may develop, including fever, chills, gastrointestinal upset, and night sweats. Symptoms that develop later (active TB) include weight loss (anorexia), nausea, vomiting, night headaches, and palpitations (chest pain). A productive cough producing odorless, Green-yellow sputum with blood (hemoptysis) is a feature of TB.

Testing for Tuberculosis

Screening of tuberculosis is done using the tuberculin skin test, which only indicates exposure to infection and does not differentiate between infection (presence of organisms, normal chest X-ray, no symptoms) and disease. An individual will give a positive tuberculin test about 4–6 weeks after inhaling enough organisms. The tuberculin skin test is based on a skin reaction to the intradermal injection of purified protein derivative (PPD) tuberculin, a protein fraction of TB. A positive reaction (48–72 hours after injection) causes local raised swelling, and induration. The PPD test is the gold standard to detect the presence of TB.

An individual with a positive skin test (PPD+) should have a chest X-ray taken. A definitive diagnosis of TB requires sputum culture. However, typical signs and symptoms, with the typical findings on chest radiograph with a positive PPD, are enough to begin therapy.

In recent years, different assays have been developed which reduce reader variability and false readings. The FDA recently approved a whole-blood interferon-release assay. Studies are needed to determine whether the responses from this test are predicative of those who have a high risk of progression to active TB.

The Centers for Disease Control and Prevention have recommended a new, more accurate blood test for tuberculosis that yields fewer false positives. Quanti-FERON-TB is a blood test that may replace the skin test in the future.

> ### Did You Know?
>
> John Henry "Doc" Holliday was trained as a dentist in Georgia of Old West fame in the 1880s. He contracted tuberculosis and could not practice dentistry so he moved to Texas where he started to gamble and engage in gunfights, which made him very famous. On the run for many years, he died of tuberculosis in 1887 in Glenwood Springs, Colorado.

Pharmacology: Treatment of TB Infection

Drugs are available to treat the disease, but unfortunately many patients are not adherent with the long-term regimens (6 to 9 months) necessary. This has led to an increase in multidrug-resistant bacterial strains, which make definitive treatment difficult. To assure adherence *directly observed therapy* is used, where the medication is given directly to the patient while someone is watching him/her swallow the antituberculosis drugs.

The goals of antituberculosis drug therapy are to cure the disease without relapse, prevent death, stop the spread of the disease, and prevent the emergence of drug-resistant TB.

Primary prevention efforts have focused on the Bacille Calmette-Guérin (BCG) vaccine. Although BCG vaccine is used commonly in many parts of the world, its efficacy is unpredictable in protecting individuals against developing TB.

Therapy begins with a multidrug (two or more) regimen which attempts to kill the tubercle bacilli rapidly and to prevent the development of drug-resistant *Mycobacterium tuberculosis*. Tuberculosis disease should never be treated with a single drug, due to increased risk of emergence of drug-resistant disease. Additionally, if a drug is failing, at least two drugs should be added.

Drugs that have been approved for the treatment of tuberculosis are classified as first- and second-line drugs (Table 20–3).

Did You Know?

Early therapy of tuberculosis includes rest, often at sanitaria. One of the first sanitaria was at Saranac Lake in New York State, started by Edward Livingston Trudeau (whose descendant draws the Doonesbury cartoon).

Latent Tuberculosis Infection

Treatment of latent tuberculosis infection (Table 20–4) is recommended in individuals with a positive PPD but no symptoms, and a normal chest X-ray. Treatment of those with latent TB infection helps eliminate a large reservoir of individuals at risk for progression to TB, and for spreading the disease.

Prophylaxis is started with isoniazid (INH), a first-line drug recommended by the American Thoracic Soci-

Table 20–3 First- and Second-Line Drugs for the Treatment of TB

First-Line Drugs (drugs of choice that are used first)

- Isoniazid (INH)
- Rifampin
- Rifapentine
- Pyrazinamide
- Ethambutol

Second-Line Drugs*
- Cycloserine
- Ethionamide
- P-Aminosalicylic acid
- Streptomycin
- Capreomycin
- Ciprofloxacin

Note: only drugs that are approved by the Food and Drug Administration are listed

ety/Centers for Disease Control and Prevention Committee on Latent Tuberculosis Infection to be taken for 9 months. Included in this category of latent TB infection are patients who have been infected recently or exposed to TB and individuals who are at increased risk of progression to TB following infection with *Mycobacterium tuberculosis* [e.g., immunosuppressed (HIV/AIDS)], although they are treated for longer periods of time. INH may be given to household contact of individuals with TB disease, though therapy may be stopped if the contact remains PPD negative after 3 months.

If drug-resistant tuberculosis infection is likely, the American Thoracic Society and the CDC recommend treatment with at least two drugs to which the organism is likely to be susceptible. These drugs are rifampin (Rifadin) and pyrazinamide (PZA), which are taken for 2 months or rifampin alone for 4 months. This treatment should not be used in HIV-positive patients. With INH and rifampin resistance, the CDC recommends ethambutol (Myambutol) with PZA. A major limitation in treating latent TB infections is poor adherence; therapy must be long enough to eradicate the organism.

The primary risk or adverse effect of isoniazid is hepatitis, characterized by abdominal pain and

Did You Know?

In colonial times, maple syrup was used to cure tuberculosis.

Table 20–4   Treatment Regimens for Tuberculosis

Drug Name	Adverse Effects	Dental Drug Interactions	Dental Notes
Latent Tuberculosis Infection			
Isoniazid (isonicotinic acid hydrazide; INH)	Drug-induced hepatitis (fatigue, weakness, nausea, vomiting), anemia, peripheral neuropathy (for prevention, pyridoxine Vitamin B_6 is used)	No significant dental drug interactions Alcohol increases incidence of INH-hepatitis Decrease metabolism of phenytoin Increased levels of carbamazepine Exaggerated histamine reaction (e.g., itching, headache, flushing, hypotension) if taken with foods containing histamine (e.g., tuna, sauerkraut juice) Decreased effects of corticosteroids, ketoconazole, fluconazole	Adults taking INH and presenting to the dental office for treatment (INH) should have a physician's consultation regarding liver enzyme levels (serum aspartate aminotransferase, alanine aminotransferase, and bilirubin levels). Avoid alcohol and alcohol-containing mouthrinses.
Rifampin (Rifadin)	Alternative treatment; cannot be taken by HIV-infected patients taking antiretroviral drugs Orange/red saliva, sweat, tears, urine, feces; hypersensitivity reactions (chills, fever); not used in pregnant women	Reduced effectiveness with combination oral contraceptives Rifampin induces P450 cytochrome enzymes (CYP3A4), which increases metabolism and results in reduced blood levels of: Macrolide antibiotics (clarithromycin, erythromycin), Benzodiazepines (diazepam, midazolam, triazolam) Lidocaine HIV protease inhibitors Idinavir, ritonavir, saquinavir, nelfinivir	Inform the patient that the saliva and other secretions will turn orange/red.

Active Tuberculosis
Two or more drugs are needed to treat active TB to reduce emergence of resistant bacterial strains. One drug alone should not be used.

Initial phase (four-drug regimen)	*Continuation Phase*
Isoniazid, rifampin, pyrazinamide and ethambutol	Isoniazid and rifampin

Pyrazinamide (PZA)	Gastrointestinal upset, hepatitis, elevated uric acid levels, arthralgias	No significant drug interactions	See above
Ethambutol (Myambutol)	Decrease in visual acuity; temporary impairment in red/green color; not used in pregnant women.	Decreased effectiveness when taken with aluminum salts (antacids)	Take with food. Dental light may not be tolerated by patient — use sunglasses.

jaundice. Risk of hepatotoxicity is increased with alcohol and acetaminophen (Tylenol) usage and is unusual before age 35. INH also causes gastrointestinal problems, peripheral neuropathy (disease involving the nerves—muscle weakness, numbness of fingers and toes), and anemia. INH causes a pyridoxine (Vitamin B_6) deficiency, which is responsible for the peripheral neuropathy. Thus pyridoxine may be given together with INH, depending on the adequacy of the patient's diet.

Treatment of Active Tuberculosis

Diagnosis of active tuberculosis must be made before treatment is started. Multiple drug therapy is used to treat adequately and to prevent drug-resistant strains from developing. A single drug should not be added to a regimen which is failing. Therapy must be long enough to eradicate the organism. There are two phases of treatment for patients with TB. The initial bactericidal phase consists of 2 months of therapy followed by the continuation phase (subsequent sterilizing phase), which lasts 4 to 7 months for patients with drug-susceptible disease in the absence of HIV infection (Table 20–4).

A four-drug regimen should be started in patients with active TB, including isoniazid, rifampin, pyrazinamide, and ethambutol. If the sensitivity of the organism becomes known, this may alter the drug regimen. After 2 months of therapy with these four drugs, the patient enters the continuation phase, where pyrazinamide and ethambutol are discontinued and isoniazid and rifampin are continued for another 4 months. Obviously, if the organism is resistant to INH and/or rifampin, this will be altered. This completes 6 months of therapy. If the patient is considered at high risk for relapse (positive TB cultures after 2 months of therapy), therapy should continue for an additional 3 months. These medications should be given together. They may be taken with food if G.I. upset occurs.

SPECIAL SITUATIONS

Generally, patients with tuberculosis and HIV infection are treated with the same drugs as patients without HIV infection; however, there is a higher risk for TB resistance. One exception is that during the continuation phase the patient should receive higher doses of INH and rifampin to prevent relapse with resistant organisms, and the recommended time of treatment is longer.

Children with tuberculosis infection have a high risk of disseminated disease, so treatment should be initiated as soon as the diagnosis is suspected. However, it is also important to remember that it is very rare for young children to spread tuberculosis. Development of drug resistance is lower in children so treatment usually starts with INH, pyrazinamide, and rifampin. Ethambutol is not routinely given to children under 13 years of age because it can cause decreased visual acuity and a temporary loss of vision. It may be difficult to detect those changes in young children. If the drug sensitivities of the source case are known, the child's therapy can be altered.

If there is INH resistance, the regimen consists of rifampin, PZA, and ethambutol; with rifampin resistance, the patient is given INH, PZA, and ethambutol.

DENTAL DRUG INTERACTIONS

Several potential drug interactions are associated with these medications. Table 20–4 reviews common drug interactions.

DENTAL HYGIENE NOTES

Adults presenting to the dental office for treatment who are currently taking isoniazid (INH) should have a physician's consultation regarding liver function studies. Patients with *active* TB should not have elective dental treatment done. Otherwise, universal precautions should be taken and the use of aerosols should be avoided.

HEPATITIS C: INTERFERONS

Hepatitis C is an infection of the liver caused by a single-stranded RNA virus that is transmitted primarily parenterally through blood and blood products, such as in blood transfusions, body piercing, electrolysis, or intravenous drug use, and sometimes through sexual contact. Many people are unaware of this disease because they may not experience symptoms until many years after they are infected. Symptoms include fatigue, flu-like symptoms, unexplained weight loss and tenderness in the abdomen. Approximately 4 million Americans have been infected with the hepatitis C virus, and about 35,000 new cases occur each year in the United States. Hepatitis C is the most common reason for liver transplantation and the leading cause of liver cancer.

Interferons are used for the treatment of chronic hepatitis C. Interferons are a group of endogenous (within the body) proteins. Interferons produce a number of side effects, including fatigue, influenza-like symptoms, and blood abnormalities. Examples of interferons include interferon alpha 2-a (Roferon-A) and peginterferon alfa-2a (Pegasys). Interferons are administered subcutaneously or intramuscularly. They work by killing the hepatitis C virus. Ribavirin (Copegus) is another antiviral drug, but it cannot be used alone and must be used with alpha interferon. These should be used with caution in pregnant women.

Milk thistle, an herbal supplement, may be beneficial in patients with liver disease by altering the physiologic markers of liver function and reducing mortality or morbidity.

HEPATITIS A AND B

Hepatitis A virus (HAV), often referred to as infectious hepatitis, is caused by an RNA virus. It is transmitted through the oral-fecal route, primarily in regions of the world having poor sanitation, or by ingestion of contaminated food or water. The introduction of hepatitis A vaccines in 1995 has led to a decrease in the number of reported HAV cases. The presence and severity of symptoms is related to the patient's age. Approximately 70 percent of infected adults develop symptoms, including jaundice, whereas approximately 30 percent of children younger than 6 years develop symptoms, which usually are flu-like, without jaundice. Treatment for HAV is pre-vention through immunization. HAV vaccine is indicated for people living in areas with high infection rates, drug abusers, or for travelers to countries with high endemic infection rates. Immune globulin, administered IM, provides short-term protection (3 to 5 months) through passive transfer of hepatitis A virus antibody.

Hepatitis B virus (HBV), often referred to as serum hepatitis, is caused by a DNA virus and is transmitted through infected blood and body fluids. Effective vaccines for HBV have been available since 1982; infant and childhood vaccination programs introduced in the 1990s has resulted in a marked decrease in new infections.

Acute HBV infection is subclinical in most adults and children. Symptoms of acute HBV include nausea, anorexia, fatigue, fever and right upper quadrant or epigastric pain. Treatment for acute infection is usually supportive.

Chronic HBV infection is defined as hepatitis B surface antigen (HB sAg) positivity for at least 6 months. There is also elevation of liver enzymes, alanine transaminase, and aspirate transaminase. Medical therapies for chronic hepatitis B include interferon alfa-2b, lamivudine, and adefovir dipivoxil.

Hepatitis B vaccine (recombinant) is administered IM to provide prophylaxis against exposure to the hepatitis B virus. Following injection, the body produces antibiodies against the virus. The Centers for Disease Control (CDC) recommends a regimen involving three doses of the vaccine, usually followed by a titer to confirm that active immunity has been achieved. Adverse effects include pain and inflammation at the site of injection. A fever may develop and the patient may feel tired and lethargic. No clinical drug interactions have been reported.

KEY POINTS

- A thorough review of patient's medical history is important.
- Many antiretroviral drugs cause dental-related side effects.
- HIV-infected patients have many opportunistic infections, including oral lesions that may be treated in the dental office with various medications.
- While the patient is being treated in the dental office, monitor the white blood cell counts.
- It is important to determine if the patient has latent or active TB infection.

- Isoniazid (INH) is the drug of choice for the treatment of latent TB infection (9 months).
- INH may cause liver problems.
- Rifampin causes red/orange saliva.
- A major problem with tuberculosis is multiple antimicrobial resistance.
- A four-drug regimen should be started in patients with active TB, including: isoniazid (INH), rifampin (Rifadin), pyrazinamide (PZA), and ethambutol (Myambutol).
- There are many drug interactions with rifampin.
- Treatment is long term and patient adherence is critical.

BOARD REVIEW QUESTIONS

1. Which of the following antiretroviral drugs may cause taste impairment? (p. 409)
   a. Enfuvirtide
   b. Nelfinavir
   c. Ritonavir
   d. Saquinavir

2. Which of the following antiretroviral drugs may cause a metallic taste in the mouth? (p. 409)
   a. Fosamprenavir
   b. Atazanavir
   c. Amprevavir
   d. Indinavir

3. Which of the following antiretroviral drugs may cause numbness in the mouth? (p. 409)
   a. Fosamprenavir
   b. Amprevavir
   c. Indinavir
   d. Saquinavir

4. Which of the following drugs decreases blood levels of ritonavir? (p. 409)
   a. Clarithromycin
   b. Warfarin
   c. Triazolam
   d. Penicillin

5. Which of the following drugs can cause dental pain? (p. 409)
   a. Fosamprenavir
   b. Atazanavir
   c. Indinavir
   d. Nelfinavir

6. Which of the following serum level parameters should be monitored in the tuberculosis patient taking INH? (p. 414)
   a. Liver
   b. Chloride
   c. Calcium
   d. Sodium
   e. Potassium

7. Which of the following drugs is also referred to as INH? (p. 413)
   a. Rifampin
   b. Isoniazid
   c. Ethambutol
   d. Fluroquinolone
   e. Pyrazinamide

8. Which of the following TB drugs causes red/orange saliva? (p. 415)
   a. Rifampin
   b. Isoniazid
   c. Ethambutol
   d. Fluroquinolone
   e. Pyrazinamide

9. Which of the following TB drugs causes a drug-induced hepatitis? (p. 414)
   a. Rifampin
   b. Isoniazid
   c. Ethambutol
   d. Fluroquinolone
   e. Pyrazinamide

10. A major problem with antituberculosis drugs is: (p. 413)
    a. Many drugs are toxic to normal cells in the body.
    b. Many drugs are not specific enough to kill the bacteria.
    c. Drug resistance
    d. Drug dependence

SELECTED REFERENCES

Blumberg, H. M., M. K. Leonard Jr., and R. M. Jasmer. 2005. Update on the treatment of tuberculosis and latent tuberculosis infection. *JAMA* 293;2776–2784.

Brundage, S. C., A. N. Fitzpatrick. 2006. Hepatitis A. *Am Fam Physician* 73:2162–2168.

Chesebro, M. J. and W. D. Everett. 1998. Understanding the guidelines for treating HIV disease. *Am Fam Physician* 57:315–322.

Dye, C., C. J. Watt, D. M. Bleed et al. 2005. Evolution of tuberculosis control and prospects for reducing tuberculosis incidence, prevalence, and deaths globally. *JAMA* 293: 2767–2775.

Friedrich, M. J. 2005. Basic science guides design of new TB vaccine candidates. *JAMA* 293:2703–2705.

Guidelines for the Use of Antiretroviral Agents in HIV-Infected Adults and Adolescents. February 4, 2002. Department of Health and Human Services (DHHS) and the Henry J. Kaiser Family Foundation.

Gulick, R. M., H. J. Ribaudo, C. M. Shikuma, C. Lalama, B. R. Schackman et al. 2006. Three- vs. four-drug antiretroviral regimens for the initial treatment of HIV-1 infection. *JAMA* 296:769–781.

Hammer, S. M., M. S. Saag, M. Schechter, J. S. G. Montaner, R. T. Schooley et al. 2006. Treatment for adult HIV infection. *JAMA* 296:827–843.

Koda-Kimble, M. A., L. Y. Young, W. A. Dradjan, and B. J. Guglielmo. 2002. Infectious diseases: Pharmacotherapy of Human Immunodeficiency Virus infection. In: *Handbook of Applied Therapeutics,* 7th ed. Philadelphia: Lippincott Williams & Wilkens, pp. 1–20.

Nelson, M. H. 2001. AIDS therapy update. *U.S. Pharmacist* 26:69–78.

Potter, B., C. K. Kraus. 2005. Management of active tuberculosis. *Am Fam Physician* 72:2225–2232.

Screening for tuberculosis and tuberculosis infection in high-risk populations: Recommendations of the Advisory Council for the Elimination of Tuberculosis. 1995. *MMWR Morb Mortal Wkly Rep* 44:19–34.

WEB SITES

www.stoptb.org/resource-center/documents.asp
www.nlm.nih.gov/medlineplus/tuberculosis
www.cddc.gov/nchstp/tb
www.tuberculosis.net
www.hivguidelines.org/public_html/p-oral/p-oral.htm
www.retroconference.org
www.aids.org

Q U I C K   D R U G   G U I D E

Antiretroviral Drugs: HIV/AIDS

Nucleoside Reverse Transcriptase Inhibitors (NRTIs)

- Abacavir (Ziagen)
- Didansoine (ddl, Videx)
- Emtricitabine (Emtriva)
- Lamivudine (3TC, Epivir)
- Stavudine (d4T, Zerit)
- Tenofovir (Viread)
- Zalcitabine (ddC, Hivid—HIVID
- Zidovudine (Retrovir): formerly azidothymidine (AZT)

NonNucleoside Reverse Transcriptase Inhibitors (NNRTI)

- Delavirdine (Rescriptor)
- Efavirenz (Sustiva)
- Nevirapine (Viramune)

Protease Inhibitors (PIs)

- Amprevavir (Agenerase)
- Atazanavir (Reyataz)
- Fosamprenavir (Lexiva)
- Indinavir (Crixivan)
- Lopinavir + Ritonavir (Kaletra)
- Nelfinavir (Viracept)
- Ritonavir (Norvir)
- Saquinavir (Fortovase)

Fusion Inhibitors

- Enfuvirtide (Fuzeon)

Antimycobacterial Drugs: Tuberculosis (TB)

First-Line Anti-TB Drugs

- Isoniazid (isonicotinic acid hydrazide; INH)
- Rifampin (Rifadin)
- Pyrazinamide (PZA)
- Ethambutol (Myambutol)

Second-Line Anti-TB Drugs

- Cycloserine (Seromycin)
- Ethionamide (Trecator-SC)
- Para-aminosalicylic acid (Paser)
- Streptomycin (Streptomycin)
- Capreomycin (Capastat sulfate)

Antiviral drugs for hepatitis C

- Peginterferon alfa-2a (Pegasys)
- Ribavirin (Copegus)

Chapter 21

Antineoplastic and Immunosuppressant Drugs

GOAL: To provide knowledge of commonly used drugs used in the treatment of cancer and organ rejection, and their oral complications.

EDUCATIONAL OBJECTIVES

After reading this chapter, the reader should be able to:

1. Discuss the role of antineoplastic agents in the treatment of neoplasms.
2. List the commonly used antineoplastic agents.
3. Discuss the common oral adverse effects of antineoplastic agents.
4. Describe the adverse effects and drug interactions of immunosuppressant drugs.

KEY TERMS

Antineoplastic drugs
Chemotherapeutic drugs
Xerostomia
Oral mucositis
Oral candidiasis
Immunosuppressant drugs

ANTINEOPLASTIC DRUGS

Actions

Antineoplastic or **chemotherapeutic drugs** are used to treat various types of cancers or neoplasms (abnormally growing cells) that cannot be treated by surgery, or are used in conjunction with surgery and radiation therapy. Neoplasms can be benign (where cells do not invade the tissues) or malignant (where cells invade and spread or metastasize to all areas of the body, including areas not affected by the cancer).

Treatment

Cancer may be treated using surgery, radiation therapy, and drugs. Radiation therapy is an effective in killing tumor cells through nonsurgical methods. High doses of ionizing radiation are aimed directly at the tumor and confined to this area as much as possible. Radiation therapy is frequently used for head and neck cancers such as squamous cell carcinoma. Cancer chemotherapy is very complex, involving the use of chemical agents that act by different mechanisms.

Antineoplastics (Chemotherapy)

Antineoplastics, the most toxic drugs in use today, act by killing cancer cells through damaging cell DNA or interfering with DNA synthesis. Unfortunately, while killing cancer cells, most drugs also affect normal cells, which contributes to a high incidence of adverse serious side effects, toxicity, and teratogenicity, even with usual dosing. The two most common adverse side effects are nausea and vomiting. Other toxic effects include bone marrow suppression (inhibition of blood cell replication in the bone marrow), resulting leukopenia (decrease in neutrophils or white blood cells) which predisposes patients to serious infections, and thrombocytopenia (decrease in platelets) which may lead to serious bleeding problems.

Some agents primarily affect cells that are actively multiplying (Table 21–1). These agents are called cell cycle-specific (CCS) antineoplastic agents. Examples include antimetabolites. Other agents, called cell cycle-nonspecific (CCNS), kill cells that are actively multiplying or at rest. These agents are more toxic to normal cells than the CCS agents, but good for slow growing neoplasms. Examples of these include alkylating agents and antitumor antibiotics. A major cause of can-cer treatment failure is drug resistance, resulting in drugs that do not work on the cells. Antineoplastic drugs are divided into the following categories:

- Alkylating agents
- Antimetabolites
- Hormones
- Antitumor antibiotics
- Immunomodulators
- Plant extracts (mitotic inhibitors)

Cetuximab (Erbitux) was FDA approved in 2006 for use in combination with radiation therapy to treat patients with squamous cell cancer of the head and neck that cannot be removed by surgery.

Some cancer cells are becoming resistant to the drugs being administered because sometimes chemotherapy has to be stopped due to low white blood cells and or infection. The oncologist's approach is to "hit hard and fast" with chemotherapy to prevent resistant cancer cells from developing.

Different agents are used to treat the various types of cancers. It is not within the scope of this textbook to review all adverse side effects particular to each drug, or to review specific features. The emphasis of this chapter will be on chemotherapeutic drugs and oral adverse side effects.

Adverse Effects

Chemotherapeutic drugs attack the faster growing cells including bone marrow, gastrointestinal tract, and skin. Many adverse reactions occur throughout the body including the following.

Blood

Bone marrow suppression is influenced by the type of drug used, the patient's age, bone marrow reserve, the patient's nutritional status, and liver and kidney function. Bone marrow suppression causes anemia (low red blood cell count), neutropenia (low neutrophil count), and thrombocytopenia (low platelet count), which can be prevented by colony-stimulating factors.

To decrease the incidence of infection (manifested by febrile neutropenia) in patients receiving myelosuppressive anticancer drugs or associated with bone marrow suppression, patients may be taking filgrastim (Neupogen), which increases neutrophil proliferation and differentiation within the bone marrow.

Table 21-1 Actions of Common Antineoplastic Drugs

Drug Name	Actions
Alkylating Agents (DNA Alkylating Drugs) Cyclophosphamide (Cytoxan) Altretamine (Hexalen) Busulfan (Myleran) Chlorambucil (Leukeran) Melphalan (Alkeran) Carboplatin (Paraplatin) Cisplatin (Platinol) Cyclophosphamide (Cytoxan) Dacarbazine (DTIC-Dome) Ifosfamide (Ifex) Mechlorethamine HCl (Mustargen) Mitomycin (Mutamycin) Carmustine (BiCNU) Lomustine (CeeNU) Procarbazine HCl (Matulane) Streptozocin (Zanosar) Thiotepa (Thioplex)	These drugs work by altering the normal biological function of cells by damaging DNA and interfering with cell replication. Use of these agents may increase the incidence of acute nonlymphocytic leukemia.
Antimetabolites (DNA Synthesis Inhibitors) Cladribine (Leustatin) Cytarabine (Cytosar-U) Floxuridine (FUDR) Fludarabine phosphate (Fludara) Fluorouracil Gemcitabine (Gemsar) Mercaptopurine (Purinethol) Methotrexate (Mexate) Pentostatin (Nipent)	These drugs are incorporated into new DNA material or combine irreversibly with enzymes in the cell, which prevents cellular division and growth.
Antitumor Antibiotics Bleomycin (Blenoxane) Daunorubicin HCl (Cerubidine) Doxorubicin HCl) (Adriamycin) Idarubicin HCl (Idamycin)	Some antibiotics are used to treat cancers instead of bacterial infections because of their cytotoxicity (toxic effect on cells). Bleomycin is used for head and neck cancer.
Plant Alkaloids or Extracts *Mitotic Inhibitors* Vinblastine (Velban) Vincristine (Oncovin) Vinorelbine (Navelbine)	These drugs inhibit cell mitosis.
Taxanes Docetaxel (Taxotere) Paclitaxel (Taxol)	These drugs inhibit cell mitosis.
Topoisomerase Inhibitors Topotecan (Hycamtin) Etoposide (VePesid) Teniposide (Vumon) Irinotecan (Camptosar)	Inhibits DNA replication Inhibits cell mitosis Inhibits DNA synthesis Inhibits DNA and RNA synthesis

Drug Name	Actions
Hormones and Antagonists Flutamide (Eulexin) Leuprolide (Lupron) Prednisone Tamoxifen (Novadex)	These drugs are mainly used in hormone-dependent cancer such as breast, prostate, and endometrial.
Immunomodulators (Cytokines) Aldesleukin (Proleukin) Interferon alfa	These drugs affect the immune system.

Did You Know?

Green tea is a natural antioxidant that is thought to have a protective effect against cancer.

Epoetin alfa (Human recombinant erythropoietin) is indicated in patients with chemotherapy-induced anemia and zidovudine-induced anemia in patients with HIV infection. Epoetin stimulates production of red blood cells (erythropoiesis).

Gastrointestinal Toxicities

Nausea, vomiting. Treatment is with antimetics before chemotherapy and after for several days.

Dermatologic Toxicities

Inhibition of epidermal mitotic activity causes alopecia (loss of hair), nail changes, dry skin, and blistering.

Other Toxicities

Chemotherapeutic drugs cause neurotoxicity, cardiac toxicities, nephrotoxicity, pulmonary toxicities, and hepatotoxicity.

Oral Toxicities: Dental Complications

Patients taking antineoplastic agents should have a medical consultation before dental treatment is started. Complications of the oral cavity occur in about 40 percent of patients treated with chemotherapy and all patients receiving radiation. Oral complications include mucositis, xerostomia, caries, bleeding, and oral candidiasis (Table 21–2).

Rapid Dental Hint

Monitor chemotherapy patients for oral conditions.

Xerostomia and caries   Xerostomia may occur due to suppression of salivary function, but it is usually not permanent, so treatment is usually palliative. Patients can become uncomfortable because there is no salivary lubrication and the mucosal tissues get "sticky." Dry mucosa may also be more prone to bleeding. Due to xerostomia, there is an increased incidence of candidiasis and dental/root caries. For prevention of caries patients should be placed on a neutral sodium fluoride rinse, such as Prevident rinse, or an acidulated phosphate rinse such as Phos-Flur. Amifostine (Ethyol), an organic thiophosphate chemoprotectant agent, is approved to reduce the incidence of moderate to severe xerostomia in patients undergoing postoperative radiation treatment for head and neck cancer.

Mucositis   Oral mucositis (OM) is an inflammation leading to ulcerations or mouth sores on the buccal, labial, and soft palate mucosa, along with the ventral surface of the tongue and floor of the mouth. Pain usually occurs in 5 to 7 days following the start of therapy. Small areas of ulceration or petechaie quickly become large areas due to the direct toxic effects of the antimetabolites; antimetabolites and antitumor antibiotics are directly toxic to the mucosa. It is caused by the suppression of epithelial cell growth, and the highest incidence is found during the lowest levels of white blood cells. It is difficult to prevent as well as treat mucositis; however, it is not permanent. Patients usually also have xerostomia. Maintenance of excellent oral care before and during cancer treatment is important to help reduce the frequency and severity of OM. Chlorhexidine is used because it is substantive and stays on the soft tissue. Refer to Table 21–3.

Rapid Dental Hint

Assess your patients for mucositis; it is difficult to prevent and treat.

Table 21–2   Dental-Related Adverse Effects in Patients Undergoing Cancer Treatment

Situation	Results	Treatment
Suppressed white blood cell count (neutropenia) (< 1000 mm³)	Infection (may be life threatening)	Contact patient's physician; use of antibiotics to prevent bacteremia (infective endocardiditis)
Thrombocyopenia < 100,000 mm³	Bleeding (gingival bleeding and mucosal surface bleeding)	Contact patient's physician before any dental treatment, including extractions. If localized bleeding occurs during dental treatment, apply a hemostatic agent such as topical thrombin solution (apply with gauze and hold in place using pressure for 30 minutes—do not remove clots that have formed).
Oral mucositis: Involves gingival tissue inflammation as well as uclerations	Pain and burning of the oral mucosa; difficult to maintain oral hygiene	Difficult to prevent and treat; treatment is palliative. Excellent oral hygiene helps reduce the frequency and severity of OM. Rinses: Chlorhexidine rinse (has substantivity so that it binds to oral tissue) Saline (salt) water, sodium bicarbonate solutions Other medications: Viscous lidocaine 2% solution (swish in mouth until pain disappears and then spit out) Diphenhydramine elixir 15.5 mg mixed with kaopectate (50% mixture by volume); rinse with one teaspoonful every Nystatin 1 ml mixed with Maalox (Ω120 ml), swish and spit out If the mucositis is localized to a specific area, use Benzocaine in Orabase (OTC – Colgate Oral) (apply by dabbing on the affected area; do not rub it on) Additional treatment: • Remove dentures and orthodontic appliances. • Gentle tooth brushing with soft brush • Avoid mouthrinses that contain alcohol. • Lubricants, such as artificial saliva, may loosen mucous and prevent membranes from sticking together • Avoid spiced, acidic, and salted foods. • Use sugar-free gum or candy to stimulate saliva.
Xerostomia: Usually not permanent	Increased caries, difficult to eat	Palliative treatment: sugarless candies, increase water intake, avoid alcohol, which further dries the mucosa Saliva substitutes (carboxymethylcellulose or hydroxyethylcellulose): Biotene Dry Mouth Relieving Gel, Optimoist, Salivart, Salix, Xero-Lube, Moi-Stir® Oral Swabsticks, MouthKote) Systemic: Cevemeline (Evoxac) Pilocarpine (Salagen) 5 mg 3–4 times a day
Oral candidiasis (thrush)	Increased growth of opportunistic fungi	Use topical/systemic antifungal agents: nystatin, clotrimazole, fluconazole
Oral biofilm accumulation	Gingival inflammation	Chlorhexidine oral rinse as an adjunct to meticulous oral hygiene

Table 21–3 Immunosuppressant Drugs: Adverse Effects/Drug Interactions

Drug Name	Adverse Effects	Drug Interactions	Dental Notes
Azathioprine (Imuran)	Bone marrow suppression (leukopenia; decreased white blood cells), hematuria (blood in urine), risk of neoplasm with chronic use, contraindicated in pregnancy (category D)	Increased bleeding with aspirin; increased azathioprine levels with allopurinol	No significant dental notes
Cyclosporine (Sandimmune, Neoral)	Gingival enlargement, hypertension, nepthrotoxic (kidney damage), tremor; pregnancy category C	Metabolized by the cytochrome P450 isoenzymes in the liver—many drug interactions. Taken with nonsteroidal anti-inflammatory agents may increase nephrotoxicity Increase plasma levels with: Erythromycin Clarithromycin Ketoconazole Fluconazole Decrease plasma levels with: Antacids Carbamazepine	Monitor blood pressure and gingival enlargement.
Tacrolimus (Prograf)	Tremor, headache, hypertension, risk of neoplasm with chronic use. Pregnancy category C	Increased plasma levels with: Erythromycin Clarithromycin Increased nephrotoxicity when taken with ibuprofen.	No significant dental notes.

Esophagitis Esophagitis is caused by damage to the mucosal lining and usually presents as dysphagia (difficulty in swallowing). Treatment involves adequate fluid intake, avoiding acidic foods, and use of drugs such as proton pump inhibitors. This is usually resolved about 1 to 2 weeks after bone marrow recovery.

Oral Candidiasis Oral candidiasis (thrush) is common due to an overgrowth of fungi because of reduced white blood cell count (leukopenia). *It may be more important to prevent rather than treat oral candidiasis.*

Bacterial Infections The primary concern with high bacteria levels is the increased incidence of bacteremia. Most patients require central line placement for administering chemotherapy. Thus, the patient may be placed on antibiotics as a prophylaxis for infective endo-

carditis. Bacterial infections are seen due to bone marrow suppression, which reduces the white blood cell count (remember that white blood cells such as neutrophils have a protective function to engulf and kill invading bacteria). Chlorhexidine gluconate oral rinse is helpful in reducing bacterial levels and help with oral hygiene.

Taste Alterations in taste are commonly seen in cancer patients which may occur due to a drug's ability to affect sensitive taste buds. Patients lose the ability to differentiate between sweet and salty foods, and are at increased risk for dental/root caries.

Bleeding and Impaired Healing Oral ulceration, petechiae, and bleeding are usually due to the thrombocytopenia (low platelet count). This generally resolves after bone marrow recovery. Impaired wound healing occurs due to neutropenia.

Limitations to Dental Treatment

There are limitations in treating patients undergoing treatment for cancer (Table 21-2). The majority of patients will have depressed white blood cells (neutrophils), which may increase the incidence of infections (signs of infection may be fever, malaise), and patients may also have low platelets, which may increase the incidence of bleeding. Antibiotics may be necessary when white blood cell counts fall below 1,500 mm^3 because of impaired healing. Bleeding becomes significant when platelets fall below 100,000 mm^3. There are some drug interactions with antineoplastic agents, but there are not any dental drug interactions. Nausea and vomiting may complicate treatment of patients.

Patients receiving intravenous bisphosphonates for cancer that has spread to the bone, and undergoing extensive dental treatment such as tooth extractions, periodontal surgery, and implant surgery can develop a condition called osteonecrosis of the jaw (ONJ). Clinical features of osteonecrosis of the jaw include areas of exposed bone that occur after dental surgery or spontaneously, that have not healed after 6 weeks. This condition is caused by a decrease in blood flow to the area. Bisphosphonates are indicated for cancer patients at high risk of hypercalcemia due to malignancy or skeletal-related events. The FDA and the drug companies have issued precautions for dentists to follow in patients receiving intravenous Acredia and Zometa. It is recommended that dental procedures requiring bone healing be done before patients are placed on bisphosphonates. Additionally, meticulous oral hygiene is important. Current treatment of ONJ includes antibiotics, oral rinses, pain control, and limited periodontal debridement (Novartis Pharmaceuticals Corporation. Updated Recommendations for the Prevention, Diagnosis and Treatment of Osteonecrosis of the Jaw in Cancer Patients, May 2006). (Refer to STI in this textbook.)

IMMUNOSUPPRESSANT DRUGS

Immunosuppressant drugs are used in patients after receiving an organ transplant from another human being to prevent rejection of the organ (e.g., kidney, heart, lung, or liver), or in the treatment of vesicular bullous conditions such as bullous pemphigoid, lupus erythrmatosus (LE), and in rheumatoid arthritis. These drugs are usually given together with glucocorticosteroids. Immunosuppressant drugs include azathioprine, cyclosporine, and tacrolimus. Patients taking an immunosuppressant will most likely develop hypertension and subsequently will also be taking an antihypertensive drug such as a calcium channel blocker (e.g., nifedipine), which may also cause gingival enlargement.

Azathioprine is a prodrug used in the treatment of bullous disorders which must be metabolized in the liver into an active form that will enter the bloodstream. In the majority of patients taking cyclosporine, the drug of choice for organ transplant donors, gingival enlargement occurs. Gingival enlargement can be controlled by frequent gingivectomy/gingivoplasty procedures and meticulous oral home care. Cyclosporine serum levels must be monitored because oral absorption is wildly variable. This drug is also used in the treatment of rheumatoid arthritis. Drugs that alter cytochrome P450 isoenzymes in the liver may alter the plasma levels of cyclosporine (Table 21-3).

Pretransplant dentistry plays a critical part in getting on a transplant list. The patient needs to be evaluated for dental infections before being placed on the list.

DENTAL HYGIENE NOTES

Many patients will present in the dental office immediately before starting cancer treatment. It is important that patients seek dental care before treatment to minimize ad-

Table 21-4 Oral Care of Cancer Patients Before, During and After Therapy

Before	*During*	*After*
• Extract all questionable/hopeless teeth • Instruct patients on proper oral home care regimens • Treat any infections	• Medical consultation before any dental treatment • May require antibiotic coverage • Treatment depends on neutrophil count (treatment only if ≥ 1000 mm^3) • Examine and monitor patients' oral status: development of ulcerations	• Resume normal dental care

verse effects and provide preventative therapy (e.g., fluoride-reducing tooth erosion caused by nausea/vomiting). It is best for patients to achieve a stable periodontium and extract any teeth that are hopeless or will present with problems later on during treatment (Table 21–4).

Lab values should be monitored and the patients' oncologist should be contacted if dental treatment is needed during therapy. At this time white blood cell and platelet counts are generally normal and will not present with any complications following dental treatment. Neutrophil counts below 500–1,000 mm^3 place patients at risk for life-threatening infections. Platelet counts below 20,000 mm^3 can lead to bleeding, usually from the gastrointestinal tract.

It is important at this time to review with the patient home care regimens that will be followed during treatment. The dental clinician should monitor for the development of xerostomia, caries, oral candidiasis, and mucositis. It is important to schedule maintenance appointments with patients during treatment and monitor the patients' gingival and tooth conditions.

KEY POINTS

- Complications of the oral cavity occur in about 40 percent of patients treated with chemotherapy and all patients receiving radiation.
- Oral adverse effects include mucositis, xerostomia, caries, and bleeding.
- Cyclosporine, a drug used to prevent rejection of an organ transplant, causes gingival tissue enlargement.
- Patients may have suppressed white blood cells, and platelets which can influence when to perform dental procedures.
- Meticulous oral hygiene is important.

BOARD REVIEW QUESTIONS

1. Which of the following treatments is started for patients who complains of burning mouth? (p. 424)
   a. Rinse with warm salt water
   b. Chew sugarless gum
   c. Rinse with viscous lidocaine
   d. Suck on xylitol-containing lozenges

2. Which of the following drugs may cause gingival enlargement? (p. 425)
   a. Azathioprine
   b. Methotrexate
   c. Cyclosporine
   d. Bleomycin

3. All of the following are adverse effects of antineoplastic treatment *except* one. Which one is the exception? (pp. 423–425)
   a. Mucositis of dorsum of tongue
   b. Gingival bleeding
   c. Xerostomia
   d. Stomatitis
   e. Thrush

4. Which of the following signs should be monitored in the dental office in a patient taking cyclosporine? (p. 425)
   a. Temperature
   b. Dilatation of pupils
   c. Respiration
   d. Blood pressure

5. Which of the following drugs should not be given to a patient taking cyclosporine? (p. 425)
   a. Tetracycline
   b. Doxycycline
   c. Clarithromycin
   d. Penicillin VK
   e. Metronidazole

SELECTED REFERENCES

Brenner, G. M. *Pharmacology.* 2000. Philadelphia: W.B. Saunders Company.

Clarkson, J. E., H. V. Worthington, and O. B. Eden. 2004. Interventions for treating oral candidiasis for patients with cancer receiving treatment. Cochrane Review Abstracts.

Koda-Kimble M. A., L. Y. Young., W. A. Kradjan, and J. Guglielmo. 2002. *Handbook of Applied Therapeutics:* Lippincott Williams & Wilkins.

Ramachandran A. 2000. *Pharmacology Recall.* Lippincott Williams & Wilkins.

Ruggiero S., Gralow J., Marx R. E., Hoff A.O., Schubert M.M., and Huryn J. M., et al. 2006. Practical guidelines for the prevention, diagnosis, and treatment of osteonecrosis of the jaw in patients with cancer. *J Oncology Practice* 2(*1*):7–14.

WEB SITES

www.medscape.com
www.cancer.gov/cancertopics/pdq/supportivecare/oralcomplications/patient

QUICK DRUG GUIDE

Alkylating Agents (Also Called DNA Alkylating Drugs)

- Cyclophosphamide
- Altretamine (Hexalen)
- Busulfan (Myleran)
- Chlorambucil (Leukeran)
- Melphalan (Alkeran)
- Carboplatin (Paraplatin)
- Cisplatin (Platinol)
- Cyclophosphamide (Cytoxan)
- Dacarbazine (DTIC-Dome)

- Ifosfamide (Ifex)
- Mechlorethamine HCl (Mustargen)
- Mitomycin (Mutamycin)
- Carmustine (BiCNU)
- Lomustine (CeeNU)
- Procarbazine HCl (Matulane)
- Streptozocin (Zanosar)
- Thiotepa (Thioplex)

Antimetabolites (Also Called DNA Synthesis Inhibitors)

- Cladribine (Leustatin)
- Cytarabine (Cytosar-U)
- Floxuridine (FUDR)
- Fludarabine phosphate (Fludara)
- Fluorouracil (Adrucil)

- Gemcitabine (Gemsar)
- Mercaptopurine (Purinethol)
- Methotrexate (Mexate)
- Pentostatin (Nipent)

Antitumor Antibiotics

- Bleomycin (Blenoxane)
- Daunorubicin HCl (Cerubidine)

- Doxorubicin HCl) (Adriamycin)
- Idarubicin HCl (Idamycin)

Plant Extracts (Mitotic Inhibitors)

- Docetaxel (Taxotere)
- Paclitaxel (Taxol)
- Vinblastine (Velban)

- Vincristine (Oncovin)
- Vinorelbine (Navelbine)

Hormones and Antagonists

- Flutamide (Eulexin)
- Leuprolide (Lupron)

- Prednisone
- Tamoxifen (Novadex)

Immunomodulators (Cytokines)

- Aldesleukin (Proleukin)
- Interferon alfa

Antibody

- Cetuximab (Erbitux): newest drug for head and neck cancer.

Immunosuprressants

- Azathioprine (Imuran)
- Cyclosporine (Neoral, Sandimmune)
- Tacrolimus (Prograf, Protopic)

Chapter 22

Nutraceuticals

GOAL: To introduce the dental hygienist to the actions, drug interactions, and concerns of common herbal and nutritional supplements seen in the dental practice.

EDUCATIONAL OBJECTIVES

After reading this chapter, the reader should be able to:

1. Discuss the views of complementary and alternative medicine.
2. Describe the actions of various herbal products used in dentistry.
3. List common adverse effects and drug–herb interactions.
4. Discuss the role of herbal medicine in dentistry.

KEY TERMS

Alternative medicine
Nutritional supplements
Herbal supplements
Homeopathy

HOMEOPATHY AND NATURAL PRODUCTS

Plants have been used for their medicinal value for thousands of years. Most early medications, and approximately 25 percent of our current prescriptions, are plant based. An herb is technically a botanical without woody tissue such as stems or bark. In Europe the treatment of diseases using plant-based therapies has achieved the status of an accepted discipline.

Complementary and **alternative medicine** refers to the use of products that are not considered to be part of conventional healthcare. Essentially, these "natural" products focus on the mind and body of the individual as well as emphasizing self-care. The term pharmacognosy refers to the study of natural products that are the results of plant and animal metabolism. For example, cannabis (marijuana) consists of the dried flowering tops of the plants of *Cannabis sativa,* and calcium alginate used for dental impressions is extracted from seaweed.

Alternative healthcare deals with **homeopathy,** naturopathy, and chiropractic therapy. Samuel Hahnemann founded the practice of homeopathy. Physicians used homeopathy in the late eighteenth and early nineteenth centuries. Essentially, the basis of homeopathy is that the cause of disease is the disturbance of a spiritual vital force which manifests as specific symptoms. In today's conventional medicine treatment of symptoms from diseases involves using medicines that oppose the action of the symptoms; for instance, the use of antipyretics such as aspirin or acetaminophen for patients with fever will lower the fever but causes fever in toxic doses. Nitroglycerin treats angina but causes angina in toxic doses. Hahnemann recognized that many natural products produce pharmacological effects which he called "symptoms." He believed that using these substances in toxic doses in healthy individuals produces symptoms similar to a given disease. Patients' symptoms disappear following a minimal dose of the substance that has a toxicology profile matching the symptoms patients display. So, homeopathy deals with "like cures like." Hahnemman did recognize that giving these substances could aggravate the condition and present with other side effects. So he decided to dilute the substance to the point where the symptoms were no longer present. Dilutions of the substance reduce the concentration of the active substance to very low levels. Homeopathic medicines have official compendial status in the United States. The Homeopathic Pharmacopoeia of the United States/Revision Service (HPRS) is recognized as the official compendium of homeopathy.

The use of **herbal** and **nutritional supplements** to treat diseases is considered to be biologically based therapies. Beginning in the late 1970s and continuing today, herbal medicine has experienced a comeback, with nearly 60 million Americans taking nonprescription herbal medicines every day. These people have the impression that natural substances have more healing power than synthetic medications. Also, these products are readily available at a reasonable cost. The percentage of people aged 45 to 64 who take herbal supplements increased about 50 percent between 1998 and 2002. Billions of dollars are spent yearly on herbal medicines. Many people take over-the-counter herbal products alone or with prescription medicines without informing their physician.

SAFETY CONCERNS

One of the major skepticisms is whether these products are safe and effective. In 1990, the Food and Drug Administration classified herbal medicines as food supplements. The Dietary Supplement and Health Education Act (DSHEA) of 1994 classifies vitamins, minerals, amino acids, and herbs as dietary supplements, which allows the marketing of these "food supplements" without the approval of any government agency for testing for safety, efficacy, or standards of manufacturing. The FDA is only required to prove that these products are unsafe. Dietary supplements do not have to be tested prior to marketing, and the effectiveness of the product does not have to be demonstrated by the manufacturer. The product label must include a disclaimer that the product is not FDA evaluated or approved and it is not intended to diagnose, treat, or prevent any disease. The DSHEA does not regulate the accuracy of the label; the product may or may not contain the product listed in the amounts claimed. Herbal products therefore cannot be marketed for the diagnosis, treatment, cure, or prevention of disease. However, these products can be labeled explaining their proposed effect on the human body (e.g., alleviation of fatigue) or their role in promoting general well-being (e.g, enhancement of mood). Dietary supplement labeling requires the wording "dietary supplement" as part of the product name, and it must include a "supplement facts" panel on the ingredients. Also, products derived from plants must designate the plant part and the Latin binomial.

It must be emphasized that herbal products can be beneficial but also have harmful effects. Patients using herbs should make their physicians aware of this. Herbs should not be used by patients with serious medical conditions, pregnant women, nursing women, or young children unless under the care of a physician. It is recommended to start with the lowest recommended dose and then to increase if needed.

ACTIVE INGREDIENTS

The two primary formulations of herbal products are solid and liquid. Solid formulations include tablets, capsules, salves, and ointments. Liquid formulations are made by extracting the active chemicals from the plants using solvents such as water, alcohol, or glycerol. The liquids are then concentrated in various strengths. Extracts are concentrated formulations of fluids, powders, solids, and oils. Teas are prepared by drying the herb, which is marketed in its coarse cut form or in tea bags.

Herbal products are made from natural chemicals extracted from a plant and are produced either in the original form or refined, where the essential extract is removed from the plant, concentrated, and then added back into the original form to make it more concentrated. The active ingredients in an herbal product may be present in only one specific part of the plant or in all parts. For example, the active ingredient in ginger is composed of roots found below ground, whereas in St. John's wort it comes from leaves and stems which are above the ground. Every herb contains many active chemicals rather than just one, like in conventional medicines. Most of these chemicals have not been isolated and identified so that the strength of the product varies considerably, which makes standardization difficult. Additionally, the chemical composition of herbal supplements is unpredictable. Some standardizations, which are printed on the product label and may differ from one manufacturer to another, have been documented, including:

- *Kava kava,* which contains about 40–45% kavalactones
- *Ginkgo biloba* contains 24% ginkgo flavone glycosides, 60 mg ginkgo biloba extract and 6% terpene lactones

- *St. John's wort,* which contains 0.3–0.5% hypericins and 3-5% hyperforin

Adverse Effects

Adverse reactions are relatively uncommon. Most reactions are due to filler substances added to the herbal product but not on the label.

More commonly encountered adverse side effects include sedation and bleeding which manifests either via direct effects on capillaries, by interfering with platelet adhesion, or by increasing fibrinolytic activity. Caution should be used when prescribing aspirin or other NSAIDs to patients taking herbs that could increase bleeding, including ginger, garlic, and ginkgo. Another adverse side effect is an allergic reaction to the herb which can manifest in the oral cavity (e.g., gingival, tongue).

NUTRACEUTICALS

There are many herbal products on the market. Some common herbs are listed in Table 22–1.

DENTAL IMPLICATIONS

Various herb or dietary supplements are used to treat various oral conditions/lesions. Table 22–2 lists some supplements commonly used.

DENTAL HYGIENE NOTES

The increasing popularity of over-the-counter nutraceuticals demands that dental clinicians be more knowledgeable about the effects that these supplements have on oral health and treatment. Patients' medical history should include the use of nutraceuticals, since many have adverse side effects and drug interactions that may affect dental treatment. Most of these effects are associated with sedative, hepatotoxic, and antiplatelet properties of the herbs. Many nutraceuticals can increase the risk of bleeding, especially when taken with anticoagulants or NSAIDs. Products that cause bleeding may have to be discontinued before surgical procedures.

Table 22-1 Nutraceuticals

Herbal Product	Uses	Adverse Effects	Drug Interactions
Betel nut (Areca catechu)	Masticatory stimulant	Oral leukoplakia, stained teeth and gingival, bronchoconstriction	May interact with antipsychotics, causing bradykinesia and jaw tremor
Chamomile (different species) (flower of plant)	Reduces flatulence, diarrhea, upset stomach, common cold, mild sedation	Allergic reactions	Aspirin: Increased bleeding Benzodizepines: CNS depression
Dong guai (Radix Angelicae Sinensis) (root of plant)	Gynecologic conditions, muscle relaxant, high blood pressure, constipation, ulcers, arthritis	Photosensitivity, bleeding	Aspirin: Increased bleeding
Echinacea (Echinacea pupurea) (different plant parts)	Strengthens immune system, prevents colds and flu	Fever, nausea, vomiting, hepatoxicity if used longer than 8 weeks	Increase liver toxicity: Acetaminophen, Ketoconazole
Ephedra (E. sinica)	Respiratory conditions, weight loss	Hypertension, cardiac arrhythmias, anxiety	Can increase sympathomimetic actions of drugs
Garlic (Allium sativum) (comes from garlic bulbs)	Decreases cholesterol levels, lowers blood pressure, and is an anticoagulant	Bleeding; topical garlic may cause the appearance of a chemical burn	Increase bleeding: Aspirin, NSAIDs, warfarin; Insulin: additive hypoglycemic effect reduces saquinavir (Fortovase) serum levels
Ginger (comes from the ginger root)	Antiemetic (nausea), vertigo	Bleeding	Aspirin, NSAIDs, warfarin: Additive anticoagulant effects
Ginkgo (Gingko biloba) (comes from leaves and seeds)	Improvement of cognitive functioning in Alzheimer's disease (dementia) Also used for sexual dysfunction caused by selective serotonin reuptake inhibitors (SSRIs)	Bleeding	Additive bleeding effects: Warfarin, NSAIDs/aspirin
Ginseng (Panax spp.) (plant root)	Increases vitality, elevates energy levels	Bleeding, hypoglycemia, hypertension	Increase bleeding: Aspirin Diuretics: increase diuresis Insulin and oral hypoglycemics: Increase hypoglycemic effect Digoxin: May increase toxicity
Glucosamine and chondroitin (glucosamine derived from chitin, but synthetic is best)	Arthritis	Bleeding	Increased bleeding: Anticoagulants, NSAIDs
Green tea (fresh or dried tea leaves)	Prevent cancer, cause weight loss	Caffeine-related irritability, irregular heartbeat, diarrhea, vomiting, headache	Atropine
Kava kava (piper methysticum) (comes from the root of the plant)	Treatment of anxiety, insomnia, and muscle tension Possesses antipyretic (fever reducer) and local anesthetic properties	Sedation, oral and lingual dyskinesia, rash, painful twisting movement of the trunk, liver problems	May increase the effects of local anesthetics Increased CNS depression with alcohol, opiates, barbiturates, benzodiazepines Levodop/carbidopa: Worsening of Parkinson's symptoms

(continued)

Herbal Product	Uses	Adverse Effects	Drug Interactions
			Phenothiazines: Increased risk of tardive dyskinesia
Licorice (*Glycyrrhiza glabra*)	Stomach ulcer	Hypertension	Increased levels of digoxin; increased blood pressure with ACE inhibitors
Melatonin (endogenous hormone secreted by the pineal gland)	Jet lag, insomnia, anticancer	Drowsiness	Unknown
Saw palmetto (*Serenoa repens*) (comes from fruit and berries)	Treatment of symptoms of benign prostate hyperplasia	Bleeding Gastrointestinal upset	Additive effect with oral contraceptives; decreased iron absorption
St. John's wort (*hypericum perforatum*) (comes from flowers, leaves and stems)	Mild to moderate depression	Xerostomia, gastrointestinal upset, allergic reactions, fatigue, dizziness, confusion, photosensitivity	Reduced effectiveness of oral contraceptive may reduce digoxin serum levels; serotonin syndrome (tremors, seizures, hypertension) in patients taking SSRIs tricyclic antidepressants, MAOIs for depression NSAIDs: Increased anticoagulant effect Efavirenz: Decreased antiretroviral activity Cyclosporine: May decrease cyclosporine levels
Valerian root (*Valeriana officinalis*) (root of the plant)	Insomnia, restless motor syndrome	Headaches, dizziness, G.I. upset	CNS depression: Benzodiazepines, opioids, CNS depressants

Table 22–2 Oral Conditions and the Appropriate Herbal Supplement

Oral Condition	Supplement
Aphthous ulcers (canker sores)	Aloe vera, red raspberry
Oral fungal infections (thrush)	Tea tree oil, cinnamon
Periodontal disease	Coenzyme Q10, sanguinaria, goldseal
Caries	Licorice root (glycyrrhiza glabra)
Oral inflammation (mucositis) in cancer patients	Chamomile, vitamin E

KEY POINTS

- Nutraceuticals are not FDA approved; however, many dental patients take various dietary supplements for different medical/dental conditions.
- Always ask patients, besides prescription and OTC drugs, if they are taking any type of nutraceutical.
- In a reference look up any potential drug–herb interaction.
- Many products cause bleeding which may interfere with some surgical dental procedures.

BOARD REVIEW QUESTIONS

1. The two primary types of formulations for herbal products are: (p. 432)
   a. Solid and liquid
   b. Solid and suppositories
   c. Liquid and suppositories
   d. Inhaled powder and solid

2. Which of the following herbs can be used in the treatment of thrush? (p. 434)
   a. Ginger
   b. Garlic
   c. Tea tree oil
   d. Saw palmetto

3. Which of the following herbs can be used in the management of an aphthous ulcer? (p. 434)
   a. Aloe vera
   b. Garlic
   c. Kava kava
   d. St. John's wort

4. Which of the following nutraceuticals may have to be discontinued prior to periodontal surgery? (p. 433)
   a. Garlic
   b. Echinacea
   c. Green tea
   d. Kava kava

5. Which of the following nutraceuticals can be used in the treatment of periodontal disease? (p. 434)
   a. Coenzyme Q10
   b. Green tea
   c. Tea tree oil
   d. Aloe vera

SELECTED REFERENCES

Abebe, W. 2002. Herbal supplements: Any relevancy to dental practice? *NY State Dent J.* 68:26–30.

ADA Guide to Dental Therapeutics, 3rd ed. 2003. Chicago: American Dental Association.

Cheema, P., O. El-Mefty, A. R. Jazieh. 2001. Intraoperative haemorrhage associated with the use of extract of Saw Palmetto herb: A case report and review of literature. *J Intern Med* 250:167–169.

Cohan, R. P., Jacobsen P. L. 2000. Herbal supplements: Considerations in dental practice. *J Calif Dent Assoc* 28:600–610.

Cupp, M. J. 1999. Herbal remedies: Adverse effects and drug interactions. *Am Fam Physician* 59:1239–1245.

Fugh-Berman, A. 1997. Clinical trials of herbs. *Primary Care* 24:889–903.

Lambrecht, J. E., Hamilton W., Rabinovich A. 2000. A review of herb–drug interactions: Documented and theoretical. *U.S. Pharmacist* 25:42–53.

WEB SITES

www.altmed.creighton.edu/homeopathy
myvitaminguide.com
www.ars-grin.gov/duke/

Special Topic **1**

Bisphosphonates and Oral Health

GOALS:

- To familiarize the student with current information regarding the use of drugs called bisphosphonate derivatives and the development of osteonecrosis of the jaw.
- To inform the student about recommendations and guidelines for dental patients taking bisphosphonates.

EDUCATIONAL OBJECTIVES

After reading this section, the reader should be able to:

1. Describe the mechanism of action of bisphosphonates.
2. Discuss the role of bisphosphonates in the treatment of certain medical conditions.
3. Describe oral signs and symptoms of ONJ.
4. Discuss the guidelines for dental patients taking bisphosphonates.
5. List dental risk factors for ONJ.

KEY TERMS

Bisphosphonates
Osteonecrosis of the jaw

In the mid-1990s **bisphosphonates** were first introduced and prescribed as alternates to hormone replacement therapies (HRTs) for osteoporosis and to treat osteolytic tumors and possibly slow tumor development. In 1996, Fosamax® (alendronate) was the first bisphosphonate drug approved for osteoporosis (low bone mass and reduced bone strength that leads to fractures of the spine, wrist, and hip) in postmenopausal women.

Over the past five years there has been major dental concerns regarding a rare adverse reaction of *osteonecrosis of the jaw (ONJ)* induced by bisphosphonates.

INDICATIONS

Bisphosphonates are prescribed in the treatment and prevention of:

1. Corticosteroid-induced osteoporosis
2. Postmenopausal osteoporosis
3. Hypercalcemia with metastatic cancer to help decrease bone pain and fracture by reducing blood calcium levels
4. Paget's disease
5. Chronic renal disease in patients undergoing dialysis (precipitates bone fragility)

STRUCTURE

First generation bisphosphonates (Table 1) contain nitrogen on the R_2 long side chain on their chemical struc-

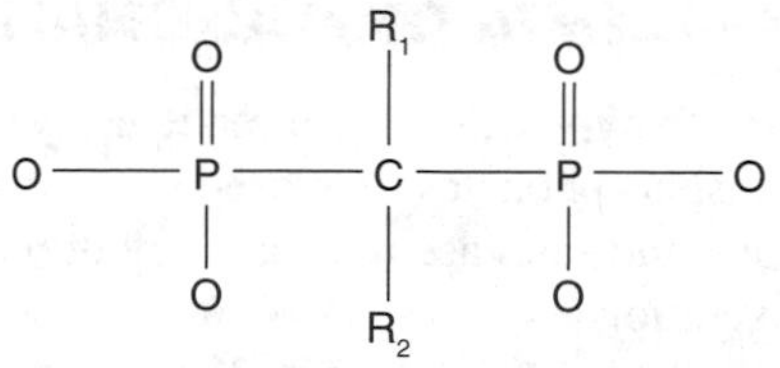

FIGURE 1   Basic structure of bisphosphonates

ture (Figure 1). The R_2 chain imparts the potency and method of affect on bone cells. These non-nitrogen containing bisphosphonates are not entirely implicated in causing ONJ. On the other hand, second and third generation bisphosphonates contain nitrogen and are more likely to cause ONJ.

Commonly prescribed bisphosphonates are listed in Table 1.

GENERAL PHARMACOLOGY

Bisphosphonates act by inhibiting bone resorption by decreasing the action of osteoclasts. The osteoclastic resorption of mineralized bone and cartilage is blocked through its binding to bone which keeps the bone more dense. Also, bisphosphonates inhibit the increased osteoclastic activity and skeletal calcium release into the bloodstream induced by various stimulatory factors released by tumors.

Table 1   Bisphosphonates

Generic Name	Trade Name	Generation 1st: nonnitrogen 2nd: nitrogen	Route of Administration	Indication	Potency Factor
Etidronate	Didronel	1st	Oral	Paget's disease	1
Tiludronate	Skelid	1st	Oral	Paget's disease	10
Clodronate	Bonefos, Loron, Ostac	1st	Oral	Hypercalcemia (bone metastases)	10
Alendronate	Fosamax	2nd	Oral	Osteoporosis	500
Risedronate	Actonel	2nd	Oral	Osteoporosis	2,000
Ibandronate	Boniva	2nd	Oral/IV	Osteoporosis	1,000
Pamidronate	Aredia	2nd	IV	Bone metastases	100
Zoledronate	Zometa	2nd	IV	Bone metastases	10,000

HYPERCALCEMIA OF MALIGNANCY

In patients with hypercalcemia of malignancy (HCM) intravenous bisphosphonates decreased serum calcium and phosphorous and increased urinary calcium and phosphorous excretion.

Generally, hypercalcemia with malignancy occurs in patients who have breast cancer, squamous cell tumors of the head and neck or lung, renal cell carcinoma and some blood malignancies such as multiple myeloma. Excessive release of calcium into the blood occurs as bone is resorbed resulting.

RISK FACTORS

Risk factors with the development of bisphosphonate induced ONJ include:

- Currently or history of taking bisphosphonates (especially IV formulations but also oral)
- History of cancer (breast, lung, prostate, multiple myeloma or metastatic disease to the bone), osteoporosis, Paget's disease, chronic renal disease on dialysis

The following are local dental risk factors for ONJ in patients taking intravenous or oral bisphosphonates:

- Periodontal surgery
- Extractions
- Dental implant surgery
- Ill-fitting dentures that are irritating to the tissues
- Less likely with: endodontic therapy, orthodontics, scaling and root planing
- Bisphosphonate ONJ can also occur spontaneously without any prior dental procedure

CLINICAL PRESENTATION

Osteonecrosis is necrosis or death of bone and can cause severe, extensive, and irreversible damage to the jaw bone (occurs more frequently in the mandible than maxilla). Oral lesions appear similar to those of radiation-induced osteonecrosis. There usually is a delayed or completely absent healing of the periodontium after dental extraction or surgery for more than 6 weeks or can occur spontaneously.

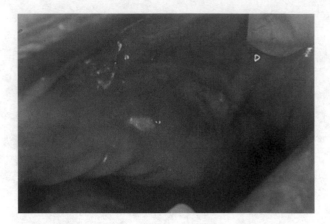

FIGURE 2 Edentulous patient with pieces of bone that became necrotic and continued to slough off after tooth extraction
(Courtesy: Jacqueline M. Plemons, DDS, MS, Baylor College of Dentistry; permission granted: US Pharmacist)

The following are signs and symptoms of ONJ (Figures 2 and 3):

- Irregular mucosal ulcer with exposed bone in the maxillofacial area
- Pain or swelling in the area
- Infection
- Pain
- Mobility of teeth
- Numbness or heavy sensation

Novartis (East Hanover, NJ), a drug company that manufactures Aredia and Zometa developed a staging criteria for ONJ:

Table 2 Staging Criteria for ONJ

Grade	Symptom Severity
1	Asymptotic
2	Mild
3	Moderate
4	Severe

MANAGEMENT

Treatment of ONJ depends on the severity of the case. Regardless of the severity, any necrotic bone should be removed. Conservative treatment of ONJ is recom-

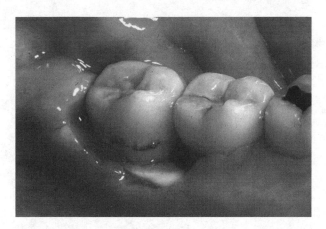

FIGURE 3   Case of ONJ that occurred spontaneously. Note the white area, which is exposed necrotic bone
(Courtesy: Jacqueline M. Plemons, DDS, MS, Baylor College of Dentistry; permission granted: US Pharmacist)

mended, including antibiotics, oral rinses (chlorhexidine), pain control and periodontal debridement where needed.

DENTAL HYGIENE NOTES

There are concerns regarding the dental management of patients currently taking or a history of taking bisphosphonates because of the development of ONJ. Although the majority of reports of bisphosphonate-associated ONJ are in patients taking IV bisphosphonates, more reports are being documented in patients taking oral bisphosphonates. Thus, patients undergoing long-term IV or oral bisphosphonate therapy should be treated with caution and close observation after dental procedures. It is important to discuss the patient's dental needs with their physician.

The Food and Drug Administration (FDA), drug companies and dental societies/associations (e.g., American Academy of Periodontology, American Association of Endodontists, American Academy of Oral Medicine and American Association of Oral and Maxillofacial Surgeons) have issued precautions and recommendations for dentists to follow regarding prevention, diagnosis and treatment guidelines for ONJ.

It is advised that patients have a dental examination and all dental procedures be completed prior to the start of bisphosphonate therapy, careful medical history is needed to determine if a patient will require or is currently on bisphosphonates. Patients should go for routine dental maintenance visits at least every 6 months and maintain good oral hygiene. Routine restorative and dental hygiene procedures may be performed. An elective dental procedure is not advised in patients on IV bisphosphonates.

SELECTED REFERENCES

www.fda.gov. March 2, 2005. Accessed August 5, 2005. Expert Panel Recommendation for the Prevention, Diagnosis and Treatment of Osteonecrosis of the Jaw.

American Association of Endodontists. Bisphosphonate-associated osteonecrosis of the jaw. Winter 2007. American Association of Endodontists. Chicago.

American Association of Oral and Maxillofacial Surgeons. Position Paper on Bisphosphonate-related Osteonecrosis of the Jaws. September 25, 2006. American Association of Oral and Maxillofacial Surgeons.

Corgel, J. O. Implants and oral bisphosphonates. J Periodontol 2007; 78:373–376.

Durie, B. G. M., M. Katz, J. Crowley, S. -B. Woo, K. Hande, P. G. Richardson, M. Maerevoet, C. Martin, L. Duck, P. Tarassoff, and Y. -J. Hei. 2005. Osteonecrosis of the jaw and bisphosphonates. *N Engl J Med.* 353:99–102. Correspondence.

Markiewicz, M. R., J. E. Margarone, III, J. H. Campbel, A. Aguirre. Bisphosphonate-associated osteonecrosis of the jaws. A review of current knowledge. JADA 2005; 136: 1669–1674.

Marx, R. E., Y. Sawatari, M. Fortin, V. Broumand. Bisphosphonate-induced exposed bone (Osteonecrosis/osteopetrosis) of the jaw: Risk factors, recognition prevention, and treatment. *J Oral Maxillofac Surg* 2005. 63(*11*):1567–1575.

Marx, R. E. Pamidronate (Aredia) and zoledronate (Zometa)-induced avascular necrosis of the jaws: A growing epidemic. 2003. *J Oral Maxillofac Surg* 61:1115–1117.

Melo, M. D., G. Obeid. Osteonecrosis of the jaws in patients with a history of receiving bisphosphonate therapy: Strategies for prevention and early recognition. *JADA* 2005;136:1675–1681.

Migliorati, C. A., M. M. Schubert, D. E. Peterson, L. M. Seneda,. Bisphosphonate-associated osteonecrosis of mandibular and maxillary bone: An emerging oral complication of supportive cancer therapy. *Cancer* 2005;104:83–93.

Ruggiero, S., J. R. E. Gralow, A. O. Marx, M. M. Hoff, J. Shubert, M. Huryn, et al. Practical guidelines for the prevention, diagnosis, and treatment of osteonecrosis of the jaw in patients with cancer. *J Oncology Practice.* 2006;2(*1*):7–14.

Ruggiero, S. L., B. Mehrotra, T. J. Rosenberg, S. L. Engroff, Osteonecrosis of the jaws associated with the use of bisphosphonates: A review of 63 cases. *J Oral Maxillofac Surg* 2004;62:527–534.

Ruggiero, S., T. J. Rosenberg. Osteonecrosis of the jaws associated with the use of bisphosphonates. *J Oral Maxillofac Surg* 2004;62:527–534.

WEB SITES

www.novartis.com
www.jop.stateaffiliates.asco.org/JanuaryIssue/Summary
Guidelines.pdf
www.aae.org
www.perio.org

Oral Manifestations of Drug Reactions

GOAL: To familiarize the dental clinician with the common oral conditions/lesions associated with certain drugs.

EDUCATIONAL OBJECTIVES

After reading this section, the reader should be able to:
1. List medications that may cause oral conditions/lesions.
2. Discuss how the dental hygienist can identify and manage these oral problems.

KEY TERMS

Drugs
Oral adverse effects

Table 1 Medications and Their Oral Side Effects

Oral Condition	Medication	Notes
Candidiasis (fungal/yeast infection) Shows up intraorally as a white, plaque-like lesion that can be wiped off with gauze. Fungal infections are found on the maxillary palatal gingival when patients do not remove their maxillary denture.	Inhalation steroids (in asthma)	Patient should rinse mouth after use of asthma drugs.
Tardive dyskinesia (abnormal mouth and tongue movements, including lip-puckering and tongue protrusion)	Antipsychotics	There is no definitive treatment; patient management is important.
Esophageal burning/ulcers	Tetracyclines	Take with full glass of water in an upright position.
Gingival enlargement	Phenytoin (Dilantin), Nifedipine (Procardia, Adalat) and other calcium channel blockers Cyclosporine	Keep meticulous oral hygiene; sometimes surgical removal of gingival is necessary, but the enlargement will return.
Gingival hemorrhages	Coumadin (Warfarin) Clopidogrel (Plavix)	Note petechiae on chart; consult with patient's physician.
Hairy tongue	Mouthrinses Antibiotics (especially broad spectrum) Steroids	Brush tongue.
Taste changes	Lithium Metrondiazole (Flagyl)	Taste changes are transient for metronidazole, but chronic for lithium because the patient will be on lithium for a long time.
Exaggerated gag reflex	Digitalis/cardiac glycosides	Patient management with impression and radiographs.
Xerostomia	Many; see table 2	Many OTC products: Orajel gel, spray, toothpaste, Biotène products, Osais moisturizing mouthrinse and saliva substitutes (e.g., Xero-Lube, Salivart). Prescription sialagogue may be beneficial; pilocarpine HCl (Salagen) and cevimeline (Evoxac).

Many **drugs** can cause **oral adverse effects,** including fungal infections, xerostomia, hairy tongue, gingival overgrowth, increased salivation, changes in taste, and bleeding. Table 1 lists drug reactions evident in the oral cavity. Table 2 lists commonly used drugs that cause xerostomia.

If the medication cannot be changed or the dose altered then increase water intake, or have the patient suck on sugarless candy or chew sugarless gum. Oral products (e.g., oral rinses, toothpaste, gel) such as Oasis and Biotène may be helpful.

Table 2 Classification of Commonly Used Drugs Causing Xerostomia

Classification	Drug
Antiacne	Isotretinoin (Accutane)
Anti-anxiety	Alprazolam (Xanax)
	Chlorazepate (Tranxene)
	Diazepam (Valium)
	Hydroxyzine (Atarax, VIstaril)
	Lorazepam (Ativan)
	Oxazepam (Serax)
Anticonvulsants	Carbamazepine (Tegretol)
	Gabapentin (Neurontin)
	Lamotrigine (Lamictal)
Antidepressants	Amitriptyline (Elavil)
	Bupropion (Wellbutrin)
	Chlomipramine (Anafranil)
	Desipramine (Norpramin)
	Doxepin (Sinequan)
	Fluoxetine (Prozac)
	Fluvoxaime (Luvox)
	Imipramine (Tofranil)
Antipsychotics	Clozapine (Clozaril), olanzapine (Zyprexa), lithium, haloperidol (Haldol)
Antihistamines	Diphenydramine (Benadryl)
	Triprolidine/pseudoephedrine (Actifed)
	Loratadine (Claritin)
	Brompheniramine (Dimetane)
	Brompheniramine/phenylpropanolamine (Dimetapp)
	Promethazine (Phenergan)
Anticholinergeric (antispasmodic/ antimotionsickness)	Belladonna alkaloids (Bellergal)
	Dicyclomine (Bentyl)
	Hyoscyamine with atropine
	Phenobarbital
	Scopolamine (Donnatal, Transderm-Scop)
Antidiarrheal	Ioperamide (Imodium AD)
	Diphenoxylate with atropine (Lomotil)
Bronchodilator	Ipratropium (Atrovent)
	Isoproterenol (Isuprel)
	Albuterol (Proventil, Ventolin)
Diuretics	Chlorothiazide (Diuril)
	Furosemide (Lasix)
	Hydrochlorothiazide (Hydrodiuril)
	Triamterene/hydrochlorothiazide (Dyazide)
Sedative/hypnotics	Temazepam (Restoril) Triazolam (Halcion)

Smoking Cessation Products

GOAL: To gain understanding about the different products used for smoking cessation in the dental office.

EDUCATIONAL OBJECTIVES
After reading this section, the reader should be able to:
1. Define the role of the dental hygienist in smoking cessation programs in the dental office.
2. List the pharmacologic agents used in smoking cessation.

KEY TERMS
Smoking cessation
Dental office
Nicotine-replacement therapy

PRACTICAL STEPS TO SMOKING CESSATION

Smoking cessation programs should be made available to patients in the dental office (Table 1). The **dental office** is the logical place to counsel patients on the effects of smoking on the periodontium and overall health. A smoking-cessation program should be a part of comprehensive preventive periodontal care.

PHARMACOLOGIC AGENTS

Acute physical withdrawal symptoms following smoking cessation are not usually long lasting (not more than 1 to 2 weeks), but the success rates of smoking-cessation programs may be augmented by weaning smokers from nicotine gradually through the use of nicotine-replacement therapy.

Nicotine-replacement therapy by itself will not be as successful as when accompanied by counseling and behavior modification, including hypnosis and biofeedback. Pharmacologic agents used for smoking cessation include nicotine gum, transdermal nicotine patches, nasal spray, and systemic bupropion. Nicotine-replacement drugs work by replacing the nicotine that is absorbed in the body while smoking, and act as a substitute for the cigarette. The manufacturers claim to reduce the cravings for nicotine. Nicotine therapy should not be used in patients who continue to smoke. The nicotine gum should be chewed slowly and then placed or "parked" between the cheek and the gums for about 30 minutes. Nicotine patches and gum are available over the counter without a prescription.

Bupropion HCl (Zyban) is an oral medication prescribed by dentists or physicians to help decrease the withdrawal symptoms and the urge to smoke that accompany smoking cessation. An advantage to oral medication is that it is nicotine free and helps the patient to quit while still smoking. Adverse side effects include xerostomia and insomnia (difficulty sleeping). Varenicline (Chantix), the newest drug, works differently than Zyban in that it makes the patient produce more dopamine, which is supposed to help lower nicotine cravings. It acts at sites in the brain affected by nicotine.

FDA-approved in May 2006, varenicline (Chantix) is an oral tablet that binds to nicotinic receptors, where it acts as a partial agonist and blocks nicotine from binding to the receptor.

Drug Interactions

The following medications may need dosage adjustment when taking nicotine patch, gum, lozenge or spray:

- Acetaminophen (Tylenol)
- Beta-blockers (atenolol, pindolol, metoprolol, timolol, nadolol, and propranolol)
- Caffeine (coffee, tea, colas)
- Furosemide (Lasix)
- Phenylephrine (Neo-Synephrine)
- Prazosin (Minipress)
- Theophylline
- Tricyclic antidepressants (amitriptyline, nortriptyline, imipramine)

SELECTED REFERENCES

Cabral, L. 2005. Smoking cessation within the U.S. Hispanic community: Caring for Hispanic Patients. *American Academy of Family Physicians.* 2:9–12.

Carr AB, Ebbert JO. Interventions for tobacco cessation in the dental setting. The Cochrane Collaboration. Cochrane Reviews, January 25, 2006

National Cancer Institute, U.S. Department of Health and Human Services. 1996.

Tobacco effects in the mouth, edited by R. E. Mechlenburg, D., Diane Pub. Co. 2004

WEB SITES

www.ahrq.gov
www.nic.nih.gov
www.cdc.gov/tobacco
www.ada.org/public/topics/smoking–tobacco.asp

Table 1 Pharmacologic Agents Used for Smoking Cessation

Product	Directions for Use	Supplied	Adverse Effects	Rx or OTC
Nicotine Gum Nicorette gum	Do not smoke during treatment because of risk of nicotine overdose. Chew one piece of gum every 1–2 hours for weeks 1–6; every 2–4 hours for weeks 7–9; and every 4–8 hours for weeks 10–12. Do not eat or drink for 15 minutes before chewing gum, and do not eat or drink while chewing gum.	2 mg, 4 mg gum; starter kit has 108 pieces and refill kits have 48 pieces	Mouth soreness, sore jaw, dyspepsia (stomach pain or discomfort)	OTC
Nicotine Transdermal System (nicotine patch) Nicoderm CQ Nicotrol Habitrol Prostep	Do not smoke during treatment because of risk of nicotine overdose. Nicoderm CQ: Use one patch daily; start at 21 mg/day for 6 weeks, then 14 mg/day for 2 weeks, then 7 mg/day for 2 weeks. Maximum therapy is 3 months.	Nicoderm CQ: (28-day supply): 21 mg, 14 mg, 7 mg patches Nicotrol: 15 mg (worn only while awake), 10 mg and 5 mg patches Habitrol: 21 mg, 14 mg, 7 mg Prostep: 22 or 11 mg patches	Local skin irritation, insomnia (difficulty in sleeping)	Rx and OTC
Nicotine Lozenge Commit	Allow lozenge to dissolve slowly over 20 to 30 minutes, swallow as little as possible	2 mg (72 pieces), 4 mg (72 pieces)	Sore teeth and gingival, indigestion and irritated throat	OTC
Nicotine Nasal Spray Nicotrol NS	Start with two sprays in each nostril every hour, which may be increased to 80 sprays per day for heavy smokers; maximum therapy is 6 months. Can cause nasal irriation.	Prescription product Easy spray delivers 0.5 mg nicotine; available in 10-ml bottles	Irritation of nasal mucosa	Rx (prescription only)
Nicotine Inhalation System Nicotrol Inhaler	Less nicotine per puff is released with the inhaler than with a cigarette. Best effect is achieved by frequent continuous puffing for about 20 minutes. The recommended treatment is up to 3 months and, if needed, a gradual reduction over the next 6–12 weeks. Total treatment should not exceed 6 months.	Prescription product Inhaler uses nicotine cartridges (10 mg/cartridge) that provides about 20 minutes of active puffing, or approximately 80 deep draws	Irritation of mouth and throat	Rx (prescription only)

Product	Directions for Use	Supplied	Adverse Effects	Rx or OTC
Oral Medications (Non-Nicotine Drugs) Bupropion HCl (Zyban)	Start initial dose while the patient is still smoking to allow for higher blood levels; initial dose is 150 mg/day for 3 days. Maximum daily dose is 300 mg. Patient should stop smoking within 2 weeks of start of therapy. Continue drug therapy for 7–12 weeks after the patient stops smoking. Can be used with nicotine patches.	Prescription 150 mg sustained-release tablets	Insomnia, xerostomia	Rx (prescription only)
Chantix (varenicline)	FDA-approved in May 2006. Not used in patients younger than 18 years old. Caution in patients with renal impairment. Packs: first month: 1 card—0.5mg × 11 tabs and 3 cards—1mg × 14 tabs Bottles: 0.5 mg, 1.0 mg	1 mg bid 11 weeks, following a 1-week titration. Days 1-3: 0.5 mg qd days 4-7: 0.5mg bid days 8-end of treatment: 1 mg bid	Nausea, trouble sleeping, headache, changes in dreams	Prescription

Medical Emergency Drugs in the Dental Office

GOAL: To introduce the basic principles for handling a medical emergency in the dental office.

EDUCATIONAL OBJECTIVES

After reading this section, the reader should be able to:

1. List the steps to follow in case of a medical emergency in the dental office.
2. Discuss the management of certain medical conditions.
3. Describe the various drugs used in the treatment of medical emergencies.

KEY TERMS

Medical emergencies
Dental office
Emergency drugs

448

INTRODUCTION

Every office should have an emergency kit based on the office patient population, distance to the nearest hospital, rapid availability of skilled EMS services, and the dental clinician's skill and comfort in using the medications and equipment. Many **medical emergencies** can occur in the dental office. The most frequent emergencies in the dental office are syncope, mild allergy, angina, postural hypotension, seizures, acute asthma, hyperventilation, epinephrine reaction, and hypoglycemia. Emergencies that are not managed properly initially have the potential for becoming fatal. The best way to minimize medical emergencies in the dental office is to prevent them. This can be accomplished by taking thorough medical histories, vital signs, and observing the patient's physical condition.

PREPARATION OF DENTAL STAFF

The **dental office** and staff must be familiar with recognizing and managing all medical emergencies. Important phone numbers including the nearest hospital emergency department, physician and emergency medical services (911) should be posted in an assessable area. Management of medical emergencies that occur in the dental office involves:

- Discontinuing dental treatment
- Call for assistance
- Accurate diagnosis
- Basic life support (BLS)
- Activation of an emergency response team
- Requesting assistance—call 911 for emergency medical services (EMS)
- Availability of emergency drugs and equipment

BASIC LIFE SUPPORT

Basic life support (BLS), also referred to as cardiopulmonary rescuscitation (CPR), consists of the ABCs: A = maintaining airway; B = administering oxygen (breathing); C = monitoring vital signs; and D = defibrillation. The staff member performing CPR should not leave the victim, but should yell for help. This staff member should bring emergency equipment and oxygen, and call 911.

EMERGENCY MEDICAL KIT AND EQUIPMENT

There is no mandatory list of **emergency drugs** that must be maintained in every dental office; however, Table 1 lists some commonly occurring conditions and medications that should be in the office for treatment. The kit should be checked quarterly, and after each use, for expired medications and replacement of medications previously used.

Basic medical equipment that is needed in the dental office includes an oxygen tank and mask, manual resuscitation bag, blood pressure cuff and stethoscope, disposable syringes and needles and a tourniquet.

SELECTED REFERENCES

Malamed, S. F. 2001. Emergency medicine: Preparation and basics of management. *Dentistry Today* 64–67.

Toback, S. L. Preparing your office for a medical emergency. *Family Practice Management* 2005;12:34–35.

Table 1 Medical Emergency Drugs

Medical Condition	Medications	Notes
Allergic reaction (mild or delayed)	Diphenhydramine (Benadryl)	Oral Adult: 25–50 mg 4 times a day (qid) Child: 10–25 mg qid Patients should carry an EpiPen.
Anaphylactic shock (life-threatening, sudden onset, severe allergic reaction with decreased BP and bronchospasm) Exposure to latex gloves, or diaphragm of anesthetic cartridge	Epinephrine (adrenalin) 1 : 1,000	IM/SQ Preloaded syringe + 2–3 1 mL ampules Patients should carry an EpiPen.
Acute asthmatic attack	First use patient's inhaler [e.g., albuterol (Ventolin)]; if not effective, then inject epinephrine (Adrenalin) 1 : 1,000	Albuterol: Inhale 1–2 puffs Epinephrine: IM/SQ
Acute angina attack	Nitroglycerin	IV, sublingual or translingual spray, sublingual tabs
Anesthetic toxicity	Oxygen (assess and support airway, administer oxygen, monitor vital signs, emergency care)	Mask
Bradycardia (slow heart rate in a cardiac patient)	Atropine sulfate + CPR	IV
Acute hypotension (low blood pressure)	Levophed (norepinephrine)	IV
Hypoglycemic (low blood sugar) shock (in a diabetic)	Sugar Dextrose	Orally (orange juice, nondiet soda) IV
Reaction to the vasoconstrictor in local anesthetic	Supplemental oxygen	Use mask
Seizures	Diazepam (Valium)	IV
	Diazepam (Diastat)	Rectal suppositories
	Lorazepam (Ativan) (recline and position to prevent injury, ensure open airway and adequate ventilation, monitor vital signs)	IV
Syncope (fainting)	Spirits of ammonia	Break open vial
	Oxygen (recline, feet up, loosen clothing, monitor vital signs)	
Antidotal drugs	Opioid antagonist: Naloxone Benzodiazepine Antagonist: Flumazenil	IV route recommended

Glossary

A

Absorption   Movement of a drug from its site of administration (e.g., mouth), across body membranes and into the blood stream (circulation).

Acethylcholine (ACh)   Neurotransmitter of the parasympathetic nervous system; also present at the sympathetic preganglionic neurons.

Acquired resistance   When a micro-organism is no longer affected by an anti-infective drug.

Action potential   Electrical changes in the membrane of a nerve cell due to changes in membrane permeability.

Acute   Disease that has a sudden onset, severe symptoms, and a short course.

Addiction   *See* Dependence.

Adherence   Also referred to as compliance. Obeying, following orders as it pertains to taking medications. The opposite is nonadherence.

Adrenal crisis (acute adrenocortical insufficiency)   Severe phase or attack characterized by insufficient amounts of the adrenocortical hormones and resulting in nausea, vomiting, low blood pressure, and life-threatening imbalances in electrolytes.

Adrenal glands   Two small, triangular-shaped glands located on top of each kidney; consists of the adrenal cortex, which synthesizes and secretes corticosteroids, and the adrenal medulla, which synthesizes, secretes, and stores dopamine, epinephrine and norepinephrine.

Adrenergic   Referring to nerves that release norepinephrine (NE) or epinephrine (EPI).

Adrenergic agonist   *See* Sympathomimetic drug; a drug that acts on or mimics the sympathetic nervous system.

Adrenergic blocker (antagonist)   A drug that blocks the actions of the sympathetic nervous system.

Adverse drug event   An undesirable and unexpected effect of a drug that occurs at a dose used in humans for prophylaxis, diagnosis, or therapy.

Adverse drug reaction   An effect which is noxious and unintended, and which occurs at normal doses, during normal use.

Affinity   Reversible binding of a drug with a receptor forming a drug–receptor complex. The higher the affinity of the drug to the receptor, the more binding occurs to that receptor versus another receptor.

Agonist   Binding of a drug to a receptor that results in a maximal pharmacologic response.

Agonist, full   An agonist drug that produces the greatest maximal response of any agonist acting on the same receptors on the same tissue.

Agonist, partial   An agonist drug that produces a response that is less than the maximal response produced by a full agonist acting at the same receptors on the same tissue.

Akathisia   Inability to remain still; constantly moving.

Aldosterone   A steroid hormone secreted by the adrenal cortex that regulates the salt and water balance in the body.

Allergen   A substance, such as pollen or aspirin, that causes an allergy or allergic reaction.

Allergic response   A hyperresponse of body defenses. Signs of allergic reactions include skin rash, itching, edema (swelling), and redness.

Alternative medicine (also referred to as complementary medicine)   Use of products that are not considered to be part of conventional healthcare.

Amide   Type of chemical linkage found in some local anesthetics involving carbon, nitrogen, and oxygen ($-N4-CO-$).

Analgesia   Loss of pain sensation without loss of consciousness.

Analgesic   A drug that relieves pain without the loss of consciousness (patient is awake).

Anaphylaxis   A severe type of allergic reaction that causes tachycardia (increased heart rate) and bronchospasm (spasm in lung tissue).

Androgens   Steroid sex hormones that promote the appearance of masculine characteristics.

Anesthesia   State of total or partial loss of sensation (inability to sense pain) with or without the loss of consciousness, induced by an anesthetic.

Anesthetic   A drug that causes loss of sensation. Example: Local anesthetic causes a loss of pain sensation but not a loss of conscious; general anesthetics cause a loss of pain sensation and a loss of consciousness.

Angina pectoris   Heart condition where acute chest pain occurs upon physical or emotional exertion due to inadequate oxygen supply to the heart.

Angiotensin   Converting enzyme (ACE); enzyme responsible for converting angiotensin I to angiotensin II.

Angiotensin II   Chemical released in response to falling blood pressure that causes vasoconstriction and the release of aldosterone. Angiotensin II receptor antagonists are drugs used in the treatment of hypertension.

Antacid   Drug that neutralizes acids in the stomach; used for heartburn (GERD).

Antagonist   The effect of two or more drugs is less than the effects produced by each individual drug. The antagonist diminishes the effects of an agonist.

Anti-inflammatory   Reduce inflammation.

Antibiotic   Substance produced by micro-organisms that inhibits or kills other microorganisms. Some antibiotics are semisynthetic.

Anticholinergic   See cholinergic blocker.

Anticoagulant   Drug that inhibits the formation of blood clots.

Anticonvulsant   See antiepileptic.

Antidepressant   Drug used in the treatment of depression.

Antiepileptic   Drug used in the management of seizures.

Antifibrinolytic   Drug used to prevent and treat excessive bleeding from surgical sites.

Antifungal   Drug used to treat fungal infections.

Antihistamine   Drug that blocks histamine (H1) receptors, eliminating symptoms of rhinitis.

Antimicrobial (drug) resistance   Bacteria can develop resistance to antibiotics, where the bacteria become insensitive to the antibiotic.

Antioxidant compounds (e.g., Vitamins A, C, and E)   That inhibit chemical reactions with oxygen. They protect cells in the body against damage by free radicals, which are reactive by-products of normal cell activity. Claims are that antioxidants can lower the risk of heart disease and some forms of cancer.

Antipsychotics   A group of drugs such as the phenothiazines or butyrophenones that are used to treat psychosis (mental disorder characterized by derangement of personality and loss of contact with reality).

Antipyretic   Pertaining to an agent that works against fever.

Antiretrovirals   Drugs used in the treatment of HIV/AIDS.

Antitussive   Drug used to suppress a cough.

Antiviral   Drugs used to treat viral infections (e.g., acyclovir).

Anxiety   State of apprehension, tension, or uneasiness from anticipation of danger. Treatment with anti-anxiety (anxiolytics) drugs, including benzodiazepines.

Anxiolysis   Anti-anxiety.

Anxiolytics   Drugs that have an anti-anxiety effect. The most commonly used anti-anxiety drugs are the benzodiazepines.

Apothecary System of Measurement   Older system of measurement using drams; rarely used.

Arrthymias   Irregular heart beat.

Asthma   Chronic inflammatory disease of the lungs characterized by airway obstruction.

Atherosclerosis   Condition characterized by a buildup of fatty plaque and loss of elasticity of the walls of the arteries.

Attention-deficit hyperactivity disorder (ADHD)   Disorder in children and adolescence characterized by hyperactivity, short attention span, poor concentration and behavior control problems.

Autonomic Nervous System (ANS)   Portion of the nervous system that regulates involuntary body functions including the heart, and intestines.

Autoreceptor   Binding of a drug to an autoreceptor results in a negative feedback response, whereby norepinephrine is inhibited from being released. Alpha$_2$-autoreceptors are located on postsympathetic sympathetic nerve endings.

B

Bactericidal   Antibiotic that kills the bacteria.

Bacteriostatic   Antibiotic that inhibits bacterial multiplication.

Balanced anesthesia   Use of multiple medications to rapidly induce unconsciousness, cause muscle relaxation and maintain deep anesthesia.

Benzodiazepines   A category of drugs used to treat anxiety and insomnia.

Beta-blockers   Drugs used to decrease high blood pressure.

Beta-lactam ring   Chemical structure found in most penicillins.

Beta-receptors Type of receptor found in the sympathetic nervous system.

Bile A greenish-yellow fluid produced in and secreted by the liver, stored in the gallbladder, and released into the intestine.

Bioavailability The amount of drug dose (in percentage) entering the systemic circulation after administration. It is the amount of drug absorbed into the blood. For example, a drug given IV has 100 percent bioavailability because the entire amount of drug directly enters the blood.

Bioequivalent (bioequivalence) A drug that acts on the body with the same strength and similar absorption (bioavailability) as the same dosage of a sample of a given substance.

Biotransformation Chemical alteration of a fat-soluble drug into a more water-soluble drug so that it can be easily eliminated from the body. Term is used interchangeably with Metabolism.

Bipolar disorder (Formerly known as manic-depressive disorder.) A psychiatric disorder characterized by alternating episodes of mania (excessive enthusiasm, interest, or desire) and depression.

Bisphosphonates Drugs used in the treatment of osteoporosis, metastatic cancer, Paget's disease, multiple myeloma. Concerns in dentistry because there is an association with the development of osteonecrosis of the jaws (ONJ).

Blood-brain barrier Anatomical structure that prevents or allows certain substances from gaining access to the brain.

Bradycardia Decreased heart rate.

Bradykinin Chemical released by cells during inflammation that produces pain and side effects similar to histamine.

Brand name Also called Trade name; a name used to identify a drug which may or may not be registered as a trademark.

Broad-spectrum antibiotic Antimicrobial that is effective against many different gram-negative and gram-positive organisms.

Bronchioles Part of the lungs.

Bronchoconstriction Constriction or reduction in the size of a bronchus or bronchial tube of the lung.

Bronchodilation Dilation or widening of the air passages of the lungs, which eases breathing by relaxing bronchial smooth muscle.

Bronchospasm Rapid constriction of the airways.

Buccal route Tablet is placed in the oral cavity between the gingiva and the cheek.

C

Calcium channel blocker Drug that blocks the flow of calcium ions into the heart. Used for hypertension, angina, arrhythmias. They are vasodilators.

Candidiasis Fungal (Candida; *C. albicans*) infection.

Cardiac output Amount of blood pumped by a ventricle in one minute.

Cardiovascular Relating to the heart and blood vessels.

Carotene Class of yellow-red pigments that are precursors to vitamin A.

Catecholamines A group of amines derived from catechol that are important as neurotransmitters which act in the autonomic nervous system (e.g., epinephrine, norepinephrine, and dopamine).

Ceiling effect The maximum pharmacologic effect that can be induced from a drug regardless of how large a dose is administered; increasing the dose will not enhance the pharmacologic response. Example: Once the maximum response is achieved with aspirin, increasing the dose does not increase the response.

Central Nervous System (CNS) Division of the nervous system consisting of the brain and spinal cord.

Certainly lethal dose (CLD) Five to 10 g of sodium fluoride is considered a certainly lethal dose for a 70-kg adult. One quarter of the certainly lethal dose can be ingested without producing serious acute toxicity and is known as the safely tolerated dose.

Chemical name Name (chemical formula) used for drugs that is established by the International Union of Pure and Applied Chemistry.

Cholecalciferol Vitamin D_3, formed in the skin by exposure to ultraviolet light.

Cholesterol Essential component of cell membranes and precursor to steroids that are synthesized in the body.

Cholinergic Also referred to as parasympathetic; a term relating to nerves that release acetylcholine (ACh).

Cholinergic agonist Drug that acts on or mimics the cholinergic nervous system.

Cholinergic blocker (anticholinergic) Drug that blocks the actions of the parasympathetic nervous system.

Chronic Disease that continues over a long time, showing little change in symptoms or course.

Chronic obstructive pulmonary disease Progressive lung disease process characterized by difficulty breathing, wheezing, and a chronic cough. Complications include bronchitis, pneumonia, and lung cancer.

Chronotropic effect Change in the heart rate.

Clearance The volume of body fluid removed by biotransfomation or excretion.

Coagulation Process of blood clotting.

Coenzyme A substance that enhances or is necessary for the action of enzymes. They are usually smaller than enzymes themselves.

Cold sore (also referred to as herpes labialis) Herpes infection of the vermillion boarder of the lip.

Comorbidity Presence of more than one disease or disorder.

Controlled drug substances Certain drugs (e.g., narcotics) whose use is restricted by the Controlled Substance Act of 1970. Prescribers of drugs must register with the Drug Enforcement Administration (DEA) in order to prescribe narcotics.

Convulsions Uncontrolled muscle contractions or spasms.

Corticosteroids Steroid hormones released by the adrenal cortex; include mineralocorticoids and glucocorticoids.

Cortisone A glucocorticosteroid (corticosteroid) hormone that is isolated from the adrenal cortex; used as an anti-inflammatory agent.

Cyclooxygenase Enzymes found in the body. COX-1 functions to maintain and protect the lining of the stomach from damaging acid; COX-2 is produced during inflammation.

Cytochrome P450 enzymes Enzymes in the liver that metabolize drugs.

Cytokines Proteins such as interleukins that are released by cells of the immune system and regulate the actions of other cells in the generation of an immune response.

D

Dental infection Pathological state resulting from the invasion of the dental structures by pathogenic microorganisms.

Dependence (Dependency.) Replaces the obsolete term *addiction*. A physiological or psychological need for a drug or substance.

Depot Long-acting formulation of an injectable drug that is designed to have only weekly or monthly dosing.

Depression Disorder characterized by a depressed mood with feelings of sadness, despair, and discouragement. Treatment is with antidepressants.

Diabetes mellitus Group of hormonal diseases that are characterized by alterations in carbohydrates, protein, and lipid metabolism, the primary manifestation being abnormally high blood glucose levels (hyperglycemia).

Disintegrate Break open. Example: capsules disintegrate or break open before the drug can be dissolved.

Distribution The movement of a drug after it is absorbed in the bloodstream to the tissues/organs that the drug is intended to act on.

Dopamine A neurotransmitter formed in the brain and essential to the normal functioning of the central nervous system. An intermediate substance in the synthesis of norepinephrine. A deficiency in its concentration within the brain is associated with Parkinson's disease. Also, different levels are associated with schizophrenia.

Dosage form The state in which a drug is dispensed to be used; for example, the most common dosage form of aspirin is a tablet.

Dose The amount or quantity of a drug administered. For example, 500 mg (milligrams) of penicillin is given to a patient with an oral infection. 500 mg is the dose of the drug.

Drug Also referred to as a ligand. A chemical that is used in the diagnosis, treatment, or prevention of diseases in the body.

Drug effects Drug has a specific action on different part of the body; can include intended action and side effects.

Drug laws To protect the public from deceitful and unsafe drug acts.

Drug-protein complex Drugs will bind reversibly to plasma (blood) proteins and circulate in the plasma until they are released or displaced from the drug-protein complex. While bound to the protein, drugs are not available for distribution to the body tissues. Drugs not bound to this complex are called "free drugs."

Duodenal ulcer Ulcer in the duodenum.

Duodenum Small intestine.

Dystonia Severe muscle spasms, particularly of the back, neck, tongue, and face; characterized by abnormal tension starting in one area of the body and progressing to other areas.

E

Edema "Fluid filled"; swelling. Sign of inflammation.

Effective dose (ED$_{50}$) The dose of a drug that produces a desired effect.

Efficacy The effectiveness of a drug in producing a more intense response as its concentration increases.

Elimination Drug is removed from the body.

Endogenous Produced or growing within the body.

Enteral Drugs administered orally or through a nasogastric tube into the digestive (gastrointestinal) tract. Most common route of drug administration.

Enteric-coated Tablets that have a hard, wax coating so that they dissolve in the basic environment of the small intestine rather than the acidic contents of the stomach, which can be irritating to the stomach.

Enterohepatic circulation Some large drug compounds are excreted in the bile rather than in the urine. After the bile empties into the intestines, part of the drug may be reabsorbed into the blood and eventually return to the liver. An example of a drug that undergoes enterohepatic circulation is oral contraceptives.

Enzyme A protein that accelerates the rate of chemical reactions.

Epilepsy Disorder of the CNS (central nervous system) characterized by seizures and/or convulsions.

Epinephrine A catecholamine released by the adrenal medulla upon activation of preganglionic sympathetic nerves. Causes increased heart rate (β_1-receptor stimulation), vasoconstriction in arteries and veins (α_1 and α_2-receptor stimulation) and vasodilation (β_2 stimulation), which decreases blood pressure.

Excretion The removal of drugs from the body. The primary site of excretion is through the kidney via urine. Other routes of drug elimination are lungs, sweat, milk, bile, and feces.

Exogenous Produced or growing outside the body.

Expectorant Drug used to increase bronchial secretions.

Extrapyramidal side effects Symptoms of acute dystonia, akathisia, Parkinsonism, and tardive dyskinesia, often caused by antipsychotic drugs.

F

Fight or flight response Characteristic set of signs and symptoms produced when the sympathetic nervous system is activated.

First-order kinetics Refers to the rate (time) of drug elimination from the body. The rate of elimination depends on the concentration of drug in the blood. As the blood concentration of a drug falls, the amount of drug eliminated or excreted also falls. First-order elimination accounts for elimination of most drugs.

First-pass effect Also referred to as first-pass metabolism. After a drug is swallowed, it is absorbed by the digestive (gastrointestinal) system. It then enters the liver via the portal vein. In the liver the drug is metabolized (broken down) before entering the systemic circulation (blood stream). Some drugs are so extensively metabolized by the liver that only a small amount of unchanged drug enters the systemic circulation (blood stream) to become available to the whole body. Drugs administered via the sublingual or rectal route undergo less first-pass metabolism than if given by the oral route. Examples of drugs that undergo first-pass metabolism are: methyldopa/levodopa for the management of Parkinson's disease, aspirin, estrogens, analapril (Vasotec; for hypertension).

Fluoride A binary compound of fluorine with another element; helps prevent dental caries.

Folic acid A B vitamin that is a coenzyme in protein and nucleic acid metabolism.

Food and Drug Administration (FDA) An agency of the U.S. Department of Health and Human Services. Responsible for the evaluation and approval of new drugs.

G

GABA (Gamma-aminobutyric acid.) Substance found in the central nervous system that is associated with the transmission of nerve impulses.

Ganglion (Plural, ganglia.) A collection of cell bodies of neurons located outside the central nervous system (CNS).

Gastic ulcer Ulcer in the stomach.

Gastroesophageal reflux disease (known as GERD) Condition of the upper gastrointestinal tract where there is a reflux or "backing up" of gastric contents from the stomach into the esophagus. Common complaint is heartburn.

Gastrointestinal Refers to the gastrointestinal (G.I.) tract which is part of the digestive system that includes the mouth, esophagus, stomach, and intestines.

General anesthesia A controlled state of unconsciousness, accompanied by a partial or complete loss of protective reflexes, including loss of ability to independently maintain airway and respond purposefully to physical stimulation or verbal command, produced by a pharmacologic or non-pharmacologic method or combination.

Generic name   A drug name assigned by the U.S. Adopted Name Council. Example: acetaminophen is the generic name of the drug Tylenol.

Glomerular filtration   Passive filtration (straining) of the blood as blood flows through the kidney. The extent to which a drug is filtered depends on size, protein binding, ionization, polarity, and kidney function.

Glucocorticosteroids   Synthetic steroids used as anti-inflammatories in certain medical conditions.

Glucogenolysis   Epinephrine is responsible for converting stored glycogen (carbohydrates) into glucose (in the liver).

H

Half-life (T 1/2.)   The time required for the concentration of a drug in the blood to be reduced by 50 percent (or 1/2). For example, penicillin G has a half-life of 20 minutes. This means that 50 percent of the drug remains in the blood 20 minutes after its intravenous administration.

Hemorrhage   Profuse bleeding.

Hepatic   Refers to the liver.

Hepatic cytochrome enzyme system   Enzymes found in the liver that are responsible for most biotransformation (or metabolism) of drugs. The primary action of these enzymes is to inactive drugs, which makes them more water soluble, to be excreted in the urine. Many drug–drug interactions can be explained by changes in the activity of these enzymes. Examples of some enzymes in the liver include CYP3A4 (CYP refers to cytochrome) and CYP2C9. Erythromycin and clarithromycin inhibit the CYP3A4 enzyme in the liver, which decreases the metabolism and elimination of alprazolam (Xanax; anti-anxiety drug) and ketoconazole (Nizoral; antifungal drug), resulting in increased/toxic blood levels of these drugs.

Hepatotoxicity (hepatotoxic)   Liver damage that is caused by many factors, including certain drugs.

Herbal (as in herbal supplements)   Use of medicinal herbs (plants) to prevent and treat diseases and ailments or to promote health and healing.

Herpes simplex virus   Virus that causes oropharygeal disease (eyes, lips, mouth, face) (HSV-1) and sexually transmitted disease (HSV-2).

High-Density Lipoprotein (HDL)   Lipid carrying particle in the blood that contains high amounts of protein and lower amounts of cholesterol; considered to be "good" cholesterol.

Highly Active Antiretroviral Therapy (HAART)   Drug therapy for HIV infection which includes high doses of three-drug combination regimens that are given concurrently.

Hormone   Chemical secreted by endocrine glands that act as a chemical messenger to effect homeostasis.

Host   The recipient (one that receives).

Host Flora   Normal microorganisms found in or on an individual.

Hydrophilic   "Water-loving"; refers to drugs that are water-soluble and do not dissolve easily in the lipid layer of the cell membrane. These drugs must go through pores or channels in the membrane.

Hydroxyapatite   Mineral component of bones and teeth.

Hypercholesterolemia   High levels of cholesterol in the blood.

Hyperglycemia   High glucose level in the blood.

Hyperkalemia   High potassium levels in the blood.

Hyperlipidemia   Excess amount of lipids in the blood.

Hypertension   High blood pressure.

Hypervitaminosis   Excessive intake of vitamins.

Hypnotic   Drug that induces sleep.

Hypoglycemia   Low glucose level in the blood.

Hypokalemia   Low potassium levels in the blood.

I

Immunocompetent   Normal immune systems.

Immunocompromised   Immune systems are not functioning properly; seen in medically ill patients such as HIV/AIDS.

Inotropic effect   Change on the strength of contractility of the heart.

Insulin   Hormone secreted by the beta cells of the pancreas. Keeps glucose levels within a normal range within the blood.

Insulin resistance   Decreased insulin effectiveness with a reduced sensitivity of the beta cells to respond to the insulin.

Interferons   A group of naturally occurring proteins that act as chemical messengers between cells. Three interferons, alpha, beta and gamma, have immune-modulating effects. Used in the treatment of cancer, hepatitis and autoimmune diseases.

Interleukins   A type of cytokine that regulates or stimulates immune cells.

Intradermal (ID) route   Drug is administered with a needle into the top layer (dermis) of skin.

Intramuscular (IM) route   Drug is administered with a needle into specific muscles.

Intravenous (IV) route   Drug is administered with a needle directly into the bloodstream. There is 100 percent bioavailability.

Ionized   Ionized form of a drug has a high water solubility, which means that the drug will diffuse (cross) lipid (fat) membranes with more difficulty than unionized/fat-soluble drugs. Ionized drugs are more water soluble and are more rapidly excreted in the urine than nonionized drugs.

Ischemia   Decreased blood supply to an organ or tissue.

Isoenzymes   Any of the chemically distinct forms of an enzyme that perform the same function.

L

Ligand   Refers to a molecule or drug that binds to another chemical entity to form a larger complex (e.g., a drug binding to a receptor resulting in a pharmacologic action).

Lipid   Refers to "fat."

Lipophylic   "Fat-loving"; refers to drugs that are lipid soluble and will dissolve easily in the lipid layer of the cell membrane.

Lipoproteins   Transport cholesterol, triglycerides, proteins and phospholipids in the blood (because lipids are insoluble in plasma). Different types: HDL, LDL, VLDL.

Loading dose   A high amount of drug is administered, usually as a first dose, which is intended to supply the blood with a level sufficient quickly to induce a therapeutic response. A maintenance dose is administered afterward.

Local anesthetic   Loss sensation to a limited part of the body without loss of consciousness (e.g., dental local anesthetics).

Low-Density Lipoproteins (LDL)   Lipid-carrying particle that contains relatively low amounts of protein and high amounts of cholesterol; considered to be "bad" cholesterol.

M

Maintenance dose   After a loading dose is administered and before plasma levels drop to zero, a maintenance dose is administered to keep the plasma drug concentration in the therapeutic range.

Manic   Disorder characterized by impulsive, excitable, and over-reactive actions.

Mechanism of action   How a drug exerts its effects.

Median Effective Dose (ED$_{50}$)   Dose required to produce a specific therapeutic response in 50 percent of a group of patients.

Median Lethal Dose (LD$_{50}$)   Often determined in preclinical trials, the dose of drug that will be lethal (kill) in 50 percent of a group of patients.

Median Toxicity Dose (TD$_{50}$)   Dose that will produce a given toxicity in 50 percent of a group of patients.

Megadoses   Usually referring to vitamins; doses of a nutrient that are more than the recommended amount.

Metabolism   (Metabolize; biotransformation.) *See also* Biotransformation Breakdown of fat-soluble drugs into water-soluble form. Primary site of metabolism is the liver.

Migraine   Common type of vascular headache involving abnormal sensitivity of arteries in the brain to various triggers.

Minerals   Natural compounds formed through geological processes; used as supplements in some medical conditions. Examples: calcium, magnesium.

Minimum effective concentration   The amount of a drug required to produce a therapeutic effect or response.

Miosis   Constriction of the pupil.

Moderate sedation   Formerly referred to as conscious sedation. Administration of drugs for the purpose of sleepiness (sedation), unaware of surroundings, amnesia or analgesia without loss of consciousness.

Monoamine Oxidase Inhibitors (MAOIs)   Drugs used to treat depression. Inhibit the enzyme monoamine oxidase which terminates the actions of neurotransmitters such as norepinephrine, epinephrine, dopamine, and serotonin. By inhibiting the enzyme action, the levels of these neurotransmitters are elevated.

Monotherapy   Use of one drug to treat a condition because it reduces the incidence of adverse effect, (e.g. monotherapy is the prefered treatment option in epilepsy).

Mood disorder   Change in behavior such as clinical depression, emotional swings, or manic depression.

Morbidity (rate)   The proportion of patients with a particular disease during a given year per given unit of population; the incidence or prevalence rate of a disease.

Mortality   Death rate.

Muscarinic receptor   *See* Receptors. Type of cholinergic receptor found in smooth muscle, cardiac muscle, and glands.

Mydriasis   Dilation of the pupil of the eye.

Myocardial infarction   Heart attack.

N

Narcotic (also refered to as opioids)   Natural or synthetic drug related to morphine; may be used as a broader legal term referring to hallucinogens, CNS stimulants, marijuana, and other illegal drugs.

Narrow therapeutic index   Dose of the desired or therapeutic effect is close to the toxic dose. Examples of drugs with a narrow therapeutic index are lithium and digoxin.

Narrow-spectrum antibiotic   Anti-infective (antimicrobial) drug that has an effect against only one or a small number of micro-organisms.

Negative symptoms   In schizophrenia, symptoms that subtract from normal behavior including a lack of interest, motivation, responsiveness or pleasure in daily activities.

Nephrotoxicity (nephrotoxic)   Pertaining to kidney failure.

Nerve membrane   Nerve sheath that surrounds a nerve cell. Local anesthetic must penetrate the membrane to be effective.

Nervous system

> **Autonomic Nervous System (ANS)**   Portion of the nervous system that regulates involuntary body functions including the heart and intestines.
>
> **Central Nervous System (CNS)**   Portion of the nervous system that consists of the brain and spinal cord.
>
> **Peripheal Nervous System (PNS)**   Portion of the nervous system that is outside the brain and spinal cord. The nerves in the PNS connect the CNS to sensory organs (e.g., eyes), other body organs, muscle, blood vessels and glands.

Neuralgia   Sharp, severe pain extending along a nerve or group of nerves.

Neuromuscular blocker   Drug used to cause total muscle relaxation.

Neuron   Cell that is the functional unit of the nervous system.

Neuropathic pain   Pain sustained by abnormal processing of sensory input by the peripheral or central nervous system. It is often described as burning, tingling, or shooting. Examples include: cancer-related pain, diabetic neuropathy, HIV-associated pain, postherpetic neuralgia, and trigeminal neuralgia.

Neurotransmitter   A chemical released by nerves at synapses and neuromuscular junctions.

Nicotonic receptor   *See* Receptors. Type of cholinergic receptor found in ganglia of both the sympathetic and parasympathetic nervous system.

Nitrous oxide   A colorless, sweet-tasting gas, N_2O, used as a mild anesthetic in dentistry and surgery.

Nociceptive pain   Pain arising from a stimulus (e.g., injury to tissues) that is outside of the central nervous system. Pain comes from skin, bone, joint, muscle or connective tissue. Pain is often described as throbbing and is well localized. Examples include pulpitis, postperiodontal surgery, post-extraction, and dentinal hypersensitivity.

Nonionized   Nonionized form of drugs have a high lipid (fat) solubility which easily crosses cell membranes, made of lipids. During excretion from the body, most nonionized drugs must be reabsorbed into the blood before being excreted in the urine because they need to be in a water-soluble form to be excreted.

Norepineprine (NE)   A neurotransmitter released from sympathetic nerves. Causes increased heart rate (β_1-receptor stimulation) and vasoconstriction in arteries and veins (α_1- and α_2-receptor stimulation).

O

Odontogenic   Pertaining to teeth.

Opiate   Any preparation or derivative of opium.

Opioid   A narcotic substance, either natural or synthetic.

Oral   Route of delivery in which drugs are swallowed, chewed, or dissolved in the mouth.

Oral lesion   An area of altered tissue in the mouth.

Orofacial   Pertaining to the mouth (oro) and face (facial), as in orofacial pain (pain in and around the mouth and the face).

Orthostatic hypotension Fall in blood pressure that occurs when changing position from recumbent to upright.

Osteonecrosis of the jaws (Bisphosphonate-associated osteonecrosis of the jaws) severe condition associated with the use of IV and oral bisphosphonates. Characterized by necrosis of the jawbone.

Over-the-counter drugs (OTC) Medications that can be obtained without a prescription.

P

Parasympathetic nervous system Part of the autonomic nervous system that is active during resting and digestion periods; produces a relaxation response (e.g., increases gastrointestinal movement and slows heart rate).

Parasympathomimetics Drugs that mimic the actions of the parasympathetic nervous system.

Parenteral route Delivery of a drug by all routes except oral and topical. Drug is administered with a needle into the skin, subcutaneous tissue, muscles, or veins.

Parkinson's Disease Degenerative condition of the nervous system caused by a deficiency of the brain neurotransmitter dopamine that results in disturbances of muscle movement.

Parkinsonism Having tremor, muscle rigidity, stooped posture, and a shuffling walk.

Pellagra Deficiency of niacin (vitamin B_3).

Peptic ulcer Erosion of the mucosa of the lining of the esophagus, stomach, or duodenum. Usually caused by the bacterium *Helicobacter pylori* (*H. pylori*). An ulcer in the stomach is called a gastric ulcer, a duodenal ulcer in the duodenum.

Periocoronitis Infection of the tissue (operculum) overlying a partially erupted tooth.

Peripheral Nervous System Division of the nervous system that includes all nerves outside the central nervous system, including the autonomic nervous system.

Permeability (Permeable.) The flow of a substance through a porous material.

pH A measure of the acidity or alkalinity of a solution. Involved in the absorption and solubility of drugs.

Pharmacodynamics What the drug does to the body: drug action on the body, mechanism of action of the drug.

Pharmacogenetics Convergence of pharmacology and genetics, which deals with genetic factors that influence an organism's response to a drug.

Pharmacokinetics What the body does to the drug: absorption (movement of the drug through the body); distribution, metabolism, and elimination.

Pharmacology Comes from the Greek words *pharmakos,* which means drug or medicine, and *logos,* which means study.

Photosensitivity Condition that occurs when the skin is highly sensitive to sunlight. Some drugs are photosensitive, including doxycycline and ciprofloxacin.

Placebo A pill or injection that has no pharmacologic action. It exerts no therapeutic effect and produces no side effects. Used in clinical studies. Patients often report a decrease in symptoms and side effects. This is the power of suggestion.

Plasma The fluid portion of blood. Whole blood does not clot. The red blood cells are centrifuged down.

Plasma half-life *See* Half-life.

Polar Soluble in water.

Polypharmacy (also referred to as polytherapy) Use of multiple medications.

Polytherapy See polypharmacy.

Positive symptoms In schizophrenia, symptoms that add on to normal behavior, including hallucinations, delusions, and a disorganized thought or speech pattern.

Posology Study of the dosages of medicines and drugs.

Postsynaptic neuron Neuron in the synapse that has receptors for the neurostransmitter.

Potency The strength of a drug at a specific concentration or dose.

Pregnancy category Classifying drugs based upon how safe they are for the unborn fetus. Category A, B, C, D, or X.

Prescription A prescriber's order (written or oral) to dispense a specific drug.

Prescription drugs Drugs obtained with a prescription (oral or written).

Presynaptic neuron Neuron that releases the neurotransmitter into the synaptic cleft.

Prodrug Drugs that are administered into the body as inactive compounds and must be biotransformed or metabolized in the liver to an active form that will result in a pharmacologic effect or response in the body.

Prophylaxis (Prophylactically; prophylactic.) Prevention of disease with treatment (e.g., antibiotic prophylaxis to prevent infective endocarditis).

Prostaglandins Class of hormones that promotes local inflammation and pain when released by cells in the body.

Protein A large complex molecule made up of one or more chains of amino acids. Proteins perform activities inside the cell.

Protein bound After being absorbed into the blood, a drug may become bound (bind) to proteins (albumin) in the blood. These protein-bound drugs are inactive.

Proton pump inhibitors Drugs that inhibit the enzyme H^+, K^+-ATPase. Used in the treatment of ulcers.

R

Reabsorption Elimination process whereby after being filtered out of the blood and through the kidneys nonionized, lipid-soluble drugs cross back through the kidney membrane and return to the blood (circulation), and are not eliminated, in order to be further metabolized into a more water-soluble form to be excreted. Ionized and water-soluble drugs generally do not get reabsorbed back into the circulation, but remain in the filtrate for excretion because these drugs are water soluble and are easily excreted in the urine.

Receptors Component (protein) of a cell to which a drug binds in a dose-related manner, to produce a response:

    Adrenergic Receptors on sympathetic nerves.

    Cholinergic Receptors on nerves that release acetylcholine.

    Alpha (α) Type of subreceptor found in the sympathetic nervous system.

    Beta (β) Type of subreceptor found in the sympathetic nervous system.

    Nicotinic Type of cholinergic receptor found in ganglia of both sympathetic and parasympathetic nervous systems.

    Muscarinic Type of cholinergic receptor found in/on smooth muscle, cardiac muscle, and glands.

Recommended Daily Allowance (RDA) Amount of vitamin or mineral needed each day to avoid a deficiency in a healthy adult.

Recurrent Minor aphthous ulcer (also referred to as canker sore).

Reflex tachycardia If blood pressure decreases, the heart beats faster in an attempt to raise it.

Refractory Resistant to treatment.

Renal Refers to the kidneys.

Renin-angiotensin system Series of enzymatic steps by which the body elevates blood pressure.

Retinoid Compound resembling vitamin A. Indicated in the treatment of severe acne and psoriasis.

Reye's Syndrome Potentially fatal complication of infection associated with aspirin use in children.

Rhinitis Inflammation of the nasal mucous membranes.

Risk factor An environmental, behavioral or biologic factor that definitely increases the probability that something will occur.

S

Scheduled drug Drugs (narcotics) that have a significant potential for abuse. There are five categories based on the abuse potential: Schedule I (high potential for abuse), Schedule II, Schedule III, Schedule IV, and Schedule V (lowest abuse potential).

Schizophrenia Psychosis characterized by abnormal thoughts, withdrawal from people and the outside environment, and preoccupation with one's own mental state.

Secretion (Secrete.) The passage of material from the inside of a cell to the outside.

Sedative-hypnotic Drug that produces a calming, sedative effect in low doses and sleep in higher doses.

Sedative Drug that quiets, calms or allays excitement.

Seizures Symptom of epilepsy characterized by abnormal electrical charges within the brain.

    Generalized seizures Seizures that go through the entire brain on both sides.

    Partial seizures Seizures that start on one side of the brain and go a short distance before stopping.

Selective Serotonin Reuptake Inhibitor (SSRI) Drug that selectively inhibits the reuptake of serotonin into the nerve terminal; used for the treatment of depression.

Selectivity Responses involving any given type of receptor, only elicited by a narrow range of drugs with similar structural properties.

Sensitivity Referring to receptors. Drugs producing marked effects at low doses.

Serotonin A compound formed from tryptophan and found in the brain, blood, and gastric mucous membranes. A neurotransmitter.

Serotonin syndrome A condition that is caused by taking selective serotonin reuptake inhibitors (SSRIs) with MAOIs. This results in increased serotonin levels increase in the brain. Characterized by agitation, confusion, severe hypertension and G.I. symptoms.

Serum Whole blood is allowed to clot. The red blood cells and fibrinogen are centrifuged down. The supernatant fluid is serum.

Sex hormones Any of various hormones, such as estrogen and androgen, affecting the growth or function of the reproductive organs and the development of secondary sex characteristics.

Soluble Dissolves in a solution.

Steroid Type of lipid that makes up certain hormones and drugs.

Subcutaneous (SC, SQ) route Drug is injected with a needle into the deepest layers of the skin. Insulin is given this route.

Sublingual Route (SL) Drug is placed under the tongue and allowed to dissolve slowly. Rapid onset of drug action because this area is very vascular (a lot of blood vessels).

Substance P Protein substance that stimulates nerve endings at an injury site and within the spinal cord, increasing pain messages.

Superinfection An infection, usually an fungus such as *Candida albicans,* caused by an organism different from the one causing the initial infection. It is usually an adverse side effect of broad-spectrum antibiotics.

Sympathetic The part of the autonomic nervous system (ANS) that deals with stress or "fight or flight." When stimulated, heart rate increases.

Sympatholytic A drug that blocks the actions of the sympathetic nervous system.

Sympathomimetic A drug that stimulates or mimics the sympathetic nervous system.

Synapse Junction between two neurons consisting of a presynaptic (preganglionic) neuron, a synaptic cleft, and a postsynaptic (postganglionic) neuron.

Synaptic cleft Space between two neurons that must be crossed by the neurotransmitter.

Syncope Fainting.

T

Tachycardia Increased heart rate.

Tachyphylaxis Rapidly decreasing response to a drug following initial doses; a type of tolerance.

Tardive dyskinesia Unusual tongue and face movements such as lip-smacking and wormlike motions of the tongue that occur during treatment with antipsychotic drugs.

Teratogen A chemical substance that harms a developing fetus or embryo.

Teratogenic Causing malformations of an embryo or fetus.

Testosterone Hormone produced by the testes; male sex hormone important in the development of secondary sex characteristics and masculinization.

Therapeutic Index The ratio of a drug's LD_{50} to its ED_{50}.

Therapeutic Range The plasma (blood) drug concentration between the minimum effect concentration and the toxic concentration.

Thrombocytopenia Low platelet count.

Thrombosis Enhanced formation of fibrin.

Thyroid gland Gland produces and releases thyroid hormones that are involved in the regulation of basal metabolic rate or the speed by which cells perform their functions. By increasing cellular metabolism, thyroid hormone increases body temperature. The gland also helps to maintain blood pressure and regulate growth and development.

Thyroxine (T_4) Major hormone secreted by the thyroid gland.

Tolerance Need for increased amount of a substance to achieve the same desired effect or intoxication.

Topical The route by which drugs are placed directly onto the skin or mucous membranes. Example: topical dental anesthetic.

Toxic concentration The plasma level of a drug that will result in serious adverse effects.

Trade name Drug name assigned by the company marketing the drug. Example: Tylenol is the trade name of the drug acetaminophen.

Transdermal drug delivery Drug from a patch penetrates the top layer of skin.

Tricyclic antidepressant Class of drugs used in the management of depression.

Triglycerides Type of lipid in the body and the main storage form of energy to support the generation of high-energy compounds.

Triiodothyronine (T_3) At the target tissue, thyroxine is converted to T_3 which enters the target cells and binds to receptors inside the cell; it is the active form of the thyroid hormone.

Tuberculosis   Bacterial infection affecting primarily the lungs, more common in urban areas, treatable with antibiotics.

Tyroxine   Hormone produced by the thyroid gland; important in growth and development and regulation of the body's metabolic rate and metabolism of carbohydrates, fats, and proteins.

V

Vascular   Referring to blood vessels.

Vasoconstriction   The narrowing of blood vessels; causes blood pressure to rise.

Vasoconstrictor   A drug added to local anesthetics to counteract the vasodilating effects of the anesthetic agent. Example is epinephrine.

Vasodilation (vasodiliation)   Relaxation of the smooth muscles of the blood vessels producing dilated vessels; causes blood pressure to lower.

Very Low-Density Lipoprotein (VLDL)   Lipid-carrying particle that is converted to LDL in the liver.

Vitamins   Organic compounds required by the body small amounts.

W

Withdrawal   Physical signs of discomfort associated with drug abuse.

X

Xerostomia   Dry mouth.

Appendix **A**

Controlled Substances

Schedule	Characteristics	Dispensing Restrictions	Examples
C-I	For research use only; high abuse, high dependency risk	• Approved protocol necessary	LSD, heroin, marijuana, methaqualone
C-II	High abuse, high dependency risk	• No telephone prescriptions are allowed unless an emergency, and then a written prescription must be sent to the pharmacy within 72 hours. The label states "Authorization for emergency dispensing"; no refills on prescriptions	Opium, codeine, cocaine, amphetamines, methadone, morphine (oxycodone), Percodan, hydromor- (Dilaudid), methylphenidate (Ritalin), secobarbital
C-III	Lower abuse than C-II, moderate dependency risk	• Not more than five refills in 6 months • Oral (telephone) prescriptions permitted. • Must receive a written prescription within 72 hours.	Opiates in combination with one or more active nonnarcotic ingredients: codeine + acetaminophen
C-IV	Lower potential for abuse than C-III, low-to-moderate dependency	• Same as C-III	Chloral hydrate, Phenobarbital, benzodiazepine (e.g., Valium) (in some states it is considered to be a C-II)
C-V	Lower potential for abuse than C-IV, limited dependency	• May be an OTC depending on the state law • If OTC: Purchaser must be at least 18 years of age • A bound record book shall be maintained • May be dispensed only by a pharmacist • Suitable identification required	Limited quantities of certain narcotic drugs for antitussive (anticough) and antidiarrheal purposes

Appendix B

Pregnancy and Breast Feeding

The Food and Drug Administration requires that all prescription drugs absorbed systemically or that are known to be potentially harmful to the fetus be given a pregnancy category of A, B, C, D or X. The following table lists all categories.

Category	Description	During Breast Feeding
A	Controlled studies in women fail to show a risk to the fetus	Yes
B	Animal or human studies have not shown a significant risk to the fetus. No controlled studies in pregnant women. Drugs that have been found to have adverse effects in animals but no well controlled studies of humans.	Yes
C	Drugs for which there are no adequate studies, either animal or humans, or drugs shown to have adverse fetal effects in animals but for which no human data are available.	Yes
D	Fetal risk in humans is evident.	No
X	Studies in animals or humans have shown definitive fetal risk. These drugs are contra-indicated in women who are or may become pregnant.	No

List of Common Dental Drugs: During Pregnancy and Nursing

Drug	FDA Category	Can Use During Pregnancy?	Can Use During Nursing?
Antibiotics			
Penicillin	B	Yes	Yes
Amoxicillin	B	Yes	Yes
Erythromycin	B	Yes (except for esolate form)	Yes
Clarithyromycin	C	No	No
Azithromycin	B	Yes; no human studies	Not enough information
Clindamycin	B		Yes
Metronidazole	B	Yes Not in first trimester	Discontinue breast-feeding for 12–24 hours
Tetracyclines	D	No	No
Analgesics			
Acetaminophen	B	Yes	Yes
Aspirin	C (in low dose		
Ibuprofen (all NSAIDs)	< 150 mg/day D (in standard doses) B/D (if used in third trimester)	No No (not in third trimester)	Give with caution Maybe (ibuprofen, with more information)
Codeine (e.g., acetaminophen with codeine)	C	No	
Hydrodone (e.g., Vicodin)	C/D	No	No
Antifungal Agents			
Nystatin	B	Yes	Yes
Clotrimazole (topical)	B	Yes	Yes
Antiviral Agents			
Acyclovir			
Penciclovir cream	B	Uncertain	Found in breast milk
	B	Yes	Found in breast milk
Local Anesthetics			**(It is not known whether local anesthetics are excreted in human milk.)**
Lidocaine	B	Yes	Caution
Mepivacaine	C	No	Caution

Drug	FDA Category	Can Use During Pregnancy?	Can Use During Nursing?
Bupivacaine	C	No	No
Etidocaine	B	Yes	Yes
Articaine	C	No	Caution
Marcaine	C	No	Caution
Anesthesia			
Nitrous oxide	unclassified	Not in first trimester; with caution in third trimester	Yes
Antianxiety Drugs			
Benzodiazepines (e.g., diazepam, alprazolam)	D X (Triazolam and Temazepam)	No	No

Appendix C

Drugs That Cause Photosensitivity

Some drugs may increase sensitivity to ultraviolet light, resulting in a phototoxic or photoallergic response which clinically is evident as exaggerated sunburn. Patients should avoid excessive sun exposure.

The following are some potential photosensitizing agents.

Product Class	Drug Name
Acne	Retinoic acid (tretinion), Retin-A, isotretinoin (Accutane)
Antibacterials	Sulfonamides
Antibiotics	Tetracyclines (doxycycline, minocycline)
Anticonvulsants	Carbamazepine (Tegretol)
Antidepressants	Amitriptyline (Elavid), desipramine (Norpramin), imipramine (Tofranil)
Antidiabetics	First generation sulfonylureas
Antihistamines	Diphenydramine (Benadryl)
Diuretics	Thiazides, flurosemide (Lasix)
Antipsychotics	Phenothiazines

Appendix D

Quick Drug Reference

(*Note:* not all drugs are listed, but more drugs can be found within the corresponding chapter)

Class/Generic Name	Brand (Market) Name
Analgesics	
Salicylates	
Aspirin	Generics
Salsalate	Disalcid
NSAIDS; COX-2 Inhibitors	
Celecoxib	Celebrex
Nonsteroidal Anti-Inflammatory Drugs (NSAIDs)/ Nonsalicylates	
Diclofenac	Voltaren
Diflunisal	Dolobid
Etodoloc	Generic only
Fenoprofen	Nalfon
Flurbiprofen	Ansaid
Ibuprofen	Motrin, Advil, Nuprin
Indomethacin	Indocin
Ketoprofen	Orudis, Actron
Ketorolac	Toradol
Mefenamic	Ponstel
Meloxicam	Mobic
Nabumetone	Relafen
Naproxen	Naproxyn, Aleve
Naproxen sodium	Anaprox
Oxaprozin	Daypro
Piroxicam	Feldene
Sulindac	Clinoril
Tolmetin	Tolectin
Narcotic Analgesics	
Codeine (CII)	Codeine
Codeine/acetaminophen (APAP) (CIII)	Tylenol w/codeine
Fentanyl (CII)	Duragesic
Hydrocodone/ibuprofen (CIII)	Vicoprofen
Hydrocodone/APAP (CIII)	Vicodin, Lortab, Vicodin ES, Vicodin HP

Class/Generic Name	*Brand (Market) Name*
Hydromorphone (CII)	Dilaudid
Meperidine (CII)	Demoral
Methadone (CII)	Dolophine
Morphine (CII)	Contin
Oxycodone (CII)	Oxycontin, Roxicodone
Oxycodone/APAP (CII)	Percocet, Tylox
Oxycodone/aspirin (CII)	Percodan
Oxycodone/ibuprofen (CII)	Combunox
Pentazocine/aspirin (CIV)	Talwin compound
Propoxyphene (CIV)	Darvon
Propoxyphene/Aspirin/Caffeine (CIV)	Darvon Compound-65
Propoxyphene/Acetaminophen (CIV)	Darvocet-A 500, Darvocet-N 50, Darvocet-N 100

Other Analgesics

Acetaminophen	Generics; Tylenol
Tramadol	Ultram

Anti-infectives

Antibacterials

PENICILLINS

Penicillin VK	V-Cillin K
Ampicillin	Omniphen
Amoxicillin	Amoxil, Trimox
Amoxicillin + clavulanate	Augmentin
Ampicillin + sulbactam	Unasyn
Carbenicillin	Geocillin
Dicloxacillin	Dynapen

CEPHALOSPORINS (SOME)

Cephalexin	Keflex
Cephradrine	Velosef
Cefaclor	Ceclor
Cefadroxil	Duricef
Cefepime	Maxipime
Cefotaxime	Claforan

MACROLIDES

Erythromycin	E-Mycin, Ery-Tab, PCE
Erythromycin stearate	Erythrocin

Class/Generic Name	Brand (Market) Name
Erythromycin ethyl succinate	EES
Troleandomycin	TAO
AZALIDES	
Azithromycin	Zithromax
Clarithromycin	Biaxin
Telithromycin	Ketek
LINCOMYCINS	
Clindamycin	Cleocin
TETRACYCLINES	
Tetracycline HCl	Generics-sumycin
Doxycycline hyclate	Vibramycin, Doryx
Doxycycline hyclate, 20 mg	Periostat, generic
Doxycycline hyclate, topical	Atridox
Minocycline HCl	Minocin
Minocycline HCl, topical	Arestin
Metronidazole	Flagyl
FLUROQUINOLONES (SOME)	
Ciprofloxacin	Cipro
Gatifloxacin	Tequin
Levofloxacin	Levaquin
Ofloxacin	Floxin
SULFONAMIDES (SOME)	
Sulfamethoxazole/trimethroprim	Bactrim
Sulfisoxazole	Gantrisin
Mycobacterial Infections (TB)	
Isoniazid	INH
Ethambutol	Myambutol
Pyrazinamide	PZA
Rifampin	rifadin
Ciprofloxacin	Cipro
Antifungals (Topical)	
Clotrimazole	Mycelex
Nystatin	Mycostatin
Antifungals (Systemic)	
Fluconazole	Diflucan
Griseofulvin	Fluvicin, Grifulvin

Class/Generic Name	Brand (Market) Name
Itraconazole	Sporanox
Ketoconazole	Nizoral
Nystatin	Mycostatin
Terbinafine	Lamisil

Antiretroviral Agents (AIDS)

Fusion Inhibitors

Enfuvirtide	Fuzeon

Nonnucleoside Reverse Transcriptase Inhibitors

Delavirdine	Rescriptor
Efavirenz	Sustiva

Nucleoside Reverse Transcriptase Inhibitors

Abacavir	Ziagen
Abacavir/lamivudine/zidovudine	Trizivir
Didanosine	Videx
Emtricitabine	Emtriva
Lamivudine	Epivir
Lamivudine/zidovudine	Combivir
Stavudine	Zerit
Zalcitabine	HIVID
Zidovudine	Retrovir
Tenofivir	Viread

Protease Inhibitors

Amprenavir	Agenerase
Atazanavir	Reyataz
Fosamprenavir	Lexiva
Indinavir	Crixivan
Lopinavir	Kaletra
Nelfinavir	Viracept
Ritonavir	Norvir
Ritonavir	Norvir
Saquinavir mesylate	Invirase

Antivirals (herpes)

Acyclovir	Zovirax
Docosanol	Abreva
Famciclovir	Famvir
Penciclovir	Denavir
Valacyclovir	Valtrex

Class/Generic Name	Brand (Market) Name
BISPHOSPHONATES	
Alendronate	Fosamax
Clodronate	Bonefos
Etidronate	Didronel
Ibandronate	Boniva
Pamidronate	Aredia
Risedronate	Actonel
Tiludronate	Skelid
Zoledronic acid	Zometa

Cardiovascular Agents

Angina Pectoris

BETA$_1$-BLOCKERS/CARDIOSELECTIVE

Acebutolol	Sectral
Atenolol	Tenormin
Betaxolol	Kerlone
Bisoprolol	Zebeta
Esmolol	Brevibloc
Metoprolol	Lopressor

BETA-BLOCKERS/NONCARDIOSELECTIVE (β_1, β_2)

Carteolol	Cartrol
Nadolol	Corgard
Pindolol	Visken
Propranolol	Inderal

CALCIUM CHANNEL BLOCKERS (DIHYDROPYRIDINE)

Amlodipine	Norvasc
Nicardipine	Cardene
Nifedipine	Procardia, Adalat

CALCIUM CHANNEL BLOCKERS (NONDIHYDROPYRIDINES)

Bepridil	Vascor
Diltiazem	Cardizem, Dilacor XR
Verapamil	Calan

VASODILATORS

Isosorbide	Isordil
Nitroglycerin	Nitro-Dur, Notro-Bid, Nitrostat, Nitrolingual Spray

Anti-arrhythmics

GROUP 1A

Disopyramide	Norpace

Class/Generic Name	Brand (Market) Name
Moricizine	Ethmozine
Procainamide	Procanbid, Pronestyl
Quinidine	Quinidex
GROUP 1B	
Lidocaine	Xylocaine
Mexiletine	Mexitil
GROUP 1C	
Flecainide	Tambocor
Propafenone	Rhythmol
GROUP II	
Acebutolol	Sectral
Propranolol	Inderal
GROUP III	
Amiodarone	Cordarone
Sotalol	Betapace
GROUP IV	
Verapamil	Calan
Digoxin	Lanoxin
Heart Failure	
ANGIOTENSIN CONVERTING ENZYME	
(ACE) INHIBITORS	
Captopril	Capoten
Enalapril	Vasotec
Fosinopril	Monopril
Lisinopril	Zestril, Prinivil
Quinapril	Accupril
Ramipril	Altace
ALPHA/BETA BLOCKERS	
Carvedilol	Coreg
ANGIOTENSIN II RECEPTOR ANTAGONISTS	
Valsartan	Diovan
BETA-BLOCKERS	
Metoprolol	Toprol
DIURETICS (LOOP)	
Bumetanide	Bumex
Ethacrynic acid	Edecrin

Class/Generic Name	*Brand (Market) Name*
Furosemide	Lasix
DIURETICS (POTASSIUM SPARING)	
Amiloride	Midamor
Spironolactone	Aldactone
Triamterene	Dyrenium
DIURETICS (POSTASSIUM SPARING/THIAZIDE)	
Amiloride/hydrochlorothiazide	Moduretic
Spronolactone (HCTZ)	Aldactazide
Triamterene/HCTZ	Dyzide
DIURETICS (THIAZIDES)	
Chlorothiazide	Diuril
Chlorthalidone	Thalitone
Methyclothiazide	Enduron
INOTROPIC AGENTS	
Digoxin	Lanoxin
Hypertension	
ACE INHIBITORS	
Benazepril	Lotensin
Captopril	Capoten
Enalapril	Vasotec
Fosinopril	Monopril
Lisinopril	Prinivil, Zestril
Quinapril	Accupril
Ramipril	Altace
ACE INHIBITORS/CALCIUM CHANNEL BLOCKERS	
Benazepril/amiodipine	Lotrel
Trandolapril/verapamil	Tarka
ALPHA-ADRENERGIC BLOCKERS	
Clonidine	Catapres
Doxazosin	Cardura
Methyldopa	Aldomet
Prazosin	Minipress
Reserpine	Generics
Terazosin	Hytrin
ALPHA-BETA BLOCKERS	
Carvedilol	Coreg
Labetalol	Normodyne

Class/Generic Name	*Brand (Market) Name*
ANGIOTENSIN II RECEPTOR ANTAGONISTS	
Candesartan	Atacand
Eprosartan	Teveten
Irbesartan	Avapro
Losartan	Cozaar
Valsartan	Diovan
ANGIOTENSIN II RECEPTOR ANTAGONISTS/THIAZIDES	
Candesartan/hydrochlorothiazide	Atacand HCT
Irbesartan/HCTZ	Avalide
Losartan/HCTZ	Hyzaar
Valsartan/HCTZ	Diovan HCT
BETA-BLOCKERS	
Acebutolol	Sectral
Atenolol	Tenormon
Betaxolol	Kerlone
Bisoprolol	Zebeta
Carteolol	Cartrol
Esmolol	Brevibloc
Metoprolol tartrate	Lopressor
Nadolol	Corgard
Propranolol	Inderal
Timolol	Blocadren
CALCIUM CHANNEL BLOCKERS (DIHYDROPYRIDINES)	
Amlodipine	Norvasc
Felodipine	Plendil
Isradipine	DynaCirc
Nicardipine	Cardene
Nifedipine	Adalat, Procardia
Nisoldipine	Sutar
CALCIUM CHANNEL BLOCKERS (NONDIHYROPYRIDINES)	
Diltiazem	Cardiazem
Verapamil	Calan, Isoptin, Verelan
DIURETICS (LOOP)	
Furosemide	Lasix
DIURETICS (POTASSIUM SPARING)	
Amiloride	Midamor
Sprironolactone	Aldactone
Triamterene	Dyrenium

Class/Generic Name	Brand (Market) Name
DIURETICS (THIAZIDES)	
Chlorothiazide	Diuril
Hydrochlorothiazide	Hydrodiuril
Methyclothiazide	Enduron
Antilipidemic Agents	
Bile acid sequestrants	
Chloestryramine	Questran
Colestipol	Colestid
Cholesterol absorption inhibitor	
Ezetimibe	Zetia
Fibric acids	
Clofibrate	Atromid-s
Fenofibrate	Tricor
Gemfibrozil	Lopid
HMG-CoA Reductase inhibitors (statins)	
Atorvastatin	Lipitor
Fluvastatin	Lescol
Lovastatin	Mevacor
Pravastatin	Pravachol
Rosuvastatin	Crestor
Simvastatin	Zocor
Nicotinic Acid	
Niacin (nicotinic acid; vitamin B_3)	Nicobid
Platelet aggregation-adhesion inhibitors	
Aspirin	Ecotrin, Bayer Aspirin
Clopidogrel	Plavix
Dipyridamole	Persantine
Aspirin/dipyridamole	Aggrenox
Anticoagulants	
Heparin	Hep-Lock
Warfarin	Coumadin
Central Nervous System	
Anticonvulsants for seizure	
Clonazepam CIV	Klonopin
Diazepam CIV	Valium
Lorazempam CIV	Ativan

Class/Generic Name	*Brand (Market) Name*
Phenytoin	Dilatinin
Ethosuximide	Zarontin
Levetiracetam	Keppra
Methsuximide	Celontin
Carbamazepine	Tegretol, Carbatrol
Divalproex	Depakote
Gabapentin	Neurontin
Primidone	Mysoline
Valproic acid	Depakene
Lamotrigine	Lamictal
Tiagabine	Gabitril
Pregabalin	Lyrica
Zonisamide	Zonegran
Migraine Triptans	
Almotriptan	Axert
Eletriptan	Relpax
Frovatriptan	Frova
Naratriptan	Amerge
Rizatriptan	Maxalt
Sumatriptan	Imitrex
Zolmitriptan	Zomig
Anticonvulsants (migraine)	
Levetiracetam	Keppra
Topiramate	Topamax
Valproic acid	Depakene
Zonisamide	Zonegran
NSAIDs	
Ibuprofen	Advil, Motrin, Nuprin
Naproxen	Naprosyn
Naproxen sodium	Aleve, Anaprox
Endocrine System	
Topical Corticosteroids	
Amcinonide	Cyclocort
Betamethasone valerate	Betarex, Beta-Val
Clobetasol propionate	Cormax, Temovate
Desoximetasone	Topicort
Fluocinolone acetonide	Synalar
Fluocinonide	Lidex

Class/Generic Name	Brand (Market) Name
Flurandrenolide	Cordan
Halcinonide	Halog
Hydrocortisone	Cortaid, Hytone, Hydrocort
Triamcinolone acetonide	Aristocort A, Kenalog
Systemic Corticosteroids	
Betamethasone	Celestone
Cortisone acetate	Cortisone
Dexamethasone	Decadron
Hydrocortisone	Cortef
Methyprednisolone	Medrol
Prednisolone	Prelone
Prednisone	Deltasone
Trimacinolone	Aristocort
Antidiabetic Agents	
Biguanides	
Metformin	Glucophage
Glucosidase Inhibitors	
Acarbose	Precose
Miglitol	Glyset
Meglitinides	
Nateglinide	Starlix
Repaglinide	Prandin
Sulfonylureas (first generation)	
Chlopropamide	Diabinese
Tolazamide	Tolinase
Tolbutamide	Tol-Tab
SULFONYLUREAS (SECOND GENERATION)	
Glimepiride	Amaryl
Glipizide	Glucotrol
Glyburide, micronized	Glynase
Glyburide	Diabeta, Micronase
Thiazolidinediones	
Pioglitazone	Actos
Rosiglitazone	Avandia
Sulfonylurea/biguanide	
Glipizide/metformin	Metaglip
Glyburide/metformin	Glucovance

Class/Generic Name	*Brand (Market) Name*
Thiazolidinediones/biguanide	
Rosiglitazone/metformin	Avandamet
Rosiglitazone/glimepiride	Avandaryl
Insulins	
Insulin glargine, human	Lantus
Insulin Lispro, human	Humalog
Insulin, NPH	Humulin N
Insulin, regular	Humulin R, Novolin R
Insulin aspart (rDNA origin)	Novolog
Antithyroid Agents	
Methimazole	Tapazole
Prophylthiouracil	PTU
Potassium iodide	SSKI, Lugol's solution
Thyroid Agents	
Levothyroxine sodium, T4	Synthroid
Liothyronine, T3	Cytomel
Thyroid, desiccated	Armour Thyroid
Contraceptives	
Ethinyl estradiol/norelgestromin patch	Ortho Evra
Levonorgestrel	Norplant
Medroxyprogesterone acetate	Depo-Provera
Oral Contraceptives	
MONOPHASIC	
Ethinyl estradiol/levonorgestrel	Alesse, Levite
Ethinyl estradiol/desogestrel	Ortho-Cept, Desogen, Apri
Ethinyl estradiol/norethindrone	Brevicon, Modicon
Ethinyl estradiol/ethynodiol diacetate	Demulen
Ethinyl estradiol/norgestrel	Lo/Ovral
Ethinyl estradiol/norethindrone	Ortho-Novum
Ethinyl estradiol/norgestrel	Ovral
Ethinyl estradiol/drospirenone	Yasmin
BIPHASIC	
Ethinyl estradiol/norethindrone	Ortho-Novum
Ethinyl estradiol/desogestrel	Mircette
Triphasic	
Ethinyl estradiol/northindrone	Ortho-Novum 10/11

Class/Generic Name	Brand (Market) Name
Ethinyl estradiol/norgestimate	Ortho Tri-Cyclen

Gastrointestinal Agents

Antidiarrheals

Atropine sulfate/diphenoxylate CV	Lomotil
Bismuth subsalicylate	Kaopectate, Pepto-Bismol
Loperamide	Imodium A-D

Antispasmodics

Atropine sulfate/hyoscyamine sulfate/ phenobarbital/scopolamine	Donnatal
Dicyclomine HCl	Bentyl

Antiulcer Agents

HELICOBACTER PYLORI TREATMENT REGIMENS

PPI + 1 gm amoxicillin bid + 500 mg clarithromycin bid	—
PPI + 500 mg metronidazole + 500 mg clarithromycin	—
400 mg ranitidine bismuth citrate + 500 mg clarithromycin + 1 gm amoxicillin or 500 mg metronidazole or 500 mg tetracycline	—
BSS qid + 500 metronidazole tid + 500 mg tetracycline qid + PPI qd	—
BSS + 250 mg metronidazole qid + 500 mg tetracycline qid + H_2 receptor antagonist qd	—
(PPI = esomeprazole 40 mg qd, lansoprazole 30 mg bid, omeprazole 20 mg bid, rabeprazole 20 mg bid, or pantoprazole 40 mg bid)	—
(BSS = bismuth subsalicylate 525 mg)	—

Protective barrier drug

Sucralfate	Carafate

H_2 Antagonists

Cimetidine	Tagamet
Famotidine	Pepcid
Nizatidine	Axid
Rantidine	Zantac

Prostaglandin E_1 Analog

Misoprostol	Cytotec

Proton Pump Inhibitors (PPI)

Lansoprazole	Prevacid

Class/Generic Name	*Brand (Market) Name*
Omeprazole	Prilosec
Rabeprazole sodium	Aciphex

GERD (gastrointestinal reflux disease)

DOPAMINE ANTAGONIST/PROKINETIC

Metoclopramide	Reglan

H₂ antagonists

Cimetidine	Tagamet
Famotidine	Pepcid
Nizatidine	Axid
Rantidine HCl	Zantac

Proton Pump Inhibitors

Esomeprazole magnesium	Nexium
Lansoprazole	Prevacid
Omeprazole	Prilosec
Pantoprazole sodium	Protonix
Rabeprazole sodium	Aciphex

Laxatives

Bowel evacuants

Polyethylene glycol with electrolytes	Colyte
Sodium phosphate/disodium phosphate	Visicol

Bulk-forming agents

Calcium polycarbophil	FiberCon
Methylcellulose	Citrucel
Psyllium	Metamucil

Emollient Laxative

Mineral oil	Mineral oil

Osmotic agent

Polyethylene glycol	MiraLax

Saline Laxatives

Magnesium citrate	Citrate of magnesia
Magnesium hydroxide	Milk of magnesia

Irritable Bowel Syndrome

Antidepressants

Amitriptyline	Elavil
Fluoxetine	Prozac
Paroxetine	Paxil

Class/Generic Name	Brand (Market) Name
Sertraline	Zoloft
Trazodone	Desyrel
Antidiarrheal agents	
Loperamide	Imodium
Cholestryramine	Questran powder
Antispasmodics	
Hyoscyamine	Levsin
Dicyclomine	Bentyl
Donnatal	Phenobarbital, hyoscyamine, atropine and scopolamine
Librax	Chlordiazepoxide/clidinium bromide
Narcotic Analgesics	
Codeine, acetaminophen, caffeine, butalbital	Fioricet
Botulinum Toxin	
Botulinum toxin Type A	Botox
Attention Deficit Hyperactivity Disorder (ADHD)	
NOREPINEPHRINE REUPTAKE INHIBITOR	
Atomoxetine	Strattera
Prodrug stimulant	
Lisotexamfetamine	Vyvanase
SYMPATHOMIMETICS	
Amphetamine and dextroamphetamine mixture CII	Adderall, Adderall XR
Dextroamphetamine CII	Dexedrine
Methamphetamine CII	Desoxyn
Methylphenidate CII	Concerta, Ritalin
Alzheimer's Therapy	
Donepezil	Aricept
Galantamine	Razadyne
Memantine	Namenda
Rivastigmine	Exelon
NMDA-RECEPTOR ANTAGONIST	
Memantine	Namenda
Anti-Anxiety/Hypnotic Agents	
BENZODIAZEPINES	
Alprazolam CIV	Xanax
Chlordiazepoxide CIV	Librium
Chlorzepate CIV	Tranxene

Class/Generic Name	Brand (Market) Name
Diazepam CIV	Valium
Estazolam CIV	ProSom
Flurazepam CIV	Dalmane
Lorazepam CIV	Ativan
Midazolam CIV	Versed
Quazepam CIV	Doral
Temazepam CIV	Restoril
Triazolam CIV	Halcion

Antidepressants

SELECTIVE SEROTONIN REUPTAKE INHIBITORS (SSRIs)

Escitalopram	Lexapro
Fluoxetine	Prozac
Paroxetine	Paxil
Sertraline	Zoloft

SEROTONIN/NE REUPTAKE INHIBITORS (SNRIs)

Venlafaxine	Effexor

MISCELLANEOUS

Buspirone	BuSpar
Chloral hydrate CIV	Noctec
Zaleplon CIV	Sonata
Soldiem CIV	Ambien

SEROTONIN/ALPHA₁ ANTAGONISTS

Nefazodone	Serzone

DOPAMINE/NOREPINEPHRINE REUPTAKE INHIBITORS

Bupropion	Wellbutrin

MONOAMINE OXIDASE INHIBITORS (MAOIs)

Isocarboxazid	Marplan
Phenelzine	Nardil
Tranylcypromine	Parnate

SERONTONIN/NE REUPTAKE INHIBITORS

Venlafaxine	Effexor

SSRIs

Citalopram	Celexa
Escitalopram	Lexapro
Fluoxetine	Prozac
Paroxetine	Paxil
Sertraline	Zoloft

Class/Generic Name	Brand (Market) Name
TETRACYCLICS	
Mirtazapine	Remeron
TRICYCLIC ANTIDEPRESSANTS	
Amitriptyline	Elavil
Amoxapine	Asendin
Desipramine	Norpramin
Doxepin	Sinequan
Imipramine	Tofranil
Nortriptyline	Pamelor
Protriptyline	Vivactil
Trimipramine	Surmontil
Miscellaneous	
Trazodone	Desyrel
Antiparkinson's Agents	
Amantadine	Symmetrel
Benztropine	Cogentin
Trihexyphenidyl	Artane
Entacapone	Comtan
Rasagiline	Azilect
Tolcapone	Tasmar
Bromocriptine	Parlodel
Pergolide	Permax
Pramipexole	Mirapex
Levodopa	Larodpa, Dopar
Carbidopa + levodopa	Parcopa
Carbidopa + levodopa + entacapone	Stalevo
Ropinirole	Requip
Antipsychotics	
Atypical (serotonin dopamine receptor antagonists)	
Clozapine	Clozaril
Olanzapine	Zpyrexa
Quetiapine	Seroquel
Risperidone	Resperdal
Ziprasidone	Geodon
PHENOTHIAZINES	
Chlorpromazine	Thorazine
Fluphenazine	Prolixin

Class/Generic Name	*Brand (Market) Name*
Mesoridazine	Serentil
Perphenazine	Trilafon
Thioridazine	Mellaril
Thiothixene	Navane
Trifluoperazine	Stelazine

DIHYDROINDOLONE DERIVATIVE

Molindone	Moban

BUTYROPHENONE DERIVATIVE

Haloperidol	Haldol

PARTIAL DOPAMINE/SEROTONIN ANTAGONIST

Aripiprazole	Abilify

Bipolar Disorders

Divalproex sodium	Depakote
Lamotrigine	Lamictal
Lithium carbonate	Eskalith
Olanzapine	Zyprexa
Resperidone	Risperdal

Obsessive-Compulsive Disorder

Fluoxetine	Prozac
Fluvoxamine	Luvox
Paroxetine	Paxil
Sertraline	Zoloft
Chlomipramine	Anafranil

General Anesthetics

Inhalational anesthetics: nonhalogenated

Nitrous oxide	—

Inhalational anesthetics: halogenated

Desflurance	Suprane
Enflurane	Ethrane
Halothane	Fluothane
Isoflurane	Florane
Sevoflurance	Ultane

Parenteral anesthetics

Fentanyl	Duragesic, Sublimaze
Ketamine	Ketalar
Midazolam	Versad
Propofol	Diprivan
Thiopental	Pentothal

Class/Generic Name	Brand (Market) Name
Local Anesthetics	
Ester type	
Benzocaine	Hurricaine
Cocaine	—
Tetracaine + benzocaine	Cetacaine
Amide type	
Articaine	Septocaine, Zorcaine, Ultracaine
Bupivacaine	Marcaine
Etidocaine	Duranest
Lidocaine	Xylocaine, Octocaine
Mepivacaine	Carbocaine
Prilocaine	Citanest
Lidocaine gel	Denti Patch
Lidocaine + prilocaine	Oraqix
	Citanest
Salivary Agents: for xerostomia (prescription)	
Cevimeline	Evoxac
Pilocarpine	Salagen
Fluoride Products	
Neutracare	
Respiratory Drugs	
Anaphylaxis Treatment	
Epinephrine	Epipen
Long-Term Control of Asthma	
CORTICOSTEROIDS (INHALED): FOR INFLAMMATION	
Beclomethasone	QVAR
Budesonide	Pulmicort
Flunisolide	Aerobid
Fluticasone	Flovent, Advir
Mometasone	Asmanex
Triamcinolone	Azmacort
SELECTIVE β_2-AGONISTS (LONG-ACTING): BRONCHODILATOR	
Salmeterol	Serevent
Formoterol	Foradil
METHYLXANTHINES	
Theophylline	TheoDur

Class/Generic Name	Brand (Market) Name
MAST CELL STABILIZERS	
Cromolyn sodium	Intal
Nedocromil	Tilade
LEUKOTRIENE MODIFIERS	
Zafirlukast	Accolate
Montelukast Singulair	
Zileuton	Zyflo
Quick-Relief Medications	
SELECTIVE β_2-ADRENERGIC (SHORT-ACTING) BRONCHODILATORS: FOR BRONCHOSPASM	
Albuterol; Drug of choice	Ventolin, Proventil
Pirbuterol	Maxair
Terbutaline	Brethine
Metaproterenol	Alupent
Levalbuterol tartrate	Xopenex
ANTICHOLINERGICS: BRONCHODILATORS	
Ipratropium bromide	Atrovent
Ipratropium bromide and albuterol sulfate	Combivent
Tiotropium bromide	Spiriva
CORTICOSTEROIDS (ORAL): ANTI-INFLAMMATORY	
Dexamethasone	Generics
Hydrocortisone	Generics
Methylprednisolone	Medrol, generics
Prednisolone	Generics
Prednisone	Generics
Expectorant/Antitussive	
Guaifenesin	Generic, Mucinex
Dextromethorphan	Generics
Benzonatate	Tessalon
Antineoplastics (prototype drug in each category)	
Alkylating agent: Cyclophosphamide	Cytoxan
Antibiotic: Doxorubicin	Adriamycin
Antimetabolite: Fluorouracil	Adrucil
Hormone, anti-estrogen: Tamoxifen	Novadex
Mitotic inhibitor: Vincristine	Oncovin
Monoclonal antibody: Erbitux	Cetuximab

Class/Generic Name	Brand (Market) Name
Immunosupressants	
Azathioprine	Imuran
Cyclosporine	Neoral, Sandimmune
Tacrolimus	Prograf, Protopic
Antihistamines (sedating)	
Diphenhydramine	Benadryl
Chlorpheniramine	Chlor-Trimeton
Clemastine	Tavist
Cyproheptadine	Periactin
Dexbrompheniramine	Drixoral
Antihistamines low/nonsedating	
Cetririzine	Zyrtec
Fexofenadine	Allegra
Loratadine	Claritin
Steroid (Nasal) Inhalers	
Beclomethasone	Beconase, Vancenase
Budesonide	Rhinocort
Flunisolide	Nasalide
Fluticasone	Flonase
Mometasone	Nasonex
Triamcinolone	Nasacort AQ
Nasal Decongestants	
Epinephrine	Primatene
Oxymetazoline	Afrin
Phenylephrine	Neo-Synephrine
Pseudoephedrine	Sudafed
Other Agents	
Benign Prostatic Hypertrophy	
Finasteride	Proscar
Doxazosin	Cardura
Terazocin	Hytrin
Tamsulosin	Flomax
Erectile Dysfunction	
Yohimbine	Adhrodyne
Sildenafil	Viagra

Class/Generic Name	*Brand (Market) Name*
Tadalafil	Cialis
Vardenafil	Levitra
Smoking Cessation	
Varenicline	Chantix
Bupropion	Zyban
Nicotine polacrilex	Nicorette gum
Nicotine transdermal	Habitrol, Prostep, Nicoderm
Nicotine Lozenge	Commit
Nicotine Nasal spray	Nicotrol NS
Nicotine inhalation	Nicotrol inhaler

Case Studies

A 62-year old male presents to the dental office with a chief complaint of bleeding gums. The patient is very anxious about going to the dentist. The dentist administers midazolam (Versed) for the patient about 30 minutes before the procedure.

Height: 5' 10" Weight: 185 lbs
BP: 140/90

The patient is a smoker and is allergic to penicillin and tetracycline (gets a rash).

Medical History

1. Diabetes mellitus
2. Hypertension
3. Depression
4. Facial pain

Medication history

1. Glyburide (Micronase)
2. Atenolol (Tenormin)
3. Paroxetine (Paxil)
4. Gabapentin (Neurontin)
5. Hydrochlorothiazide (Hydrodiuril)

Self-Quiz

1. Which of the following substance should the patient not take for at least 24 hours before taking midazolam?
   a. Peanut butter
   b. Sugar-free soda
   c. Grapefruit juice
   d. Ice cream

2. The patient has an endodontic abscess with lymphadenopathy. Which of the following antibiotics is recommended?
   a. Penicillin VK
   b. Erythromycin
   c. Clarithromycin
   d. Clindamycin
   e. Trimox

3. The patient had a maxillary first molar extracted and is in pain. Which of the following analgesics is best for this patient?
   a. Aspirin
   b. Acetaminophen
   c. Ibuprofen
   d. Naproxen sodium

4. Which of the following statements is correct concerning the administration of a local anesthetic to this patient?
   a. 2% lidocaine 1 : 100,000 epinephrine can be administered safely
   b. Benzocaine 20% can be used for profound anesthesia
   c. Lidocaine topical can be used for profound anesthesia
   d. 2% lidocaine 1 : 50,000 epinephrine can be administered but use only five cartridges

5. After the dental procedure is finished, the patient should remain sitting in the dental chair and then arise slowly because he is taking which of the following drugs?
   a. Atenolol
   b. Gabapentin
   c. Glyburide
   d. Paroxetine

6. The patient is taking gabapentin. Which of the following dental management techniques is necessary?
   a. Antibiotic prophylaxis is required.
   b. Do not administer epinephrine.
   c. No special precautions
   d. An antimicrobial mouthrinse is recommended.

7. In which of the following classifications does the antidepressant the patient is taking belong?
   a. Tricyclic antidepressant
   b. Monoamine oxidase inhibitor (MAO)
   c. Anticonvulsant
   d. Selective serotonin reuptake inhibitor (SSRI)

8. The dentist prescribed Bupropion to this patient. What is the indication for this drug?
   a. Smoking cessation
   b. Analgesic

c. Anti-anxiety
d. Heartburn

9. Which of the following periodontal adjunctive therapies can be used in this patient?
   a. Periostat
   b. Arestin
   c. Atridox
   d. PerioChip

10. Which of the following drugs the patient is taking is a diuretic?
    a. Glyburide (Micronase)
    b. Atenolol (Tenormin)
    c. Paroxetine (Paxil)
    d. Hydrochlorothiazide (Hydrodiuril)

Answers and Explanations To Self-Quiz

Disease	Medications With Potential Dental Drug Interactions	Dental Management
Diabetes	Glyburide	Do not recommend any form of aspirin.
	Aspirin	Acetaminophen is recommended as long as the patient does not take alcohol, which together increase liver toxicity
Hypertension	Atenolol Epinephrine in local anesthetic? Hydrochlorothiazide NSAIDs	Atenolol is a selective β-blocker. There is minor concern (with increasing blood pressure) about using epinephrine (vasoconstrictor) with selective β-blockers. There is more concern using EPI with a nonselective β-blocker such as propranolol (Inderal) where epinephrine acts on both β_1 and β_2 receptors
Depression	Paroxetine Epinephrine in local anesthetic? Grapefruit juice	Paxil is a selective serotonin reuptake inhibitor (SSRI), not a tricyclic antidepressant. Only two cartridges of 1 : 100,000 epinephrine should be given to a patient taking a tricyclic antidepressant because epinephrine utilizes the NE reuptake pump, as tricyclic antidepressants do. Thus, EPI will accumulate, resulting in hypertension and cardiac arrythmias. Selective serotonin reuptake inhibitors (SSRIs) have a different mechanism of action so that epinephrine can be given without any precautions.
Facial pain	Gabapentin	No special dental precautions
Anxiety	Midazolam Grapefruit juice	Do not take these two drugs together. Grapefruit juice has effects up to 24 hours. Excessive sedation occurs.

1. c: Grapefruit juice inhibits the CYP3A4 enzyme in the liver, which breaks down (biotransforms) midazolam. Thus, increased midazolam levels will result in excessive sedation.

2. d: The patient is allergic to penicillin, so penicillin and amoxicillin (Trimox) are contraindicated. Midazolam interacts with erythromycins and clarithromycin, resulting in prolonged sedation. Thus, clindamycin is the only antibiotic that can be used.

3. b: Aspirin with glyburide may increase the risk of hypoglycemia. Five days or more taking nonsteroidal anti-inflammatory drugs (NSAIDs; ibuprofen, naproxen sodium) can reduce the antihypertensive effects of beta-blockers (Atenolol). Acetaminophen is acceptable as long as the patient does not drink alcohol before or during treatment.

4. a: 1:100,000 epinephrine given to a patient taking a cardioselective β-blocker such as atenolol is of minor concern because epinephrine has a greater affinity to β_2 receptors. This patient is taking an antidepressant called paroxetine. It is not a tricyclic antidepressant but a selective serotonin reuptake inhibitor (SSRI), which does not have any affect on epinephrine because epi uses the NE (norepinephrine) reuptake pump, which is how tricyclic antidepressants work.

5. a: Atenolol, a beta-blocker, as well as other antihypertensive drugs cause orthostatic hypotension. If the patient gets up quickly from the dental chair he can faint (syncope).

6. c: Gabapentin is prescribed for facial pain.

7. d: Paroxetine (Paxil) is an SSRI.

8. a: Bupropion is used for smoking cessation as well as an antidepressant.

9. d: The patient is allergic to tetracyclines. Periostat is doxycycline 20 mg, Arestin contains minocycline, and Atridox containes doxycycline. Periochip contains chlorhexidine.

10. d: Hydrochlorothiazide is the diuretic. Atenolol is a beta-blocker, glyburide is an antidiabetic drug, and paroxetine is an antidepressant.

CASE II

A 54-year old male patient presents to the dental office with a chief complaint of "My front teeth are moving"?

    Height: 5' 7"   Weight: 165 lbs.
    Blood pressure: 130/80
    Allergies: None
    Social history: Drinks occasionally

Medical history

1. Asthma
2. Hypertension
3. Hyperlipidemia

Medications

1. 81 mg aspirin/day (without physician's approval)
2. albuterol (Proventil) (oral inhalation)
3. Beclomethasone dipropionate (Beclovent) (oral inhalation)
4. nifedipine (Procardia)
5. simvastatin (Zocor)

Self-Quiz

1. Which of the following advice should be given to this patient concerning his asthma medication and dental care?
   a. Drink orange juice after each inhalation dose.
   b. Rinse mouth with water after each inhalation dose.
   c. Eat grapefruit before each inhalation dose.
   d. Gargle with sodium bicarbonate before each inhalation dose.

2. The patient complains of her gingiva being overgrown and bulbous. Which of the following drugs the patient is taking is the cause of this?
   a. Aspirin
   b. Albuterol
   c. Beclomethasone dipropionate
   d. Nifedipine
   e. Simvastatin

3. The patient requires an antibiotic for a dental infection. Which of the following antibiotics should not be given to this patient?
   a. Clarithromycin (Biaxin)
   b. Penicillin VK
   c. Metronidazole (Flagyl)
   d. Clindamycin (Cleocin)

4. The patient is taking 81mg of aspirin per day. The patient is taking this drug and dosage to:
   a. Increase the effectiveness of nifedipine
   b. Keep himself pain free
   c. Prevent strokes
   d. Keep his urine acidic

5. What advice should the dental hygienist give this patient concerning the aspirin he is taking?
   a. He should contact his physician and only take medications under the supervision of his physician.
   b. Tell him not to take it.
   c. Take it with water.
   d. Take it in the morning.

6. Which of the following analgesics is best for this patient after a tooth extraction?
   a. Aspirin
   b. Advil

   c. Motrin
   d. Acetaminophen with codeine (No. 3)

7. Which of the following foods should be avoided in this patient?
   a. Orange juice
   b. Grapefruit juice
   c. Calcium supplements
   d. Antacids

8. Regarding the use of lidocaine in this patient with 1:100,000 epinephrine, which of the following statements is true?
   a. Epinephrine is contraindicated in this patient because he has hypertension and is taking a calcium channel blocker.
   b. Epinephrine is contraindicated in this patient because he has asthma.
   c. Epinephrine can be used in this patient, but limit the number of cartridges to two because he has hypertension.
   d. Epinephrine can be used in this patient with no special precautions taken.

9. Which of the following precautions should the dental hygienist take regarding the patient's asthmatic medications?
   a. Tell the patient to keep the inhaler within easy reach.
   b. There is no need to bring the medicine if he has not had an attack in the last 3 months.
   c. Keep the medicine in the patient's pocket because it is not under OSHA regulations to keep it on the dental cart.
   d. The dental hygienist should hold the medicine in her/his pocket until the patient requires it.

10. Which of the following should the dental hygienist do before any dental procedures are started on this patient?
    a. Tell the patient to rinse his mouth with chlorhexidine before the dental procedure.
    b. Take vital signs because he is hypertensive
    c. Limit the appointment time.
    d. Avoid shining the dental light on the patient because nifedipine is a photosensitive drug.

Answers and Explanations to Self-Quiz

Disease	Medications with Potential Dental Drug Interactions	Dental Management
Asthma	Albuterol (Proventil) Aspirin NSAIDs	There is a high percentage of aspirin sensitivity in asthma patients where aspirin as well as nonsteroidal anti-inflammatory drugs (NSAIDs) such as ibuprofen (Advil, Motrin, Nuprin) can cause bronchospasm and induce an asthma attack.
		Patients with asthma or nasal polyps should not take aspirin or other NSAIDs. Aspirin-sensitive asthma (ASA) and NSAID sensitivity occurs in up to 10–15% of asthmatics and up to 30–40% of asthmatics with nasal polyps. Thus, asthmatics are much more sensitive to aspirin and NSAIDs.
Hypertension	Nifedipine (Procardia) No significant dental drug interactions	There are no precautions regarding antibiotics or other dental drugs.
		Gingival overgrowth is the only significant side effect of this drug.
Hyperlipidemia	Simvastatin (Zocor) Grapefruit juice Erythromycin and clarithromycin	Grapefruit juice inhibits the metabolism of simvastatin. Avoid grapefruit juice. Erythromycin and clarithromycin inhibit the metabolism of simvastatin, increasing blood levels. Avoid using these antibiotics.

1. b: Beclomethasone dipropionate (Beclovent) is administered through oral inhalation. It is a corticosteroid and can cause oral candidiasis (fungal infection). Thus the dental hygienist should instruct the patient to rinse the mouth with water after each dose.

2. d: Nifedipine is a calcium channel blocker used for the treatment of hypertension. It causes gingival enlargement. Teach the patient the importance of good oral hygiene and frequent maintenance appointments. Surgical removal of the enlarged gingival may be necessary.

3. a: Erythromycin and clarithromycin inhibit the metabolism of simvastain, increasing blood levels. Avoid using these antibiotics.

4. c: 81 mg (baby) aspirin is taken for the prevention of strokes and heart attacks. This patient is also an asthmatic. The hygienist should inform the patient to go to his physician.

5. a: Tell the patient to inform his physician that he is taking aspirin. He is also an asthmatic and if he is sensitive to aspirin, an asthmatic attack may be precipitated.

6. d: Since there is a chance of this patient being sensitive to aspirin and NSAIDs, acetaminophen, or acetaminophen with codeine, are acceptable analgesics.

7. b: Grapefruit juice inhibits the breakdown of simvastatin.

8. c: The patient has hypertension so epinephrine can be used, but limit the dose to 0.04 mg, which is two cartridges of 1 : 100,000.

9. a: Ask the patient when his last asthmatic attack was. The patient should always keep the inhaler on hand.

10. b: The hygienist should take vital signs on all patients before treatment is started.

Answers to Board Review Questions

Chapter 1

1. a
2. d
3. a
4. d
5. d

Chapter 2

1. b
2. a
3. a
4. a
5. a

Chapter 3

1. c
2. b
3. a
4. b
5. b
6. b
7. b
8. c
9. b
10. a

Chapter 4

1. a
2. c
3. a
4. b
5. b

Chapter 5

1. a
2. a
3. c

4. c
5. b
6. d
7. d
8. d
9. c
10. d
11. a
12. c
13. a
14. a
15. c

Chapter 6

1. c
2. d
3. b
4. a
5. c
6. b
7. c
8. c
9. a
10. d
11. c
12. d
13. b
14. a
15. c
16. c
17. d
18. c
19. a
20. c

Chapter 7

1. d
2. a
3. a

4. b
5. c
6. b
7. a
8. a
9. c
10. b

Chapter 8

1. d
2. b
3. a
4. e
5. b
6. a
7. a
8. d
9. b
10. a

Chapter 9

1. a
2. a
3. b
4. a
5. c
6. c
7. b
8. b
9. c
10. c

Chapter 10

1. a
2. e
3. d
4. d
5. d

Chapter 11

1. c
2. a
3. a
4. a
5. c

Chapter 12

1. a
2. c
3. a
4. b
5. a

Chapter 13

1. d
2. c
3. d
4. c
5. e
6. a
7. b
8. c
9. c
10. c
11. d
12. a
13. a
14. d
15. b

Chapter 14

1. c
2. a
3. c
4. a
5. b
6. c
7. d
8. a
9. b
10. b

Chapter 15

1. c
2. a
3. a
4. a
5. c
6. c
7. c

8. a
9. b
10. c

Chapter 16

1. c
2. c
3. a
4. a
5. a

Chapter 17

1. a
2. d
3. b
4. a
5. b

Chapter 18

1. c
2. d
3. a
4. d
5. d

Chapter 19

1. c
2. b
3. b
4. a
5. d
6. b
7. c
8. a
9. a
10. c
11. b
12. b

13. c
14. b
15. a
16. a
17. b
18. a
19. a
20. a
21. a
22. c
23. e
24. a

Chapter 20

1. c
2. d
3. a
4. a
5. b
6. a
7. b
8. a
9. a
10. c

Chapter 21

1. c
2. c
3. a
4. d
5. c

Chapter 22

1. a
2. c
3. a
4. a
5. a

Index